EDIBLE MEDICINAL PLANTS

of CANADA

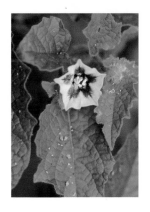

NEW EDITION

MacKinnon · Kershaw · Arnason

Owen · Karst · Hamersley Chambers

LONE
PINE

Distributed by: Canada Book Distributors
www.canadabookdistributors.com
www.lonepinepublishing.com
Tel: 1-800-661-9017

Cataloguing in Publication Data

MacKinnon, A. (Andrew), 1956-, author
     Edible and medicinal plants of Canada / Andrew MacKinnon,
Linda Kershaw, John Arnason, Patrick Owen, Amanda Karst,
Fiona Hamersley Chambers.

Co-published by: Lone Pine Publishing Inc.
New Edition. Originally published: Edmonton : Lone Pine Pub., c2009.
Includes bibliographical references and index.
ISBN 978-1-77213-002-7 (paperback)

1. Medicinal plants—Canada. 2. Plants, Edible—Canada.
3. Medicinal plants—Canada—Identification. 4. Plants, Edible—
Canada—Identification. I. Title.

QK98.5.C3M34 2015   615.3'210971   C2015-906971-8

Illustrations: All illustrations are by Ian Sheldon, except: Frank Burman 54, 89, 112, 122, 123, 132, 154, 158, 173, 178, 183, 191, 202, 204, 223, 224, 236, 249, 259, 266, 270, 276, 284, 290, 293, 294, 296, 299, 301, 338, 339, 341, 349, 356, 373, 375, 377, 379, 413; Linda Kershaw 418–23.

Photos: All photos in this book are reproduced with the generous permission of their copyright holders. See p. 434 for a full list of credits.

Cover Photographs: Linda Kershaw

Map: From the publication *The Forests of Canada* by Ken Farr, published by Natural Resources Canada, Canadian Forest Service and Fitzhenry & Whiteside, 2003. Reproduced with the permission of Natural Resources Canada, Canadian Forest Service. © Her Majesty the Queen in Right of Canada, 2008.

DISCLAIMER: This guide is not meant to be a "how-to" reference guide for consuming wild plants. We do not recommend experimentation by readers, and we caution that many of the plants in Canada, including some traditional medicines, are poisonous and harmful.

We acknowledge the financial support of the Government of Canada.
Nous reconnaissons l'appui financier du gouvernement du Canada.

Funded by the Government of Canada
Financé par le gouvernement du Canada | Canadä

Printed in China

PC: 38-16

Contents

The following people are thanked for their valued contributions to this book:

Ian Sheldon and Frank Burman, for their delicate and beautiful illustrations;

the many photographers who allowed us to use their incredible photographs, especially Linda Kershaw;

Lone Pine's talented editorial and production staff;

and finally, the native peoples, settlers, botanists and writers who kept written records or oral accounts of the many uses of plants across Canada.

PICTORIAL GUIDE

TREES

Spruces p. 30	Two-needled pines p. 32	Ponderosa pine p. 33	Five-needled pines p. 34	Firs p. 36
Larches p. 38	Hemlocks p. 40	Douglas-fir p. 42	Cedars p. 44	Tree junipers p. 46
Yellow-cedar p. 48	Trembling aspen p. 49	Balsam poplar p. 50	Cottonwoods p. 51	Birches p. 52
Red alder p. 54	Hop hornbeam p. 55	Oaks p. 56	American chestnut p. 60	American beech p. 61
Hickories p. 62	Walnuts p. 63	Elms p. 64	White ash p. 65	Maples p. 66

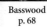

Basswood
p. 68

Kentucky coffee tree
p. 70

Cascara
p. 71

Apples
p. 72

Arbutus
p. 74

PICTORIAL GUIDE

Shrub junipers
p. 76

Yews
p. 78

Hawthorns
p. 80

Mountain-ashes
p. 82

Wild roses
p. 84

Cherries
p. 86

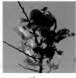
Plums
p. 88

Indian-plum
p. 89

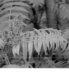
Sumacs
p. 90

Skunkbush
p. 91

Devil's club
p. 92

Blackberries
p. 93

Raspberries
p. 94

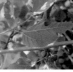
Mulberries
p. 96

Barberries
p. 98

Oregon-grapes
p. 100

Pawpaw
p. 101

Spicebush
p. 102

Sassafras
p. 103

Currants
p. 104

Gooseberries
p. 106

Prickly currants
p. 108

Saskatoon
p. 109

Dogwoods
p. 110

Black huckleberry
p. 112

Huckleberries
p. 113

Blueberries
p. 114

Cranberries
p. 116

False-wintergreens
p. 118

Bearberries
p. 120

PICTORIAL GUIDE

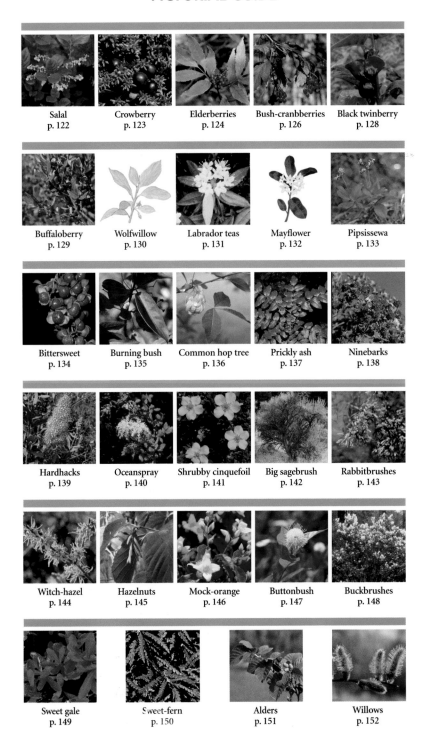

Salal
p. 122

Crowberry
p. 123

Elderberries
p. 124

Bush-cranberries
p. 126

Black twinberry
p. 128

Buffaloberry
p. 129

Wolfwillow
p. 130

Labrador teas
p. 131

Mayflower
p. 132

Pipsissewa
p. 133

Bittersweet
p. 134

Burning bush
p. 135

Common hop tree
p. 136

Prickly ash
p. 137

Ninebarks
p. 138

Hardhacks
p. 139

Oceanspray
p. 140

Shrubby cinquefoil
p. 141

Big sagebrush
p. 142

Rabbitbrushes
p. 143

Witch-hazel
p. 144

Hazelnuts
p. 145

Mock-orange
p. 146

Buttonbush
p. 147

Buckbrushes
p. 148

Sweet gale
p. 149

Sweet-fern
p. 150

Alders
p. 151

Willows
p. 152

PICTORIAL GUIDE

VINES

F. Virginia creeper
p. 154

Grapes
p. 155

Honeysuckles
p. 156

Manroot
p. 158

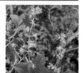
Wild cucumber
p. 159

HERBS

Hops
p. 160

Greenbrier
p. 162

Jack-in-the-pulpit
p. 163

Am. skunk-cabbage
p. 164

Skunk-cabbage
p. 165

Sweetflags
p. 166

Clintonia
p. 168

Twisted-stalks
p. 169

Lilies-of-the-valley
p. 170

F. Solomon's-seals
p. 171

Fairybells
p. 172

Trilliums
p. 173

Asparagus
p. 174

Pokeweed
p. 175

Blue cohoshes
p. 176

Mayapple
p. 177

Strawberries
p. 178

Indian strawberry
p. 180

Prickly-pear cacti
p. 181

Ginsengs
p. 182

Sarsaparillas
p. 184

Bunchberry
p. 185

Partridge berry
p. 186

Horse-gentian
p. 187

Cow-lilies
p. 188

PICTORIAL GUIDE

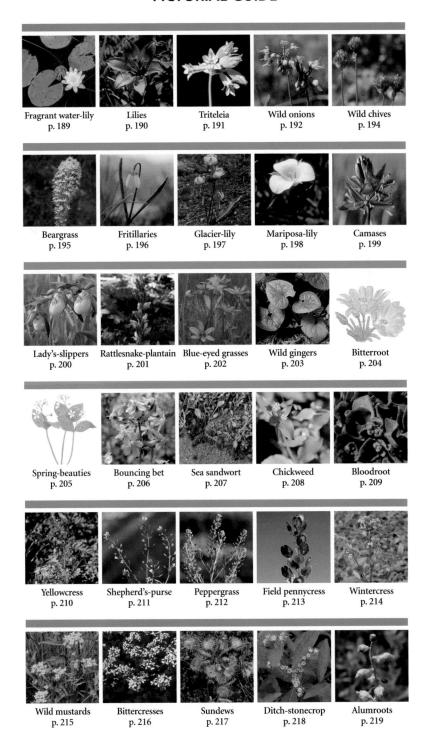

Fragrant water-lily
p. 189

Lilies
p. 190

Triteleia
p. 191

Wild onions
p. 192

Wild chives
p. 194

Beargrass
p. 195

Fritillaries
p. 196

Glacier-lily
p. 197

Mariposa-lily
p. 198

Camases
p. 199

Lady's-slippers
p. 200

Rattlesnake-plantain
p. 201

Blue-eyed grasses
p. 202

Wild gingers
p. 203

Bitterroot
p. 204

Spring-beauties
p. 205

Bouncing bet
p. 206

Sea sandwort
p. 207

Chickweed
p. 208

Bloodroot
p. 209

Yellowcress
p. 210

Shepherd's-purse
p. 211

Peppergrass
p. 212

Field pennycress
p. 213

Wintercress
p. 214

Wild mustards
p. 215

Bittercresses
p. 216

Sundews
p. 217

Ditch-stonecrop
p. 218

Alumroots
p. 219

PICTORIAL GUIDE

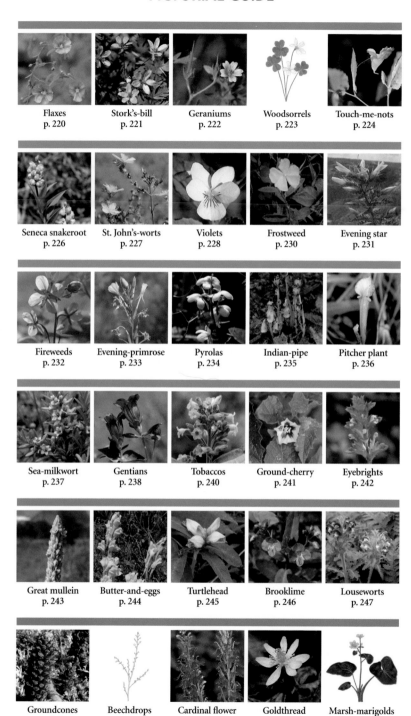

Flaxes p. 220	Stork's-bill p. 221	Geraniums p. 222	Woodsorrels p. 223	Touch-me-nots p. 224
Seneca snakeroot p. 226	St. John's-worts p. 227	Violets p. 228	Frostweed p. 230	Evening star p. 231
Fireweeds p. 232	Evening-primrose p. 233	Pyrolas p. 234	Indian-pipe p. 235	Pitcher plant p. 236
Sea-milkwort p. 237	Gentians p. 238	Tobaccos p. 240	Ground-cherry p. 241	Eyebrights p. 242
Great mullein p. 243	Butter-and-eggs p. 244	Turtlehead p. 245	Brooklime p. 246	Louseworts p. 247
Groundcones p. 248	Beechdrops p. 249	Cardinal flower p. 250	Goldthread p. 252	Marsh-marigolds p. 253

PICTORIAL GUIDE

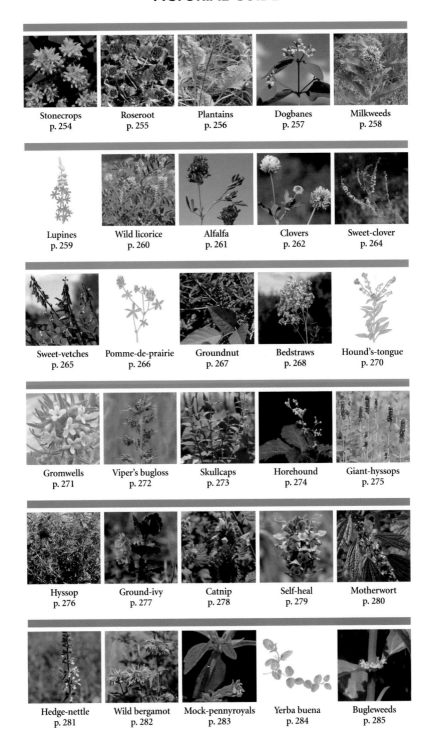

Stonecrops
p. 254

Roseroot
p. 255

Plantains
p. 256

Dogbanes
p. 257

Milkweeds
p. 258

Lupines
p. 259

Wild licorice
p. 260

Alfalfa
p. 261

Clovers
p. 262

Sweet-clover
p. 264

Sweet-vetches
p. 265

Pomme-de-prairie
p. 266

Groundnut
p. 267

Bedstraws
p. 268

Hound's-tongue
p. 270

Gromwells
p. 271

Viper's bugloss
p. 272

Skullcaps
p. 273

Horehound
p. 274

Giant-hyssops
p. 275

Hyssop
p. 276

Ground-ivy
p. 277

Catnip
p. 278

Self-heal
p. 279

Motherwort
p. 280

Hedge-nettle
p. 281

Wild bergamot
p. 282

Mock-pennyroyals
p. 283

Yerba buena
p. 284

Bugleweeds
p. 285

PICTORIAL GUIDE

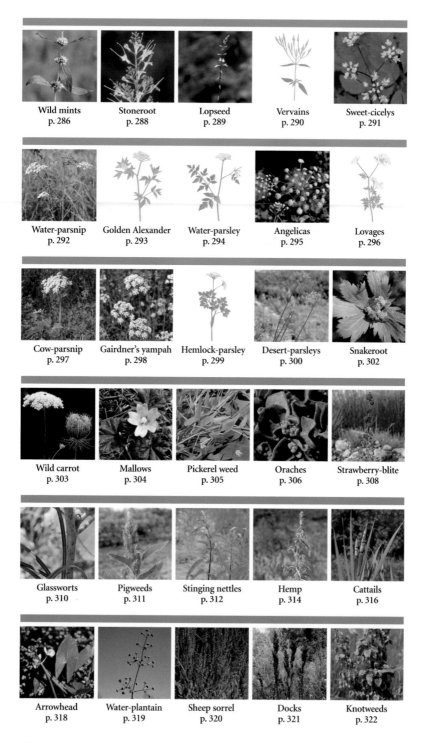

Wild mints
p. 286

Stoneroot
p. 288

Lopseed
p. 289

Vervains
p. 290

Sweet-cicelys
p. 291

Water-parsnip
p. 292

Golden Alexander
p. 293

Water-parsley
p. 294

Angelicas
p. 295

Lovages
p. 296

Cow-parsnip
p. 297

Gairdner's yampah
p. 298

Hemlock-parsley
p. 299

Desert-parsleys
p. 300

Snakeroot
p. 302

Wild carrot
p. 303

Mallows
p. 304

Pickerel weed
p. 305

Oraches
p. 306

Strawberry-blite
p. 308

Glassworts
p. 310

Pigweeds
p. 311

Stinging nettles
p. 312

Hemp
p. 314

Cattails
p. 316

Arrowhead
p. 318

Water-plantain
p. 319

Sheep sorrel
p. 320

Docks
p. 321

Knotweeds
p. 322

PICTORIAL GUIDE

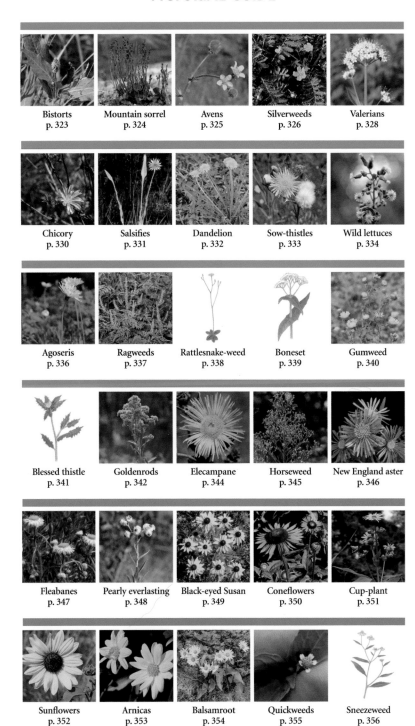

Bistorts
p. 323

Mountain sorrel
p. 324

Avens
p. 325

Silverweeds
p. 326

Valerians
p. 328

Chicory
p. 330

Salsifies
p. 331

Dandelion
p. 332

Sow-thistles
p. 333

Wild lettuces
p. 334

Agoseris
p. 336

Ragweeds
p. 337

Rattlesnake-weed
p. 338

Boneset
p. 339

Gumweed
p. 340

Blessed thistle
p. 341

Goldenrods
p. 342

Elecampane
p. 344

Horseweed
p. 345

New England aster
p. 346

Fleabanes
p. 347

Pearly everlasting
p. 348

Black-eyed Susan
p. 349

Coneflowers
p. 350

Cup-plant
p. 351

Sunflowers
p. 352

Arnicas
p. 353

Balsamroot
p. 354

Quickweeds
p. 355

Sneezeweed
p. 356

PICTORIAL GUIDE

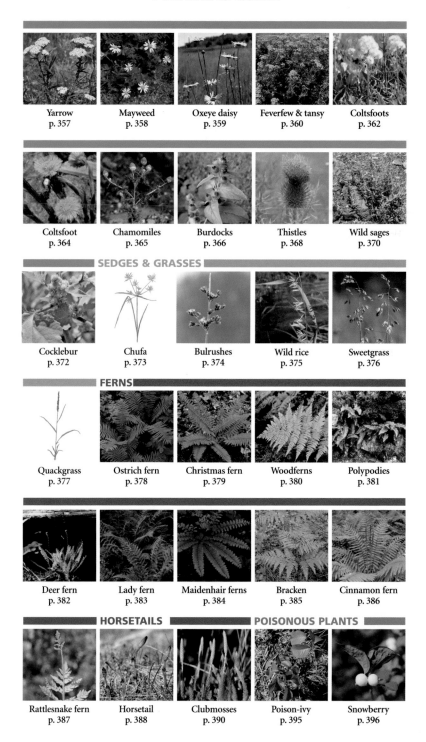

Yarrow
p. 357

Mayweed
p. 358

Oxeye daisy
p. 359

Feverfew & tansy
p. 360

Coltsfoots
p. 362

Coltsfoot
p. 364

Chamomiles
p. 365

Burdocks
p. 366

Thistles
p. 368

Wild sages
p. 370

SEDGES & GRASSES

Cocklebur
p. 372

Chufa
p. 373

Bulrushes
p. 374

Wild rice
p. 375

Sweetgrass
p. 376

FERNS

Quackgrass
p. 377

Ostrich fern
p. 378

Christmas fern
p. 379

Woodferns
p. 380

Polypodies
p. 381

Deer fern
p. 382

Lady fern
p. 383

Maidenhair ferns
p. 384

Bracken
p. 385

Cinnamon fern
p. 386

HORSETAILS   POISONOUS PLANTS

Rattlesnake fern
p. 387

Horsetail
p. 388

Clubmosses
p. 390

Poison-ivy
p. 395

Snowberry
p. 396

PICTORIAL GUIDE

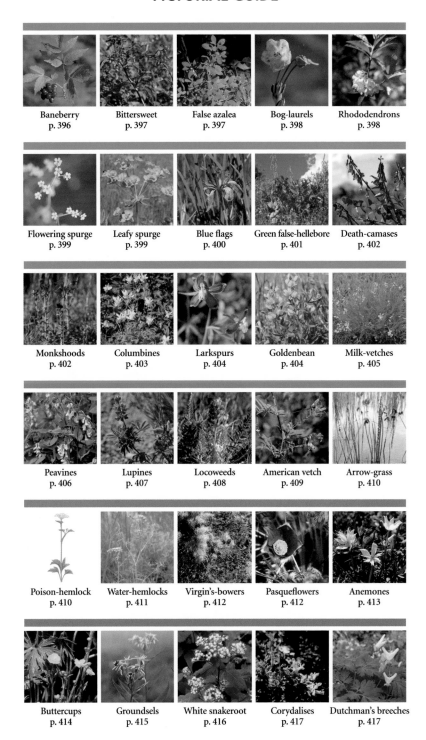

Baneberry
p. 396

Bittersweet
p. 397

False azalea
p. 397

Bog-laurels
p. 398

Rhododendrons
p. 398

Flowering spurge
p. 399

Leafy spurge
p. 399

Blue flags
p. 400

Green false-hellebore
p. 401

Death-camases
p. 402

Monkshoods
p. 402

Columbines
p. 403

Larkspurs
p. 404

Goldenbean
p. 404

Milk-vetches
p. 405

Peavines
p. 406

Lupines
p. 407

Locoweeds
p. 408

American vetch
p. 409

Arrow-grass
p. 410

Poison-hemlock
p. 410

Water-hemlocks
p. 411

Virgin's-bowers
p. 412

Pasqueflowers
p. 412

Anemones
p. 413

Buttercups
p. 414

Groundsels
p. 415

White snakeroot
p. 416

Corydalises
p. 417

Dutchman's breeches
p. 417

15

FOREST REGIONS OF CANADA

Legend:
- BOREAL FOREST
- GREAT LAKES–ST.LAWRENCE FOREST
- ACADIAN FOREST
- CAROLINIAN FOREST
- SUBALPINE FOREST
- COLUMBIA FOREST
- MONTANE FOREST
- COASTAL FOREST
- TUNDRA
- GRASSLANDS

From the publication *The Forests of Canada* by Ken Farr, published by Natural Resources Canada, Canadian Forest Service and Fitzhenry & Whiteside, 2003. Reproduced with the permission of Natural Resources Canada, Canadian Forest Service. © Her Majesty the Queen in Right of Canada, 2009.

Introduction

All animals, including humans, depend on plants for survival. Throughout human history, plants have provided us with food, clothing, medicine and shelter. Our ancestors needed to know which of their local plants were edible or poisonous, which could heal or harm and which could provide materials for making implements, clothing and shelters. Today, many of us spend our lives in artificial environments, isolated from our natural surroundings. Most of life's necessities

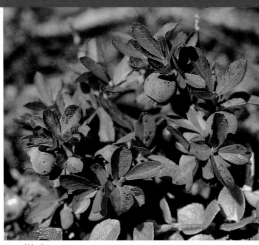

Dwarf blueberry

are mass produced elsewhere and purchased as needed. We no longer forage for food, build our shelters or gather fuel for heating and cooking. Instead, we depend on hundreds of people in our society to supply the knowledge, materials and skills necessary to feed, clothe and house us. As we grow increasingly isolated from our natural surroundings, it is easy to forget that the air we breathe, much of the food we eat and many of the drugs we use come from plants. Recognizing wild plants and knowing how they have been used in the past increases our appreciation of our environment.

With an ever-growing human population and the introduction of aggressive weed species from around the world, fewer and fewer areas remain where natural, native plant communities persist. Wild plant communities cannot support the large numbers of people now living on this continent, so vast tracts of land have been converted into cultivated fields, pastures and plantations. The remaining wilderness needs to be treated with care and consideration.

The main goal of this book is to illustrate the great variety of ways in which plants have been used by humans. Much of the information on Canadian species comes from ethnobotanical accounts written in collaboration with First Nations healers. Other sources are pioneer and modern herbal and scientific literature. To date, fewer wild plants have been studied as medicines or foods by scientists than were known to the traditional healers and

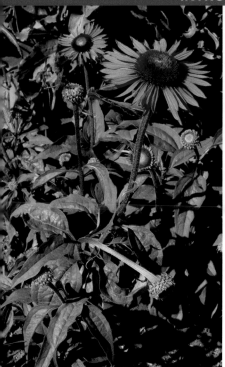

Purple coneflower

herbalists. Collection of plants should be made with respect and only after consideration of their abundance or rarity. Following First Nations tradition, a gift of tobacco or a prayer is offered in exchange for the gift of healing.

Sources of Information

The information in this book has been collected from many publications (see References, p. 432) and is not based on personal experimentation. No judgment has been made regarding the validity of most reported uses. Instead, a wide range of information is included for your interest.

Many sources disagree about how a plant should be used. One book says that a plant has been used for food, while another reports that it contains toxins and needs special preparation or perhaps should not be eaten at all. Controversy is even greater over medicinal herbs. One author says that a plant was used to treat diarrhea and dysentery, while another reports that it was used to relieve cold symptoms and soothe sore throats. All reports are included in the text to give some idea of the wide range of uses over the years.

Of course, not all reported uses are valid. Some "edible" species may have been used for food only during famines, when tastier, more nutritious plants were not available. What won't fatten will fill. Medicinal herbs were not necessarily effective or safe. During the smallpox or measles epidemics that swept across North America, most plants were tried at one time or another as a cure. Also, many "powerful medicines" are lethal poisons when used improperly. More detailed discussions of herbal medicines and food preparation can be found in some of the books listed in the references section.

Using Wild Plants

With growing populations and dwindling areas of natural vegetation, visitors to wilderness regions can no longer expect to collect wild plants. The use of wild resources must be viewed as a privilege rather than a right. If everyone decided to "harvest nature's crop," many species and many plant communities would soon disappear. No one has seeded or tended these wild plants, so neither "harvest" nor "crop" apply, though both terms are often used. Many populations of wild medicinal plants have disappeared as a result of uncontrolled harvesting, especially around densely populated areas. However, many common plants, in the wild and in fields or on roadsides closer to home, can be gathered without threatening natural ecosystems. Gathering wild plants simply requires common sense and respect for the environment. It also requires respect for the intellectual property rights that may rest with local First Nations based on their traditional uses of these plants. Commercial use of plants traditionally used by First Nations without benefit sharing is a highly controversial issue that readers interested in such commerce need to become aware of.

A Few Gathering Tips

1. Gather only common plants, and never take more than five percent of the population (e.g., one plant in 20, one berry in 20). Even then, a cautious personal quota will still deplete the plants if too many people gather them in one area. Remember, plants growing in harsh environments (e.g., arctic, alpine, desert) might not have enough energy to produce flowers and fruits every year. Also, don't forget the other local wildlife. Survival of many animals can depend on access to the roots, shoots and fruits that you are harvesting.

2. Never gather plants from protected and/or heavily used areas such as parks and nature preserves. Doing so is not only wrong, but is also often illegal. Be sure to check the regulations for the area you are visiting.

3. Know which part of the plant you need. It isn't always necessary to kill a plant to use it. Don't pull up an entire plant if you are only going to use the flowers or a few of the younger leaves. Take only what you need, and damage the plant as little as

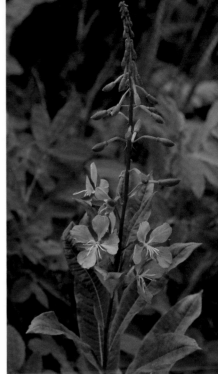
Common fireweed

possible. If you are gathering bulbs or rhizomes, leave smaller pieces buried in the ground to produce new plants. If you want to grow a plant in your garden, try propagating it from seed rather than transplanting it from the wild.

4. Take only as much as you need. If you are gathering a plant for food, taste a sample. You may not like it, or the berries at this site may not be as sweet and juicy as the ones you gathered last year. Don't take more than you will use.

5. Gather plants only when you are certain of their identity. Many irritating and poisonous plants grow wild in Canada, and some of them resemble edible or medicinal species. If you are not positive that you have the right plant, don't use it. It is better to eat nothing at all than to be poisoned.

6. Gather plants carefully. Always take care not to accidentally mix in the leaves or rhizomes of nearby plants, which could be poisonous.

No Two Plants Are the Same

Wild plants are highly variable. No two individuals of a species are identical and many characteristics can vary. Some of the more easily observed characteristics include the colour, shape and size of stems, leaves, flowers and fruits. Other less obvious features, such as sweetness, toughness, juiciness and concentrations of toxins or drugs, also vary from one plant to the next.

Many factors control plant characteristics. Time is one of the most obvious. All plants change as they grow and age. Usually, young leaves are the most tender, and mature fruits are the largest and sweetest. Underground structures also change throughout the year. Rhizomes, bulbs, tubers and corms are storage chambers for nutrients. During the growing

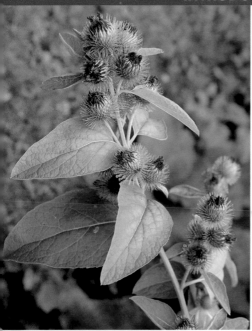

Common burdock

season, these underground structures become smaller, tougher and spongier as their supplies are moved up to support rapidly growing stems, leaves, flowers and fruits. In late summer, the roots and underground stems swell once again as the aging upper plant sends nutrients back down for storage in preparation for next year's growth. Crisp, firm rhizomes remain swollen with starches and sugars through winter and early spring, which are often the best time of year to gather these parts.

Habitat also has a strong influence on plant growth. The leaves of plants from moist, shady sites are often larger, sweeter and more tender than those of plants on dry, sunny hillsides. Berries may be plump and juicy one year, when shrubs have had plenty of moisture, but they can become dry and wizened during a drought. Without the proper nutrients and environmental conditions, plants cannot grow and mature.

Finally, the genetic make-up of a species determines how the plant develops and how it responds to its environment. Wild plant populations tend to be much more variable than domestic crops, partly because of their wide range of habitats, but also because of their greater genetic variability. Humans have been planting and harvesting plants for centuries, repeatedly selecting and breeding plants with the most desirable characteristics. This process has produced many highly productive cultivars—trees with larger, sweeter fruits, potatoes with bigger tubers and sunflowers with larger, oilier seeds. These crop species are more productive, and they also produce a specific product each time they are planted. Wild plants are much less reliable.

Wild species have developed from a broader range of ancestors growing in many different environments, so their genetic make-up is much more variable than that of domestic cultivars. One population may produce sweet, juicy berries while the berries of another population are small and tart; one plant may have low concentrations of a toxin that is plentiful in its neighbour. This variability makes wild plants much more resilient to change. Although their lack of stability may seem to reduce their value as crop species, it is one of their most valuable features. Domestic crops often have few defenses and must be protected from competition and predation. As fungi, weeds and insects continue to develop immunities to pesticides, we repeatedly return to wild plants for new repellents and, more recently, for pest-resistant genes for our crop plants.

The Species Accounts

This book includes common plants that have been used by people from ancient times to the present. Species are organized by growth form—trees, shrubs, vines, herbs, sedges and grasses and ferns—with closely related or similar plants grouped together for comparison. A section on poisonous plants is at the end of the book. Many entries focus on a single species, but if several similar species (e.g., several violets, *Viola* spp.) have been used in the same ways, two or more species may be described together.

Plant Names

Both common and scientific names are included for each plant. Scientific names are from Flora of North America, for families already completed (Flora of North America is a work in progress). For other plant families, scientific names follow Flora of Canada (Scoggan 1978–1979). Common names are also largely from the Floras of North America and Canada.

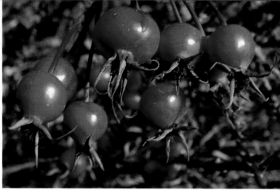

Prairie rose

Food

Although many common plants in Canada are edible, all are not equally palatable. Present-day diets have much more sugar and salt and many more highly refined ingredients than were found in the foods of our ancestors. Consequently, many of the plants and fruits that were eaten in the past are quite bitter by modern standards, and many fibre-rich wild foods can cause digestive upset, at least at first. When trying a wild food for the first time, it is best to take only a small amount. See if you like it and if it agrees with your system before you go to the trouble of preparing a larger amount.

Many wild greens are much more nutritious than the domestic vegetables that commonly fill our salad bowls, but just because a plant is wild doesn't mean that it is better. The edible parts of wild plants (e.g., tubers or fruits) are usually much smaller than those of domestic varieties (though some people would argue that a small wild strawberry contains all the flavour of a large domestic one). Many wild plants are more bitter and fibrous than their domestic counterparts. Also, wild species are more variable than cultivated varieties, so you may need to sample as you go in order to assess the sweetness or tenderness of the plants you are gathering.

This guide is not a cookbook, and there are no specific recipes in the Food sections. However, some notes on preparation are included if special techniques have been used to improve the flavour or texture of a food or to reduce its toxicity. Food plants have been prepared and served in many different ways.

Raw plants provide salad greens, garnishes and trail-side nibbles. Sweet, tender parts, such as young leaves and shoots, flowers and fruits, are often eaten raw. Sharp-tasting or peppery plants are usually mixed with milder greens or used as garnishes in sandwiches and salads, but they can also provide a refreshing, thirst-quenching snack along the trail.

When eating raw plants, make sure that they are free of contaminants. This preparation may involve careful peeling and washing. Never eat plants from areas that may have been contaminated with pesticides, engine exhaust, sewage or other pollutants. Always use clean water for washing. If you wouldn't drink the water, don't use it to wash foods that are going to be eaten raw.

Boiling improves the palatability of many wild foods. It breaks down plant fibres to tenderize tough plants, and it can also improve flavour.

Bitter, astringent plants are often cooked in one or more changes of water to remove undesirable, water-soluble compounds. This process involves pouring boiling water over the vegetable in a pot, returning the water to a boil, draining, adding fresh hot water, and bringing the water to a boil again. Sometimes, a pinch of baking soda is added to the water to tenderize tough plants. Boiling can also remove water-soluble toxins, which are then

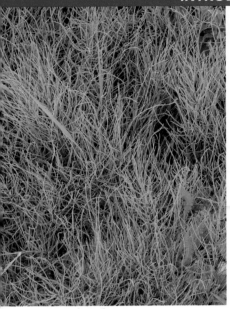

Common horsetail

discarded with the cooking water. The heat from cooking may break down some poisons, making certain toxic foods safe to eat.

Most tender plants are cooked as little as possible if they are going to be served as a hot vegetable, but they can also be simmered for long periods in soups as thickeners. Many cooked greens are chilled, mixed with vinegar, oil and seasonings and used in salads.

Baking and roasting can also improve texture and palatability. Often, this type of cooking breaks down relatively indigestible carbohydrates, producing sugars that make the food sweeter and easier to digest.

Many First Nations used cooking pits to slowly roast food. A pit was dug and lined with stones that had been heated in a fire. The stones were covered with green leaves, followed by a layer of the food to be cooked, a layer of leaves and matting and finally about 15 cm of firmly packed soil. Often, sticks were placed vertically in the pit during the layering, and when the pit was complete, they were removed and water was poured down to the hot rocks to steam the contents. The holes were then plugged, and a hot fire was built on top of the pit and maintained until cooking was complete. Cooking lasted from several hours to a few days. Large amounts of food could be cooked in pits for social gatherings or for storage for later use.

Foods with tough, outer coverings were often placed on, or covered with, hot coals and left to roast. The burned outer layers were then peeled away, and the edible inner parts were eaten.

Drying was the traditional way of preserving many plant foods. Roots and berries were cleaned and spread on leaves in well-ventilated areas, often in the sun, where they dried in a few days. Smoke and heat from slow-burning fires often kept insects away and increased the rate of drying. Larger, thicker plant parts were usually sliced to speed the drying process. Sometimes fruits or roots were first mashed and/or boiled into mush and then spread in a thin layer (like fruit leather) or formed into cakes and dried. Leaves were usually dried by hanging bundles of plants in a warm, dry place.

Today, fruits and vegetables can be dried in dehydrators or in ovens with the door propped open a crack to allow ventilation. Ovens must be set at very low heat, or the food may cook and thus change its flavour and texture. Many dried foods, especially berries and other sweet fruits, can be eaten dry as snacks or trail food, but most dried vegetables are best softened by soaking and/or boiling.

Preserving and canning have also been widely used to prepare wild foods for storage. Many fruits, including a large number of berries that are too sour to enjoy fresh, make excellent jams and jellies. Basically, fruits are boiled with sugar and water until they thicken to make jam and then strained to make jelly. Some fruits thicken on their own, but others need additional pectin in order to jell. Even fruits that are low in pectin can provide tasty sauces for desserts, but they usually require large amounts of additional sugar. Pickling is a preserving technique that uses vinegar instead of sugar to maintain the quality of the food. Basically, fruits or vegetables are packed in jars with a mixture of spices, covered with boiling vinegar and left to pickle for several weeks. Most cookbooks have recipes and instructions for canning and for making jams, jellies and pickles.

Flours and cereals are prepared from starchy fruits (e.g., grains and acorns), rhizomes, tubers, bulbs and corms. This preparation usually involves cleaning and thoroughly drying the plant part and then grinding the product into meal or flour.

Seed cleaning involves removing tough outer parts such as the small bracts that surround grass grains and the thick hulls that enclose acorn nut meats. First, the outer parts must be broken free from the seed. In some cases, gently rubbing the fruits between your hands will break and remove the outer shell, but in other cases, it is necessary to crack and lightly grind the fruits. Once the grains or meats have been freed, the mixture is repeatedly tossed into the air, poured back and forth between containers or covered with water so that breezes or buoyancy can separate the heavy, starchy grains from their lighter outer coverings.

Cleaning underground plant parts such as rhizomes usually involves thorough washing and the removal of rootlets and tough outer layers. The cleaned, starchy parts are then dried thoroughly and ground

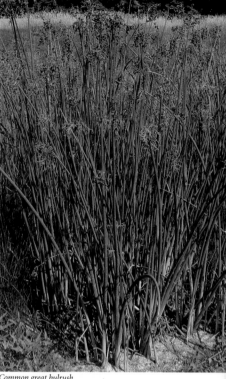
Common great bulrush

into meal or flour. Sometimes, large, starchy rhizomes are peeled and then broken apart under water to free starch from the tough central fibres. The fibres are then discarded, the heavy starch is allowed to settle and the water is poured off. This starchy residue can be used immediately as a wet dough, or it can be dried and ground into flour.

Traditionally, grinding involved crushing grains between two rocks, but blenders and electric mills have greatly simplified this task. Starchy meal or flour can be eaten alone or mixed with fats, cooked in water as mush, added to soups and stews as a thickener or used alone or (usually) with other flours in breads, muffins, pancakes, etc.

Parching can greatly improve the flavour of many grains and nutlets. Slightly roast dried seeds or seed-like fruits at low temperatures until they are lightly browned. The ones with hairs or other coverings that are difficult to remove may be lightly burned to remove their outer layers, while at the same time parching the seed within. Sometimes, parching will split open the tough outer shells of fruits, and in a few cases (e.g., cow-lilies, p. 188), it pops the seeds, as with corn seeds to produce popcorn.

Steeping, decocting and juicing all produce beverages. Many wild plants can be used to make caffeine-free teas, coffees and cold drinks.

Most teas are made by pouring boiling water over leaves, flowers, bark or fruits and leaving the mixture to steep for five to ten minutes to make an infusion. Sometimes, plants are boiled in water to make decoctions. The strength of the tea increases with the length of steeping or boiling time and with the amount of plant material used.

Coffees are made by drying and roasting rhizomes, grains or nutlets until they are brown and then grinding them into meal or powder. These mixtures can be perked or dripped as they are, but often they are mixed with domestic coffee as a coffee-stretcher or flavour-enhancer.

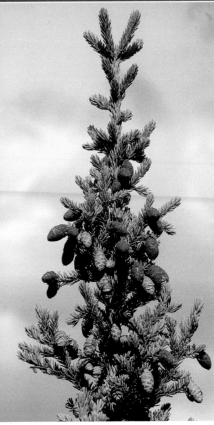

Black spruce

Some teas and coffees make excellent cold drinks. A few are chilled and served plain, but most are sweetened with sugar and/or mixed with ginger, lemon, raspberries or other fruit for flavouring. Delicious cold drinks can also be made by mixing mashed fruits with sugar and soda water. Similarly, sour-tasting leaves may be bruised, soaked in water and sweetened to make a refreshing drink similar to lemonade.

Fermentation can transform a great variety of wild fruits, flowers, roots, leaves and barks into delicious beers, wines and vinegars. Generally, this process requires steeping or boiling selected plant parts in water and straining off the liquid, but sometimes the sweet spring sap of trees is used. The plant extract is sweetened with sugar, yeast is added and the mixture is left to bubble (ferment) in a warm place until much of the sugar has been converted into alcohol and carbon dioxide. Sometimes, when the fermenting liquid is contaminated with certain bacteria, vinegar is produced instead. The quality of homemade wine, beer and vinegar varies greatly from plant to plant and batch to batch. Success requires knowledge of wine-making techniques and the use of proper equipment combined with a certain amount of experimentation. Many books are available on this topic.

Sugar extraction can be a long, tedious task. The best-known source of wild sugar is the sweet, watery sap of maple and birch trees. Large quantities of sap (about 10–15 times the final volume, depending on sugar content) must be collected in early spring and boiled for many hours to remove the water and concentrate the sugars. At times in the past, sugar from sweet plants was dissolved in water, and the liquid was then boiled like sap to produce syrup. Sugar extraction is a lengthy, laborious task, and it is understandable that the traditional diets of native peoples relied largely on berries and other naturally sweet foods for sweetening.

Oil extraction from plants can be time consuming. Most tribes relied on animal fat because very few wild plants contain enough oil to merit refining. However, some oil-rich seeds (e.g., sunflower seeds) were boiled in water, and the oil that rose to the surface was skimmed off and stored for later use. Water in narrow containers has a small surface area and so a thicker layer of oil, which makes skimming easier.

Seasonings are strong-flavoured or salt-rich plants that may not be edible by themselves but that can be used to add flavour to other foods. Plants used for seasoning were often dried and stored for later use. Some salt-rich plants were burned slowly on rocks or in clay balls, and their ashes were then used as seasoning. Flavour and salt content can vary greatly with the habitat and age of a plant, so amounts added are usually based on personal taste and experimentation. Some strong-flavoured plants are mixed with vinegar to make condiments, such as mustard and mint sauce.

Medicine

Plants have been used to cure, or at least to relieve the symptoms of, human diseases and injuries for thousands of years. Ancient medicinal uses were often based more on superstition and folklore than on fact. In Europe, the "Doctrine of Signatures" decreed that the plant's form revealed its use, so hairy plants were good for stimulating hair growth, and plants with kidney-shaped leaves were used to treat kidney problems. Many of the uses recorded in ancient herbals were probably short lived. When one medicine failed, another was tried, but the first may still have been recorded as a treatment. In some parts of North

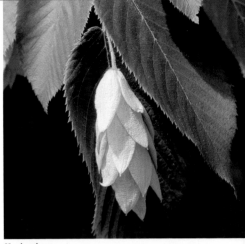

Hop hornbeam

America, it seems as though every common plant has been used to treat measles, smallpox, tuberculosis or syphilis. The historical use of a plant does not imply that it was effective. It could have been just one in a long series of failed experiments.

Many plants have persisted as medicines through years of trial and error because they proved effective. Some of these may have strengthened the patient by supplying important minerals and vitamins, but some contained powerful drugs that acted alone or in combination with other compounds. Modern medicine approaches drug plants from a different point of view, demanding standardized tests on the treatment of specific symptoms (rather than general, personal anecdotes) and analyzing the structure and action of the chemicals involved (rather than basing use on the knowledge passed down from earlier generations). This scientific approach has discredited many natural medicines, but there are also cases where research supports traditional uses. Most plants have yet to be studied.

Preparations for herbal medicines are not described in detail in this book. Medicinal information is presented for interest's sake, not as a how-to guide for a home pharmacy. Some plants can be used safely for treating minor injuries and illnesses, but many medicinal plants are poisonous if prepared improperly or taken in large doses. A person who is truly ill should consult a health-care professional rather than experiment with possible cures at home. Also, if you are taking medication, always check with your doctor before trying herbal remedies to avoid dangerous chemical interactions; the drugs in the herbs could counteract the drugs in your medication, they could supplement your dose and raise it to dangerously high levels or they could cause complications by creating antagonistic side effects. It takes years of study to understand the actions and interactions of medicinal herbs before safely using them. If you are interested in learning more about the uses of medicinal plants, there are many books on this subject (see p. 432).

Plants are prepared and administered in many different ways as medicines. Drugs to be taken internally are usually prepared as medicinal teas. Water extracts are prepared by pouring boiling water over selected plant parts and then either leaving the mixture to steep for a short time to make an infusion or boiling it to produce a decoction. When the active ingredient is not water-soluble, it is usually extracted by soaking the plant parts in alcohol (usually ethanol or vodka) for several hours or days to produce a tincture. Many plant extracts are applied externally to combat infection and to treat a wide range of skin diseases, injuries, aches and pains. Some medicinal teas are used as washes to clean and heal injuries.

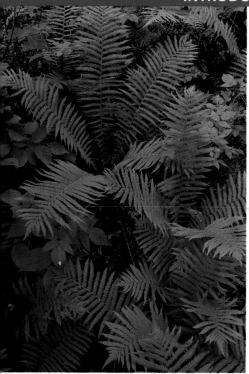

Ostrich fern

Many plants (fresh or dried) are crushed, moistened and applied to injuries as hot or cold compresses or poultices.

The concentration of active chemicals in a plant can vary greatly with its habitat and age. Some compounds are most concentrated in young shoots, while others increase as the plant ages and are most concentrated in mature plants. Many drugs are strongest in specific parts of the plant (e.g., in the roots, leaves or seeds) and are absent or much less concentrated elsewhere.

The way in which a plant material is prepared also affects the strength and effectiveness of the medicine produced. Many medicinal herbs are dried and stored for future use. Drying usually involves placing thin layers of plant parts on a well-ventilated surface (e.g., a screen or loosely woven fabric) in a warm, dry, dark place to ensure rapid drying and to reduce chemical breakdown from exposure to light (photolysis). Thoroughly dried plants are then stored in airtight containers to reduce the loss of volatile compounds.

Plant material is often ground to produce herbal medicines. Traditionally, grinding involved crushing material between two rocks or with a mortar and pestle, but modern blenders, grain mills and coffee mills have greatly simplified the process. Some dried plants can be simply rolled into powder using a rolling pin.

Other Uses

Plants provide most of our foods and medicines, but they can also be used in many other ways. Plant fibres produce paper, clothing, thread and twine. Wood provides building materials and fuel. Light, airy plants and seed-fluff can provide insulation, bedding, tinder and absorbent padding for diapers and dressings. Even plant toxins can be used to our advantage for killing or repelling insects, rodents and other pests. Many plants are used for pleasure—chewed like gum, smoked like tobacco (p. 240) or used to make toy flutes and dolls for children. These applications are discussed under the heading Other Uses.

Warning

Many plants have developed very effective protective mechanisms. Thorns and stinging hairs discourage animals from touching, let alone eating, many plants. Bitter, often poisonous compounds in leaves and roots repel grazing animals. Many protective devices are dangerous to humans. The Warning boxes throughout the book include notes of potential hazards associated with the plant(s) described. Hazards can range from deadly poisons to airborne pollen that may cause allergic reactions. These Warning boxes may also include descriptions of poisonous plants that could be confused with the species being discussed and notes about factors affecting toxicity (e.g., seeds or roots may be more toxic than other parts of the plant; young plants may be more dangerous than old plants).

The Poisonous Plants section (pp. 392–417) includes toxic species that have not been widely used by humans. Many plants discussed in the main body of the book are also poisonous, but they are included with the useful species because they have been gathered as foods or medicines or used in other ways.

The fine line between delicious and dangerous is not always clearly defined. Many of the plants that we eat every day contain toxins. Broccoli, asparagus and spinach all contain carcinogenic alkaloids, but you would have to eat huge amounts in a short time to be poisoned. Almost any food is toxic if you eat too much of it. Personal sensitivities can also be important. People with allergies may die from eating common foods (e.g., peanuts) that are harmless to most of the population. Most wild plants are not widely used today, so their effects on a broad spectrum of society remain unknown.

As with many aspects of life, the best approach is "moderation in all things." Enjoy a varied diet with a mixture of different fruits, vegetables and grains. When trying something for the first time, take only a small amount to see how you like it and how your body reacts. Enjoy the wonderful array of foods that nature has provided, but sample wisely!

Description

The plant description and the accompanying photos and illustrations are important parts of each species account. If you cannot correctly identify a plant, you should not use it. Identification is more critical with some plants than with others. For example, most people recognize strawberries (p. 178) and raspberries (p. 94), and all of the species in

Bristly black currant

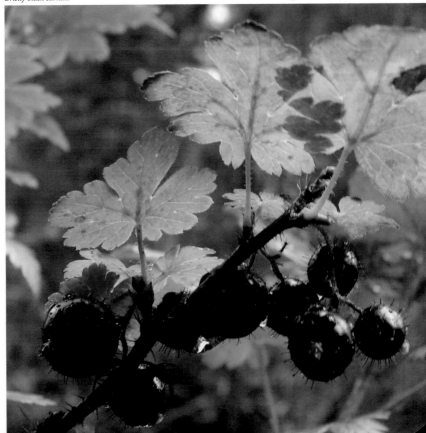

these two groups are edible, though not all are equally palatable. However, plants in the Carrot family (pp. 291–303, 410–412) are much more difficult to distinguish from each other, and some species contain deadly poisons, so confusion can have fatal results. Using a plant in this group without positive identification has been called herbal roulette.

Each plant description begins with a general outline of the form of the species or genus named at the top of the page. Detailed information about diagnostic features of the leaves, flowers and fruits is then provided. Flowering time is included as part of the flower description to give some idea of when to look for blooms and, by extension, when fruits can be expected. If two or more species of the same genus have been used for similar purposes, several of the most common species in Canada may be illustrated and their distinguishing features described.

As discussed earlier, plant characteristics such as size, shape, colour and hairiness vary with season and habitat and with the genetic variability of each species. Identification can be especially tricky when plants have not yet flowered or fruited. If you are familiar with a species and know its leaves or roots at a glance, you may be able to identify it at any time of year (from very young shoots to the dried remains of last year's plants), but sometimes a positive ID is just not possible.

General habitat information is provided for each species to give you some idea of where to look for a plant. The habitat description provides information about general habitat (e.g., in moist, mossy forest), elevation (e.g., low to montane elevations) and range (e.g., Saskatchewan to Nova Scotia). If you are hiking along the British Columbia coast, you probably won't find a plant whose habitat is described as "dry slopes on the prairies," but the habitat information included for each species is meant as a general guide only. Common plants often grow in a variety of habitats over a broad geographical range.

The origin of non–North American species is also noted. The flora of many areas in Canada has changed dramatically over the past 200 years, especially in and around human settlements. European settlers brought many plants with them, either accidentally (in ship ballast, packing and livestock bedding) or purposely (for food, medicine, fibre, etc.). Many of these introduced species have thrived, and some are now common weeds on disturbed sites across much of Canada.

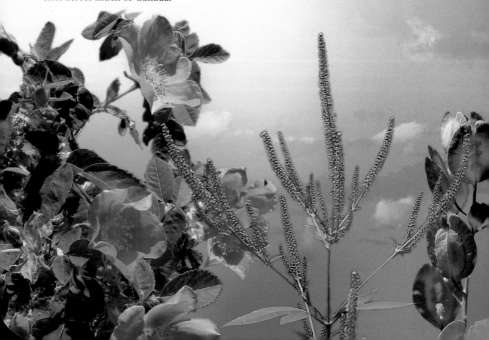

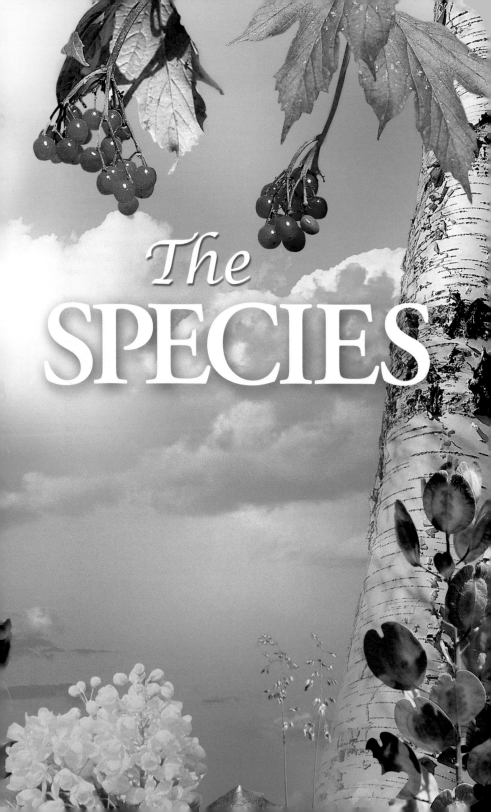

The
SPECIES

Spruces
Picea spp.

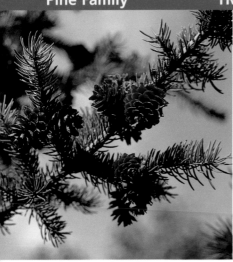

Engelmann spruce (all images)

FOOD: Spruce beer was popular among early northern travellers and was important in preventing scurvy; it is said to taste like root beer. The cambium (inner bark) was harvested in spring and either eaten fresh or dried into cakes and eaten with berries. Dried inner bark can be ground into a nutritious meal for extending flour during times of food shortage. Tender young shoots, stripped of their needles, can be boiled as an emergency food. The branches were made into a tea. As with fir, spruce needles are an exceptional source of vitamin C in winter, and the flavonoids have antioxidant properties as well.

MEDICINE: Spruce is among the top 10 medicinal plants used by First Nations. The sticky sap or moist inner bark was used in poultices on slivers, sores and inflammations. Similarly, sap mixed with fat provided salves for treating skin infections, insect bites, chapped hands, cuts, scrapes, eczema, burns, rashes, blood poisoning, heart trouble, syphilis and arthritic joints; it was also placed on the eyes for snowblindness. Melted sap was used as plaster when setting bones. Spruce gum was chewed or boiled and taken like cough syrup to relieve coughs and sore throats. It was also taken to help digestion, to treat gonorrhea and as a laxative. Some sources recommend spruce pitch as a sunscreen, but it seems like a rather sticky solution, not easily removed. Emerging needles were boiled to make an antiseptic wash or chewed to relieve coughs. Medicinal teas, made from the inner bark, were believed to cure rheumatism, kidney stones and stomach problems. Hot spruce needle tea was used to stimulate sweating and to treat scurvy and cancer, and the vapour was inhaled to relieve bronchitis. The cone was used for toothaches, venereal disease, pain, urinary problems and to assist women after childbirth. The bark was used for respiratory ailments, tuberculosis and diarrhea and as a sweat bath for rheumatism and backaches. Rotten, dried, finely powdered wood was used as baby powder and for skin rashes. The roots were used to treat trembling and fits, stomach pain and diarrhea.

OTHER USES: Spruce was an exceptionally important utility plant for Aboriginal cultures. Spruce bark was sometimes used to make canoes, baskets and utensils and to thatch the roofs of lodges; the trunks were sometimes used to make tepee poles. Lumps of hardened pitch were chewed for pleasure and to keep teeth white; it was applied to the

WARNING

Always use evergreen teas in moderation. Do not eat the needles or drink the teas in high concentrations or with great frequency. Some people develop rashes from contact with spruce resin, sawdust or needles.

ends of redcedar torches used in night fishing. Melted pitch was used to caulk canoe seams and to stick sheets of birch bark or strands of willow-bark twine together. It was also used to preserve and waterproof strips of hide (babiche) in ropes, snares, harpoons and snowshoes. Fresh or soaked spruce roots were peeled and split to make cord for stitching canoes, sewing snowshoes, baskets, tools, mats, hats and fish nets. Split roots were also woven into watertight bags for cooking. The roots were also used to make headgear and masks for ceremonies, trays and buckets. Spruce wood is generally strong and uniform. The wood was used to make canoe paddles, ribs and gunwales for birchbark canoes, canoe or kayak stringers, cabins and caches, fish traps, scrub brushes, arrows, digging sticks and bark peeling tools. It is used for lumber, plywood, mine timbers, poles and railway ties. Its long fibres, light colour and low resin content make it excellent pulp wood (black spruce is best). Because of its resonance, Engelmann spruce wood is used to make piano sounding boards and violins. The boughs were used for pillows, bedding, camp mattresses, dog bedding and rituals, often for purification and initiation rituals or as protection from death and illness. A yellow-brown dye can be obtained from the rotten wood and was used to dye white goods or to smoke tanned hides.

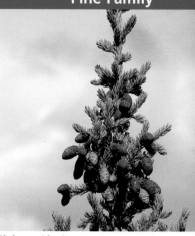

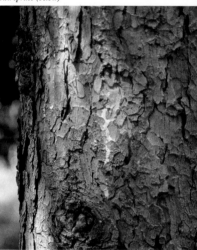

Black spruce (above)
Red spruce (below)

DESCRIPTION: Coniferous, evergreen trees, 20–95 m tall, with thin, scaly bark. Leaves pointed, 4-sided needles, 1–3 cm long, borne on persistent stubs and spirally arranged on all sides of the branches. Cones male or female, with both sexes on the same tree. Seed (female) cones with thin, flexible scales, hanging, produced from May to July, open in autumn and fall intact.

Engelmann spruce (*P. engelmannii*) grows to 50 m tall; usually has minutely hairy young twigs, and the scales of its 3–8 cm long female cones have jagged upper edges. Grows on cool, moist montane and subalpine slopes in BC and AB.

White spruce (*P. glauca*) grows to 30 m tall; has hairless young twigs, and the scales of its 2.5–5 cm long seed cones have smooth, broadly rounded edges. Grows in muskeg, bogs and on riverbanks to montane slopes in all provinces and territories. White spruce and Engelmann spruce often hybridize. White spruce is the provincial tree of MB.

Black spruce (*P. mariana*) grows to 25 m tall; its young twigs have tiny, rusty hairs, and its small (1–3 cm long) seed cones persist on the tree for several years. This is a northern species found in all provinces and territories. Black spruce is the provincial tree of NL.

Red spruce (*P. rubens*) grows to 40 m tall; has stout twigs, yellow-brown, hairy or smooth. Found in upper montane to subalpine forests in ON, QC, NB, NS and PEI. Red spruce is the provincial tree of NS. See p. 424 for conservation status.

Sitka spruce (*P. sitchensis*) grows to 95 m tall; has smooth, pinkish brown, stout twigs. Found in coastal forests in BC.

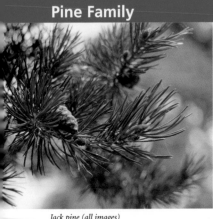

Jack pine (all images)

Two-Needled Pines

Pinus spp.

FOOD: The inner bark is succulent and sweet when the sap is running in spring. It was eaten fresh or dried into cakes. The seeds are high in fat and protein, and they often have a resinous flavour. Evergreen tea made from pine needles is best sweetened with sugar, honey, molasses or maple syrup, or spiced with cinnamon, nutmeg and orange peel. The pitch was sometimes chewed like gum.

MEDICINE: Pine needle tea is high in vitamins A and C and was taken in winter to prevent or cure scurvy. The inner bark was used as a dressing for scalds, burns and skin infections. Pine pitch was chewed to soothe sore throats and sweeten bad breath; it was taken internally to treat kidney problems, stomachaches and tuberculosis and as a purgative and diuretic. Warmed sap was applied to sore muscles, arthritic joints, insect bites, swellings, skin infections, sore eyes and the chest for heart trouble. It was also heated until it turned black, mixed with bone marrow (1 part marrow to 4 parts sap) and used as a salve for burns.

OTHER USES: The straight, slender trunks of lodgepole pine were used as poles for travois, tepees and lodges (hence the name). Each tepee required 25–30 poles, 7–8 m long. These usually had to be replaced almost every year, and Aboriginal people from the prairies sometimes travelled hundreds of kilometres to the mountains to get new poles. Lodgepole pine wood is light coloured and straight grained, with a soft, even texture. The wood was used to make story sticks, fire tongs, cedar bark peelers and digging sticks. The Blackfoot used to make lodgepole pine wind chimes: these were presented to newly married couples. The pitch, mixed with bear tallow, rose petals and red ochre, was used as a face cream or for blemishes, or rubbed on the skin of newborn babies. The pitch was also used as a glue in headdresses and bows or applied to moccasins for waterproofing. Today, pine lumber is used to frame homes and construct moldings and furniture.

DESCRIPTION: Coniferous trees, 12–30 m tall, with 2–6 cm long, evergreen needles in bundles of 2. Seed cones thick-scaled, oval, mature in 2 years, but may remain closed on branches or on the ground for many years.

Jack pine (*P. banksiana*) grows to 20 m tall; has seed cones with no spines, or with tiny prickles only, that point toward branch tips. Found in boreal forests, tundra transition, dry flats and hills from northeastern BC to Labrador, including the Maritimes, but not in YT. See p. 424 for conservation status.

Lodgepole pine (*P. contorta* var. *latifolia*) grows to 30 m tall; has seed cones with spine-tipped scales that point straight out or backward along the stem. Widespread in foothill and montane zones in BC, AB, extreme southwestern SK, NT and YT. Lodgepole pine is the provincial tree of AB. A shorter variety, **shore pine** (*P. contorta* var. *contorta*), grows along BC's coast.

Red pine (*P. resinosa*) grows to 25 m tall; has reddish to pinkish bark, with oval cones. Found on fresh to dry, sandy to loamy sites from MB to the Maritimes.

WARNING
Large amounts of evergreen tea can be toxic. Pregnant women should not drink this tea.

Ponderosa Pine

Pinus ponderosa

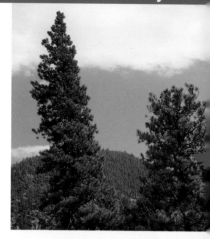

FOOD: The sweet inner bark (cambium) was said to taste something like sheep fat. It was collected on cool, cloudy days when the sap was running. The bark was removed from 1 side of a tree only (to avoid killing the tree), and the edible inner bark was then scraped from the tough outer layer. This inner bark was usually eaten immediately, but it could also be kept moist, rolled in bags, for a few days. Some pines still bear large scars from the traditional harvest of the cambium; these are known as "culturally modified trees" (CMTs). CMTs provide valuable information about human activities extending far back in time. The oil-rich seeds are also edible. They were shaken from the cones and ground into meal that was used to make bread. The young, unopened male cones can be boiled as an emergency food. When finely chopped, the young needles can be used to make tea. Some say that ponderosa pine makes the best pine tea, whereas others say that it is the most potentially toxic.

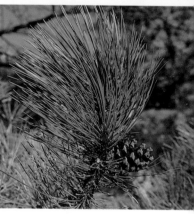

MEDICINE: The resin was applied alone or in salves to boils, carbuncles, abscesses, rheumatic joints and aching backs. A dubious method for treating dandruff involved jabbing the pointed ends of the needles into the scalp to "kill the germs." The needle tea is rich in vitamins A and C.

OTHER USES: The pitch was chewed as gum, plastered in hair, used as glue, burned in torches and used to waterproof woven containers. The light, soft wood has been used to make dwellings, fence posts, saddle horns, snowshoes and baby cradles. Today, it is used as lumber and made into moldings, cabinets and crates.

DESCRIPTION: Coniferous tree, to 35 m tall, with evergreen needles 10–25 cm long, usually in bundles of 3. Bark orange-brown to cinnamon with jigsaw-like plates outlined by deep, black fissures. Seed cones oval, 8–14 cm long, with thick, spine-tipped scales, maturing in 2 years. Grows on dry sites in foothill and montane zones in southern BC; introduced in AB.

> **WARNING**
> Large amounts of pine tea can be toxic, and extended use irritates the kidneys. Pregnant cows that eat ponderosa pine needles may abort their calves in 2 days to 2 weeks. Pregnant women should not drink this tea.

Five-Needled Pines

Pinus spp.

FOOD: The inner bark (cambium) is sweet and edible in spring, and young needles can be steeped to make pine tea. The oil-rich, nutritious seeds were eaten by Aboriginal peoples and early settlers. Unopened cones were burned in a large fire, which cooked and released the seeds at the same time. The seeds were then eaten, ground into meal for making breads or stored for later use (sometimes mixed with dried berries).

MEDICINE: The tender young needles are a good source of vitamin C and have been used to treat scurvy. This tea is said to stimulate urination and help bring up phlegm and mucous from the lungs, so it is often used for respiratory problems such as coughs and tuberculosis. Pine resin has been used for many years in cough syrups and in ointments for burns and skin infections. The resin was often applied externally to treat cuts, sores, bruises, scabs and boils, for drawing out thorns and slivers and as a skin cosmetic. It is used both internally and as a rub and steam bath in the treatment of rheumatic affections. It has been used for stomach and kidney troubles, as a spring emetic, blood purifier and fertility aid. The inner bark was applied to the chest to treat strong colds. The powdered wood was used on babies to treat chafing and sores or on improperly healed navels.

Eastern white pine (all images)

OTHER USES: Eastern white pine is the sacred tree and symbol of the Ojibwa. The pitch was used as a protective coating for whaling and fishing equipment and as a waterproofing and cleansing agent. The boughs of eastern white pine wood were used on the ground or floor as bedding. Western white pine wood is the most important western source for matchwood. The wood has been used to make small totem poles, canoes and baskets. A tan or green dye can be obtained from the needles. Western white pine populations have been seriously affected by white pine blister rust, a fungus that was introduced from Europe. Resistance to this fungus is genetic, so some individuals are relatively unaffected by the rust. Eastern white pine is an important timber tree and is grown widely in plantation

WARNING

Large amounts of evergreen tea can be toxic. Pregnant women should not drink this tea. Extended use irritates the kidneys.

forestry; it was a valued source for ship masts in the past.

DESCRIPTION: Coniferous trees, 20–50 m tall, with evergreen needles 4–7 cm long, in bundles of 5. Seed cones thick-scaled, containing large (1 cm long) seeds.

Whitebark pine (*P. albicaulis*), at high elevations, grows as a spreading, prostrate shrub; at lower elevations and in favourable conditions, grows to 20 m tall; has purplish brown, 5–8 cm long cones that usually remain closed and gradually break apart. Grows on exposed slopes near the timberline in southern BC and western AB (Rocky Mountains). See p. 424 for conservation status.

Western white pine (*P. monticola*) grows to 50 m tall; has larger (10–25 cm long), creamy brown to yellowish cones that shed their seeds and fall soon after. Grows in lowland and montane, moist forests in southern BC and western AB (Rocky Mountains). See p. 424 for conservation status.

Eastern white pine (*P. strobus*) grows to 30 m tall; has grey-brown to pale brown cones, 8–20 cm long, that shed their seeds and fall quickly after. Grows in mesic to dry sites from southeastern MB across to NL and grew to exceptional size as emergents in eastern Canadian forests. Eastern white pine is the provincial tree of ON. See p. 424 for conservation status.

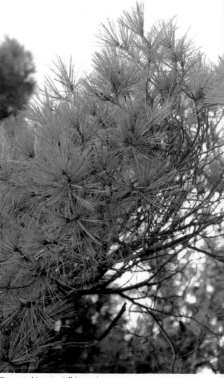

Eastern white pine (all images)

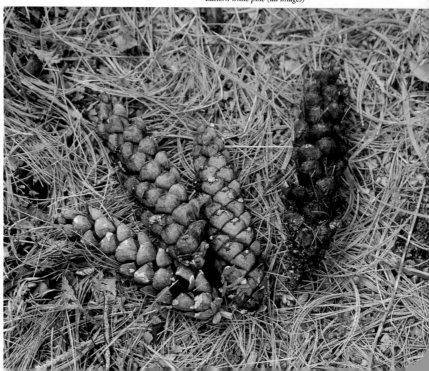

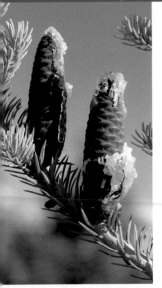

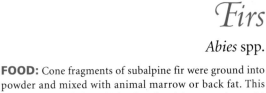

Firs

Abies spp.

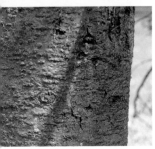

Balsam fir (all images)

FOOD: Cone fragments of subalpine fir were ground into powder and mixed with animal marrow or back fat. This mixture was cooled until it hardened and then served at social events as a delicacy that had the added benefit of aiding digestion. Inner bark of balsam fir was used for food, sometimes grated and eaten or dried and ground into a nutritious (though not very tasty) meal and mixed with flour to extend food supplies in times of shortage. The hardened pitch of Pacific silver fir was chewed like candy. The bark of balsam fir and the gum or branch tips from grand fir were used to make a beverage.

MEDICINE: Balsam fir was the most widely used medicinal plant by eastern First Nations, who used it to make various preparations for treating cuts, wounds, ulcers, sores, bleeding gums and skin infections. The needles are high in antioxidant flavonoids, and their vitamin C content is exceptionally high in winter months. Needles are also said to stimulate urination and to help bring phlegm up from the lungs. Fir needle tea was taken for colds and as a laxative; a poultice made from the needles was used to induce sweating and treat fevers and chest colds. Smoke from burning fir needles was inhaled as a treatment for headaches, fainting, swollen faces associated with venereal disease and to prevent sickness. Fir pitch was taken alone or in teas as a treatment for coughs, sore throats, colds, asthma, tuberculosis, menstrual irregularity, fractures, kidney troubles, diarrhea, loss of appetite, ulcers, cancer (balsam fir gum with dried beaver kidneys), gonorrhea, general feelings of weakness or any type of illness. In stronger doses, it was said to induce vomiting and act as a purgative. Fir pitch provides a handy antiseptic for wounds, cuts, insect bites, sores, infections, bruises, scabies and boils. The pitch was also chewed to clean the teeth and as a cure for bad breath. Pacific silver fir bark was taken for stomach ailments such as ulcers, for internal injuries (when mixed with red alder [p. 54] and hemlock [p. 40] bark) and as a general tonic. The roots of balsam fir were taken for heart disease or used in an herbal steam for rheumatic joints or during childbirth.

OTHER USES: Fir needles (in tea or dried and powdered) or the gum was mixed with deer or bear grease to produce a pleasant-smelling hair tonic, as a treatment for dandruff or to prevent hair loss. Powdered needles were also used as baby powder, put in

WARNING
Fir resin can cause skin reactions in some people. Always use evergreen teas in moderation. Do not eat the needles or drink the teas in high concentrations or with great frequency.

moccasins as a foot deodorant or rubbed on the body and on clothing as perfume and insect repellent. Fir needles were burned as incense (smudging), and fir boughs were hung on walls as air-fresheners. Fir incense was thought to chase away bad spirits and ghosts and to revive the spirits of people near death. The needles and wood were stuffed into pillows and used for good health. The boughs were used for pillows, bedding, as mats on tent floors or to make a brush shelter. The boughs of Pacific silver fir were used to line eulachon ripening pits and to make bush sleighs to pull cargo across deep snow. The wood was used for kindling and to make shingles on roofs, canoes, paddles and chairs and to insect-proof storage boxes for dancing regalia. Roots were used to make thread, and the resin was used to make canoe pitch (for waterproofing seams). Fir was also used for ceremonial purposes: the pitch was applied to the faces of mourners, the needles were used in sweats, and branches and pollen were used in purification ceremonies. The long, hard knots in the wood were used to make halibut hooks. Ground needles were used in horse medicine bundles, an infusion of bark was given to horses for diarrhea and a needle smudge was used to fumigate sick horses. Burning fir wood was believed to give protection and renewed confidence to people who were afraid of thunder and lightning. On grand fir, black conks (hoof-shaped, "woody" fungal growths) called Indian paint fungus were used as a source of red pigment. Canada balsam is used in the manufacture of glues, candles and as a cement for mounting microscope slides. Firs are a traditional Christmas tree in many areas because they hold their needles well and have a wonderful fragrance.

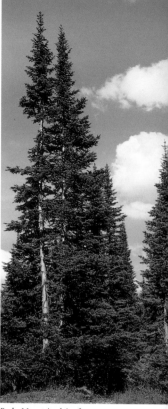

Rocky Mountain alpine fir

DESCRIPTION: Fragrant, evergreen, coniferous trees, 20–75 m tall, with whorled branches and thin, smooth young bark, with bulging resin blisters. Leaves flattened needles, spirally arranged but sometimes twisted upward or into 1 plane. Cones male or female, with both sexes on the same tree. Seed (female) cones cylindrical, stiffly upright, shedding scales with seeds and leaving a slender central core, appearing from May to July and maturing in 1 season.

Balsam fir (*A. balsamea*) grows to 25 m tall; needles 1.2–2.5 cm long, twisted into 1 row or spiralled. Groove on upper surface. Found in boreal and northern forests from AB to NL. Balsam fir is the provincial tree of NB.

Subalpine fir (*A. lasiocarpa*) reaches 20 m tall; thick, short (2.5–3 cm long), sometimes pointed needles curve upward, giving the branch tips a rounded appearance. Grows in subalpine forests in western YT and BC. Subalpine fir is the territorial tree of YT.

Rocky Mountain alpine fir (*A. bifolia*) reaches 30 m in height. It is difficult to distinguish from subalpine fir, but it grows in different places: continental subalpine forests in or near the Rocky Mountains.

Two other common west coast firs, grand and Pacific silver, have leaves twisted into 2 opposite rows, giving the branches a flattened, spray-like appearance. Both species have white lines (stomates) on lower surface only.

Grand fir (*A. grandis*) grows to 80 m tall; has 3–4 cm long needles flattened into 1 plane. Grows in moist, coastal, coniferous forests and mountain slopes in BC.

Pacific silver fir (*A. amabilis*) grows to 55 m tall; has shorter (1–2.5 cm long) needles, with some pressed against the upper surface of the branch. Found in moist, coastal, coniferous forests in BC.

Larches
Larix spp.

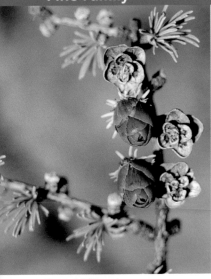

Tamarack (all images)

FOOD: Some tribes hollowed out cavities in western larch trunks to collect the trees' sweet sap. About 4 litres could be taken from a good tree, once or twice a year. This sap was evaporated to the consistency of molasses; more recently, it was mixed with sugar to make syrup. The sweet inner bark was eaten in spring, and sweet lumps of dried sap were chewed like gum year-round. The gum is said to taste like candy. Larch sap contains galactan, a natural sugar with a flavour like slightly bitter honey. Dried, powdered larch gum was used as baking powder. Tender young larch shoots can be cooked as a vegetable, and the inner bark can be dried, ground into meal and used to extend flour.

MEDICINE: Larch gum was chewed to aid digestion and to relieve sore throats, internal bleeding and enlarged, hardened livers. The gum and/or the soft inner bark were used in poultices to treat insect bites, cuts, bruises, wounds, frostbite, infections, ulcers and persistent skin problems such as eczema and psoriasis. They were also applied externally and taken internally in teas to relieve rheumatism and arthritis. The pitch was valued as a bone-setter for broken bones that would not heal. Larch bark tea was taken to treat jaundice, colds, coughs, bronchitis, tuberculosis, asthma, physical weakness, fevers, vomiting and ulcers and to stimulate the appetite; tea made from the bark and needles was said to cure both diarrhea and constipation. The bark is known to contain immune-enhancing arabinogalactans that are now commercially used. The plant tops were taken as a blood purifier, to treat cancer or used as an antiseptic for cuts and sores. The leaves or bark were used as a wash for infants to make them strong and healthy.

OTHER USES: Old larch logs were often a preferred source of fuel for smoking hides because the finished buckskins were neither too dark nor too light. The wood was used to make toboggans and arrow shafts and as kindling. Because larch wood was reputed not to rot, it was often used in boat-building. The roots were used to make bags and sew canoes. The pitch was heated, rubbed into a fine powder, mixed with grease and used as red paint on girls' faces. Today, the straight, relatively branch-free trunks, with their heavy, durable wood, are often used for telephone poles, railway ties, posts, construction timbers and mine timbers. Water-soluble gums (arabinogalactans) are extracted from larch

WARNING
Larch resin and sawdust cause skin reactions in some people. Always use evergreen teas in moderation. Do not eat the needles or drink the teas in high concentrations or with great frequency. Some tribes warned that eating too much of the sweet inner bark would purge the intestines.

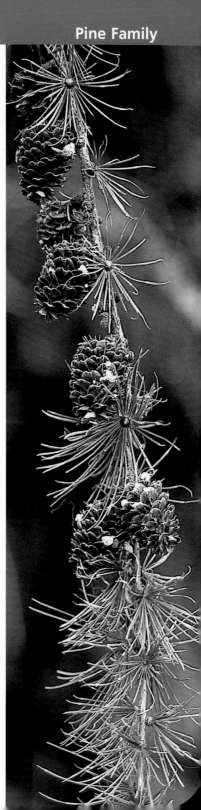

bark for use in paint, ink and medicines. The changes in leaf colour of western larch signalled the coming of autumn and the movement of pregnant bears to their dens for winter.

DESCRIPTION: Slender, coniferous trees, 12–70 m tall, with short, well-spaced, sparsely leaved branches. Leaves soft, deciduous needles, 2.5–4.5 cm long, in tufts on stubby twigs, bright yellow in autumn and shed in winter. Cones male or female, but both sexes on the same tree. Seed (female) cones with slender bracts between the thin, woody scales, red or purplish when young, produced from May to July, mature by autumn.

Tamarack (*L. laricina*) grows to 25 m tall; has hairless young twigs and very small (1–2 cm long) seed cones, with flat-topped needles that are strongly ridged beneath. Grows in boreal forests in wet, poorly drained sphagnum bogs and muskegs in all provinces and territories. Tamarack is the territorial tree of NT.

Subalpine larch (*L. lyallii*) grows to 15 m tall; has woolly young twigs, larger (3.5–4.5 cm long) cones and 4-sided needles. Usually grows at elevations near the timberline in southern BC and southwestern AB (Rocky Mountains).

Western larch (*L. occidentalis*) grows to 70 m tall; has essentially hairless young twigs and small (2.5–3 cm long) seed cones, and its needles are flat-topped but strongly ridged beneath. Grows on well-drained, upper foothill and montane slopes in southern BC and southwestern AB (Rocky Mountains). See p. 424 for conservation status.

Western larch (all images)

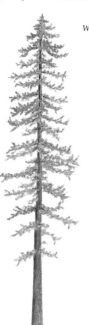

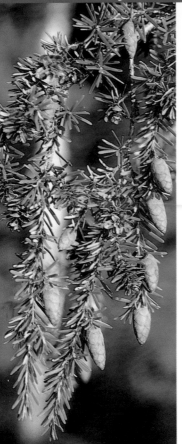

Hemlocks

Tsuga spp.

FOOD: The sweet inner bark (cambium) was a staple food for some First Nations in BC. It was scraped from the trunk and baked or steamed in underground pits. The cambium was then pressed into cakes and eaten with fish oil or cranberries, or it was dried in the sun for future use. In winter, some tribes enjoyed the dried bark whipped together with snow and fish grease. Hemlock cambium can also be eaten raw in an emergency (though it is harder to digest) or dried, ground into meal and added to flour to extend it. The fresh needles were sometimes combined with maple sap and eaten; they make a fragrant evergreen tea that was widely drunk. The leaves or branch tips were sometimes eaten to relieve hunger if one was without food in the woods.

MEDICINE: Hemlock bark was boiled to make medicinal washes for treating burns, rashes, cuts and wounds. It was also applied externally for bruises, broken bones, internal injuries, eczema and other skin conditions. Teas made from the bark were used to treat flu, coughs, colds, sore throats, tuberculosis, rheumatic fever, grippe, scurvy, abdominal pains and diarrhea. The needles are rich in vitamin C, especially in winter, and they were used in teas to cure colds and relieve congestion. Branches were formed into a poultice to treat arthritis or an infant's infected navel; they were taken as a tea to treat fevers or as an emetic. Ground bark was used as a powder for prickly heat and for chafed babies. A poultice containing hemlock gum was applied to treat heart trouble, sores on the face and sunburn. Hemlock oil was used for cholera, fatigue, consumption and bowel, stomach and internal troubles, and as a liniment to relieve rheumatic pain.

OTHER USES: The soft, fragrant boughs were used for bedding, as a disinfectant and deodorizer and as camouflage and for making temporary shelters or huts; they were also immersed in water to collect herring eggs and wrapped over food in earth ovens. Boiled hemlock bark produced a preservative and a red-brown, rosy-tan or black dye for tanning hides, colouring wooden articles (e.g., spears, paddles) and making nets less visible to fish; it was also used on traps to remove rust and give them a clean smell. The pitch was used to waterproof baskets and to protect skin from chapping and sunburn. Traditionally, the wood was used to make digging sticks, mallets, masks,

Western hemlock (all images)

WARNING
Do not eat evergreen needles or drink evergreen teas in high concentrations or with great frequency.

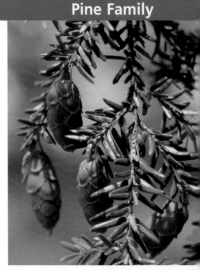

dishes, spoons, rattles, halibut hooks (knots), spears, fuel and kindling. Today, the hard, strong wood, with its even grain and colour, is used to make doors, windows, staircases, moldings, cupboards and hardwood floors. It also provides construction lumber, pilings, poles, railway ties, pulp and cellulose for making paper, cellophane, rayon and some plastics. This attractive, feathery tree is a popular ornamental, and several cultivars have been developed.

DESCRIPTION: Graceful, coniferous, evergreen trees, 15–50 m tall, with feathery, down-swept branches and flexible, nodding crown-tips. Leaves small needles, about 1–2 cm long, unequal, borne on small stubs. Cones male or female, with both sexes on the same tree. Seed (female) cones with thin, brownish scales, hanging, produced from May to June, opening in autumn and shed intact.

Eastern hemlock (*T. canadensis*) grows to 30 m tall; has 1.5–2.5 cm long seed cones, with white lines on the lower needle surface only. Grows on moist, rocky ridges, ravines and hillsides in southern ON, QC, NB, NS and PEI.

Western hemlock (*T. heterophylla*) grows to 50 m tall; has 1.5–2.5 cm long seed cones and flat needles with white lines (rows of stomata) on the lower surface only. Grows on moist foothill and montane slopes in BC and southwestern AB (Rocky Mountains). See p. 424 for conservation status.

Mountain hemlock (*T. mertensiana*) grows to 35 m tall; has 3–7 cm long seed cones and rounder needles with white lines on both sides. Grows on subalpine slopes in coastal BC; less common in southeastern BC.

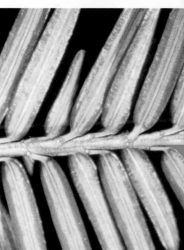

Eastern hemlock (all images)

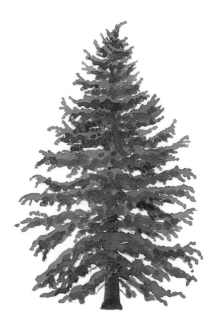

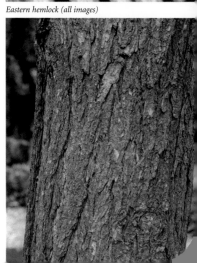

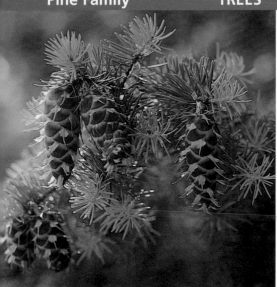

Douglas-Fir
Pseudotsuga menziesii

FOOD: The soft inner bark was used for survival food, and the small, pitchy seeds were also eaten. Young twigs and needles can be used as a substitute for coffee or tea. This mixture is usually sweetened with sugar. Sometimes, on hot, sunny days when photosynthesis and root pressure are high and transpiration is slow, white crystals of sugar appear at the needle tips and over the branches. This rare treat was usually eaten as a sweet nibble, but when quantities warranted, it was collected and used to sweeten other foods, such as arrow-leaved balsamroot (p. 354) seeds.

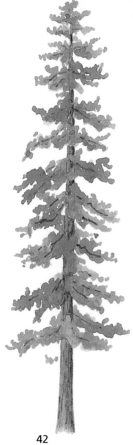

MEDICINE: Dried sap was chewed to relieve cold symptoms, and sticky buds were chewed to heal mouth sores. Liquid pitch and the soft inner bark can be used on cuts, boils, sores and other skin problems to aid healing and prevent infection. The pitch was also chewed for sore throats and applied as a poultice for injured or dislocated bones. Tea made from the gum or inner bark was used to treat colds or taken as a diuretic and for gonorrhea. Young Douglas-fir needles contain vitamin C and were used in teas to treat scurvy. A decoction made with the first year's growth shoots was taken as an emetic for anemia, intestinal pains, diarrhea and high fevers. Shoots were placed in the tips of moccasins to keep the feet from perspiring and to prevent athlete's foot. The bark was boiled to make a laxative tea or burned and pulverized to treat diarrhea. An infusion of green bark was taken for bleeding bowels, stomach troubles and excessive menstruation. A decoction of twigs was taken as a kidney and bladder remedy, diuretic and tonic. Rheumatism was treated through a moxa (burning an herb just above or on the skin as a counterirritant) of ashes, heated branches, bough tips or needles.

OTHER USES: Fragrant Douglas-fir boughs were often used for bedding and floor coverings for lodges and sweat houses. Hunters would scrub themselves with boughs before hunting so deer could not smell them, and boughs were placed under deer

> **WARNING**
> Always use evergreen teas in moderation. Do not eat the needles or drink the teas in high concentrations or with great frequency.

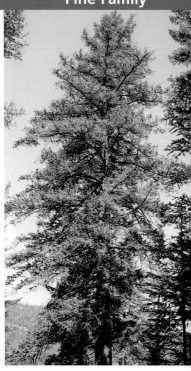

while butchering. Chewing branch tips helped freshen the breath. Rotted wood from old logs was burned slowly to smoke hides, and the bark was used in tanning or boiled with nets to make them brown and less visible to fish. The wood was used as a valuable fuel and to make bows, herring and eulachon rakes, halibut and cod hooks, tepee poles, spear shafts, seal spears and poles for placing codfish lures. Young saplings were made into dipnet hoops, snowshoe frames and handles, while peeled twig bundles served as whippers for soapberries (p. 129). The pliable roots have been used to weave baskets. The resin was sometimes burned as a fumigant and used to patch canoes and water vessels, and resinous branches provided torches. The pollen-shedding cones indicated that ponderosa pine (p. 33) cambium was ripe. Strong, durable Douglas-fir wood provides excellent lumber, plywood, poles and railway ties. These fragrant trees are popular Christmas trees.

DESCRIPTION: Coniferous, evergreen tree, to 80 m tall, with spreading or drooping branches. Mature trees with very open crowns. Buds pointed, shiny and reddish brown. Young bark thin, smooth and resin-blistered. Older bark ridged and fissured. Leaves flat, blunt needles, 2–3 cm long, spirally arranged, but sometimes twisted into 2 rows. Cones male or female, with both on the same tree. Seed (female) cones 4–10 cm long, hanging, with 3-toothed bracts projecting beyond stiff scales, produced from April to May, opening in autumn and falling intact. Douglas-fir grows on foothill, montane and subalpine slopes in coniferous and mixed forests in southern BC and southwestern AB (Rocky Mountains). Two varieties are recognized: **coast Douglas-fir** (*P. menziesii* var. *menziesii*), with larger cones (6–10 cm long) and deep green foliage; and **Rocky Mountain Douglas-fir** (*P. menziesii* var. *glauca*), with shorter cones (4–7 cm long) and bluish green foliage.

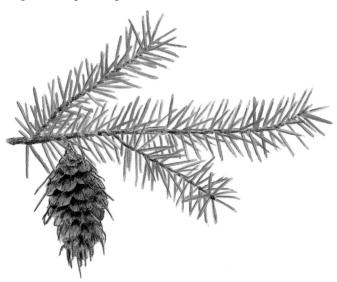

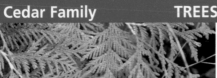

*C*edars
Thuja spp.

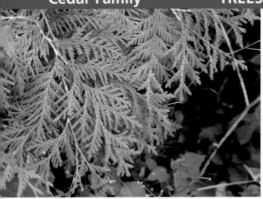

FOOD: The moist, inner bark (cambium) was collected in spring and eaten fresh, or dried and ground into a powder, then used with wheat and other cereals in bread-making. The pleasantly sweet pith of young white-cedar shoots was cooked and added to soups.

MEDICINE: The bough tea, sweetened with honey, was used to relieve diarrhea, coughs, colds, sore throats, bronchitis and other respiratory problems. Tea made from the bark and twigs was used to treat kidney problems. The sprays are strongly antifungal and antibacterial. Alcoholic extracts are said to cure fungal skin infections such as athlete's foot, ringworm, jock itch and nail fungi. Redcedar teas and tinctures are reported to stimulate smooth muscles and vascular capillaries, so they are recommended by some herbalists for the treatment of problems associated with mucous accumulations or sluggishness in the respiratory, urinary, reproductive and digestive tracts. White-cedar has established antiviral activity and is used in modern herbalism to treat warts and polyps. Steam from boiling sprays of redcedar was sometimes inhaled by pregnant women to induce labour, and that of white-cedar for rheumatism, arthritis and colds. The green buds were chewed to relieve toothaches. Oil from the leaves has been applied to warts, hemorrhoids, fungal infections and *Herpes simplex* sores (watery blisters on the skin and mucous membranes).

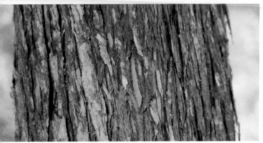

Eastern white-cedar (all images)

OTHER USES: Redcedar was the most important and widely used plant for western First Nations. The bark peels off easily in long, fibrous strips. Native peoples twisted, wove and plaited the soft inner strips to make baskets, blankets, clothing, ropes, mats and other items. Sometimes the bark was boiled with wood ash to make the fibres softer, more easily separated and easier to work. Bark was also pounded until fluffy and used in diapers, sanitary pads and mattresses. Sheets of bark were formed into

> **WARNING**
> Pregnant women and people with kidney disorders should not take redcedar teas and extracts internally.

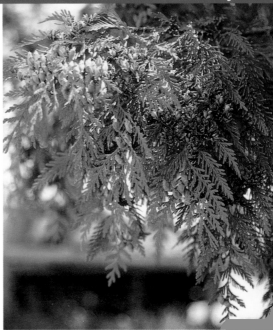

containers. Fine roots were split and peeled to make watertight baskets for cooking. Coiled larger roots were alternately bound together in twos with split roots to make baskets. Dugout canoes, rafts and frames for birch-bark canoes were made from redcedar trunks. The light, easily worked wood splits readily and resists decay. It was made into totem poles, cradle boards, bowls, masks, roofing, siding and many implements. Today it is widely used for siding, roofing, panelling, doors, patio furniture, chests and caskets. Cedar oil is extracted commercially for medicinal rubs and salves, and cedar sprays make a lovely incense.

Western redcedar (all images)

DESCRIPTION: Evergreen trees, 20–60 m tall, with stout trunks with short branches, fibrous bark and opposite, scale-like leaves, 3 mm long, that form flat, yellowish green, fan-like sprays. Both male and female cones appear on the same tree: female cones 8–10 mm long, green becoming brown; male cones tiny, reddish. Seeds, produced from April to May, have 2 lateral wings that almost surround them. These handsome trees are usually called white-cedar or redcedar to distinguish them from the true cedars (*Cedrus* spp.), which occur in Canada only as cultivated ornamentals.

Western redcedar (*T. plicata*) grows to 60 m tall in rich, moist to wet, low elevation to montane sites in BC and southwestern AB. Western redcedar is the provincial tree of BC. See p. 424 for conservation status.

Eastern white-cedar (*T. occidentalis*) is a smaller tree, to 20 m tall. Grows in wet forests, swamps and cool, rocky streambanks from southeastern MB to the Maritimes. See p. 424 for conservation status.

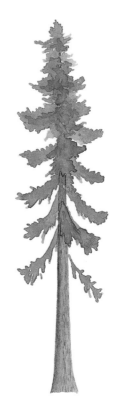

WARNING
Both western redcedar and eastern white-cedar produce an essential oil that is toxic to rats at 120 mg/kg. It has a very high content of thujone, a neurotoxin that is also found in the banned alcoholic drink absinthe. Cedar oil can cause low blood pressure, convulsions and even death. Essential oils are especially not recommended for use with infants.

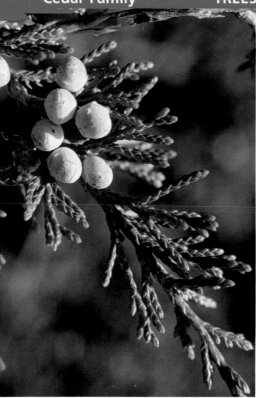

Eastern redcedar

Tree Junipers
Juniperus spp.

FOOD: Some tribes cooked juniper berries into a mush and dried them in cakes for winter use. The berries were also dried whole and ground into meal for making mush and cakes. Small pieces of the bitter bark or a few berries were chewed in times of famine to suppress hunger. Dried, roasted juniper berries were ground and used as a coffee substitute. Teas were occasionally made from the stems, leaves and/or berries, but they were usually used as medicines rather than beverages. Juniper berries are well known for their use as a flavouring for gin, beer and other alcoholic drinks. "Tricky Marys" can be made by soaking juniper berries in tomato juice for a few days and then following your usual recipe for Bloody Marys, but omitting the gin. The taste is identical and the drink is non-alcoholic.

MEDICINE: Juniper berry tea has been used to aid digestion, stimulate appetite, relieve colic and water retention, treat diarrhea and heart, lung and kidney problems, prevent pregnancy, stop bleeding, reduce swelling and inflammation and calm hyperactivity. Juniper berries were chewed to relieve cold symptoms, settle upset stomachs and increase appetite. Tea made from the branches and cones was used to treat fevers, colds, coughs and pneumonia. This tea was also heated to soak arthritic and rheumatic joints, or it was mixed with a bit of turpentine and applied as a liniment. Oil-of-juniper, diluted with less-irritating oils, was often used in liniments. It is still found in some patent medicines.

OTHER USES: Juniper berries were sometimes dried on strings, smoked over a greasy fire and polished to make shiny black beads for necklaces. Some tribes scattered berries to be used for necklaces on anthills. The ants would eat out the sweet centre, leaving a convenient hole for stringing. The durable wood of Rocky Mountain juniper was used in lance shafts, bows and other items. It was admired for its dark red, seemingly-dyed-in-blood colour. Today, this attractive plant is often grown as an ornamental. Juniper branches were sometimes boiled to produce an anti-dandruff hair rinse. The bark, berries and needles produced a brown dye, using ash from burned green needles as a mordant.

> **WARNING**
> Large and/or frequent doses of juniper can result in convulsions, kidney failure and an irritated digestive tract. People with kidney problems and pregnant women should never take any part of a juniper internally. Juniper oil can cause blistering.

DESCRIPTION: Coniferous, evergreen shrubs or small trees, to 20 m tall, with opposite rows of small (1–1.5 mm long), scale-like leaves. Fruits small, 5–9 mm wide, bluish purple to bluish green "berries" (fleshy cones), produced from May to June on female plants only and maturing the following year.

Rocky Mountain juniper (*J. scopulorum*) is an erect shrub or small tree that grows to 15 m tall. Young leaves often 5–7 mm long and needle-like, but mature leaves tiny and scale-like. Grows on dry, rocky ridges, open foothills and bluffs from BC to southwestern SK. (These junipers growing in southwestern BC and the Puget Sound have recently been recognized as a separate species, *J. maritima*.) See p. 424 for conservation status.

Eastern redcedar (*J. virginiana*) is a small tree growing to 20 m tall. Leaves green but sometimes turning reddish brown in winter, 1–3 mm long, overlapping by more than a quarter of their length. Grows in upland to low woods, old fields, glades and river swamps in southern ON and southwestern QC. See p. 424 for conservation status.

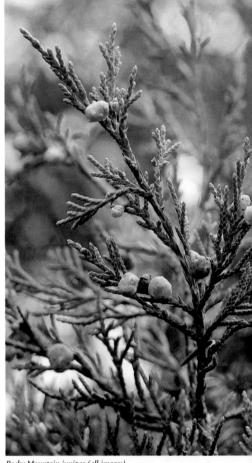

Rocky Mountain juniper (all images)

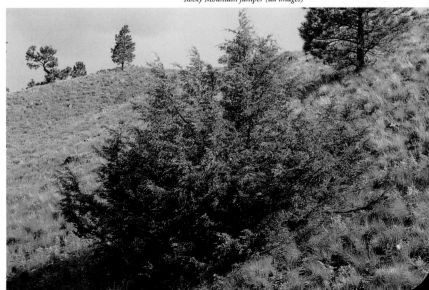

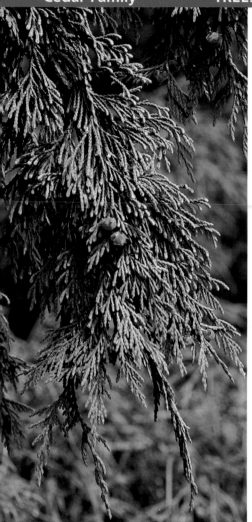

Yellow-Cedar
Chamaecyparis nootkatensis

MEDICINE: The crushed foliage and freshly cut wood has a rather rank odour. It was sometimes used in sweat baths for arthritis and rheumatism. Although an infusion of the branch tips was sometimes taken internally for general illnesses, the plant was most often used topically. The soft bark was used as a cover for poultices. A poultice of chewed leaves was applied to sores, and an infusion of the branch tips was used as a wash for sores and swellings. The sharp boughs were rubbed on sores and swellings until the skin broke, and the leaves, mixed with other ingredients, were applied externally to treat swelling of the kidney in women. The bark was burned, and the ash mixed with oil and used as a lotion to give strength to the very ill.

OTHER USES: The tough, straight-grained wood was used by nearly every Northwest Coast First Nation for construction and tool-making. It was ideal for making bows, canoe paddles, boat ribs, ceremonial masks, headdresses, totem poles, chests, storage containers, dishes, digging sticks, adze handles and fish-net hoops. The fibre of the inner bark is fine and was used for cordage, weaving capes, loincloths, mats, blankets, hats, baby clothing, skirts, face towels and fine clothing for the nobility. Today the wood is used for furniture, fine carpentry and boats. Because of its sometimes slow growth (it may require over 200 years to reach a marketable size), it is hard, durable, resistant to weather, insects and splintering and wears smoothly over time. The oldest specimen recorded in BC to date is 1834 years old, though some individuals almost certainly live more than 2 millennia.

DESCRIPTION: Medium-sized tree, 20–40 m tall, occasionally taller, with a broadly buttressed and often fluted base, tapered trunk and sharply conical crown of spreading and drooping branches bearing loosely hanging branchlets. Bark thin, greyish brown, scaly on young trees, with narrow, intersecting ridges in more mature trunks. Leaves dark bluish green, opposite, 3–5 mm long, pointed, scale-like, with the tips often diverging. Male and female cones occur on the same tree: female cones spherical, 10–14 mm in diameter when mature at the end of the second season, scales thick, 4–6, umbrella-shaped; male cones to 4 mm long. Seeds have 2 lateral wings about twice as wide as the seeds. Grows in cool, wet forests from sea level to subalpine in coastal BC, and a few spots in southeastern BC.

Trembling Aspen
Populus tremuloides

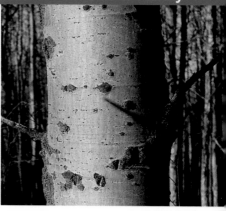

FOOD: In spring when the sap began to flow, the pulpy inner bark (cambium) provided a sweet treat for children of many First Nations. It was scraped off in long strips and eaten raw. The bitter leaf buds and young catkins are edible and rich in vitamin C. The Montagnais steeped the bark to make a tea. The Fisherman Lake Slave people used the ashes from trembling aspen wood as a salt source before contact. The leaves were eaten by the Great Lakes peoples as a famine food.

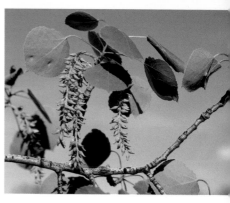

MEDICINE: Bark tea has been used to treat skin problems, intermittent fevers, urinary tract infections, jaundice, debility and diarrhea and to kill parasitic worms. Some tribes believed that the bark had to be collected by stripping it downward from the tree; otherwise the patient would vomit it out! The leaves and inner bark contain salicin, a compound related to aspirin, which relieves pain, fever and inflammation. Syrup made from the inner bark was taken as a spring tonic and as a cough medicine.

OTHER USES: Aspen trunks were used occasionally as tepee poles. The light, odourless wood shreds and splits easily, so it has been used to make paddles, bowls, wooden matches, vegetable crates, wallboard and excelsior for packing. Today, aspen wood is primarily harvested for pulp and particleboard and for making chopsticks. Because it does not splinter, it is a preferred wood for sauna benches and playground equipment. The wood is also used to smoke fish and meat. Aspen is an attractive, fast-growing tree, but it is seldom used in landscaping because it is susceptible to many diseases and insects, and its spreading root system tends to invade sewers, yards and drainpipes. In spring, when the bark can be slid from the branches, short sections can be used to make toy whistles.

DESCRIPTION: Slender, medium-sized, deciduous tree that grows to 25 m tall, with smooth, greenish white bark marked with blackened spots and lines. Buds small, not resinous. Leaves 2–8 cm long, with slender, flattened stalks that cause them to tremble in the slightest breeze. Flowers tiny, in hanging, 2–10 cm long clusters (catkins), with male and female catkins on separate trees, appearing from March to May, producing cone-shaped capsules that release many tiny seeds tipped with soft, white hairs. Grows in dry to moist forests, openings and disturbed sites (including burned areas) in all provinces and territories. See p. 424 for conservation status.

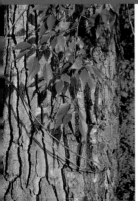

Balsam Poplar

Populus balsamifera ssp. *balsamifera*

FOOD: Many First Nations across Canada relished the thick, juicy and sweet inner bark (cambium) of balsam poplar in spring and early summer when the sap was running. After the thick outer bark had been removed, a buffalo or elk rib was used to scrape off the translucent inner bark in long, ribbon-like strips. This treat spoils easily, so it was generally eaten as it was gathered or brought home and eaten immediately, sometimes with eulachon grease (on the west coast) or other oil. Hollows were sometimes carved in trunks to collect the sap. The young catkins were also considered tasty. The Blackfoot peoples sometimes used the inner bark in smoking mixtures. The wood has been used to smoke fish.

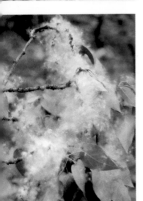

MEDICINE: Balsam poplar leaves were applied to bruises, sores, boils and aching muscles and to sores on horses that had become infected with maggots. The bark was chewed to relieve colds or was used in teas for treating tuberculosis and whooping cough. Some tribes boiled the bark tea to make a thick syrup that was spread on cloth to make casts for supporting broken bones. Bark ashes, mixed with water and cornmeal, provided a poultice for boils. Resins from the sticky, aromatic buds (gathered in late winter and spring) have been used for centuries in salves, cough medicines and painkillers. Salves, made by mixing the buds with fat, were used to relieve congestion from colds and bronchitis, to heal skin infections and to soothe aching muscles. Poplar contains a variety of salicin derivatives with analgesic properties.

OTHER USES: Balsam poplar wood was said to be ideal for tepee fires because it did not crackle and it made clean smoke. However, poplar trunks are often punky from fungal infections, and this wood does not burn as well as uninfected wood. In spring, buds mixed with blood produced a permanent black ink that was used to paint records on traditional hide robes. Twigs and bark were occasionally fed to horses when forage was limited. When stealing horses, war parties carried balsam poplar bark with them to feed the animals, and some warriors rubbed themselves with the sap to mask their scent. These fast-growing trees with relatively low lignin content are now sometimes grown as a crop for pulp.

DESCRIPTION: Deciduous tree, to 25 m tall, with deeply furrowed mature bark and large, resinous, fragrant buds. Leaves 5–12 cm long, round-stalked, dark green above and paler beneath. Flowers tiny, in hanging clusters (catkins), with 2–3 cm long male catkins and 4–10 cm long female catkins on separate trees, appearing from April to May and producing oval capsules that release fluffy masses of tiny seeds tipped with soft, white hairs. Found in moist woods, riversides (often pioneer species on gravel bars) and prairie parklands across Canada. See p. 424 for conservation status.

WARNING
Some sources report that the bark tea may be slightly toxic. The bud resin may irritate sensitive skin.

Cottonwoods

Populus spp.

FOOD: Many First Nations ate the sweet inner bark, cambium tissues and sap in spring and early summer. As with balsam poplar, these needed to be eaten immediately after they were harvested so they would not ferment. Also eaten were the buds, seed capsules and seeds of cottonwoods.

MEDICINE: Some western tribes, such as the Ditidaht and Nuu-chah-nulth, picked the buds in spring and boiled them in deer fat to make a fragrant and healing salve that was molded into the bulbous float of bull kelp. The Nuxalk used

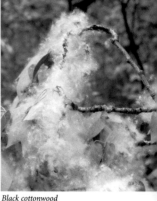

Black cottonwood

the gum from the buds in preparations to treat baldness, sore throats, whooping cough and tuberculosis. The buds were used as a poultice for lung pains and rheumatism, and the old, rotten leaves were boiled and used in a bath for body pains, rheumatism and stomach trouble. The Tahltan used cottonwood as a fuel for smoking fish. In eastern Canada, the Cree ate the young inner bark and also used a bark decoction as a purgative. The Ojibwa cooked the spring buds in grease to make a salve used to treat cuts, wounds, bruises, colds, bronchitis, sores and inflammation. This tribe also used a poplar root decoction to treat back pain and female complaints. The Iroquois used a decoction of the bark as a vermifuge.

OTHER USES: The inner bark was used to reinforce other plant fibres in spinning, and the young branches to make sweat lodge frames. Buckets and temporary houses could also be made using slabs of the bark. The supple roots were twisted into rope for tying house planks together and for making fish traps. The Coast Salish occasionally made small dugout canoes from black cottonwood, a practice more common among interior BC tribes. The aromatic gum from the spring buds was used to waterproof baskets and boxes and as a glue for securing arrowheads and feathers to shafts and, mixed with other plants and grease, as a paint. Although the Okanagan and some coastal peoples made friction-fire sets using dried cottonwood roots for the hearth and dried branches for the drill, the Chehalis believed that the tree had a life of its own because it shakes when there is no wind, and never used it as firewood. The Okanagan used the ashes to make soap and a hairwash. The sticky resin on the buds and newly opened leaves has a powerful, sweet, balsamic fragrance that permeates whole river valleys in spring and early summer. Bees collect the resin (which contains propolis) as an anti-infectant for their hives to prevent decay and to seal them up to keep intruders such as mice out.

DESCRIPTION: Open-crowned, deciduous trees, 20–50 m tall, with resinous, fragrant buds. Leaves alternate, simple, finely toothed and hairy. Flowers tiny, in separate male and female catkins on separate trees. Fruits oval capsules.

Eastern cottonwood (*P. deltoides*) is a smaller tree, to 20 m tall, with triangular leaves (the base squared-off) that are not resinous. Grows on streambanks and disturbed sites at low elevations from southern AB to southwestern QC, and planted elsewhere. See p. 424 for conservation status.

Black cottonwood (*P. balsamifera* ssp. *trichocarpa*) is a larger western species, to 50 m tall, with oval to lance-shaped, resinous leaves (the bases rounded or heart-shaped). Grows at low to medium elevations on moist to wet sites; forms extensive stands on islands and floodplains along major rivers and disturbed upland sites in BC and southwestern AB.

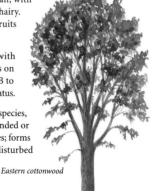

Eastern cottonwood

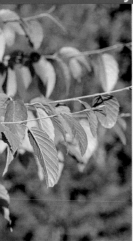

Birches

Betula spp.

FOOD: These trees produce large amounts of sap in spring that can be used straight from the tree as a beverage. The sap has also been boiled to make syrup, although it contains only about half as much sugar as maple sap. Thin syrup or the sap mixed with sugar or honey was fermented to make birch beer, wine or vinegar. Young twigs and bark were boiled to make tea. A very delightful tea was made from the twigs and leaves of yellow and sweet birch, which contain an essential oil that has the flavour of wintergreen. The tea was also sweetened with sugar or honey and made into beer or vinegar. The sweet inner bark was added to soups and stews or was dried and ground into flour for making bark bread. However, inner bark flour was generally regarded as a famine food and used only when other forms of starch were unavailable or in short supply. Young leaves and catkins were sometimes used to flavour salads, meat dishes and cooked vegetables.

MEDICINE: Sweet birch, the most fragrant of the birches included here, was widely used by First Nations for fevers, stomachaches, kidney stones and respiratory complaints. The bark tea was also used to expel worms, to induce sweating and urination and as a tonic in cases of dysentery. A decoction of yellow birch bark was used by First Nations as a blood purifier because of its emetic and cathartic actions. The essential oil (methyl salicylate) from sweet and yellow birches is an anti-inflammatory and analgesic, useful in the treatment of rheumatism, gout, scrofula, bladder infections and neuralgia. It was rubbed topically to alleviate pain or sore muscles. A commercial preparation of the essential oil (once called oil of wintergreen) is now produced synthetically using menthol as a precursor. The bark

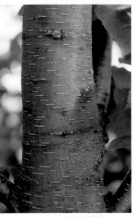

Sweet birch (all above)
Yellow birch (below & right)

contains large amounts of the triterpene betulin and a small amount of betulinic acid. Recent research indicates that betulinic acid from paper birch may be useful for treating skin cancer. It was also found to be active against malignant brain tumours, ovarian carcinoma, leukemia and certain squamous cell carcinomas. It is presently

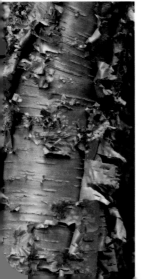

WARNING
The essential oil of sweet birch bark contains 97–99 percent methyl salicylate, which is very toxic when taken internally. It can also be absorbed through the skin, and fatalities have been reported. As little as 4.7 g can be fatal to children.

undergoing development by the National Cancer Institute and could become an ingredient in future sunscreens and tanning lotions. Betulinic acid has also demonstrated anti-HIV, antimalarial and anti-inflammatory properties.

OTHER USES: The thin, paper-like bark of paper birch was an extremely important material, widely used by First Nations to make canoes, baskets, storage containers, cups and platters. The barks of all birches are waterproof and were used as the outer skin of canoes and as roofing material on dwellings. Heating makes it amazingly pliable. Thin strips of birch bark make excellent kindling, and the wood produces long-burning, sweet-smelling fires. Birch wood is extremely hard. It was traditionally

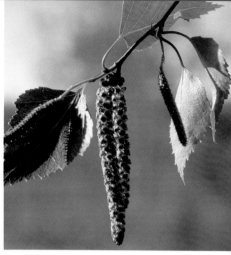

Paper birch

used to make sleds, snowshoes, paddles, canoe ribs, arrows, tool handles and even needles. Birch trunks were sometimes used as poles for making tepees and drying racks. Do not cut birch bark from living trees; bark removal can permanently scar and even kill birches. The essential oil of sweet birch is used commercially as a food flavouring and as an ingredient in cosmetics and shampoos. It is also used as an insect repellent.

DESCRIPTION: Small to medium trees, to 30 m tall, recognizable by their paper-like bark, characteristically marked with long, horizontal lenticels. Bark smooth on young trees, peels off in thin, papery layers as the tree gets older. Leaves alternate, doubly serrate and feather-veined, sometimes appearing paired on older branchlets. Leaf buds on elongated twigs show only 3 bud-scales, whereas the bud on the dwarf twig has 5–7 scales. Flowers fully developed as the leaves begin to appear, male and female on the same tree, borne on 3-flowered clusters in the axils of the scales of drooping or erect aments. Fruit a very small nut with a thin wing (samara) on each side and borne on minute, 3-lobed, leaf-like scales attached to slender stems.

Yellow birch (*B. alleghaniensis*) grows to 25 m tall, has thin, dark reddish brown bark on young trunks, turning to tan, yellowish, lustrous, smooth bark producing thin, papery shreds. Twigs have an odour and taste of wintergreen. Leaves oval with coarse, irregularly serrate teeth, 6–10 cm long. Flowers from April to May, but remain intact after the release of the fruits in late autumn. Grows in moist, well-drained soils in rich woodlands and streambanks at lower elevations from ON to NL. Yellow birch is the provincial tree of QC. See p. 424 for conservation status.

Sweet birch or **black birch** (*B. lenta*) grows to 20 m tall and is very similar to yellow birch but bark on mature trees is light greyish brown and not freely peeling, and leaves have fine, sharp teeth. Grows in rich, moist, cool forests in southern ON. See p. 424 for conservation status.

Alaska paper birch (*B. neoalaskana*) grows to 25 m tall and is similar to paper birch, but its twigs and leaf stalks have wart-like resin glands on them. Found in boggy sites, often with black spruce, from northeastern BC to northwestern ON and in YT and NT.

Paper birch (*B. papyrifera*) grows to 30 m tall, has smooth, white to yellowish bark that peels off in papery sheets. Leaves 4–9 cm long, yellow in autumn. Pollen (male) catkins 5–10 cm long, loosely hanging. Seed (female) catkins 2–4 cm long, erect, shedding winged nutlets and 3-lobed scales, from April to May. Common and familiar tree in dry to moist, upland forests throughout Canada. Paper birch is the provincial tree of SK. See p. 424 for conservation status.

Scrub birch (*B. glandulosa*) is a many-branched, densely glandular, hairy shrub, to 2 m tall, included here to keep it with its birch cousins. Grows in generally wet sites (wetlands, streamsides, meadows) from montane to alpine elevations in all provinces and territories.

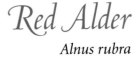

Red Alder
Alnus rubra

FOOD: The inner bark of red alder was a popular springtime food for many First Nations on the Pacific coast. It was eaten fresh, mixed with oil, or dried for later use. Buds and young catkins are not very tasty, but they are edible and high in protein and can be eaten in an emergency.

MEDICINE: Alder bark tea was an important medicine within the range of the species, especially for respiratory ailments (including tuberculosis). A wash of alder bark has been applied to wounds and swellings and seems to have antibiotic properties. Red alder bark tea was also widely used as a spring tonic.

OTHER USES: Red alder wood was, and is, a preferred fuel for smoking salmon and other fish. The soft wood is easily carved and was used to make masks, feast bowls and other items. The bark yields an orange or red dye, which was used for dyeing many things, including the inner bark of western redcedar (p. 45). The dye colour varies with preparation method and steeping time: darker colours were used to dye fish nets, to make them less visible to fish. Red alder (and shrubby alders, p. 151) make nodules in their roots to house cyanobacteria, micro-organisms that can pull (fix) gaseous nitrogen out of the air and make it available for the alders. Red alder can thus grow on disturbed sites where few other plants could, and the mulch from its fallen leaves enriches the soil for other plants and soil organisms.

DESCRIPTION: Deciduous tree, to 25 m tall, with thin, grey, smooth bark, which becomes white with age as it becomes covered with lichens. Leaves alternate, elliptic, to 15 cm long, sharp-pointed at the tip, the margins wavy with coarse, blunt teeth, rusty-hairy underneath. Flowers tiny, in dense clusters (catkins), with male and female catkins on the same branch. Pollen (male) catkins slender and loosely hanging, 5–12 cm long; seed (female) catkins woody, cone-like, 1–2 cm long; both produced before the leaves. Fruits tiny, oval, winged nutlets in the seed cones. Grows along streams, on low-lying floodplains and other frequently disturbed sites at low elevations along the BC coast.

Hop Hornbeam

Ostrya virginiana

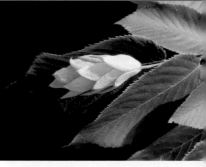

FOOD: Although not fit for human consumption, buds and catkins are the preferred food for a variety of wildlife, including grouse, wild turkey, bobwhite, red and grey squirrels, cottontails, white-tail deer, ring-necked pheasant, purple finch, rose-breasted grosbeak and downy woodpecker.

MEDICINE: An infusion of the bark was used by First Nations as a blood medicine to strengthen the cardiovascular system, to treat dysentery and as a mouthwash to relieve toothaches. The bark was also used as a decoction to bathe sore muscles and for cancer of the rectum. Mixed with other ingredients, it was used as a tonic and a remedy for tuberculosis. The root was used in compound medicines as a tonic and as a gynecological aid. A tea made from the heartwood was considered beneficial for lung hemorrhages, coughs, colds, catarrh and kidney disorders. Heartwood tea, mixed with other herbs, was poured onto hot rocks and the steam used to relieve rheumatic pain.

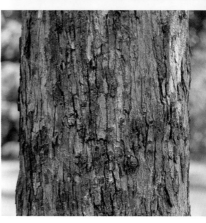

OTHER USES: The wood of hop hornbeam is close-grained, very hard, very strong and durable. Up to the turn of the century, it was used for runners on sleighs. It is used for posts, mallets, tool handles and other purposes where a strong, tough wood is required. The wood is of superior quality; however, the tree's scattered occurrence and small size prevent it from becoming important as a commercial species. The tree is sometimes planted as a street tree or ornamental.

DESCRIPTION: Small tree to 18 m tall, with a crown often as wide as it is high. Bark greyish brown, broken into longitudinal, narrow strips peeling at both ends. Leaves alternate, simple, oval or elliptic to oblong or lance-shaped, in 2 rows along the twig, with irregular, double-toothed margins. Flowers fully developed as the leaves begin to appear, with male and female flowers borne in separate clusters on the same tree. Clusters consist of slender, flexible stems with closely spaced flowers. Male flowers, 2–5 cm long, visible in winter as slender, cylindrical catkins; female catkins, 8–15 mm long, from April to May. Fruit a flattish nut, 4–8 mm long, fully enclosed in a papery white husk, 1–1.5 cm long, with 10–30 nuts on a catkin. Grows in moist, open to forested hillsides to dry, upland slopes at low elevations from MB to NS. See p. 424 for conservation status.

Oaks

Quercus spp.

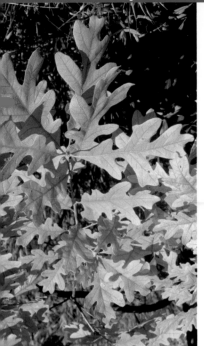

White oak (all images)

FOOD: Acorns were eaten raw, boiled, roasted in ashes or dried and ground into meal. White acorns, such as those of white oak, are sweetest, but even they were often too bitter to eat fresh from the tree. The outer shells were removed and the inner kernels (fresh or dried, crushed or whole) were placed in a mesh bag in water and soaked for several hours (or weeks). Many eastern First Nations groups such as the Iroquois and Ojibwa collected white oak acorns in autumn, cracking them open with a pair of rounded stones containing a pitted centre to hold the acorn in place. Sometimes wood ashes (that contain lye) were added to speed the process, or kernels were boiled in several changes of water until the water no longer turned brown. Leaching removes the tannin, but most of the important food components remain. Some tribes added special clays to mask the bitterness, and others buried the acorns in moist ground for long periods of time to reduce the tannin levels. Powdered gelatin may also work. Acorn meal was a staple food of some tribes. It was used to make mush, breads, muffins and pancakes and to thicken soups. Roasted acorn kernels taste much like other nuts and can be eaten as a snack, baked in cookies and cakes or dipped in syrup and eaten like candy. Dried kernels and meal keep for several months. Acorn shells and/or kernels were roasted, ground and brewed to make a coffee-like drink. Despite their relatively high tannin content, the acorns of Garry oak were eaten by a number of Coast Salish peoples in BC. The acorns were prepared by extended steaming, boiling or roasting, thereby removing much of the offending tannins. Northern red oak and black oak acorns, which are also very bitter-tasting, were used mostly as a famine food by the Iroquois, Huron, Ojibwa, Potawatomi and other peoples. Oak acorns are an important food source for many wildlife species.

MEDICINE: Oak bark tea is high in tannins and quercin, and swellings on the twigs (insect-caused galls) contain 2–3 times as much of these compounds as regular bark. Oak bark teas have

> **WARNING**
> The bark, leaves and shoots of many oaks are poisonous because of their relatively high level of tannins, toxic compounds implicated in some forms of cancer, and should not be consumed. Take care to remove these bitter-tasting tannins in acorns by first boiling the acorns in many changes of fresh water or by leaching.

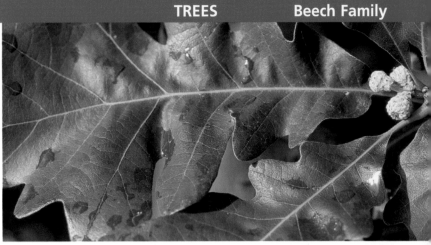

Bur oak (all images)

been widely used in washes and gargles for treating inflamed gums, sore throats, burns, cuts, scrapes, insect bites and rashes and in medicines and enemas for treating diarrhea, hemorrhoids and menstrual problems. Quercin is said to strengthen capillaries, and tannic acid is antiviral and antibacterial. Pieces of oak bark were chewed to relieve toothache pain. Oak root bark was boiled to make medicinal teas for purging the system, speeding delivery of afterbirth, relieving pain after childbirth and regulating bowel problems (especially in children). Northern red oak bark has been used to treat bronchial infections and as an astringent, disinfectant and cleanser. The bark of Garry oak was one of the ingredients in the BC Saanich First Nation's "4 barks" medicine used against tuberculosis and other ailments. The inner bark of white oak in particular is naturally astringent, antibacterial and anti-inflammatory and has been used to treat hemorrhoids, diarrhea and varicose veins as well as ulcers, strep throat and various skin afflictions. Bark gathered in early spring contains the highest level of tannins. Of all the native oak species, white oak is the most recommended for its medicinal qualities.

OTHER USES: Oak wood, being heavy, moisture-resistant, close-grained and hard, is valued for cabinets, flooring, veneers, and exterior uses such as fence posts, shipbuilding, cooperage, railway ties, agricultural tools and construction. The bark of a number of species was used to produce tannins on

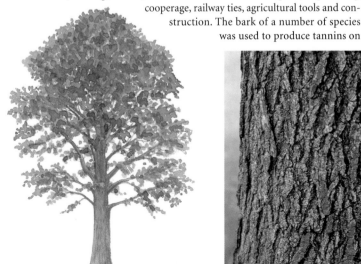

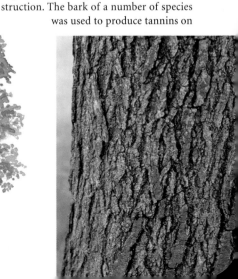

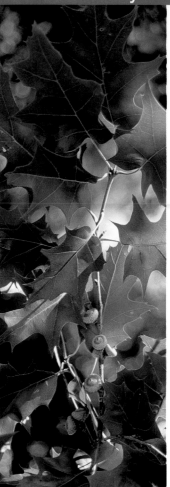

a commercial level. First Nations uses for the wood included combs, digging sticks, fuel, weaving tools, bows and arrows, baby cradles and ceremonial bullroarers. The inner bark of black oak contains a yellow pigment, quercitron, which was sold commercially as a dye as late as the 1940s and produced colours ranging from buff, orange and gold to soft brown. The genus name *Quercus* comes from the Celtic words *quer*, meaning "fine" and *cuea*, meaning "tree." Oaks have a long history of being a sacred tree for Druids and are symbolic of fertility and immortality.

DESCRIPTION: Deciduous trees, 20–40 m tall, with alternate, usually pinnately lobed or toothed leaves. Flowers tiny, without petals, either male or female, but with both sexes on the same plant. Male (pollen) flowers in dense, elongated clusters (catkins) and female (seed) flowers single, clumped or in catkins. Fruits 1-seeded nuts (acorns), each seated in a thick, scaly cup.

White oak (*Q. alba*) is a large, deciduous tree, to 35 m tall, with pale grey, scaly and fissured bark. Leaves oval, to 20 cm long and 10 cm wide, tapered at the base, deeply cut into 2–4 lobes on each side, pink-tinged and downy white becoming bright green above, blue-green beneath, turning a decorative purple-red in autumn. Fruit to 3 cm long, egg-shaped to pointed, held in a rough-textured scaly cap covering at most half of the nut. Inhabits moist to dry, deciduous forests at low to montane elevations from southern ON to southwestern QC and NS. See p. 424 for conservation status.

Swamp white oak (*Q. bicolor*) is a large, deciduous tree that grows to 30 m tall, with dark grey, scaly or flat-ridged bark. Leaves oval to elliptic, to 20 cm long and 12 cm wide, tapered at the base, variously toothed and/or lobed, dark green and glossy above, light green and minutely hairy below. Fruit small (to 5 mm long), the cap covering half to three-quarters of the nut. Found in swampy ground and streambanks at low to montane elevations from southern ON to southwestern QC. See p. 424 for conservation status.

Garry oak (*Q. garryana*) is a sprawling, deciduous tree that grows to 20 m tall with heavy limbs, but sometimes it grows as a shrub. Leaves dark green and glossy on top, lighter in colour and usually hairy beneath; generally 7–15 cm long, 5–10 cm wide, elliptic, blunt or rounded at both ends; deeply lobed halfway or more to midvein. Bark light grey or whitish, thin, scaly or furrowed into broad ridges. Acorns 2.5–3 cm long, elliptic, enclosed by a shallow, thin, scaly cup. Found in dry prairies, foothills and rocky bluffs in southwestern BC, particularly southern Vancouver Island and the Gulf Islands. Garry oak is the only oak native to BC.

Bur oak (*Q. macrocarpa*) is a large, deciduous, broadly spreading tree, to 40 m tall, with grey, deeply furrowed bark. Leaves oval, to 25 cm long and 12 cm wide, deeply cut with a distinctive wide space between the lobes near the base of the leaf. Acorns to 5 cm long, half covered by the cup, which is rimmed with a fringe of scales. Found in moist woods and bottomlands to dry prairie slopes and sand-hills from southeastern SK eastward (except PEI and NS).

Northern red oak (all images)

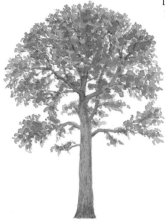

Northern red oak (*Q. rubra*) is a large, grey-barked, deciduous tree that grows to 30 m tall. Leaves alternate, elliptic, to 20 cm long and 12 cm wide, divided less than halfway to midvein into 7–11 shallow, wavy lobes with a few irregular, bristle-tipped teeth. Leaves dull green above, light, dull green below with tufts of hairs in vein angles. Acorns mature in the second year, with approximately three-quarters of the acorns held by shallow, saucer-shaped cups. Found in dry to mesic, upland woods in southern ON and QC, PEI, NS and NB. The common name of this species refers to the red colour of the petioles and autumn foliage and the reddish tinge of the interior wood. Northern red oak is the provincial tree of PEI.

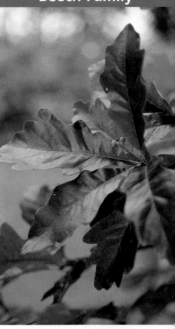

Black oak (*Q. velutina*) is a large, deciduous tree growing to 25 m tall in an often irregular shape, with dark brown to black, ridged bark. Leaves oval to elliptic, alternate, to 25 cm long and 15 cm wide, with 5–7 bristle-tipped lobes separated by deep, U-shaped notches. The upper leaf is dark, shiny green, the lower yellowish brown. Acorns small and oval, to 2.5 cm long, with the top half outside of the deep cup and covered in a cap of loose scales that form a characteristic fringe around the nut. Has a limited range in Canada, inhabiting dry woods in southern ON, where it prefers moist, rich, well-drained soil. The species name of this oak, *velutina*, refers to the underside of the leaves, which are covered with distinctive, fine hairs.

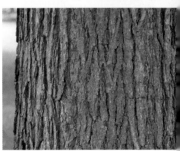

Swamp white oak (all above)
Garry oak savannah (below)

The Garry oak savannah is one of Canada's most endangered ecosystems, with an estimated 1 percent of its original range remaining. Garry oak is the signature plant of this ecosystem, intermixed with a beautiful parkland carpet of spring wildflowers—blue camas, white fawn lilies, yellow spring gold and buttercups, brown chocolate lilies and purple shooting stars in a gorgeous tapestry. When the first Europeans arrived on the west coast, they marvelled at this magnificent park-like landscape, which they thought to be untouched by human hands (James Douglas described it in 1843 as "a perfect Eden in the midst of the dreary wilderness"). What they did not know is that the Garry oak savannah is essentially a cultural artifact, the result of an estimated 5000 years of controlled burning, digging, weeding, pruning and other practices by local First Nations. This "cultivation" enhanced the productivity of key food plants growing in the meadows: camas bulbs, chocolate lily and other bulbs and roots were an important source of carbohydrates; the oaks provided edible acorns (needing leaching of tannins); there were wild strawberries, trailing blackberries and other edible fruits; and deer and other game fattened on the native grasses. The ongoing threats to this ecosystem are introduced species and habitat loss because of urban development.

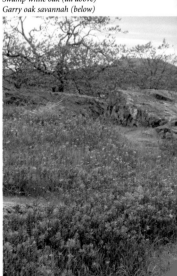

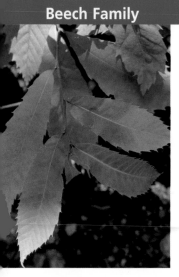

American Chestnut
Castanea dentata

FOOD: Before the decline of this species (see sidebar), the nuts of this tree were an important food source for many First Nations of eastern Canada. The Iroquois ate the nuts both raw and cooked, and also dried and pounded them into a flour. The nuts can also be roasted and made into a coffee-like drink, or added to soups, stews and puddings. Early European settlers greatly valued this tree for its wood, bark and nuts, which they found to be much sweeter and more palatable than those of the European chestnut.

MEDICINE: The leaves were traditionally used to treat snakebites, inflammation, whooping cough and burns.

OTHER USES: American chestnut wood was highly valued because it split well and was very rot-resistant, light and easy to work. It was used in great volumes for furniture, fence posts, musical instruments, cooperage, flooring, utility poles and many other products. The wood is naturally high in tannins, compounds that retard rotting and that were also commercially extracted (from the bark) for use in the tanning process. Some eastern First Nations used large slabs of the bark to cover their shelters and the wood to make canoes. The nuts and leaves of this tree were an important food source for domestic animals such as pigs.

DESCRIPTION: Broadly columnar, deciduous tree to 30 m tall. Leaves oblong, to 25 cm long and 5 cm wide, alternate, simple, straight-veined, sharply toothed or lobed. Leaves smooth on both sides, matte dark green above, paler beneath. Bark dark brown, rough, shallowly fissured, with broad, scaly ridges. Both male and female flowers small and creamy yellow, in catkins to 20 cm long, blooming from June to July. Nuts flattened on 1 or both sides, 2–4 (usually 3) in each bur. On dry, gravelly or rocky, mostly acidic soils in southern ON woods.

This tree is becoming increasingly rare (see p. 424) because of a fungus (*Cryphonectria parasitica*) that causes chestnut blight. The disease first appeared on Chinese chestnut trees in the Bronx Zoo in New York in 1904, likely introduced from Asia. This fungus kills the trees by girdling the branches and trunks and was so virulent that up to 99 percent of American chestnut trees in the US had been killed by 1937. In Canada, one survey in 1949 found not a single mature tree left old enough to bear nuts, but found many smaller saplings, suggesting that the blight eradicates trees when they have reached 2 m in height or so. Some living roots of this species still remain and are strong enough to produce suckers, which are sometimes mature enough that they produce seeds. However, the resulting seedlings are invariably killed by the blight within their first few years of life. Although this species is considered extirpated in its native range in eastern Canada, healthy plantings are found in western Canada, so far disease-free. A non-profit group, the Canadian Chestnut Council, is attempting to re-introduce American chestnut seedlings that show tolerance to the blight to restore the tree's population in its native range.

American Beech

Fagus grandifolia

FOOD: The nuts of this tree, which are considered sweet and highly edible, were consumed in large quantities by First Nations and early settlers. The Iroquois, Ojibwa, Mi'kmaq , Maliseet, Algonquin and Potawatomi all consider these nuts a traditional food. The Iroquois also rendered the oil for cooking.

MEDICINE: A lotion to treat skin irritations caused by poison-ivy (p. 395) was made by steeping the bark in salt water. Beech wood can be distilled to produce an antiseptic creosote, which has been used commercially in medicinal soaps and salves for skin conditions. A decoction of the leaves or bark was also applied topically to treat ulcers, sores and burns.

OTHER USES: Beech wood is strong, heavy and highly valued for making handles for hand tools, as charcoal and as a fuel. It lends itself easily to steaming and bending and is therefore commonly used in flooring, furniture, veneers, plywood and baskets. The nuts are an important food source for many species of wildlife. Because American beech grows best in rich, loamy soils with good drainage, early settlers looked for healthy, large trees as a sign of good farmland.

DESCRIPTION: Deciduous, slow-growing, rough-barked tree growing to 30 m tall in a broadly spreading shape. Leaves oval to oblong, shallowly serrated, to 12 cm long and 6 cm wide, ending in a tapered point. Leaf colour dark glossy green above, paler beneath, turning yellow in autumn. Female flowers green, males yellow, both growing in separate clusters on the same plant from April to June. Nuts held in a prickly husk, sharply triangular in shape, usually growing in pairs, 2 cm long and enclosing 1–3 small nuts. Found in rich woods at low to montane elevations from southern ON to QC, NB, PEI and NS. This is the only species of this genus native to North America.

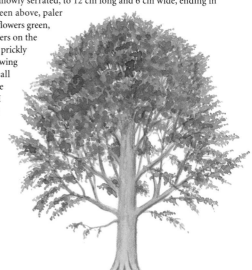

WARNING

Beechnuts should be consumed in moderation because the nuts contain a saponin-like substance that can cause gastrointestinal upset if consumed in large quantities.

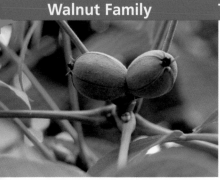

Shagbark hickory

Hickories
Carya spp.

FOOD: Shagbark hickory nut was a valued food source for indigenous peoples who lived within its range. Bitternut hickory was also gathered in times of need, but, as the name suggests, the seed was quite bitter and had to be boiled in lye to remove the bitterness before it could be eaten. Nuts were gathered in autumn, mostly by women and children; the hulls were cracked open with rounded stones with pitted centres. The nuts were prepared in a variety of ways; they could be eaten plain or with honey, and the fresh nut meats were crushed and added to soups (e.g., corn soup) or hominy, mixed with corn pudding, cornmeal and beans or berries and made into bread. Sometimes the oil would be skimmed off after fresh nut meats were crushed and boiled slowly in water. The oil was used as baby food or seasoned with salt and used as gravy. The nut meats left after skimming off the oil were seasoned and mixed with mashed potatoes. Fresh nut meats were also used as a drink, after being crushed and boiled into a liquid.

MEDICINE: A shagbark hickory decoction was taken internally or applied externally as a poultice for arthritis or rheumatism. Fresh, small shoots were steamed over hot rocks as an inhalant for headaches. A compound decoction with inner bark was taken to treat worms in adults. Shagbark hickory was also used as a gynecological aid and tonic. Bitternut hickory was known for its diuretic and laxative properties and was used as a cure-all.

OTHER USES: The nutmeat oil of hickory was formerly used either alone or mixed with bear grease for hair, and used as a mosquito repellent. Hickory wood has substantial commercial value because of its strength and shock resistance. It was used to make bows, tool handles, wheel spokes, sporting goods, baskets, chairs, etc. Hickory bark is also a valuable fuel because it gives off a lot of heat and produces excellent charcoal. Shagbark hickory is grown extensively in central Europe for timber. A yellow dye can be obtained from the inner bark. Not only of value to humans, hickory nuts are also a high quality food source for wildlife. The wood of bitternut hickory is said to give the best flavour to smoked hams and bacon.

DESCRIPTION: Large, deciduous trees, to 50 m tall, with grey or brownish bark. Leaves pinnately compound, with oval leaflets, the leaflets pointed and finely toothed near the tip. Male and female flowers borne in separate clusters on the same tree, male catkins in bunches of 3 from first- or second-year twigs, females in few-flowered spikes at the end of the branch, in spring. Nuts enclosed in husks. Outer husks split apart to the base at maturity.

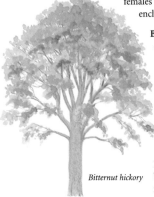

Bitternut hickory

Bitternut hickory (*C. cordiformis*) grows to 25 m tall and has grey or brownish bark that splits into shallow crevices or plates when mature. Twigs tan. Leaves 20–40 cm long, 7–11 leaflets, winter buds bright orange. Husk of nut winged; seeds bitter. Found in river floodplains, limestone glades and on well-drained hillsides in southern ON and southwestern QC.

Shagbark hickory (*C. ovata*) grows to 25 m tall and has light grey bark that eventually separates into long strips that remain on the trunk, the ends often curling away. Twigs greenish, reddish or orangish brown. Leaves 30–60 cm long, 3–7 leaflets. Husk of nut wingless; seeds sweet. Found in rich woods and bottomlands in southern ON and southwestern QC. See p. 424 for conservation status.

Walnuts

Juglans spp.

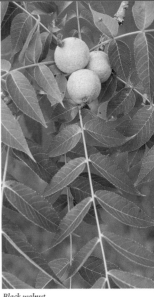

FOOD: Walnuts were a valued food source for indigenous peoples in eastern Canada. The nuts were often prepared in similar ways to bitternut hickory (p. 62).

MEDICINE: Walnuts are high in antioxidants and omega-3 fatty acids; they are known to lower cholesterol and may reduce the risk of Alzheimer's disease. Black walnut was used to treat a wide variety of medical ailments. A compound decoction of the plant was taken for pain during urinatation, as a blood purifier, for venereal disease and "when the skin becomes thin." A compound decoction with bark was taken to kill worms in adults, to induce pregnancy and as a laxative, physic, tonic and cathartic. The chewed bark was used as a poultice on bleeding wounds, infected and swollen tubercular glands and headaches. The plant was also used as a purgative and to treat yellow skin and too much gall. A compound infusion of the buds was used as a mouthwash for ulcers, and the juice was also used to

Black walnut

treat toothaches. Combined with brandy, a decoction was taken as a blood purifier. Butternut has been shown to have pronounced antifungal and antibacterial activity against a wide variety of fungi and bacteria.

OTHER USES: The nut oil, either alone or mixed with bear grease, was traditionally put in the hair and used as a mosquito repellent. Black walnut is valued for its attractive wood. The wood has been used for furniture, cabinetry, instrument cases, interior woodwork and altars. The Ojibwa used the nut hull to make a brown dye, and early settlers used the fruit husks and inner bark to make orange or yellow dye. Black walnut produces a toxin known as "juglone" that inhibits the growth of other plants around it. The fungal disease "butternut canker" is killing butternut across its range. The name "butternut" refers to mature nut kernels, which are sweet and oily, like butter.

DESCRIPTION: Medium to large, deciduous trees, to 50 m tall, with stiff, upright branches, wide, spreading crown and smoothly ridged, brownish grey bark. Pinnately compound, alternate leaves, with pointed, lance-shaped leaflets with finely toothed margins. Male and female flowers in separate areas on same tree: male catkins greenish, drooping, 6–14 cm long; female flowers in short clusters (6–8 flowers each). Fruit husks do not split apart when mature. Kernels rich and flavourful.

Butternut (*J. cinerea*) is a medium-sized tree, 20–30 m tall, with greyish or grey-brown bark that is smooth or divided into scales. Young twigs, stems and leaflets have sticky, oily hairs. Leaflets 11–17. Fruits egg-shaped to cylindrical, in clusters of 2–5; husk thick, with sticky, glandular surface. Found on river terraces, rocky slopes and in rich woods in southern ON, QC and NB. See p. 424 for conservation status.

Black walnut (*J. nigra*) is a large tree, 40–50 m tall, with bark that has deep furrows and narrow, forking ridges. Twigs light brown to orangish. Leaflets 15–19. Fruits round, in groups of 2–3 or solitary, the thick, semi-fleshy husk yellowish green and covered in short hairs. Found in fields and rich woodlands in southern ON, QC and NB and introduced elsewhere (e.g., MB, NS).

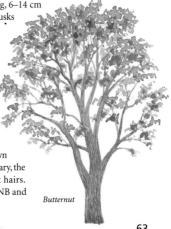

Butternut

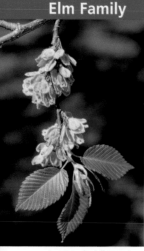

American elm (all images)

Elms
Ulmus spp.

FOOD: The Iroquois ate the inner bark as a famine food. The inner bark of slippery elm was sometimes chewed to quench thirst.

MEDICINE: The Iroquois treated hernias with a tea made from the barks of elm and oak (p. 56). The bark infusion was an important treatment for summer (or choleraic) diarrhea, internal hemorrhage and piles. The inner bark of slippery elm was often steeped into a tea to treat sore throats and fevers. Bark poultices were used to treat inflammations and burns. Slippery elm was also used to soothe heartburn and ease the labour of pregnant women. Today, slippery elm is an important commercial medicinal because of its mucous-like polysaccharides.

OTHER USES: Elm wood is heavy with an attractive grain, durable, flexible and water-resistant, all of which make it excellent for wharves, boat frames, wheel hubs and spokes, hockey sticks, tool handles, furniture and panelling. It is also relatively odourless, so it is ideal for crates and barrels destined to hold food such as cheese, fruits and vegetables. Elm wood is difficult to split, and thus not often used for firewood.

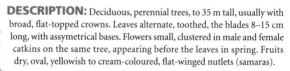

DESCRIPTION: Deciduous, perennial trees, to 35 m tall, usually with broad, flat-topped crowns. Leaves alternate, toothed, the blades 8–15 cm long, with assymetrical bases. Flowers small, clustered in male and female catkins on the same tree, appearing before the leaves in spring. Fruits dry, oval, yellowish to cream-coloured, flat-winged nutlets (samaras).

American elm (*U. americana*) has light brown to grey bark, leaves hairless or nearly so, and fruits hairy and longer than broad. Prefers moist bottomlands and protected slopes from southeastern SK to NS and is used as an ornamental elsewhere.

Slippery elm (*U. rubra*) has brown to reddish bark, leaves hairy and rough, and fruits hairless and about as long as broad. Grows in moist, wooded sites and disturbed areas in southern ON and QC.

These elms were common in parks and along roads and fence lines until Dutch elm disease essentially eliminated the species in eastern Canada. This plague, caused by the fungi *Ophiostoma ulmi* and *O. novo-ulmi*, arrived in Canada in 1944 in infected wooden crates. Within 15 years, 600,000 to 700,000 elms had died. The fungal spores are carried from tree to tree by small beetles (*Scolytus scolytus* and *Hylurgopinus rufipes*), which tunnel under the bark to breed. The fungus can also spread from an infected tree to neighbours via their root systems, which, being shallow and extensive, are often "grafted" together. The fungus blocks the flow of water and nutrients in the trunk, killing the tree within a few years. Many methods have been tested to control Dutch elm disease, but all have proven either ineffective or too expensive and labour intensive. Attempts to breed disease-resistant trees have had some success, and clones of these trees are available for landscaping. Dutch elm disease has still not been introduced to most of AB (one tree was found to have the disease in 1998 but was destroyed and a quarantine area established) and west of the Rocky Mountains to BC. Both provinces prohibit the importation of firewood as a control measure.

White Ash

Fraxinus americana

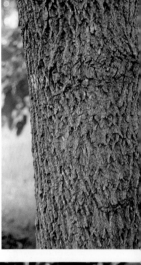

FOOD: The Ojibwa ate the cambium layer after scraping it down in long, fluffy layers and cooking it.

MEDICINE: White ash was used by First Nations in eastern Canada (Iroquois, Abenaki, Mi'kmaq , Maliseet, Ojibwa) for female ailments, wounds and as a general tonic. An infusion of bark was taken by women to induce or assist menstruation, a compound decoction of the roots and bark was taken to induce pregnancy, and the leaves were used for "cleansing" after childbirth. An infusion of the bark was applied as a poultice to syphilitic lumps and neck sores, to stop bleeding in wounds and cuts and to treat snakebites. The bark was also taken for stomach cramps and as a laxative. An infusion of the plant combined with another

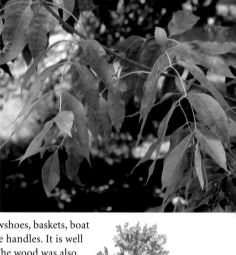

(unspecified) plant was used as ear drops for earaches, and an infusion of the reduced sap combined with goldthread (*Coptis groenlandica*) root was taken to treat deafness. White ash was also used as a blood medicine (to treat bad blood). The bark was chewed as a medicine to induce vomiting and purge the insides before deer hunting. The leaves and roots contain betulin, which has been shown to have anticancer, anti-inflammatory and antiviral properties.

OTHER USES: The wood of white ash is highly valued for its strength, hardiness and elasticity. It is the most valuable timber of all the ashes. The wood was used by eastern First Nations to make the frames of snowshoes, baskets, boat frames, chair backs, canoes and axe and knife handles. It is well known for its use in wooden baseball bats. The wood was also mixed with feed and fed to horses as a laxative. White-tailed deer and cattle browse white ash. Beavers, porcupines and rabbits eat the bark of young trees. The seeds are eaten by many birds and small mammals.

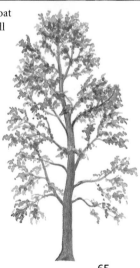

DESCRIPTION: Deciduous tree, to 30 m tall, with grey, furrowed bark, often in a diamond pattern. Twigs grey to olive green. Leaves 20–30 cm long, opposite, pinnately compound with 5–9 leaflets; leaflets smooth or serrated, lance-shaped, 6–13 cm long, dark green above, paler below. Flowers numerous, light green to purplish, from April to May; male and female flowers on separate plants, male flowers appear in tighter clusters than females. Fruit 1-winged and flat with 1 seed, maturing in autumn and dispersing over winter. Found in deep, well-drained soils in full to partial sun with other hardwoods in ON, QC, NB, NS and PEI.

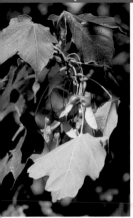

Black maple
(all images)

Maples
Acer spp.

FOOD: Maples are famous worldwide for their sweet sap, well known for its use in making syrup and sugar. The sugar maple, found only in eastern Canada, produces the highest amount of syrup; other species produce sap, but it is not as sweet. Traditionally gathered by First Nations by "tapping" the tree with a wooden peg set into the trunk supporting a birch-bark pail or sack made of deer stomach, the watery sap would drip from the tree along the peg and collect into the pail or sack. The sap would later be reduced to syrup by boiling and used as a sweetener. Maple syrup continues to be celebrated in spring festivals and is currently prepared using reverse-osmosis as well as evaporators. It is common to find syrup, cookies and taffy made with sugar maple sap for sale at maple sugar producers in eastern Canada (called sugar shacks or *cabanes à sucre*). Bigleaf maple sap is also used to produce maple syrup and was used fresh from the tree or dried for cooking and flavouring. Some First Nations made chewy taffy and others made candies by mixing syrup with animal hide shavings. Sugar maple sap can also be fermented to make wine, beer or vinegar. The sweet inner bark of Rocky Mountain maple and of striped maple were gathered in spring and used to make wine and other sweet beverages. Dried leaves of Rocky Mountain maple and bigleaf maple were used to spice meats. Bark from sugar maple was dried, pounded and sifted into flour that was used to make bread. De-winged or sprouted bigleaf maple seeds were cooked in milk and butter as a vegetable, but they are not very palatable and are not recommended (see **Warning**).

MEDICINE: Maple bark is the main part of the tree or shrub that was used as a medicine. Infusions made from bigleaf maple bark were used to treat tuberculosis, and decoctions of inner bark from black maple helped relieve diarrhea. Bark from striped maple and the inner bark of sugar maple were both traditionally used as a cough remedy and expectorant. Striped maple bark was also steeped and applied as a poultice to broken bones. Silver maple bark was used as a cough remedy and for boils. Branches of Rocky Mountain maple were used to make medicinal teas and also used externally to wash and help reduce swelling from snakebite wounds. Saskatoon (p. 109) branches were added to these teas and given to young mothers to help stimulate milk flow and heal internal injuries caused by childbirth. Vine maple wood charcoal, mixed with water and brown sugar, was taken internally for dysentery and polio.

OTHER USES: The wood of Rocky Mountain maple, bigleaf maple, black maple, striped maple, sugar maple and vine maple is very strong when dried and was used to make arrows, spear handles, tongs for cooking, bowls, screens for smoke drying, drum hoops, cradle frames and canoe paddles and oars. Large burls or knots on the lower trunks of Manitoba maple trees as well as black maple roots

WARNING
Seeds from some maple species are reportedly poisonous. Ingestion of wilted maple leaves may reduce red blood cell count and cause acute anemia in horses. Note that decoctions and infusions (teas) prepared with the bark or inner bark of Manitoba maple and striped maple cause vomiting. Teas prepared with Rocky Mountain maple bark have cathartic properties. Red maple contains potentially toxic digallates.

were used to make bowls, dishes and drums, and smaller branches were carved into pipe stems. Sugar maple and bigleaf maple wood were used in construction, lumber and crafting furniture. They also produce hot, long-lasting fires with good coals for cooking meat, were used as ceremonial incense, and their charcoal was used for ceremonial painting and tattooing. Young Rocky Mountain maple and vine maple tree trunks and twigs were made into bows and fish-net hoops, and those of Manitoba maple were used as prayer twigs. In spring, bigleaf maple bark could be crafted into rope and the inner bark into baskets. Vine maple stems were used for making strong utility baskets and to make handles for axes and frames.

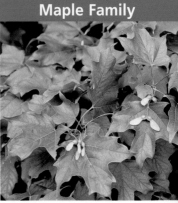

Sugar maple

DESCRIPTION: Deciduous shrubs or trees with opposite branches and hanging, V-shaped pairs of winged seeds (samaras).

Vine maple (*A. circinatum*) is a tall shrub or small tree, to 10 m tall, with 7- to 9-lobed, round or heart-shaped leaves to 9 cm long, becoming yellow to bright red (full sun) in autumn. It has white flowers and smooth, green bark that becomes bright reddish brown. Winged seeds in pairs, 2–4 cm long, green becoming reddish brown. Grows in moist forests and streamsides at low to montane elevations along BC's southwestern coast, rare on southern Vancouver Island.

Rocky Mountain maple (*A. glabrum*) is a clumped shrub, to 10 m tall, with typical maple leaves 2–10 cm wide that turn orange in autumn. Its yellowish green, 8 mm wide flowers (male and female on separate plants) produce 2–3 cm long, greenish brown, wrinkled samaras. Grows in moist foothill and montane sites in BC and AB.

Bigleaf maple (*A. macrophyllum*) is a large tree, to 30 m tall, with simple, opposite leaves 15–30 cm wide. It produces fragrant, yellow flowers and yellowish brown, paired fruit 3–6 cm long, and has deeply furrowed, reddish brown bark. Found in moist forests at low to montane elevations along the south-coastal areas of BC.

Manitoba maple (*A. negundo*) is a small tree, to 20 m tall, with either male or female flowers. Its ash-like leaves are divided into 3–5 leaflets and are opposite and turn yellow in autumn. Widespread garden escapee, and in Canada can be found in various habitats from AB to NS.

Black maple (*A. nigrum*) is a large tree, to 35 m tall, with paired, opposite, palmate leaves, 10–14 cm long, with 3–5 long-pointed lobes. The lower surface of the leaf is yellow-green with soft hairs. It has a bell-shaped flower with a 5-lobed, yellow calyx, and its dark grey or black bark is deeply furrowed. Found in moist soils in southern ON and southwestern QC. See p. 424 for conservation status.

Striped maple (*A. pensylvanicum*) is a small tree, to 10 m tall, with unique white, vertical stripe markings on its green bark. It has 3-lobed leaves to 20 cm wide. Bears small, greenish flowers. Grows in rich forests from ON to the Maritimes.

Red maple (*A. rubrum)* is a small tree, to 10 m tall, with irregularly toothed, sharply notched leaves with 3–5 palmate lobes. Small, red to orange, short-stalked flowers appear in tassel-like clusters from March to April. Pairs of reddish or yellow, winged samaras spread at a 50–60 degree angle. Grows in moist to wet forests, streamsides and swamps from ON to NL.

Sugar maple (*A. saccharum*) is a large tree, to 35 m tall, with coarsely toothed, dark green leaves, 5–11 cm wide, that turn intensely red, orange or yellow in autumn. Widely distributed in hilly forests from MB to the Maritimes.

Silver maple (*A. saccharinum*) is a tall tree, to 35 m tall, with a broad, open crown. Opposite leaves silvery white underneath and have 5–7 palmate lobes, separated by deep, concave notches. Clusters of greenish yellow or reddish flowers from February to April. Winged samaras spread at a 90 degreee angle. Found on moist to wet sites, often near streams in ON, QC and NB (and planted elsewhere).

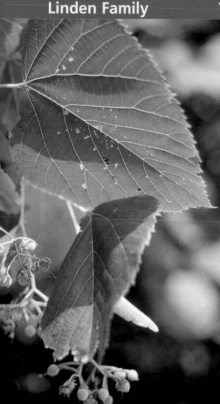

Basswood
Tilia americana

FOOD: The Ojibwa ate the inner bark, young buds and twigs of basswood, either raw or cooked. The bark, which is said to be tender like half-cooked radishes, was also well cooked, pounded and then added to fish broth or mixed with fish oil for making stews. The inner bark of basswood was eaten by the Iroquois, but only as a famine food. Basswood (also called linden) and European linden flowers produce a sweet, honey-flavoured herbal tea that is one of the most popular teas in Europe and is also commonly available in Canada. Basswood honey is valued for its rich taste and possible health benefits (see below).

MEDICINE: Basswood is poor in essential oil, but rich in mucilage (which soothes and reduces inflammation), sugars, flavonoids (antioxidants) and tannins (astringents). The flavonoids as well as the p-coumaric acid content of the lignan are what give basswood its sweat-inducing and antispasmodic properties. The wood, bark, leaves and flowers are all considered to have medicinal value. Closely related trees (*T. cordata, T. platyphylos*) have a long tradition of being used in Europe as diuretics, appetite stimulants, sedatives, sweat-inducers and blood purifiers. Children were also given an evening bath infused with basswood to calm them and help them sleep soundly. Used externally, basswood is effective as a mouthwash and a gargle for sore throats and is often employed in the manufacture of European cosmetics. Honey from basswood flowers is valued as a cough suppressant, sudorific and digestive aid. The Iroquois used the bark to treat wounds and gave an infusion of the twigs with staghorn sumac (p. 90) bark to women before giving birth. The Algonquin made a poultice of the boiled leaves as an eyewash, and the Maliseet used an infusion of the roots as a vermifuge. A decoction of basswood leaves can be used to promote sweating and reduce fevers. First Nations wrapped the bark around weak arms and legs to provide splint-like support. A solution made from boiled bark was applied to burns and sores to ease discomfort. The most unusual but very culturally important "medicinal" use of basswood was the carving of "false face" masks from the trunk of living trees by the Iroquois. Members of the "false face" society, a traditional medicine society, wore the masks during a ritual and spiritual ceremony to purify the long houses.

OTHER USES: Basswood was an important utility plant. Its inner bark fibre could be made into twine, fine string or thread and was used for mat-weaving, bag-making or with birch bark in the building of wigwams. First Nations also made troughs of basswood to use in maple syrup processing. The soft, light wood, which sands easily and does not crack or warp, is valued for handcarving, modelling, turnery and furniture parts. Basswood is a beautiful tree, especially when flowering, and makes a wonderful and useful addition to a garden.

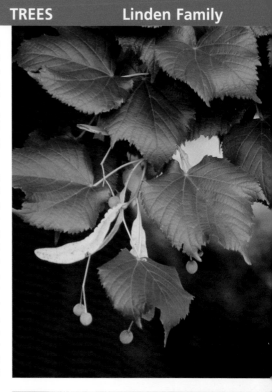

DESCRIPTION: Large, long-lived (some research indicates up to 1000 years), hardwood, deciduous tree, to 25 m tall (occasionally over 30 m). Trunk straight, to 75 cm in diameter; crown rounded; branches slender, arching upward or spreading outward and turning upward near tips; root system deep, wide-spreading. Bark dark greyish brown, in long, flat ridges; sprouts from the base of old stumps. Twigs stout, yellowish brown, hairless; buds broad, clearly asymmetrical at base, hairless, often reddish. Leaves alternate, stalked, simple, heart-shaped, 11–12 cm wide and slightly longer, hairless to sparsely hairy, with tufts of hair in axils of veins beneath; margins with gland-tipped, sharp teeth. Flowers creamy yellow, 1.3 cm wide, very fragrant, 5-petalled; in small, flat-topped, long-stalked clusters from the centre of elongate, leafy bracts in leaf axils; appear from June to July. Fruits nut-like, hard, woody, round, 6 mm across, brown-hairy, 1- to 2-seeded; remain on tree over winter. Inhabits dry to moist, sandy to clayey upland sites, as an associate of sugar maple, eastern hemlock, yellow birch and other hardwoods from southeastern SK to NB. See p. 424 for conservation status.

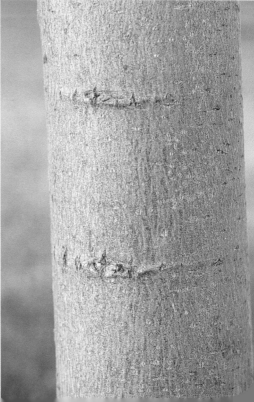

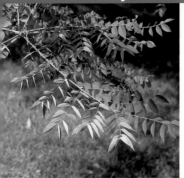

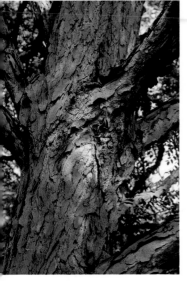

Kentucky Coffee Tree
Gymnocladus dioicus

FOOD: Although early settlers used the roasted and ground seeds of this tree as a coffee substitute, this practice is not recommended because the saponin compounds in the beans are known to be poisonous in large quantities. In addition, people who have tried this coffee-like drink in more modern times report it to be foul-tasting and nothing at all like the real thing. First Nations ate the seeds after roasting them. The seeds are considered poisonous when raw.

MEDICINE: A tea made from the leaves and bean pulp of this tree was reportedly used as a laxative, and tea made from the bark was administered as a cough medicine.

OTHER USES: Like its close relative the honey locust, the Kentucky coffee tree is valued as a fast-growing shade tree that adapts well to urban conditions. The wood is strong and has been used for railway ties and fence posts, which are reported to last as long as 50–80 years in the ground. This tree is horticulturally striking, as it has the largest leaves of any native Canadian tree.

DESCRIPTION: Deciduous tree, to 30 m tall, in a broadly columnar shape. Bark dark brown and rough with scaly ridges. Leaves bipinnate and very large, to 1 m long, with numerous oval leaflets to 7.5 cm long, untoothed, becoming dark green above, bluish beneath. Flowers whitish, fragrant, about 2.5 cm across and 10–30 cm long. Male and female flowers usually on separate trees. Fruits large, leathery, red-brown legumes (pods) 15–25 cm long, containing 6–9 dark brown, rounded, hard-coated seeds, produced on female trees only. This species prefers sunny locales in rich, moist woodlands and at the edges of marshes. However, it tolerates a wide variety of growing conditions in full sun. In Canada, it occurs only in extreme southwestern ON, at the northern limits of its natural range. However, trees planted for horticultural purposes survive far beyond this limited area. This species is considered rare throughout its range, with fewer than 20 natural stands of mature trees (containing less than 200 mature individuals) in southwestern ON. See p. 424 for conservation status.

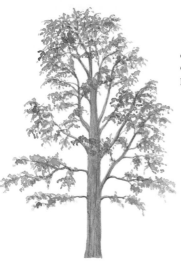

WARNING

The leaves, seeds and pulp of this tree are known to be poisonous to sheep, cattle, horses and humans. Sprouts eaten by livestock in spring have produced toxicosis, while pods and seeds on the ground eaten in autumn or winter have resulted in poisoning. The toxin is highest in the leaves, young sprouts and seeds with the gelatinous pulp around them.

Buckthorn & Cascara

Rhamnus spp.

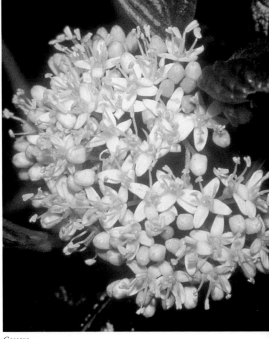
Cascara

FOOD: Some sources report that the purple berries of these small trees or shrubs were eaten by native peoples, but possibly in modest amounts given their strong purgative effects. A bark extract of cascara, with the bitterness removed, is often used for flavouring soft drinks, baked goods and ice cream.

MEDICINE: These species have been used as a source of laxatives for hundreds of years. The bark of alder-leaved buckthorn contains a laxative, but cascara has been much more widely used. Indigenous peoples collected the bark in spring and summer, by scraping either downward (if the patient needed a laxative) or upward (if the patient needed to vomit). It was then dried and stored for later use. Ingesting fresh bark and berries could have very severe effects, but curing the bark for at least 1 year or using a heat treatment reduced the harshness. The dried bark was traditionally used to make medicinal teas, but today it is usually administered as a liquid extract or elixir, or in tablet form. Each year, 0.5–1.4 million kg of bark are collected, mainly from wild trees in BC, WA, OR and CA. Some tribes used these plants to induce vomiting when poisons had been eaten. The chewed bark was used for children with worms, to treat rheumatism and arthritis and as a blood purifier and physic. This genus contains large amounts of anthraquinones, which are responsible for the emetic properties.

OTHER USES: A green dye is obtained from cascara bark. Cascara wood is also used to make the handles of small tools.

DESCRIPTION: Erect or spreading shrubs or small trees, 50 cm–10 m tall, with alternate, oval to elliptic, prominently veined, 5–12 cm long leaves. Flowers greenish yellow, all male or all female in 1 cluster, forming flat-topped clusters in leaf axils, from June to July. Fruits black to bluish black, berry-like drupes, 6–9 mm long.

WARNING

These small trees or shrubs can cause severe vomiting and diarrhea. A few rare cases of mild poisoning have been reported. They are best avoided when gathering sticks for roasting hot dogs.

Alder-leaved buckthorn (*R. alnifolia*) is a medium-sized shrub, 50 cm–1.5 m tall, with 2- to 5-flowered, stalkless flower clusters and 10- to 14-veined leaves. Grows in moist, open to shady meadows and on streambanks at steppe to montane elevations in all provinces. See p. 424 for conservation status.

Cascara (*R. purshiana*) is generally a small tree, to 10 m tall, with 8- to 30-flowered, stalked clusters and 20- to 24-veined leaves. Grows on streamsides and in open to closed forests at low to montane elevations in southern BC.

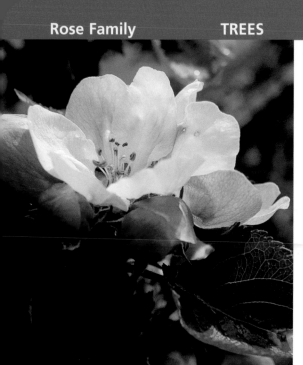

Common apple (all images)

Apples
Malus spp.

FOOD: The berries of Pacific crab apple served as an essential food item traditionally, and they are also an important food for First Nations in BC today. Large quantities were harvested in the past and are still picked every year. They were typically collected from late summer into autumn, after the first frost. One method of harvest was to pick the berries when they were still green and leave them to soften in baskets. They were either eaten fresh with eulachon oil or stored for winter. Traditionally, they were placed, raw or cooked, in bentwood cedar boxes or large watertight baskets lined with skunk-cabbage (p. 165) leaves and covered with water and a layer of animal grease. They are preserved today by canning, freezing or being made into jelly. For some Aboriginal people, crab apples were used only in ceremonial situations, such as potlatches or large feasts. Boxes of Pacific crab apples were a common trade item in the past and were also used as gifts at events such as weddings. The fruit of Pacific crab apple is rich in pectin, so it can be added to low-pectin fruits when making jams and jellies. The common apple was one of the first fruits to be cultivated, and it is the most widely cultivated fruit tree. There are now thousands of varieties of apples, several of which are sold commercially across Canada.

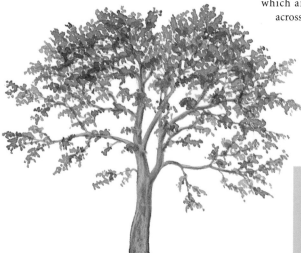

> **WARNING**
> Apple bark contains cyanide-producing compounds, so it should be used with caution.

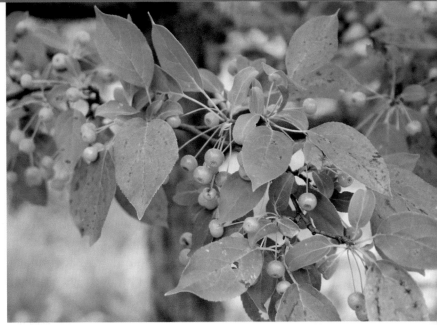

Pacific crab apple

MEDICINE: The bark of Pacific crab apple (trunk, branches or inner bark) was used to treat a number of ailments and was considered by some to be a cure-all tonic. It was valued for its laxative and diuretic properties and used to treat problems such as stomach disorders, diarrhea, dysentery, blood spitting, ulcers, heart troubles, intestinal disorders, consumption, coughs, fractures, rheumatism and sciatica. It was also used for sore eyes, eczema or skin troubles and wounds. Pacific crab apple was considered a fattening medicine and blood purifier. The leaves were chewed for lung trouble. After a long day of hunting, the fruit was eaten to "kill poison in muscles." The plant was used as a tonic for young men in training and was also chewed by hunters to suppress thirst.

OTHER USES: The wood of Pacific crab apple is hard, close-grained and durable and was used to make a number of items, including bows, digging sticks, sledgehammer handles, mallet heads, axe handles, spoons, halibut hooks, fishing floats, mauls (for driving stakes) and seal spear prongs. The sticks were used to strike rods of cedar while hunting, which would make noise to drive animals into the open. The sticks were also used to retrieve special cooking stones used for cooking edible seaweed. The crab apples are eaten by grouse, which were sometimes hunted during crab apple harvesting.

DESCRIPTION: Deciduous trees, 3–12 m tall, with brown or greyish bark. Leaves alternate, elliptic to lance-shaped, toothed and sometimes lobed, dark green to yellow-green above and paler, slightly hairy below. Flowers fragrant, white to pinkish with 5 showy petals, in rounded clusters, blooming late April. Fruits apples and crab apples, fleshy pomes.

Pacific crab apple (*M. fusca*) is a tall shrub or small tree, usually 3–8 m tall, with leaves with 1–3 irregular lobes and small fruit (crab apples) 10–15 mm long. Found in estuary fringes, wetlands, on streambanks and upper beaches along the BC coast.

Common apple (*M. pumila*) is a small tree, 4–12 m tall, with leaves toothed but not lobed, and larger fruit (apples) more than 2 cm long. This widely cultivated and highly variable fruit tree, native to central Asia, escapes cultivation in disturbed sites across southern Canada.

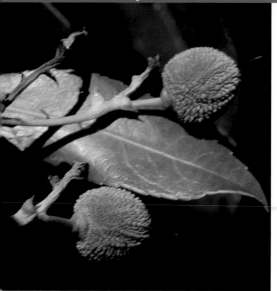

Arbutus
Arbutus menziesii

FOOD: Arbutus (also called madrone or madrona) is the only broad-leaved evergreen tree native to Canada. Its berries were eaten by Pacific First Nations, but because of their high tannin content, they are particularly astringent, so they were often roasted first on top of an open fire, or chewed and spit out, never swallowed. The crushed berries were also made into a sweet cider or preserved as jellies. To store them over winter, they were first boiled or steamed, and then dried. They were then soaked in warm water before being eaten.

MEDICINE: Most of the medicinal applications of arbutus can be attributed to its astringency. The bark and leaves were useful as an infusion to treat bladder infections, stomachaches, cramps, colds, as a folk remedy for diabetes and as a postpartum contraceptive. As a mouthwash, it was gargled for sore throats. The infusion was also given to horses with sore backs. Bad colds and sore throats were treated by chewing the fresh leaves and swallowing the juice. Arbutus bark was part of a 10-ingredient bark medicine used for treating tuberculosis and the spitting up of blood. Externally, an infusion of the bark was used as a sitz bath for skin sores and impetigo and applied to wounds, sores and cuts. Women rubbed it on their skin to close the pores and make their skin appear soft and lustrous. Fresh leaves were applied to burns. A cider made from the berries was employed to create an appetite.

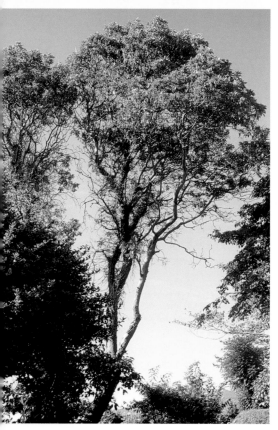

OTHER USES: The tannins in the bark were used as a preservative on wood and ropes, to tan paddles and fish hooks and as a source of brown dye. First Nations dipped camas bulbs (p. 199) into a boiling infusion of the bark to turn them pinkish in colour. The leaves were used to test the temperature of pitch: leaves would turn black when the pitch was ready to be used. Arbutus was the tree that at least one west coast Salish First Nation tied their canoes to following the Great Flood; to this day some Saanich people will not burn arbutus wood because of the service it provided. Leaves were sometimes smoked like tobacco. The wood is very hard, heavy, moderately strong and durable in water; it is used as fuel and to build lodge poles, saw handles and other tools and for small cabinet work and turnery. It is ideal for carving because it will not split upon drying. A fine grade charcoal is obtained from the wood. Traditionally, the inner bark was sewn together to make clothing, and the leaves and scarlet berries were used to make necklaces and decorations.

DESCRIPTION: Small to medium, broadleaf, evergreen tree, to 30 m tall (but usually much shorter). Bark thin, smooth, reddish brown, peels in papery flakes and strips, with newly exposed surfaces yellowish green, soon reddening, thickening on old trunks and breaking into many small flakes. Leaves alternate, simple, thick and leathery, oval to elliptic, 7–15 cm long and 4–8 cm wide. Flowers greenish white to white (sometimes pinkish), 6–8 mm long, with a sweet honey-like fragrance, in drooping, branched clusters at the ends of the branchlets, from April to May. Fruit an orange-red berry with a glandular surface, about 6.5 mm wide, containing several seeds. Grows in well-drained soils in dry, open forests and on exposed, rocky bluffs near sea level along the Pacific coast in extreme southwestern BC. It is rarely found more than 10 km inland or at heights above 300 m.

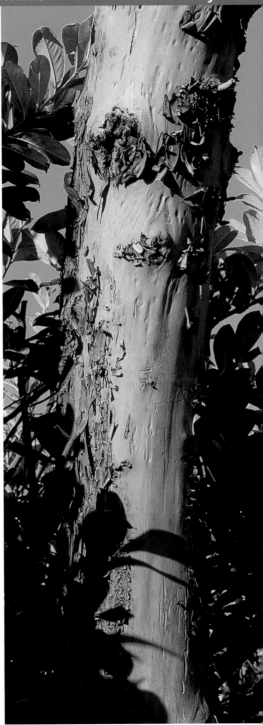

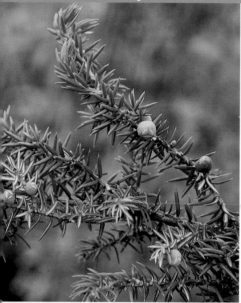

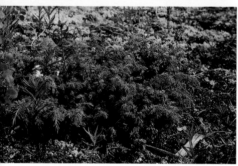

Common juniper (all images)

Shrub Junipers
Juniperus spp.

FOOD: Juniper is most famous as the flavouring for gin. Berries can be quite sweet by the end of their second summer or the following spring, but they have a rather strong, pitchy flavour that some people find distasteful. They are usually added as flavouring to meat dishes (recommended for venison and other wild game, veal and lamb), soups and stews, either whole, crushed or ground and used like pepper. For more information, see tree junipers (p. 46).

MEDICINE: Oil-of-juniper prepared by steam distillation is used today in aromatherapy or direct topical application for a variety of conditions, including nervous conditions, cellulitis and arthritis. Traditionally, oil from juniper berries was mixed with fat to make salves for protecting wounds from irritation by flies. Juniper berries stimulate urination by irritating the kidneys and give the urine a violet-like fragrance. They are also said to stimulate sweating, mucous secretion, production of hydrochloric acid in the stomach and contractions in the uterus and intestines. Some studies have shown juniper berries to lower blood sugar caused by adrenaline hyperglycemia, suggesting that they may be useful in the treatment of insulin-dependent diabetes. Juniper berries also have antiseptic qualities. Strong juniper tea was used to sterilize needles and bandages, and during the Black Death in 14th-century Europe, doctors held a few berries in their mouths to avoid being infected by patients. During cholera epidemics in North America, some people drank and bathed in juniper tea to prevent infection. Juniper tea was often given to women in labour to speed delivery, and after the birth, it was used as a cleansing, healing agent. Juniper needles were dried and powdered as a dusting for skin diseases, and juniper smoke or steam was inhaled to relieve colds and chest infections. The components of juniper oil are a-pinene, camphene,

WARNING
Large and/or frequent doses of juniper can result in convulsions, kidney failure and an irritated digestive tract. People with kidney problems and pregnant women should never take any part of a juniper internally. Juniper oil can cause blistering.

b-pinene, sabinene, myrcene, a-phellandrene, a-terpinene, y-terpinene, 1,4-cineole, b-phellandrene, p-cymene, terpinen-4-ol, bornyl acetate and cayophyllene.

OTHER USES: Juniper branches were often burned in smudges to repel insects. Smoke from the berries or branches of junipers was used in religious ceremonies or to bring good luck (especially for hunters) or protection from disease, evil spirits, witches, thunder, lightning and so on. If a horse was sick, it was made to inhale smoke from juniper needles 3 times for a cure. The berries make a pleasant, aromatic addition to potpourris, and vapours from boiling juniper berries in water were used to purify and deodorize homes affected by sickness or death. Juniper boughs were sometimes hung in tepees for protection from thunder and lightning.

DESCRIPTION: Evergreen shrubs with small, 5–9 mm, bluish purple to bluish green "berries" (actually fleshy cones), produced from April to May and maturing the following year.

Common juniper (*J. communis*) is a spreading, 30 cm–3 m tall, evergreen shrub. Leaves sharp, 5–12 mm long needles, in whorls of 3. Grows on dry, open sites and in rocky, infertile soils throughout Canada.

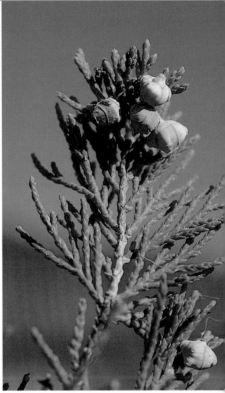

Creeping juniper (all images)

Creeping juniper (*J. horizontalis*) is a low shrub (seldom over 25 cm tall) with trailing branches, bearing tiny, scale-like leaves in 4 vertical rows. Grows in dry, rocky soils in sterile pastures and fields throughout Canada. See p. 424 for conservation status.

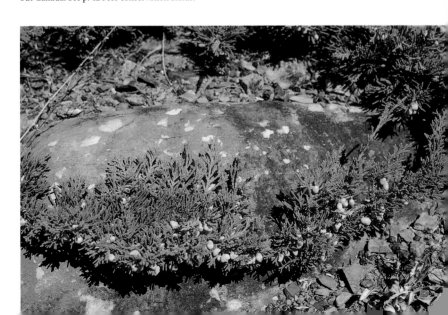

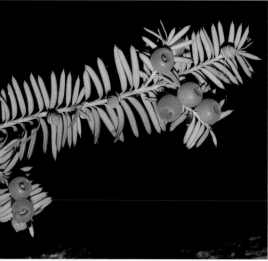

Yews

Taxus spp.

FOOD: The fleshy red part of the fruit is said to be edible, but the seeds are extremely poisonous, so this fruit is not recommended for consumption (see **Warning**). The leaves are also toxic.

MEDICINE: The bark of western yew is an original source of the anticancer drug taxol. After a long period of development by the National Cancer Institute and pharmaceutical partners, this drug was approved for use in treating a variety of cancers and

Western yew (all images)

was particularly successful in treating breast and ovarian cancers. The slow growing western yew quickly became depleted by demand, and more recently, taxane derivatives are obtained from managed harvest of the more common Canada yew in eastern Canada, from which the drug is prepared by extraction and semi-synthesis. Some native peoples used yew bark for treating illness (indeed, this is how modern researchers first knew to research this plant) and applied the wet needles as poultices on wounds—do not try this remedy (see **Warning**). The Ojibwa treated rheumatism by boiling Canada yew and eastern redcedar (p. 47) twigs together and either drinking the resulting decoction or sprinkling it on hot rocks to produce steam. The Algonquin boiled the needles, sometimes with pin cherry (p. 87), to treat rheumatism and to take as a tea after childbirth. The Montagnais used a tea of Canada yew to treat fevers and general weakness, and the Cree used the tea to treat stomachaches and menstrual cramps. The bark was used by the Micmac to treat bowel and internal troubles, and a tea of the needles for fever.

OTHER USES: The heavy, fine-grained wood of western yew is extremely durable and was prized by all First Nations within the plant's range to make items such as bows, wedges, clubs, paddles, digging sticks, halibut and other fish hooks, tool handles and harpoons that experienced great stress. Western yew was also used to make mat-sewing needles, awls, dipnet

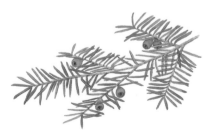

frames, knives, dishes, spoons, boxes, dowels and pegs, canoe spreaders, bark scrapers, fire tongs, combs and snowshoe frames. The Saanich people of Vancouver Island inventively fitted a spear to a young yew sapling, pulled it back and released it as a lethal catapult during times of war. The Kwakwaka'wakw bound yew branches together to make a sort of "nest" that they lowered into deep water to entrap sea urchins, and young men tested their strength by trying to twist a yew tree from its bottom to top. The wood was a valuable trade item to exchange with other peoples where the tree does not naturally grow. The Okanagan made a red paint by mixing fish oil with dried yew wood. Two ancient spears, dating from the early Stone Age, were found to be made of yew wood. Bows, carved from seasoned yew wood, were varnished with boiled animal sinew and muscle. The wood is still prized today by carvers, but it is relatively scarce because of the tree's slow growth and reproduction, which requires a male and female tree. With their dark, evergreen needles and scarlet berries, yews make lovely ornamental shrubs, but their poisonous seeds, branches and leaves are dangerous to children and horses (see **Warning**).

DESCRIPTION: Evergreen shrubs or trees with reddish brown, scaly bark. Leaves usually appear to be arranged in 2 rows. Fruits berry-like, orange to scarlet arils containing a single bony seed.

Western yew (*T. brevifolia*) is a small, western tree, to 15 m tall (sometimes to 25 m). Male and female cones are on separate trees, the male cones inconspicuous, the female fruits scarlet "berries" (arils), 4–5 mm across, with a cup of fleshy tissue around the seed. Grows in moist, shady sites such as streambanks at low to montane elevations in BC and southwestern AB. See p. 424 for conservation status.

Canada yew (*T. canadensis*) is an eastern shrub rarely over 2 m tall. Male and female cones are usually on the same shrub, the male cones inconspicuous, the female fruits scarlet arils about 7.5 mm long. Grows in dry to moist, rich forests and wetlands (swamps, bogs) at low to subalpine elevations from southeastern MB to NL. See p. 424 for conservation status.

Canada yew

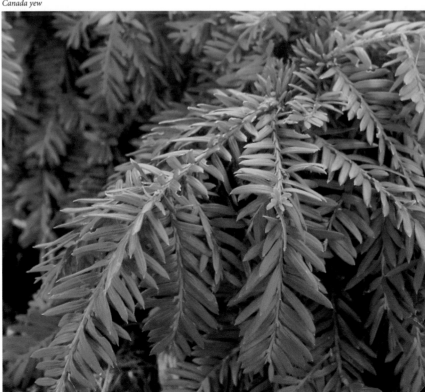

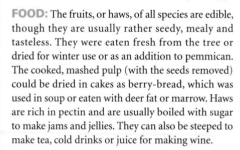

Hawthorns

Crataegus spp.

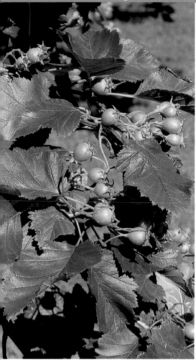

FOOD: The fruits, or haws, of all species are edible, though they are usually rather seedy, mealy and tasteless. They were eaten fresh from the tree or dried for winter use or as an addition to pemmican. The cooked, mashed pulp (with the seeds removed) could be dried in cakes as berry-bread, which was used in soup or eaten with deer fat or marrow. Haws are rich in pectin and are usually boiled with sugar to make jams and jellies. They can also be steeped to make tea, cold drinks or juice for making wine.

MEDICINE: Hawthorn flowers and fruits are famous in herbal medicine as heart tonics, though not all species are equally effective. Studies have supported the use of hawthorn extracts as a treatment for high blood pressure associated with a weak heart, angina pectoris (recurrent pain in the chest and left arm owing to a sudden lack of blood in the heart muscle) and arteriosclerosis (loss of elasticity and thickening of the artery walls). Hawthorn is said to slow the heart rate and reduce blood pressure by dilating the large arteries supplying blood to the heart and by acting as a mild heart stimulant. However, it has a gradual, mild action and must be taken for extended periods to produce noticeable results. Hawthorn tea has also been used to treat kidney disease and nervous conditions such as insomnia. Dark-coloured haws are especially high in flavonoids and have been steeped in hot water to make teas for strengthening connective tissues damaged by inflammation. The haws were sometimes eaten in moderate amounts to relieve diarrhea (some indigenous peoples considered them very constipating), and diets high in hawthorn have also been recommended

Downy hawthorn (above)
Cockspur hawthorn (all below)

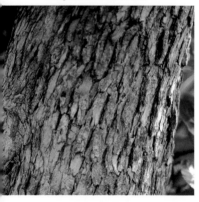

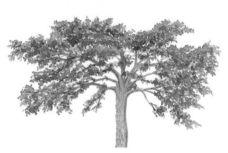

> **WARNING**
> Eye scratches from these thorns often cause blindness. Ingesting too many haws may cause nausea, vomiting and diarrhea. Hawthorns contain compounds that affect blood pressure and heart rate. People with heart conditions should use these shrubs only under the guidance of a doctor. Children and pregnant or nursing women should avoid using hawthorns.

in weight-loss programs. Tea made from the inner bark was used for treating dysentery.

OTHER USES: Hawthorn wood is very hard and makes excellent walking sticks. These tough, hardy shrubs have been planted on highway medians to prevent cars from swerving across into oncoming traffic. The thorns have been used as awls and fish hooks. Predatory songbirds called northern shrikes display their hunting prowess by impaling prey on the thorns. This behaviour may also serve as a means of storing excess food during times of plenty.

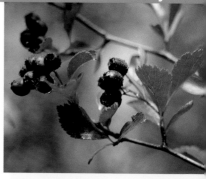

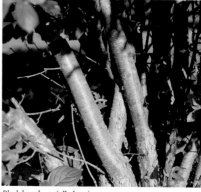

DESCRIPTION: Deciduous shrubs or small trees that grow 6–11 m tall with strong, straight thorns. Leaves alternate, generally oval, with a wedge-shaped base. Flowers whitish, 5-petalled, unpleasant-smelling, forming showy, flat-topped clusters, from May to June. Fruits "haws," small, pulpy, red to purplish pomes (tiny apples) containing 1–5 nutlets.

Fireberry hawthorn (*C. chrysocarpa*) is a shrub or small tree, to 6 m tall, with a crooked trunk. Stout branches usually have numerous shiny black thorns, 2–6 cm long, and dull yellowish green, toothed, lobed leaves. Small, 1–1.5 cm wide, white flowers appear from May to June. Haws usually deep red and hairy and often persevere through winter. Found on open, gravelly sites near water throughout southern Canada. See p. 424 for conservation status.

Black hawthorn (all above)

Red hawthorn (*C. columbiana*) is a shrub or small tree, to 6 m tall, with 4–7 cm long thorns and red haws. Grows on open prairies, meadows, streambanks and forest edges in steppe and montane zones in BC and AB.

Cockspur hawthorn (*C. crus-galli*) is a small tree, to 10 m tall, with large thorns (to 6 cm long), flowers ranging from white to red and haws that are dull red or green. Found in openings, fencerows and old fields in southern ON and southwestern QC. See p. 424 for conservation status.

Black hawthorn (*C. douglasii*) is a small tree, to 11 m tall, with 1–2 cm long thorns, toothed to shallowly lobed leaves and black, 1 cm long, purplish black haws. Grows in forest edges, thickets, streamsides and roadsides in lowland to montane zones from BC to ON. See p. 424 for conservation status.

Downy hawthorn (*C. mollis*) is a small tree, to 10 m tall, with leaves hairy underneath, 2.5–5 cm long thorns and large (2.5 cm long), scarlet or crimson haws. Found in open woods and thickets in the lowland zone in southern ON.

Fleshy hawthorn (*C. succulenta*) is a shrub or multistemmed, shrubby tree, to 8 m tall, with thorns 3–4.5 cm long and bright red haws 7 mm–1.2 cm long. Found in thickets, pastures and woodland edges from southern SK to the Maritimes. See p. 424 for conservation status.

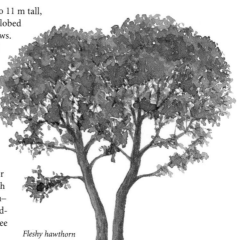

Fleshy hawthorn

81

Mountain-Ashes

Sorbus spp.

FOOD: The bitter fruits of these trees can be eaten raw, cooked or dried, but many Aboriginal groups considered them inedible. They were sometimes stored fresh underground, added to other berries or used to marinate meat such as marmot. The green berries are too bitter to eat, but the ripe fruit, mellowed by repeated freezing, is said to be quite tasty. Mountain-ash fruit is usually cooked and sweetened. It has been used to make jams, jellies, pies, ale and a bittersweet wine. The berries have also been dried and ground into flour. In northern Europe, this flour was fermented and used to make a strong liquor.

MEDICINE: Indigenous peoples boiled the peeled branches or inner bark to make teas for treating back pain, colds, headaches, rheumatism, sore chests and internal bleeding (perhaps associated with tuberculosis). American mountain-ash buds

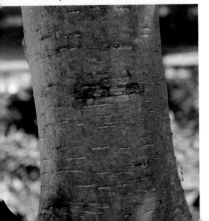

European mountain-ash (above & below)

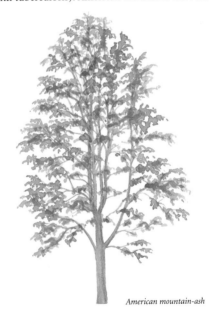

American mountain-ash

WARNING
The fruits are said to be somewhat toxic because they contain cyanide-related compounds and parascorbic acid (reported to be a cancer-causing compound).

and inner bark were used as a tonic and to treat depression and general weakness. A poultice made from the bark was used to treat boils. The branches of mountain-ashes were boiled and then the steam was inhaled to relieve colds, headaches and sore chests and to make labour easier for women. The berries can be used to make a juice rich in vitamin C. The astringent berry tea has been used as a gargle for relieving sore throats and tonsillitis. European mountain-ash fruit was used to make medicinal teas for treating indigestion, hemorrhoids, diarrhea and problems with the urinary tract, gallbladder and heart. Teas made from its bark and leaves have been used to treat malarial fevers, ulcers, hemorrhoids and sores.

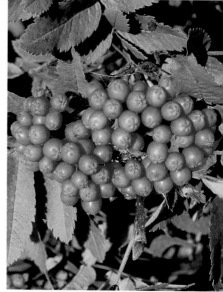

OTHER USES: European mountain-ash is a popular ornamental tree, and the native mountain-ashes make attractive garden shrubs, easily propagated from seed sown in autumn. The scarlet fruit clusters attract many birds. Some indigenous peoples rubbed the berries into their scalps to kill lice and treat dandruff.

Western mountain-ash (above)
Sitka mountain-ash (below)

DESCRIPTION: Clumped, deciduous shrubs or trees with pinnately divided, sharply toothed leaves. Flowers white, about 1 cm across, 5-petalled, forming flat-topped, 9–15 cm wide, smelly clusters from June to July. Fruits berry-like pomes, about 1 cm long.

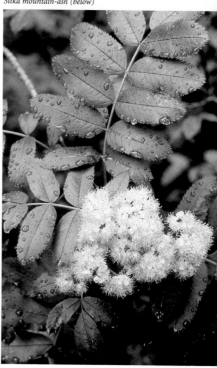

European mountain-ash or **Rowan tree** (*S. aucuparia*) is a widely planted ornamental tree, to 15 m tall, with white-hairy buds, leaf stems and leaves (underneath at least), and orange to red fruit. This Eurasian species is widely cultivated, and just as widely escaped, in all provinces.

American mountain-ash (*S. americana*) is a small tree, to 10 m tall, much less hairy than European mountain-ash, the buds, leaf stems and leaves hairless or nearly so, with bright coral-red fruits. Grows in moist sites along swamps, wet forests and rocky hillsides from ON across to NL. See p. 424 for conservation status.

Western mountain-ash (*S. scopulina*) is a tall shrub, to 4 m tall, with sticky twigs and buds, 9–13 shiny green, pointed leaflets, with teeth almost to the base, and orange fruit. Grows in moist to wet, open forests, glades and on streambanks at higher elevations in YT and NT and from BC to SK. See p. 424 for conservation status.

Sitka mountain-ash (*S. sitchensis*) is a tall shrub, to 4 m tall, with rusty-hairy (but non-sticky) twigs and buds, 7–11 dull bluish green, round-tipped leaflets without teeth near the base, and crimson to purplish fruit. Grows in foothill to subalpine zones in YT, BC and western AB. See p. 424 for conservation status.

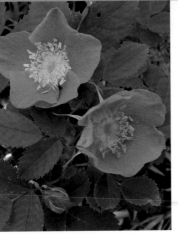

Prickly rose

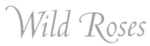

Wild Roses
Rosa spp.

FOOD: Most parts of rose shrubs are edible. The hips remain on the branches throughout winter, so they are available when most other fruits are gone. Hips can be eaten fresh or dried or used in tea, jam, jelly, syrup and wine. Usually only the fleshy outer layer is eaten (see **Warning**). Because they are so seedy, some indigenous peoples considered rose hips famine food. Rose petals may be eaten alone as a trail nibble, added to salads, teas, jellies and wines or candied. Rose leaves, roots and peeled twigs have also been used in teas. Buds, young shoots and young leaves may be eaten raw or cooked.

MEDICINE: Rose hips are rich in vitamins A, B, E and K and are one of the best sources of vitamin C. Three hips can contain as much vitamin C as an orange. During World War II, when oranges could not be imported, British and Scandinavian people collected hundreds of tonnes of rose hips to make syrup. The vitamin C content of fresh hips varies greatly, but that of commercial "natural" rose hip products can fluctuate even more. Stem or root bark tea was taken to treat diarrhea, stomach upset or syphilis and to reduce labour pain. It was also used as an eyewash for treating snow-blindness. Root decoctions were used in hot compresses for reducing swelling, gargled to treat mouth bleeding, tonsillitis and sore throats or mixed with sugar to make a syrup for soothing sore throats. The leaves were boiled to make a wash for strengthening babies. Rose petals were taken to relieve colic, heartburn, headaches and mouth sores. They were also ground and mixed with grease to make a salve for mouth sores or mixed with wine to make a medicine for relieving earaches, toothaches and uterine cramps. The cooked seeds were eaten to relieve sore muscles. The bark of Nootka rose was used as a wash for sore eyes, and the chewed leaves were applied as a poultice to bee stings.

OTHER USES: Dried rose petals have a lovely fragrance and have been used in potpourri. The inner bark was sometimes smoked like tobacco (p. 240), and the roots were boiled to make hair rinse. Pithy stems were occasionally used for pipe stems, handles or arrow shafts, and heavy, split wood was used to make cradle hoops. Rose sprigs were hung on cradle boards to keep ghosts away from babies, and on the walls of haunted houses and in graves to prevent the dead from howling. During pit cooking, the leaves of Nootka rose were placed under and over food to add flavour and prevent burning. The roots were combined with gooseberry (p. 106) and cedar (p. 44) roots to

Prairie rose

> **WARNING**
> The dry inner "seeds" (achenes) are not palatable, and their sliver-like hairs can irritate the digestive tract and cause "itchy bum." All members of the *Rosa* genus have cyanide-like compounds in their seeds that can be destroyed by drying or cooking.

Prickly rose

make reef nets. Hunters made a wash wash was made from Nootka rose branches to get rid of their human scent.

DESCRIPTION: Thorny to prickly, deciduous shrubs, 30 cm–2 m tall, with leaves pinnately divided into about 5–7 oblong, toothed leaflets. Flowers light pink to deep rose, 5-petalled, fragrant, from June to August. Fruits scarlet to purplish, round to pear-shaped, berry-like hips, 1.5–3 cm long, with a fleshy outer layer enclosing many stiff-hairy achenes.

Prickly rose (*R. acicularis*) grows to 1.5 m tall, with bristly, prickly branches and small clusters of 5–7 cm wide flowers or 1–2 cm long hips. Grows in open woods, thickets and on rocky slopes from BC to NB, and in YT and NT. Prickly rose is AB's floral emblem. See p. 424 for conservation status.

Arkansas rose (*R. arkansana*) is a small shrub, to 50 cm tall, with densely bristly stems with prickles of various sizes, flowers clustered at end of branches, and apple-like hips 8–13 mm across. Grows in prairies and open forests from northeastern BC to MB.

Baldhip rose (*R. gymnocarpa*) grows 50 cm–2 m tall and has few to abundant soft prickles, with clusters of small flowers 2–3 cm wide, and 5–10 mm wide hips. Grows in open forests and open areas in southern BC.

Nootka rose (*R. nutkana*) is a small shrub, to 1.5 m tall, with well-developed thorns at its joints, large (4–8 cm wide), mostly single flowers and 1.5–2 cm long hips. Grows in moist, open areas (shorelines, forest edges, streambanks, roadsides) in southern BC.

Large-hip rose (*R. rugosa*) is a shrub, 1.2–1.8 m tall, with stems hairy beneath with bristles and fine thorns, single, large (to 10 cm across) flowers from white to purple and red hips 1.3–3.8 cm across. Asian species naturalized in sand dunes and disturbed sites from ON to NL.

Prairie rose (*R. woodsii*) is a small shrub, 20–50 cm tall, with well-developed thorns at its joints, no small bristles or prickles on upper stems, small clusters of 3–5 cm wide flowers or 6–10 mm long hips. Grows in thickets, prairies and on riverbanks in southern YT and NT, and from BC to ON. See p. 424 for conservation status.

Prairie rose

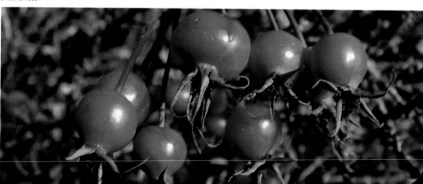

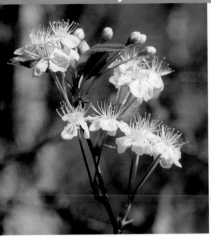

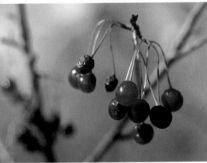

Cherries
Prunus spp.

FOOD: Wild cherries may be eaten raw as a tart nibble, but the cooked or dried fruit is much sweeter, and additional sugar further improves the flavour. Usually these cherries are cooked, strained and made into jelly, syrup, sauce or wine. The fruit seldom contains enough natural pectin to make a firm jelly, so pectin must be added. Although wild cherries are small compared to domestic varieties, they can still be collected in large quantities. The cherry flesh can be used in pies, muffins and pancakes, but pitting such small fruits is a tedious job. Traditionally, wild cherries were eaten fresh, cooked into a sauce or dried (whole or as cakes) for winter storage. Choke cherries are among the fruits most used by indigenous peoples in Canada. They were sometimes eaten with grease or added to pemmican (with meat, such as buffalo, and fat), soups and stews. For winter storage, they would be dried in the sun, sometimes crushed on a stone or left to dry whole. Choke cherries have been used to make beer and wine as well.

MEDICINE: Choke cherry bark was traditionally made into tea to treat coughs, colds, sore throats, pneumonia and diarrhea. The bark tea was also taken by women after childbirth as a strengthening tonic. Mashed choke cherry seeds were used as stomach medicine, and the branches were taken as a laxative, for influenza and by nursing mothers to pass medicinal qualities to the baby. Choke cherry was listed in the US Dispensary from 1800 to 1975. The bark has been used to make cough drops and syrups. The bark has also been used in folk medicine to expel worms or treat abscesses or ulcers. The Cree used the bark of pin cherry to

Pin cherry (all above)
Black cherry (below)

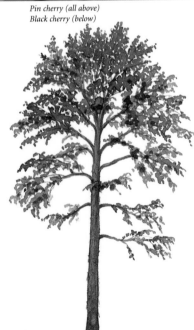

WARNING
Cherry leaves, bark, wood and seeds (stones) produce hydrocyanic acid and so can cause cyanide poisoning. The flesh of the cherry is the only edible part. The stone should always be discarded, but cooking or drying will destroy the toxins. Cherry leaves and twigs are poisonous to browsing animals.

treat sore eyes, and a poultice of the mashed leaves was applied to oral abscesses. The Maliseet and Micmac used black cherry bark for colds, coughs, consumption and smallpox, while the inner bark was taken for chest pains and soreness. This bark contains several flavonoids, including narigenin.

OTHER USES: Crushed leaves or thin strips of bark will kill insects in an enclosed space. Cherry wood is very hard. Seasoned branches make excellent canes and walking sticks, and black cherry is used for furniture. Choke cherry wood has been used to make digging sticks, tent pegs and other tools. Bitter cherry and choke cherry wood was split into strips to ornament baskets and was used for making watertight baskets that resist decay. Black cherry has been used as rootstock for several varieties of cultivated plums in North America. Ripening choke cherry fruits signalled to the Okanagan-Colville that the spring salmon were coming up the river to spawn. Dried choke cherries were an important trade item for some indigenous peoples in Canada. The berries were used as a paint for painting pictographs by the Shuswap of BC.

DESCRIPTION: Deciduous shrubs or small trees, 1–25 m tall, with raised horizontal pores (lenticels) on reddish brown branches. Leaves 3–10 cm long, with 2 small glands near the stalk tip. Flowers white, about 1 cm across, 5-petalled, from May to June. Fruits fleshy drupes (cherries) with large stones (pits).

Bitter cherry (*P. emarginata*) grows to 15 m tall, with blunt-tipped, blunt-toothed leaves and red to dark purple cherries, 8–12 mm long. Grows in moist, sparsely wooded areas along streams or cleared areas in BC.

Pin cherry (*P. pensylvanica*) grows to 10 m tall, with slender-pointed, sharp-toothed leaves and bright red cherries, 4–8 mm long. Grows in moist, forested areas, clearings and burned areas in all provinces and NT. See p. 424 for conservation status.

Sand cherry (*P. pumila*) is a low, slender shrub, to 1 m tall, with fine-toothed, lance-shaped leaves and dark purple fruit, 13–15 mm long. Grows in sandy spots (dunes, beaches) and open areas in calcareous soils from southern SK to NL.

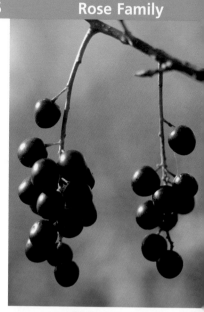

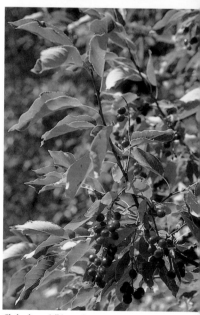

Choke cherry (all images)

Black cherry (*P. serotina*) is a medium-sized tree, to 25 m tall, with sharp-pointed, lance-shaped leaves with elongated, incurved teeth and a narrow mat of hair on either side of the midvein. Fruits dark purple or black, 8–10 mm across. Grows in dry, open areas and open forests from ON to the Maritimes and is introduced in BC (around Vancouver).

Choke cherry (*P. virginiana*) grows to 8 m tall, with broadly oval leaves with a sharp tip and red to crimson to black fruits, 8–12 mm across. Grows along fencerows, streams and forest edges in all provinces and NT.

Plums

Prunus spp.

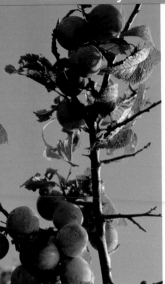

FOOD: The fruits of both plums described here are edible, though a bit tougher and not as sweet as commercially cultivated plums. They can be dried or cooked, sweetened and made into preserves (but see **Warning**). The Iroquois boiled the sun-dried fruits of American plum to make a sort of coffee. Dried American plum fruit cakes would be soaked in warm water, cooked as a sauce and mixed with corn bread.

MEDICINE: An infusion of the inner bark of Canada plum has been used to treat colds and unsettled stomachs. The scraped inner bark of American plum has been used as a tea to treat mouth sores, as a wash to treat skin disorders and as a poultice to treat cuts (antiseptic). An infusion of the bark of American plum has been employed to treat diarrhea and disorders of the kidney and bladder.

American plum (all images)

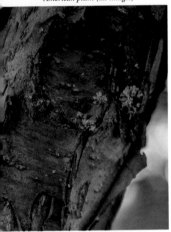

OTHER USES: Both species are used for dyeing. The leaves yield a green dye, the fruits a grey to green dye and the roots (of American plum at least) a red dye. American plum is commonly used as a rootstock for commercially cultivated plums.

DESCRIPTION: Deciduous tall shrubs or small trees, 2–10 m tall, often in thickets. The stems and branches bear raised, horizontal pores (lenticels). Leaves alternate, simple, oval to elliptic, 7–10 cm long, the margins toothed. Flowers white to pink, fragrant, in bundles, and bloom from April to May, often before the leaves. Fruits yellow or red drupes (plums), 2–3 cm long, and contain a compressed seed (pit).

American plum (*P. americana*) has young leaves with sharp, glandless teeth, leaf stalks mostly without apical glands and petals that remain white as they age. Grows in thickets and forest edges from southern SK to southwestern QC. See p. 424 for conservation status.

Canada plum (*P. nigra*) has young leaves with rounded, glandular teeth, leaf stalks with 2 apical glands and petals that are white but become pinkish with age. Grows on forest edges and in thickets from southeastern MB to NB and NS.

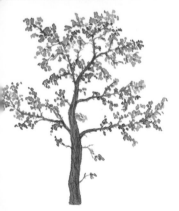

> **WARNING**
> Plum leaves, bark, wood and seeds (stones) contain hydrocyanic acid and so can cause cyanide poisoning. The flesh of the plum is the only edible part. The stone should always be discarded. Plum leaves and twigs are poisonous to browsing animals.

Indian-Plum

Oemleria cerasiformis

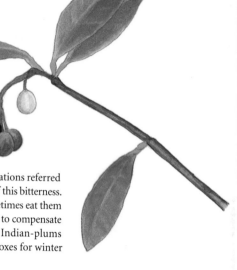

FOOD: The berries of Indian-plum were eaten in small quantities by some indigenous peoples in BC. They were eaten fresh, dried or cooked, typically at family meals or at large feasts, and stored over winter. The smashed fruit can be made into bread. The fruits are very bitter before they become fully ripe. Some First Nations referred to Indian-plum as "choke cherry" because of this bitterness. Those unfamiliar with the fruits would sometimes eat them with large quantities of oil (but never water) to compensate for their dryness and puckering potential. Indian-plums were covered with oil and stored in cedar boxes for winter eating.

MEDICINE: The wood of the Indian-plum was used for medicinal purposes. The twigs were applied to "sore places" after being chewed or burned and mixed with fish oil. A tea made from the bark was taken as a purgative and tonic; it has mild laxative effects. The bark was also taken to treat tuberculosis and used as a healing agent.

OTHER USES: The species name, *cerasiformis*, means "cherry-like." Another common name for Indian-plum is oso-berry; "oso" means "bear," and bears are known to eat these berries. Ground squirrels and other rodents, birds, deer, foxes and coyotes also eat the berries. The flowers are an early nectar source for bees and other insects.

DESCRIPTION: Deciduous shrub or small tree, 1.5–5 m tall, with purplish brown bark. Leaves alternate, the blades 5–12 cm long, lance-shaped to oblong, smell like cucumber or watermelon rind when crushed, light green and smooth above, paler below. Flowers greenish white, 1 cm across, male and female flowers on separate plants, often appear before leaves, in clusters hanging from leaf axils, strong smelling (male flowers are said to smell like cat urine while female flowers smell like cucumber or watermelon rind), blooming from April to May. Fruit a fleshy drupe about 1 cm long, peach-coloured when unripe, bluish black when ripe, with a large pit, borne on a red stem. Found in dry to moist, open woods, along rivers and streambanks and clearings in southwestern BC.

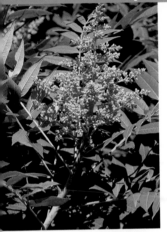

Sumacs
Rhus spp.

FOOD: Sumac's showy, red fruit clusters can be made into a refreshing pink or rose-coloured drink with a lemon-like flavour. The crushed berries can be soaked in cold water and then strained to remove the hairs and other debris. The juice is best sweetened with sugar and served cold. Boiling fruit in hot water releases tannins and produces a bitter-tasting liquid. The fruits have also been used to make jellies or "lemon" pies. When chewed as a trail nibble, sumac fruits relieve thirst and leave a pleasant taste in the mouth.

Smooth sumac (above)
Staghorn sumac (all below)

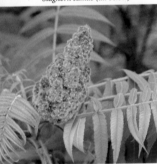

MEDICINE: The fruits were boiled to make a wash to stop bleeding after childbirth. The root tea was taken to treat fluid retention and painful urination. Roots were also chewed and the juice swallowed to soothe sore throats. Root bark was used in poultices for healing ulcers and open wounds. Sumac branches were used to make medicinal teas for treating tuberculosis, and the bark, steeped in hot water, produced an astringent tea that was applied to skin problems, gargled to relieve sore mouths and taken internally to relieve diarrhea, dysentery, gonorrhea and syphilis. The bruised, moistened leaves were applied to rashes and to skin reactions associated with plant irritants such as poison-ivy (p. 395). The berries, steeped in hot water, made a medicinal tea for treating diabetes, bowel problems and fevers. This tea was also used as a wash for ringworm, ulcers and skin diseases such as eczema.

OTHER USES: The leaves, bark and roots yield a yellow-tan, grey or black dye, depending on the part used and the mordant. The red autumn leaves were sometimes rolled and smoked.

DESCRIPTION: Deciduous shrub or small tree, 1–6 m tall, usually forming thickets. Branches exude milky juice when broken. Leaves pinnately divided into 11–31 lance-shaped, 5–12 cm long, toothed leaflets, bright red in autumn. Flowers cream-coloured to greenish yellow, about 3 mm across, with 5 fuzzy petals, forming dense, pyramid-shaped, 10–25 cm long clusters, from May to July. Fruits reddish, densely hairy, berry-like drupes, 4–5 mm long, in persistent, fuzzy clusters. Fruits mature July to August and may remain through winter.

Smooth sumac (*R. glabra*) grows 1–3 m tall with hairless twigs and leaves; buds with whitish hairs. Grows on dry forest openings, prairies, fencerows, roadsides and burned areas from southern BC to southwestern QC (except in AB). See p. 424 for conservation status.

Staghorn sumac (*R. typhina*) grows to 6 m tall with flat-topped crowns. Branches have velvety hair; leaflets have hairy, reddish central stalks; buds densely hairy. Colonizes open, sandy or rocky areas from southern ON to the Maritimes. See p. 424 for conservation status.

WARNING
People who are hypersensitive to the poisonous members of this genus (e.g., poison-ivy, p. 395) may also be allergic to these "safe" sumacs.

Skunkbush

Rhus trilobata

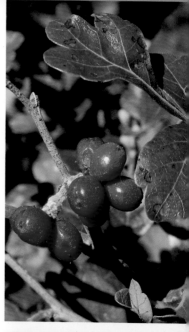

FOOD: Skunkbush fruits were eaten raw (sometimes ground with a little water) or boiled, or they were dried and ground into meal. The berries and meal were often mixed with other foods, especially sugar and roasted corn. Skunkbush berries can be crushed, soaked in cold water and strained to make a pink lemonade-like drink. Soaking in hot water produces a bitter-tasting liquid. The inner bark was also eaten.

MEDICINE: The leaves were chewed to cure stomachaches or boiled to make a contraceptive tea that was said to induce impotence. Skunkbush leaves were also used in poultices to relieve itching. Tea made by boiling the root bark was taken to aid delivery of the afterbirth. The fruits were boiled and their oil, skimmed from the surface, was used to prevent hair loss.

OTHER USES: Skunkbush branches were split lengthwise (usually 3 times) and woven into baskets and water bottles. Sun shades or hats were woven from the smaller branches, but they were for adults only. It was said that if children placed skunkbush on their heads, they would stop growing. Large stems (about 2 m long) were used to make bows or spear shafts tipped with points made of harder wood or iron. Twigs from the east side of the shrub were woven into the form of an owl, which was hung on the west side of the tepee smoke hole. The owl, moving up and down in the smoke, was used to scare children and make them behave. Making an owl was a sure sign that it would rain. The leaves were boiled to produce a black dye for baskets, leather and wool, and the ashes were used to set dyes.

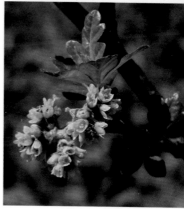

DESCRIPTION: Strong-smelling, 1–2 m tall shrub with bright green leaves divided into 3 broad-tipped, lobed leaflets that taper to wedge-shaped bases. Flowers yellowish green, about 3 mm across, with 5 fuzzy petals, forming close clusters of spikes near the branch tips, from May to July, before the leaves appear. Fruits sticky, fuzzy, reddish orange, berry-like drupes, 6–8 mm long, in small, fuzzy clusters, from June to October. Grows along streams and in open areas in prairies, shrublands and foothills in southern AB and SK. See p. 424 for conservation status.

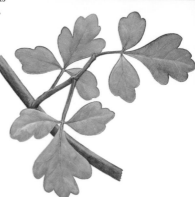

> **WARNING**
>
> People who are hypersensitive to the poisonous members of this genus (e.g., poison-ivy, p. 395) may also be allergic to this "safe" sumac.

Devil's Club
Oplopanax horridus

FOOD: Roots and young, fleshy stems were cooked and eaten (see **Warning**). Young leaves, collected before the spines stiffen, may be eaten raw or cooked in soups and casseroles.

MEDICINE: Throughout its range, devil's club is considered to be one of the most powerful and important of all medicinal plants. The root tea has been reported to stimulate the respiratory tract and to help bring up phlegm when treating colds, bronchitis and pneumonia. It has also been used to treat diabetes because it helps regulate blood sugar levels and reduce the craving for sugar. Although this tea is recommended for binge-eaters who are trying to lose weight, some tribes used it to improve appetite and to help people gain weight. In fact, it was said that a patient could gain too much weight if it was used for too long. Devil's club extracts have lowered blood sugar levels in laboratory animals. Crushed, fresh stems were steeped in hot water to make teas for relieving indigestion and constipation, or they were boiled to make a blood purifier, tonic and laxative. A strong decoction induced vomiting in purifying rituals preceding important events such as hunting or war expeditions. This decoction was also applied to wounds to combat *staphylococcus* infections, and ashes from burned stems were sometimes mixed with grease to make salves for healing swellings and weeping sores. Like many members of the Ginseng family, devil's club contains glycosides that are said to reduce metabolic stress and thus improve one's sense of well-being.

OTHER USES: The light-coloured wood was widely used for carving fishing hooks and lures. Possibly because of its diabolical spines, devil's club was considered a highly powerful plant that could protect one from evil influences of many kinds. Devil's club sticks were used as protective charms, and charcoal from burned devil's club was used to make a protective face paint for dancers and others who were ritually vulnerable to evil influences. The aromatic roots were smoked with tobacco (p. 240), and the dried, powdered bark was ground to make sweet-smelling baby powder and deodorant. Devil's club berries were rubbed into hair to combat dandruff and lice and to add shine.

DESCRIPTION: Strong-smelling, deciduous shrub, 1–3 m tall, with spiny, erect or sprawling stems. Leaves broadly maple-like, 10–40 cm wide, with prickly ribs and long, bristly stalks. Flowers greenish white, 5–6 mm long, 5-petalled, forming 10–25 cm long, pyramid-shaped clusters, from May to July. Fruits bright red, berry-like drupes, 5–8 mm long, in showy clusters. Grows in moist, shady foothill and montane sites in YT, BC, AB and ON (Porphyry and Slate Islands). See p. 424 for conservation status.

WARNING
Devil's club spines break off easily and often cause infections. Some people have an allergic reaction to their scratches.

Blackberries

Rubus spp.

Blackberries and relatives (raspberries, salmonberry, thimbleberry and cloudberry, p. 94) are all closely related members of the genus *Rubus*. The best way to distinguish blackberries from raspberries is by looking at their fruits: if they are hollow, they are raspberries, and if they have a solid core, they are blackberries.

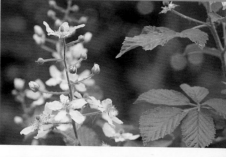

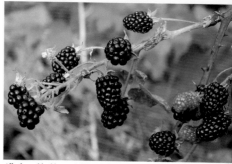

Allegheny blackberry (all images)

FOOD: Blackberries were traditionally gathered by indigenous peoples in Canada and are still enjoyed today. They were typically gathered in large quantities and both eaten fresh and stored (usually dried) for winter. Common, traditional methods of eating the berries were to combine them with other berries or with oil (sometimes whipped) and meat. Blackberries today are enjoyed on their own, with cream and sugar, in pies and sauces, as jam or jelly or as blackberry wine. Blackberries and raspberries are widely cultivated across Canada for their delicious fruits. Blackberry-raspberry crosses (such as loganberries and boysenberries) are also popular.

MEDICINE: Blackberry leaf tea is very popular today has been used to treat sore throats, diarrhea, dysentery, cholera, excessive menstruation, fevers, hemorrhoids and sores in the mouth. The leaves were added to bitter medicine to make the medicine sweeter.

OTHER USES: Some Coast Salish First Nations on BC's south coast have an origin myth for trailing blackberry. A woman was chased up a tree by a jealous husband. The blood of the woman fell from the tree and became blackberries. A purification rite of the same First Nation involved scrubbing trailing blackberry stems across a person's body before spirit dancing.

DESCRIPTION: Prickly, perennial shrubs, 50 cm–5 m tall. Leaves alternate, compound. Flowers white, ripening from June to July. Fruits juicy, black drupelets aggregated into clusters that fall from the shrub with the fleshy receptacle (i.e., the blackberries have a solid core).

Allegheny blackberry (*R. allegheniensis*) is a medium to large, erect shrub, to 3 m tall. Stems and leaves glandular-hairy; deciduous leaves usually have 5 leaflets arranged palmately (like the fingers on a hand). Found in dry thickets, clearings and woodland margins from southern ON to the Maritimes, and introduced in BC's lower Fraser Valley.

Himalayan blackberry (*R. armeniacus*) is a large shrub, to 5 m tall, similar to Allegheny blackberry, but its leaves are evergreen, and its leaves and stems lack glandular hairs. This introduced European species grows in open, disturbed sites in southwestern BC.

> **WARNING**
> Wilted leaves can be toxic. Only fresh or completely dried leaves should be used to make tea, but even then the tea should be taken in moderation because extended use can irritate the stomach and bowels.

Trailing blackberry (*R. ursinus*) is a trailing shrub, less than 50 cm tall but 5 m or more long, with 3 deciduous leaflets. Found in thickets, dry, open forests and disturbed sites in southwestern BC.

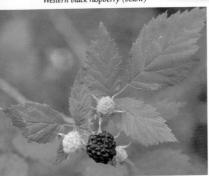

Raspberries, Salmonberry, Thimbleberry & Cloudberry

Rubus spp.

Wild red raspberry (above)
Western black raspberry (below)

Raspberries and relatives (salmonberry, thimbleberry and cloudberry) are all closely related members of the genus *Rubus*. The best way to distinguish these berries from blackberries is by looking at their fruits: if they are are hollow, they are raspberries (or relatives), and if they have a solid core, they are blackberries.

FOOD: Wild raspberries are popular fresh from the branch or added to pies, cakes, puddings, cobblers, jams, jellies, juices and wines. Because the cupped fruit clusters drop from the receptacle when ripe, they are soft and easily crushed. Tender, young shoots, peeled of their bristly outer layer, are edible raw or cooked. Fresh or dried leaves have been used to make tea (see **Warning**), and the flowers can make a pretty addition to salads. Red raspberries were a popular and valuable food of indigenous peoples across Canada. They were often gathered in enough quantities for winter storage. The berries were sometimes crushed to make a juice. Cloudberry was historically and is presently a principal food for northern indigenous peoples; these juicy berries have twice the concentration of vitamin C as an orange. They are typically stored in seal pokes, wooden barrels or underground caches in cold water or oil, with other berries or with edible greens. Black raspberries were important fruits for indigenous peoples. The young shoots of black raspberries were also eaten raw or cooked. Thimbleberry was a berry valued by some indigenous peoples in BC and was eaten fresh or gathered and stored for winter use. The young shoots of thimbleberry were also enjoyed as an edible green. Salmonberry fruits and shoots were popular foods for coastal indigenous peoples in BC. They were almost always eaten fresh, sometimes at feasts, because they do not preserve well. The shoots are peeled and eaten raw, steamed or boiled.

MEDICINE: Raspberry leaf tea has traditionally been given to women before, during and after childbirth to prevent miscarriage, reduce labour pains and increase milk flow. It has also been used to slow excessive menstrual flow. Raspberry leaf contains fragarine, a compound that acts both as a relaxant and a stimulant on the muscles of the uterus. Unfortunately, studies on the effectiveness of raspberry leaves for treating "female problems" have often proved inconclusive or contradictory.

WARNING
Wilted leaves can be toxic. Only fresh or completely dried leaves should be used to make tea, but even then the tea should be taken in moderation because extended use can irritate the stomach and bowels.

Raspberry leaf tea and raspberry juice boiled with sugar have been gargled to treat mouth and throat inflammations.

OTHER USES: The large, maple-like leaves of thimbleberry served many purposes for some indigenous peoples in BC. They were used to whip soapberries (p. 129), wipe the slime from fish, line and cover berry baskets and dry other kinds of berries. Swainson's thrush is often called the salmonberry bird because it is associated with ripening salmonberry in northwest coast native mythology.

DESCRIPTION: Armed or unarmed, perennial shrubs or herbs, 15 cm–4 m tall. Leaves deciduous, lobed or compound (divided into leaflets). Flowers white or pink, from June to July. Fruits juicy druplets aggregated into clusters that fall from the shrub without the fleshy receptacle (the raspberries and relatives have a hollow core).

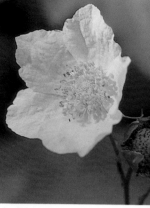

Thimbleberry (all images)

Arctic dwarf raspberry or **nagoonberry** (*R. arcticus*) is a low, herbaceous plant (sometimes a bit woody at the base), to 15 cm tall, with typically 3 leaflets, no prickles or bristles, pink to reddish flowers, and deep red to dark purple fruits. Found in bogs, wet meadows and tundra across Canada.

Cloudberry or **bakeapple** (*R. chamaemorus*) is a low, unbranched herb, to 30 cm tall, with 1–3 leaves per stem. Leaves round to kidney-shaped (not divided into leaflets), shallowly 5- to 7-lobed, no prickles or bristles. Flowers single, white at end of stem, the male and female flowers on different plants. Fruit amber to yellow when mature. Found in peat bogs and peaty forests across Canada. See p. 424 for conservation status.

Wild red raspberry (*R. idaeus*) is an erect shrub, to 2 m tall, with red fruit and slender prickles often as gland-tipped hairs. Grows in thickets, open woods, fields and on rocky hillsides across Canada.

Eastern black raspberry (*R. occidentalis*) has long, arching branches to 2 m tall, prickles, no bristles, and is covered with waxy coating. Flowers borne singly or in small clusters. Fruits reddish purple to black. Found in thickets, ravines and open woods in ON, QC and NB. See p. 424 for conservation status.

Western black raspberry (*R. leucodermis*) is very similar to eastern black raspberry, but this western species has glaucous-grey stems (vs. glaucous-purple in *R. occidentalis*) and is generally pricklier, with prickles on leaf stalks stout, broad-based and usually hooked (vs. narrow and straight in eastern black raspberry). Found in the same habitats as eastern black raspberry, in southern BC.

Thimbleberry (*R. parviflorus*) is an erect shrub, to 2.5 m tall, with no prickles or spines. Leaves large, maple-like, 5-lobed, toothed around margins, fine hairs above and below; flowers white, in clusters of 2–7; fruit shallow-cupped, bright red. Found in open sites and open forests in BC and southwestern AB, and also in southern ON.

Trailing wild raspberry or **five-leaved bramble** (*R. pedatus*) is a trailing herb from long, creeping stolons, usually less than 10 cm tall, with 5 coarsely toothed leaflets, no prickles or bristles, white flowers and red fruits. Found in bog forests, streambanks and moist, mossy forests in YT, BC and southwestern AB. See p. 424 for conservation status.

Trailing raspberry or **dewberry** (*R. pubescens*) is a trailing, soft-hairy shrub, to 50 cm tall but often more than 1 m long, with 3 leaflets, white flowers, dark red fruits and no thorns or prickles. Found on damp slopes, rocky shores and low thickets across Canada, except YT. See p. 424 for conservation status.

Salmonberry (*R. spectabilis*) is a robust, erect shrub, to 4 m tall, with reddish brown to yellowish, shredding bark. Salmonberry leaves have 3 leaflets. Magnificent rosy red to reddish purple flowers and large, raspberry-like fruits, from gold to ruby red to purplish black. Found in moist to wet forests, swampy areas and streambanks in coastal BC.

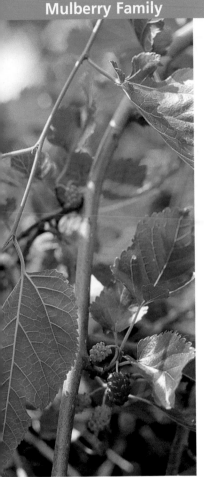

Mulberries

Morus spp.

FOOD: Juicy mulberries are an explosion of dark, fruity taste somewhat like a mix of perfectly ripe blackberry and blackcurrant. The berries are notorious for creating hard to remove stains on clothing and pavement, but the taste of the fruit is *well* worth the possible trouble! The Iroquois and Huron peoples enjoyed the berries of red mulberry fresh or preserved, but recognized that the unripe berries and milky sap were toxic and may also be irritating to the skin.

MEDICINE: White mulberry has a long history of medicinal use in China, where the leaves are considered to have antibacterial, astringent, hypoglycemic and ophthalmic properties. Leaves are gathered in autumn after the first frost and are used either fresh or dried. The stems are gathered in late spring or early summer and are used as a diuretic and to treat rheumatism.

OTHER USES: The leaves of white mulberry are the main source of food for silkworms in eastern Asia. The milky juice is rich in rubber-like compounds said to add tenacity to the silk fibres spun by the worms. The white mulberry has been cultivated for thousands of years in China as part of the silk industry, where the trees are pollarded (cut back to the trunk) to stimulate a dense head of leafy shoots to feed the silkworms. As long ago as the 3rd century BC, Chinese silk caught the eye of the Romans, who encountered it on the "silk roads" over which Chinese goods were traded to the west. In later centuries, various forces (e.g., Arab conquerors in Persia, Crusaders and Marco Polo's journeys to China) facilitated the

White mulberry (all images)

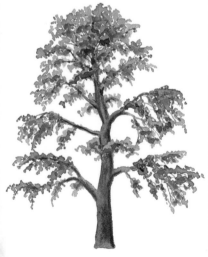

WARNING

Red mulberry is endangered in Canada and is the only mulberry native to this country. Unfortunately, red mulberry frequently hybridizes with its European cousin, white mulberry, and this genetic alteration is probably its single greatest threat. Hybrids are often difficult to identify. Some people develop skin reactions from contact with mulberry leaves, sap and branches. Unripe mulberry fruits can cause stomach upset and are considered poisonous.

growth of a silk industry in European countries such as Italy, France and Germany. Silk production flourished there for several hundred years, until WWII interrupted the flow of raw silk from Japan and effectively ended silk-making in Europe. White mulberry shrubs, along with silkworms, were brought to North America in the 1800s in an attempt to establish a western silk industry. This ambitious undertaking soon failed, but since then, these hardy trees have thrived and spread across southern ON. Mulberry is an attractive, fast-growing species that is planted as an ornamental or fruit tree, but it requires sufficient space to accommodate its spreading branches. Female trees attract many birds and small mammals to parks and yards and are planted to lure birds away from other fruit. Mulberry wood is very durable and has been used in ornamental carving and for making fences, barrels and boats.

DESCRIPTION: Deciduous shrubs or small trees, 10–20 m tall, with milky sap. Leaves alternate, simple, oval to heart-shaped, 10–15 cm long, yellow in autumn. Flowers tiny, green; male and female flowers in separate clusters. Male clusters loose and elongated; female clusters short, dense and cylindrical; appear in early spring. Fruits rounded, blackberry-like; clusters (multiple fruits) 1–3 cm long, composed of tiny, seed-like fruits (achenes), each surrounded by a small, juicy segment; mature June to July.

White mulberry (*M. alba*) has hairless leaves (or leaves with tufts of hairs underneath) and white, reddish or purplish to blackish fruits. Native to China, but naturalized in open, disturbed sites, along fences and near the edges of forests and in planted gardens in southern ON and BC.

Red mulberry (*M. rubra*) has leaves hairy beneath and fruits red to dark purple or almost black. Native to southern ON, where it grows in moist, rich forests and floodplains. See p. 424 for conservation status.

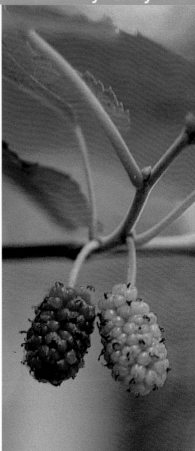

Red mulberry (all images)

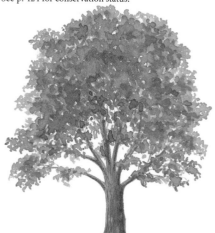

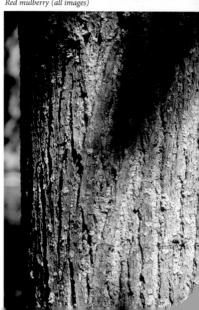

Barberries
Berberis spp.

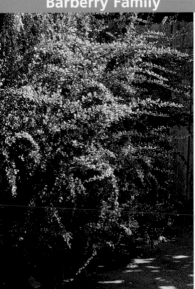

Japanese barberry

FOOD: These dense, viciously thorny shrubs provide edible and medicinal benefits that have a long history of use. Barberry fruits are acceptable raw in small quantities, but they are very acidic and instead make rather excellent preserves or jellies. In Iran, dried *Berberis* berries, called *zereshk*, are widely used and impart a tart flavour to chicken and rice dishes. A popular candy in the Ukraine of the same name is also made from the berries. A rich source of vitamin C and the soluble fibre pectin, barberry makes a refreshing lemonade-like cold beverage when sweetened. The leaves make a fine trailside nibble eaten raw, or they can be used as a flavouring agent.

MEDICINE: Used traditionally by First Nations to improve appetite and treat general debility, barberry contains a number of well-studied alkaloids, especially berberine, which has displayed a wide array of biological activities. Berberine is a good antimicrobial and possesses anti-inflammatory, astringent, hemostatic, anticonvulsant, immunostimulant, uterotonic, antitumour and hypotensive activity. It has been tested for its potential usefulness in treating diabetes, prostate cancer, cardiac arrhythmia and leukemia, although not enough research has been conducted in humans. The alkaloid stimulates bile and bilirubin secretion and has the ability to correct high tyramine levels in patients with liver cirrhosis. By itself, berberine is a relatively weak antibiotic. An extract that contains barberry's other components, such as the isoquinoline alkaloids berbamine and oxyacanthine, displays significantly stronger antibacterial activity, as well as effects against amoebas and trypanosomes. These alkaloids are poorly absorbed through the digestive tract, so they are particularly useful against enteric infections, such as bacterial dysentery, and parasite infections. In this regard, herbalists do not recommend that wild licorice (p. 260) be consumed at the same time because it is surmised that it nullifies the effects of barberry.

Despite these pharmacological properties, barberry and its alkaloids are not currently widely used. Even the crude plant material in bitter tonics is not as popular today as it once was. The clinical use of purified berberine today is mainly to counteract bacterial diarrhea, and in eye drops to treat ocular trachoma infection, hypersensitive eyes, inflamed eyelids and conjunctivitis. Berberine is found predominantly in the roots and can be poisonous if taken in large doses (see **Warning**). In low doses, a tea of the roots was used as a bitter tonic and as a treatment for ulcers, heartburn and stomach problems. Large doses were taken only to induce severe vomiting or purging. A milder laxative can be made from an infusion of the berries mixed with wine. A decoction of the berries or root bark makes an effective mouthwash or

> **WARNING**
> Berberine reportedly interferes with normal liver function in infants and should not be consumed during pregnancy and breast-feeding. Strong barberry preparations may cause intestinal discomfort. Adverse reactions can result from herb-drug interactions with the antibiotic tetracycline.

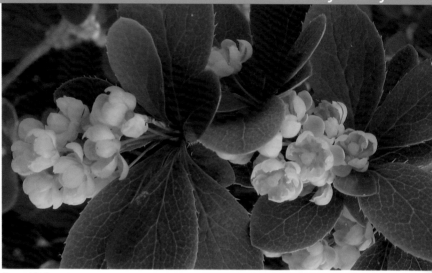

Common barberry

gargle for mouth and throat complaints. Fresh berry juice was thought to strengthen the gums and relieve pyorrhea when brushed directly on them. A tea made from the root bark promotes sweating and was used traditionally to treat jaundice, hepatitis, gallbladder pain, gallstones, fevers, hemorrhage, diarrhea and as a tincture for arthritis, rheumatism and sciatica. A tea from the leaves was used for coughs.

OTHER USES: The roots, bark and stems provide a good quality yellow dye popularly used to stain baskets, cloth and wood. The stem wood is very hard and fine grained, used to make carvings, toothpicks, mosaics and other crafts. The shrubs are sometimes planted as hedges and as barriers under vulnerable windows to deter trespassers. They tolerate trimming but cannot tolerate extreme maritime exposure. A dwarf cultivar of Japanese barberry called 'Atropurpurea nana' grows into dense groundcover if planted 30 cm apart. Barberry is the intermediate host for wheat rust and was the focus of an extensive eradication effort that lasted from 1918 to 1975. Although more than 100 million barberry bushes were destroyed in the program, the plant is making a comeback in the wild.

DESCRIPTION: Perennial, deciduous shrubs, to 3 m tall, with dimorphic shoots. Long shoots erect, branched or unbranched, with simple or 3-spined thorns 3–30 mm long. In the thorn axils are short shoots that produce leaves to 10 cm long, margins entire or spiny. Flowers produced in clusters of up to 20 per head, yellow to orange, 3–6 mm long, with 6 petals and sepals. Fruit a small berry, ripening to red or dark blue, usually long and narrow, resembling a bar (hence the name barberry).

American barberry (*B. canadensis*), 40 cm–2 m tall, has purple or brown branches, widely toothed leaves (16–20 teeth per side) to 7.5 cm long, 3-pronged thorns and yellow flowers with notched petals in few-flowered clusters (3–15 flowers), from April to May. Berries red, oblong, to 1 cm long. Grows in woods or glades near rivers and on rocky slopes in southern ON.

Japanese barberry (*B. thunbergii*), 30 cm–3 m tall, has purple or brown glabrous stems with untoothed leaves to 2.5 cm long, usually simple thorns with solitary or small clusters (1–5) of flowers in its axils, from March to May. Berries red, elliptical or round, to 1 cm long. This introduced species grows in open places (woodlands, fields, roadsides) from southern ON to the Maritimes.

Common barberry (*B. vulgaris*), 90 cm–3 m tall, has grey branches. Leaves 2.5–7.5 cm long and bristle-toothed. Pendulous clusters of 10–20 small, yellow flowers and leaves with 16–20 teeth per side. Flowers from May to June. Fruits elliptical and scarlet when mature. This introduced Eurasian species is widely naturalized in disturbed spaces (pastures, roadside thickets) in southern BC, MB and ON to NS.

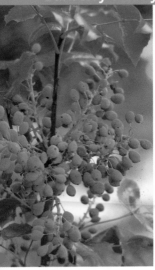

Oregon-Grapes
Berberis spp.

The western Canadian Oregon-grapes are close relatives of the eastern Canadian barberries (p. 98), but their leaves are evergreen and compound (vs. deciduous and simple in barberries), and their stems are never spiny.

FOOD: These tart, juicy berries have been eaten raw or used to make jelly, jam or wine. Mashed with sugar and served with milk, they make a tasty dessert. A refreshing drink was made with mashed berries, sugar and water. The sweetened juice tastes much like grape juice. Berry production can vary greatly from year to year, and the fruits are sometimes rendered inedible by grub infestations. Very young leaves have been used as a trail nibble or salad vegetable, and the young leaves of tall Oregon-grape were sometimes simmered until tender.

Tall Oregon-grape

MEDICINE: The plants contain the alkaloids berberine, berbamine, isocorydin and oxyacanthine, which stimulate involuntary muscles. Root tea was used to aid in delivery of afterbirth and to relieve constipation. It was also taken as cough medicine, though the stimulative effects would seem more likely to increase, rather than reduce, coughing. The crushed plants and roots have antioxidant, antiseptic and antibacterial properties. They were used to make medicinal teas, poultices and powders for treating gonorrhea and syphilis and for healing wounds and scorpion stings. The leaf tea was used as a tonic and/or contraceptive and as a treatment for kidney troubles, stomach troubles, diarrhea, dysentery, rheumatism, skin problems such as psoriasis and eczema, and persistent problems of the uterus.

OTHER USES: Boiled, shredded root bark produces a brilliant yellow dye. Tall Oregon-grape is often planted as an ornamental.

DESCRIPTION: Perennial, evergreen shrubs, to 3 m tall, with leathery, holly-like leaves pinnately divided into spiny-edged leaflets, red or purple in winter. Flowers yellow, about 1 cm across, forming elongated clusters, from April to June. Fruits juicy, grape-like berries, about 1 cm long, purplish blue with a whitish bloom.

Tall Oregon-grape (*B. aquifolium*) is 50 cm–3 m tall, with 5–11 leaflets that are shiny above and not whitened beneath. Grows in dry forests at low to montane elevations in southern BC.

Dull Oregon-grape (*B. nervosa*) is 10–80 cm tall, with 9–19 dull (not shiny) leaflets. Grows in moist to dry forests and open slopes at low to montane elevations in southwestern BC.

Creeping Oregon-grape (*B. repens*) is 10–20 cm tall, with 3–7 dull leaflets that are bluish green (at least on the lower surface). Grows in open forests, shrublands and grasslands at low to montane elevations in southern BC and AB. See p. 424 for conservation status.

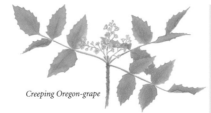

Creeping Oregon-grape

WARNING
High doses of Oregon-grape can cause nosebleeds, skin and eye irritation, shortness of breath, sluggishness, diarrhea, vomiting, kidney inflammation and even death. Pregnant women should not use this plant because it may stimulate the uterus.

Common Pawpaw
Asimina triloba

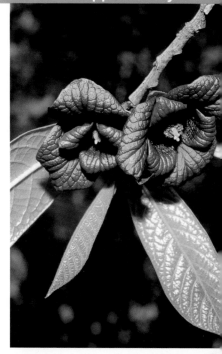

FOOD: The fruit is edible and tastes somewhat like a papaya. It is the largest edible fruit native to North America and contains a high amount of amino acids. Traditionally, it was mashed and made into small cakes, eaten raw, cooked into sauces or dried for storage.

MEDICINE: The seeds, bark and leaves were traditionally applied directly to abscesses. Twigs, leaves and seeds contain insecticidal compounds, and powdered seeds were used to treat head lice. The fruit has laxative qualities. The main active ingredients are acetogenins, which are mitochondrial inhibitors under development as insecticides and anticancer agents. Pawpaw extractives have been used commercially as dietary supplements and lice treatments in the US market.

OTHER USES: The inner bark was made into cordage by twisting it into string and strong rope.

DESCRIPTION: Perennial shrub or small tree, to 12 m tall, with drooping, pear-shaped, alternate leaves 10–30 cm long that smell like bell peppers when crushed. Leaves have a pointed tip and smooth margins, and are coated with fine hairs: white hairs on the upper surface and reddish hairs on the underside. Green flowers have 3 sepals that turn dark purple and 6 petals that curl backward. Large (7–16 cm long), yellowish green or brown, mango-shaped fruit. Grows in moist forests and streamsides in southern ON. See p. 424 for conservation status.

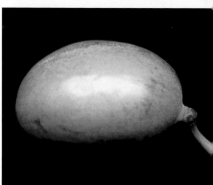

WARNING
The seeds are toxic, emetic and have narcotic properties. The acetogenin compounds found in the seeds, leaves and bark, which are responsible for the insecticidal and anti-tumour properties of pawpaw, may have irritant or toxic properties at high doses.

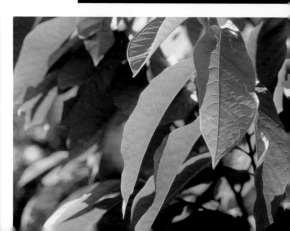

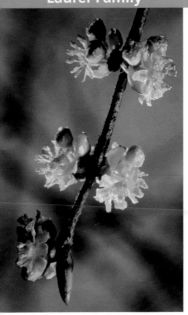

Spicebush
Lindera benzoin

FOOD: Both twigs and branches of the spicebush plant were used to make beverage teas and to season cooking meat and other foods by indigenous peoples living in southwestern ON. The young leaves, twigs and fruit all contain an aromatic essential oil, which is how it was given the common name spicebush. The fruit, dried and powdered, has been used as a substitute for allspice.

MEDICINE: Spicebush was often used by indigenous peoples in both Canada and the United States, most commonly to treat colds and fevers and as a general tonic. A decoction or infusion of stripped leaves and twigs was taken for colds and measles. A compound decoction of plants was used as a steam bath for cold sweats. Roots processed into a compound decoction were ingested as a cure-all and to treat gonorrhea and syphilis. A compound poultice of the bark was applied to lumps that remain after having syphilis. The bark has been used to treat coughs, colds, dysentery and intestinal parasites. The oil from the fruits was a remedy for bruises, rheumatism and intestinal gas. In addition to indigenous use, the twigs of spicebush have been a common household remedy for colds, fevers, worms and colic. Valued for its ability to induce perspiration, it was once widely used for typhoid and other fevers.

OTHER USES: The leaves of spicebush can be used as insect repellent and disinfectant, as they have a small amount of camphor. The oil from the leaves is said to smell like lavender. The fruit yields a spice-scented oil, and the twigs and bark produce an oil smelling of wintergreen.

DESCRIPTION: Deciduous shrub or small tree, to 5 m tall; bark brown to grey-brown. Young twigs slender, smooth or sparsely hairy, olive green to brown in colour, have a spicy peppery smell when broken. Leaves alternate, smooth or hairy, elliptical, 6–15 cm long, on stalks, strongly aromatic throughout the growing season. Flowers small, yellow, appearing in clusters before the leaves in spring (March to April). Fruit shiny, red "berry" with single seed, 10 mm long, peppery taste and scent, on short stalk, matures from August to November. Seeds dispersed by animals and birds. Found along streambanks, uplands, wet woods and margins of wetlands in southern ON.

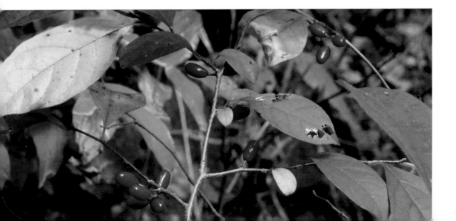

Sassafras
Sassafras albidum

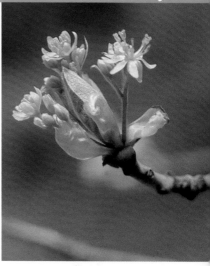

FOOD: The Iroquois nations in Canada and the United States used sassafras twigs as chewing sticks, the leaves as seasoning in meat soups and the bark and roots as a spice. Sassafras was also quite popular among all people as a tea using leaves, roots, and/or flowers. The leaves can be eaten raw (added to salads) or cooked; they have a mild, aromatic flavour. The young shoots have been used to make beer. The root has been prepared in a number of ways, such as brewing with maple syrup, to be used as a condiment, tea or flavouring. Sassafras root was one of the original ingredients of root beer; however, the essential oil is now banned as a food flavouring in America.

MEDICINE: Sassafras was widely used as a medicine by indigenous peoples and was especially valued for its tonic effects. Parts of the sassafras plant (roots, pith from new sprouts, bark) were often taken for blood ailments: for example, high blood pressure, to thin the blood, for nosebleeds, as a blood purifier, to treat watery blood or to "clear" the blood. A compound infusion of sassafras roots and whisky was taken for tapeworms and rheumatism, and the leaves were applied as a poultice for wounds, cuts and bruises. It was often used to treat female ailments such as painful menstruation, fevers after childbirth and colds in women. The roots were also applied to treat swellings on the shins and calves, and a wash was prepared from the whole plant to treat sore eyes or cataracts. As a folk medicine, sassafras tea made from root bark was renowned as a spring tonic and blood purifier; it was considered a household cure for gastrointestinal complaints, colds, kidney problems, rheumatism and skin eruptions. Sassafras root was occasionally used in commercial dental poultices.

OTHER USES: Sassafras oil has been applied externally to control lice and treat insect bites, but it can cause skin irritations. The oil has also been used in soaps, perfumery, toothpastes and soft drinks. A yellow dye can be derived from the wood and bark.

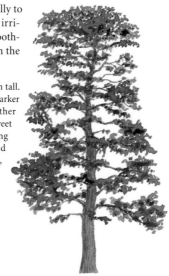

DESCRIPTION: Medium to large, deciduous tree, to 35 m tall. Bark dark red-brown, deeply furrowed. Twigs pale green with darker olive mottling. Leaf blade to 16 cm long, oval to elliptic, either unlobed or with 2–3 lobes. Flowers greenish yellow, fragrant (sweet lemony), to 5 cm across, borne in clusters, blooming in spring (April to May). Fruit develops in autumn, dark blue, 1-seeded "berry," 1 cm across, on a red stalk. Found in disturbed areas, forests, woodlands and old fields in southern ON.

WARNING
Safrole is a main component of sassafras oil (80 percent). In large doses, it can cause dilated pupils, vomiting and kidney and liver damage and is suspected of being carcinogenic and toxic to the liver as well as causing dermatitis.

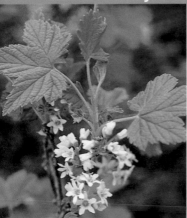

Northern black currant (above)
Golden currant (below)

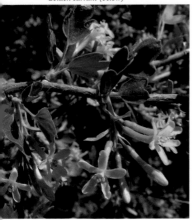

Currants

Ribes spp.

FOOD: Currants are common and widespread across Canada and were eaten by many First Nations, including the Haida, Blackfoot, Ojibwa (who cooked them with sweet corn) and probably the Micmac and Maliseet. Sticky currant berries were highly valued by the Haida and other northwest coast First Nations, who collected large quantities to eat fresh with grease or oil (some say this addition was to prevent constipation or stomach cramps). Currants have historically also been mixed with other berries and used to flavour liqueurs or fermented to make delicious wines. Raw currants tend to be very tart, but these common shrubs can provide a safe source of food in an emergency. Wax currants have been described as tasteless, bitter and similar to dried crab apples. Golden currant is one of the most flavourful currants. Some species, such as stink currant, have a skunky smell and flavour when raw but are delicious cooked. All are high in pectin and make excellent jams and jellies that are delicious with meat, fish, bannock or toast. Some tribes ate *Ribes* flowers as a nibble or cooked the young leaves and ate them with raw fat. For more information on closely-related species, see gooseberries (p. 106) and prickly currants (p. 108).

MEDICINE: Some tribes ate wax currants as a strengthening tonic and used them to treat diarrhea. In northern Canada, currants were taken to prevent heart disease. A medicinal tea was sometimes made by boiling the roots and used to treat kidney problems. In Europe, currant juice is taken as a natural remedy for arthritic pain. For more information, see gooseberries. Black currant seeds contain gamma-linoleic acid, a fatty acid that has been used in the treatment of migraine headaches, menstrual problems, diabetes, alcoholism, arthritis and eczema.

OTHER USES: Some native peoples believed that northern black currant had a calming effect on children, so sprigs were often hung on baby carriers. Currant shrubs growing by lakes were an indicator of fish, and in some legends, when currants dropped into the water, they were transformed into fish. Red flowering currant is commonly sold in garden centres in BC as a decorative native shrub, with flowers ranging in colour from pure white to dark red.

DESCRIPTION: Erect to ascending, deciduous shrubs, 1–3 m tall, without prickles, but often dotted with yellow, crystalline resin-glands that have a sweet, tomcat odour. Leaves alternate, 3- to 5-lobed, usually rather

WARNING
In the late 1700s, the Arctic explorer Samuel Hearne reported that large quantities of northern black currants could cause severe diarrhea and vomiting, but that these results would not occur if currants were mixed with cranberries. Native peoples warned that too many wax currants cause illness. Sticky currant is reported to cause vomiting, even in small quantities.

maple leaf–like. Flowers small (about 5–10 mm across), with 5 petals and 5 sepals, borne in elongating clusters in spring. Fruits tart, juicy berries (currants), often speckled with yellow, resinous dots or bristling with stalked glands.

Black currant (*R. americanum*) is a small, non-prickly shrub growing to 1 m or more in height. Leaves simple, rounded and alternate, to 10 cm wide, palmately lobed, with 3–5 pointed lobes with doubly-toothed edges. The surfaces of the leaves are scattered with resinous dots. Flowers creamy white to yellowish, bell-shaped and hanging in clusters from the leaf axils. Fruit a black berry, globular, smooth, each with a characteristic residual flower at the end. Found in damp soil along streams, wooded slopes, open meadows and rocky ground from southern AB to NB. See p. 424 for conservation status.

Golden currant (*R. aureum*) grows 1–3 m tall and is named for its showy bright yellow flowers, not its smooth fruits, which range from black to red and sometimes yellow. Its leaves have 3 widely spreading lobes and few or no glands. Inhabits streambanks and wet grasslands to dry prairies and open or wooded slopes from southern BC to southwestern SK, and introduced in southern ON and QC. See p. 424 for conservation status.

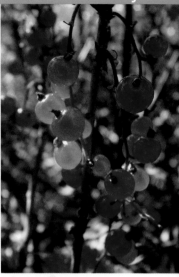

Red swamp currant

Stink currant (*R. bracteosum*) is a more or less erect, unarmed, straggly, deciduous shrub growing to 3 m tall. All parts of the plant are covered with round, yellow glands that smell sweet-skunky or catty. Leaves alternate, 5–20 cm wide, maple leaf–shaped, deeply 5- to 7-lobed, sweet-smelling when crushed. Flowers white to greenish white; many (20–40) in long, erect clusters 15–30 cm long. Fruits blue-black berries with a whitish bloom, edible, taste variable, from unpleasant to delicious. Found in moist to wet places (woods, streambanks, floodplains, shorelines, thickets, avalanche tracks) at low to subalpine elevations in coastal BC.

Wax currant (*R. cereum*) grows to 1 m tall, with small clusters of 2–6 white to pinkish flowers and red, smooth to glandular-hairy berries. Its shallowly lobed, fan-shaped leaves are glandular on both sides. Found on dry slopes and rocky places from the interior of BC to the mountains of southwestern AB.

Northern black currant (*R. hudsonianum*) grows to 1.5 m tall, with elongated clusters of 6–12 saucer-shaped, white flowers or shiny, resin-dotted, black berries. Its relatively large, maple leaf–like leaves have resin dots on the lower surface. Fruit strong-smelling and often bitter-tasting. Found in wet woods and rocky slopes in BC and central YT, northern AB, SK, MB, northernmost ON and western QC. See p. 424 for conservation status.

Sticky currant (*R. viscosissimum*) is a loosely branched shrub, to 2 m tall, with erect to spreading stems. Leaves 3- to 5-lobed, heart-shaped at the base, 2–10 cm wide and glandular-sticky. Flowers white or creamy in clusters of up to 16. Fruits bluish black, hairy and glandular berries. Grows in moist to dry forests and woodlands at montane to subalpine elevations in southern BC and AB.

Red flowering currant (*R. sanguineum*) is an erect, unarmed, 1–3 m tall shrub with crooked stems and reddish brown bark. Flowers a distinctive rose colour (varying from pale pink to deep red), rarely white, 7–10 mm long; in erect to drooping clusters of 10–20 or more flowers. Fruits blue-black, round berries with glandular hairs and a white, waxy bloom, 7–9 mm long; unpalatable. Inhabits dry to moist, open forests and openings at low to middle elevations in southern BC.

Red swamp currant (*R. triste*) is an unarmed, reclining to ascending shrub, to 1.5 m tall. Flowers reddish or greenish purple, small, several (6–15) in drooping clusters; flower stalks jointed, often hairy and glandular. Fruits bright red, smooth and sour but palatable. Found in moist, coniferous forests, swamps, on streambanks and montane, rocky slopes in all provinces and territories. See p. 424 for conservation status.

Wax currant

Gooseberries

Ribes spp.

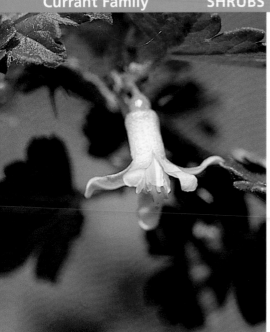

Northern gooseberry

FOOD: Gooseberries and currants occur across Canada, with almost 30 native species described. All gooseberries and currants (*Ribes* species) are edible raw, cooked or dried, but flavour and sweetness vary greatly with species, habitat and season. All are high in pectin and make excellent jams and jellies. Gooseberries are often eaten fresh, and they are delicious alone or mixed with other fruit in pies. Gooseberries were often eaten with grease or oil, and also mashed (usually in a mixture with other berries) and formed into cakes that were dried and stored for winter use. Dried gooseberries were sometimes included in pemmican, and dried gooseberry and bitterroot (p. 204) cakes were sometimes traded with other tribes. Because of their tart flavour, gooseberries can be used much like cranberries. They make a delicious addition to turkey stuffing, muffins and breads. Timing is important when picking gooseberries. Green berries are too sour to eat, and ripe fruit soon drops from the branch. The Nuxalk of BC, however, liked to pick the green berries of coastal black gooseberry and boil them to make a sauce that was much enjoyed. Sometimes green berries can be collected and left to ripen. Too many gooseberries can cause stomach upset, especially in the uninitiated. For more information on related species, see currants (p. 104) and prickly currants (p. 108).

MEDICINE: Because of the large number of species and wide distribution of gooseberries, there is a very large spectrum of uses for this genus. They were commonly eaten or used in teas for treating colds and sore throats, which may be related to high vitamin C content. Teas made from gooseberry leaves and fruits were given to women whose uteruses had slipped out of place after too many pregnancies. Gooseberry tea was also used as a wash for soothing skin irritations such as poison-ivy rashes and erysipelas (a condition with localized inflammation

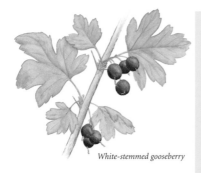

White-stemmed gooseberry

In the early 1900s, 10 million pine seedlings infected with white pine blister rust (*Cronartium ribicola*) were brought to North America from Europe, and the rust soon spread to infect the native, 5-needled pines. To reproduce, this rust must spend part of its life cycle on an alternate host. *Ribes* species are the alternate host for blister rust, so a program to eradicate these shrubs was attempted, unsuccessfully. Some provinces restrict the commercial growing of *Ribes* for the same control reason.

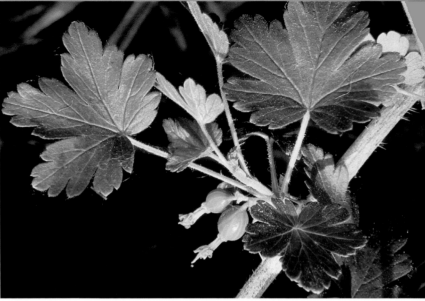

Northern gooseberry

and fever caused by a *Streptococcus* infection). Both currants and gooseberries have strong antiseptic properties. Extracts have proved effective against yeast (*Candida*) infections; roots and barks were also used, for example as a general tonic and for sore eyes.

OTHER USES: Gooseberry thorns were often used as needles for probing boils, removing splinters and applying tattoos.

DESCRIPTION: Erect to sprawling, deciduous shrubs with spiny branches. Leaves alternate, maple leaf–like, 3- to 5-lobed, about 2.5–5 cm wide. Flowers whitish to pale greenish yellow, to 1 cm long, tubular, with 5 small, erect petals and 5 larger, spreading sepals, in 1- to 4-flowered inflorescences in leaf axils, from May to June. Fruits smooth, purplish (when ripe) berries, about 1 cm across.

Coastal black gooseberry (*R. divaricatum*) is an erect to spreading shrub growing to 2 m tall. Branches arching in form, stems not prickly but have 1–3 stout spines on each node, bark greyish and smooth. Leaves small, maple leaf–shaped, with 3–5 lobes. Flowers white to more commonly red to reddish green, drooping, in clusters of 2–4. Berries round and smooth, purplish black when ripe, translucent skin, with the dried brown flowerhead attached at the bottom end of the ripe fruit. Found in open woods, meadows, moist clearings and hillsides at low elevations on southwestern Vancouver Island and adjacent islands and mainland.

White-stemmed gooseberry (*R. inerme*) is similar to coastal black gooseberry but has white to pinkish petals (vs. often reddish in coastal black gooseberry), 1–1.5 mm long (vs. 1.5–2.5 mm in coastal black gooseberry). Grows over a different range, in foothill and montane forests in southern interior BC and southwestern AB. See p. 424 for conservation status.

Sticky gooseberry (*R. lobbii*) has clusters of 3 slender spines at each node, is straggly in form and covered with soft, sticky hairs (hence the common name). Bark reddish brown and shreds with age. The fruit of this species is the largest of our native gooseberries (to 1.5 cm diameter) and most resembles the cultivated gooseberry in size and flavour. Found in lowland valleys and on streambanks to open or wooded, montane slopes in BC and YT. See p. 424 for conservation status.

Northern gooseberry (*R. oxyacanthoides*) is an erect to sprawling shrub, to 1.5 m tall, branches bristly, often with 1–3 spines to 1 cm long at nodes; older bark is whitish grey. Found in wet forests, thickets, clearings, open woods and exposed, rocky sites across Canada. See p. 424 for conservation status.

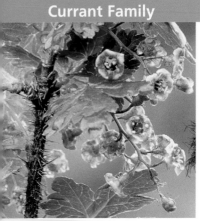

Prickly Currants
Ribes spp.

FOOD: Despite the prickly and strongly irritating stems of these plants, the fruit is quite palatable when ripe and makes delicious jam and pies (either alone or mixed with other fruit) for those who survive the spikes. Bristly black currants were widely used for food, although their flavour is sometimes described as insipid. The berries were traditionally eaten by the Stoney in AB, a number of BC First Nations and likely others within the range of the plant. They were prepared fresh, cooked or sometimes dried. Dried

Bristly black currant (all images)

currants were occasionally included in pemmican, and they make a tasty addition to bannock, muffins and breads. Currants may be boiled to make tea or mashed in water and fermented with sugar to make wine. The leaves, branches and inner bark of bristly black currant produce a menthol-flavoured tea, sometimes called "catnip tea." To make this tea, the spines were singed off, and the branches (fresh or dried) were steeped in hot water or boiled for a few minutes. Bristly fruits were rolled on hot ashes to singe off their soft spines. Both red currant jelly and the juice of green currants are said to be correctives for spoiled food (especially high, or aged and slightly decomposed, meat), but this use is not recommended. For more information on these closely related plants, see currants (p. 104) and gooseberries (p. 106).

MEDICINE: Tea made with bristly black currant stem bark was used to treat colds, and catnip tea (above) was taken to relieve cold symptoms and diarrhea. Black currants were boiled with sugar to make syrups and lozenges for treating sore throats. A spoonful of black currant jelly in a cup of hot water has a similar soothing effect. Red currant jelly has been recommended as a soothing salve for burns and is said to relieve pain and reduce blistering (especially if it can be applied immediately).

OTHER USES: Some native peoples considered the spiny branches (and by extension, the fruit) to be poisonous. However, these dangerous shrubs could also be useful—their thorny branches were thought to ward off evil forces.

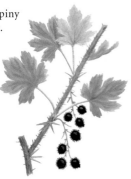

DESCRIPTION: Erect to spreading, deciduous shrubs with spiny, prickly branches and alternate, 3- to 5-lobed, maple leaf–like leaves. Flowers reddish to maroon, saucer-shaped, about 6 mm wide, forming hanging clusters of 7–15 from May to August. Fruits 5–8 mm wide berries, bristly with glandular hairs.

Bristly black currant (*R. lacustre*) is an erect to spreading shrub, 50 cm–2 m tall, covered with numerous small, sharp prickles, with larger, thick thorns at leaf nodes. Bark on older stems is cinnamon-coloured. Leaves large (2–7 cm wide) and hairless to slightly hairy. Berries dark purple. Found in moist woods and streambanks to drier forested slopes and subalpine ridges in all provinces and territories. See p. 424 for conservation status.

Mountain prickly currant (*R. montigenum*) is similar to bristly black currant but has smaller leaves (generally 1–2.5 cm wide) that are glandular-hairy on both sides, and bright red berries. Grows on rocky montane, subalpine and alpine slopes in south-western BC.

> **WARNING**
> The spines of bristly black currant can cause serious allergic reactions in some people. Eating too many currants will cause gastro-intestinal upset.

Saskatoon & Serviceberries

Amelanchier spp.

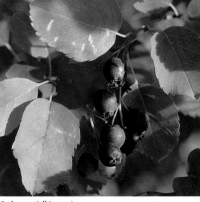
Saskatoon (all images)

FOOD: These sweet fruits were and still are extremely important to many indigenous peoples in Canada. Large quantities of the berries were harvested and stored for consumption during winter. They were eaten fresh, dried like raisins or mashed and dried. Some indigenous peoples steamed saskatoons in spruce bark vats filled with alternating layers of red-hot stones and fruit. The cooked fruit was mashed, formed into cakes and dried over a slow fire. These cakes could weigh as much as 7 kg. Dried saskatoons were the principal berries mixed with meat and fat to make pemmican or were added to soups and stews. Today, they are used in pies, pancakes, puddings, muffins, jams, jellies, sauces, syrups and wine, much like blueberries.

MEDICINE: Saskatoon juice was taken to relieve stomach upset and was boiled to make ear drops. Green or dried berries were used to make eye drops, and root tea was taken to prevent miscarriage. Tea made by boiling the inner bark was given to women to help them pass after-birth. The fruits or twigs of Canada serviceberry were given to mothers after childbirth for afterpains. The fruits were used as a blood remedy. A sharpened saskatoon stick, driven deeply into the swollen ankle of a horse, was used to drain blood and other liquids.

OTHER USES: These hard, strong, straight branches were a favourite material for making arrows, spears and pipe stems. They were also used for canes, canoe cross-pieces, basket rims, tepee stakes and tepee closure pins. The berry juice provided a purple dye. Saskatoons are excellent ornamental shrubs. They are hardy and easily propagated, with beautiful white blossoms in spring, delicious fruit in summer and colourful, often scarlet, leaves in autumn. The blossoms were an indicator to the Iroquois that it was time to plant corn.

DESCRIPTION: Shrub or small tree, to 7 m tall, with smooth, dark grey bark, often forming thickets. Leaves alternate, coarsely toothed on the upper half, yellowish orange to reddish brown in autumn. Flowers white, forming short, leafy clusters near the branch tips, from April to July. Fruits juicy, berry-like pomes, purple to black and sometimes with a whitish bloom, 6–12 mm across.

Saskatoon or **serviceberry** (*A. alnifolia*) has leaf blades 2–5 cm long, oval to nearly round. Flowers with petals to 2.5 cm long. Grows in prairies, thickets, hillsides and dry, open woods from BC to western QC, and in YT and NT. See p. 424 for conservation status.

Downy serviceberry (*A. arborea*) has leaf blades 5–13 cm long, hairy beneath. Flowers with petals to 2 cm long, in nodding clusters. Found in swampy lowlands, dry woods, rocky ridges, forest edges and open woodlands in ON, QC and NB.

WARNING

The leaves and pits contain poisonous cyanide compounds. Cooking or drying destroys these toxins.

Canada serviceberry (*A. canadensis*) has leaf blades 5–9 cm long, oblong, covered with fine, soft, grey fuzz when young, smooth when mature. Flowers with petals to 1.2 cm long, in ascending clusters. Found in moist woods, swamps and thickets in ON, QC, NB, NS and PEI. See p. 424 for conservation status.

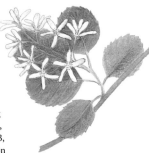

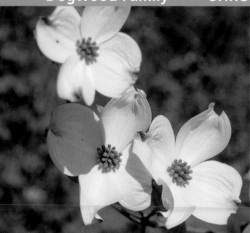

Dogwoods
Cornus spp.

FOOD: These fruits are very bitter for modern-day tastes, but many native peoples collected them for food in the past. Berries with a bluish tinge are said to be the sourest. Usually the berries were gathered in late summer and autumn and eaten fresh, either alone or mashed with sweeter fruits such as saskatoons (p. 109). Occasionally, they were dried for later use. More recently, these berries were used to make a dish called "sweet-and-sour" by mixing them with sugar and other sweeter berries. Some people separated the stones from the mashed flesh and saved them for later use. They were then eaten as a snack, like peanuts.

MEDICINE: Some First Nations used the bark tea to treat digestive disorders because of its laxative effects. The bark infusion was also used for swollen legs and venereal disease. The bark was smoked to treat sickness of the lungs. The inner bark contains an analgesic, coronic acid, so it has been used as a salicylate-free painkiller.

OTHER USES: The soft, white inner bark was dried and used for smoking. It was said to be both aromatic and pungent and to have a narcotic effect that could cause stupefaction. Usually, it was mixed with tobacco (p. 240) or common bearberry (p. 120). The inner bark from the roots was included in herb mixtures that were smoked in ceremonies. The flexible branches of red-

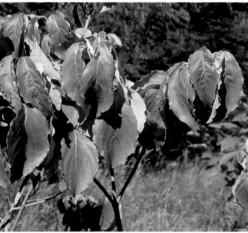

Eastern flowering dogwood (all images)

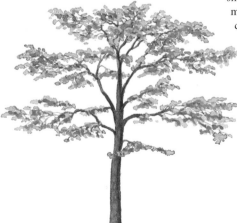

> **WARNING**
>
> All parts of these plants can be toxic, especially if they are consumed in large quantities.

osier dogwood are often used in wreaths or woven into contrasting red rims and designs in baskets. These attractive shrubs, with their lush green leaves and white flowers in spring, red leaves in autumn and bright red branches and white berries in winter, are popular ornamentals. They grow best in moist sites and are easily propagated from cuttings or by layering.

DESCRIPTION: Erect to sprawling, deciduous shrubs or small trees with opposite branches. Leaves opposite, simple, pointed, toothless, with leaf veins following the smooth leaf edges toward the tips, greenish above, white to greyish below, becoming red in autumn. Tiny flowers surrounded by petal-like bracts that resemble a single large flower. Flowers radially symmetrical with 4 sepals, petals and stamens, all attached at the top of the ovary. Fruit a fleshy, berry-like drupe.

Eastern flowering dogwood (*C. florida*) is a small tree or tall shrub, to 10 m tall, with a spreading, bushy crown and dark reddish brown bark. Clusters of small, yellowish flowers, about 30 in a cluster to 1.5 cm wide, subtended by 4 white or pinkish tinged, showy bracts. Shiny, berry-like, red drupes in clusters of 3–6. Found in wet or sandy forests and ravines in southeastern ON.

Pacific dogwood (*C. nuttallii*) is a small tree, to 20 m tall, with blackish brown, smooth bark, becoming finely ridged with age, and greyish purplish young branches. Clusters of small,

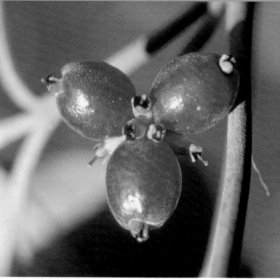

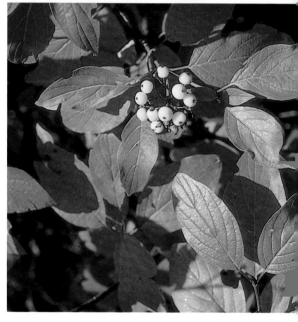

Eastern flowering dogwood (above)
Red-osier dogwood (below)

yellowish green or red flowers, about 75 in a cluster to 2 cm wide, subtended by 4–7 white or pinkish tinged, showy bracts. Fruits bright red, berry-like drupes in clusters of at least 20. Grows in moist, well-drained soils in the shade of coniferous trees in southwestern BC. Pacific dogwood is the provincial flower of BC.

Red-osier dogwood (*C. sericea*) is a shrub, to 6 m tall, with bright red twigs and branches (when young). Clusters of small flowers, 2–4 cm wide, without showy bracts, from May to August. Fruits white (sometimes bluish), berry-like drupes, to 9 mm across, containing large, flattened stones. Grows on moist sites, shores and thickets throughout Canada. See p. 424 for conservation status.

Black Huckleberry

Gaylussacia baccata

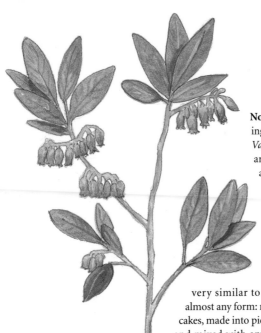

Note: Common names can be confusing. In addition to this plant, species of *Vaccinium* with fruits that aren't blue are often called huckleberries (p. 113), and *V. membranaceum* is commonly called black huckleberry, the same common name used here. Take heart, though—they're all tasty!

FOOD: There are few people who are at a loss about how to eat huckleberries. In taste, they range from tart to sweet with a flavour very similar to blueberries. They are delicious in almost any form: raw, baked in cakes, muffins and pancakes, made into pies, jams, jellies, syrups and ice creams and mixed with any other fruits. They can be frozen, canned, dried or made into wine. Dried huckleberries can be ground into a powder and mixed with cornmeal, soda and water to make bread and other baked goods. They are well suited for making bannock and pemmican.

MEDICINE: Huckleberries were considered good for the liver by some First Nations and were eaten as a ceremonial food to ensure health and prosperity for the coming season. An infusion of the leaves was recommended for acute or chronic nephritis (kidney disease) and dysentery, the latter also treated with an infusion of the bark. Herbalists prescribed the leaf tea for patients suffering from diabetes and gallbladder disease, believing that huckleberry tea purifies the kidneys. A tea made from the roots is recommended for swollen joints, scurvy and bleeding gums.

OTHER USES: Huckleberries are relished by bears and other wildlife. The small, dark, rather insignificant fruit became a metaphor in the early part of the 19th century for something humble or minor. This later came to mean somebody inconsequential, an idea that was the basis for Mark Twain's famous character, Huckleberry Finn. In an 1895 interview, he revealed that he wanted to establish the boy as "someone of lower extraction or degree" than Tom Sawyer.

DESCRIPTION: Deciduous, low, colonial shrub, 30 cm–1 m tall, similar to blueberries and other huckleberries but with resin glands on the leaves, and fruits that are berry-like drupes with only 10 seeds in each (versus fruits that are true berries with many seeds in each for *Vaccinium* spp.). Leaves simple, elliptic to oblong to lance-shaped, alternate, entire, pinnately veined, and glandular on both surfaces. Flowers pink, 5-parted, about 6 mm wide, tubular, stalked, and borne on a glandular raceme that is usually shorter than the leaves, from May to June. Fruit a black, fleshy "berry," less than 5 mm in diameter, ripening from June to September. Grows in dry, rocky or sandy soil in woods, forests and thickets from ON to NL. See p. 424 for conservation status.

Huckleberries

Vaccinium spp.

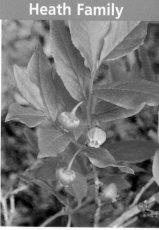

Note: Common names can be confusing. Taller species of *Vaccinium* with fruits that aren't blue (such as these three) are often called huckleberries, while shorter *Vaccinium* species with tart red berries are commonly called cranberries (p. 116). Species of *Vaccinium* with fruits that **are** blue are usually called blueberries (p. 114).

FOOD: Some people consider black huckleberry the most delicious and highly prized berry in western Canada and the Rockies, while others think blueberries are best. On the west coast, many First Nations considered evergreen huckleberry

Black huckleberry (all images)

to be the tastiest and travelled considerable distances to collect it. Huckleberries can be used like domestic blueberries—eaten fresh from the bush, added to fruit salads, cooked in pies and cobblers, made into jams and jellies or crushed and used in cold drinks. They are also delicious in pancakes, muffins, cakes and puddings. Black huckleberries are often collected in large quantities in open, subalpine sites (such as old burns), and in some regions they are sold commercially. Native peoples gathered huckleberries and ate them fresh, but they also sun-dried or smoke-dried them mainly for winter use. Red huckleberries were sometimes stored soaked in grease or oil. The berries were mashed and formed into cakes or spread loosely on mats for drying. Later, they were reconstituted by boiling either alone or with roots. Dried huckleberry leaves and berries make excellent teas.

MEDICINE: The leaves and berries are high in vitamin C. Roots and stems of black huckleberry were used to make medicinal teas for treating heart trouble, arthritis and rheumatism. The leaf tea has been taken by some diabetics to stabilize and reduce blood sugar levels (reducing the need for insulin) and to treat hypoglycemia. Huckleberry leaf tea has also been used as an appetite stimulant and as a treatment for bladder and urinary tract infections. The leaves and bark of red huckleberry were used in a decoction that was gargled for sore throats and inflamed gums.

OTHER USES: Red huckleberries were used as fish bait in streams.

DESCRIPTION: Deciduous or evergreen shrubs, 40 cm–3 m tall, with alternate, 2–5 cm long leaves. Flowers various shades of pink, round to urn-shaped, 4–6 mm long, nodding on single, slender stalks, from April to June. Fruits berries, 6–10 mm across.

Red huckleberry (*V. parvifolium*) is a deciduous shrub with bright red berries. Branches green and strongly angled. Grows in dry to moist forests in lowland and montane zones in BC, most abundantly on the coast.

Black huckleberry (*V. membranaceum*) is a deciduous shrub with purplish black berries. Branches greenish when young but greyish brown with age and at most slightly angled. Grows in dry to moist forests at montane to subalpine elevations on open or wooded slopes in YT, BC, AB and ON. See p. 424 for conservation status.

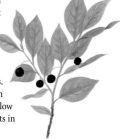

Evergreen huckleberry (*V. ovatum*) is an evergreen shrub with purplish black berries. Branches greenish when young but brown with age and at most slightly angled. Grows at low to montane elevations in dry to moist forests in coastal BC.

WARNING

Large quantities of these berries—any berries, actually—can cause diarrhea.

Blueberries

Vaccinium spp.

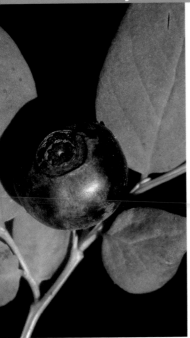

Oval-leaved blueberry

Note: Common names can be confusing here. Species of *Vaccinium* with blue fruits are usually called blueberries. Taller species of *Vaccinium* with fruits that **aren't** blue are usually called huckleberries (p. 113), and shorter *Vaccinium* species with tart, red berries are commonly called cranberries (p. 116).

FOOD: These sweet, juicy berries can be eaten fresh from the bush, added to fruit salads, cooked in pies, tarts and cobblers, made into jams, syrups and jellies or crushed and used to make juice, wine, tea and cold drinks. Bog blueberry wine is said to be especially intoxicating. Blueberries also make a delicious addition to pancakes, muffins, cakes and puddings. They were widely used by First Nations, either fresh or dried singly or in cakes. To make cakes, the berries were boiled to a mush, spread in slabs and dried on a rack in the sun or near a fire. The juice was slowly poured onto the drying cakes or was cooled to make jelly.

MEDICINE: Dubbed the "super berry," these delicious berries are rich in antioxidants, including vitamin C and 25 anthocyanins. Blueberry roots were traditionally boiled to make medicinal teas that were taken to relieve diarrhea, gargled to soothe sore mouths and throats or applied to slow-healing sores. Bruised roots and berries were steeped in gin, which was to be taken freely (as much as the stomach and head could tolerate) to stimulate urination and relieve kidney stones and water retention. The leaf or root tea of low bilberry (*V. myrtillus*) is reported to flush pinworms from the body. Blueberry leaf tea and dried blueberries have been used like cranberries to treat diarrhea and urinary tract infections. Currently, blueberry leaf tea is widely used by people suffering from type 2 diabetes to stabilize and reduce blood sugar levels and to reduce the need for insulin. Recent research confirms this activity in pharmacological models. Blueberry extracts containing anthocyanins protect against retinopathy, or degeneration of the retina, in diabetes. These compounds are most concentrated in the dried fruit, preserves, jams and jellies. Their effect is said to wear off after 5–6 hours. The antioxidant anthocyanins may reduce leakage in small blood vessels (capillaries), and blueberries have been suggested as a safe and effective treatment for water retention (during pregnancy), hemorrhoids, varicose veins and similar problems. They have also been recommended to reduce inflammation from acne and other skin problems and to prevent cataracts. Researchers have demonstrated that blueberry anthocyanins, proanthocyanins, flavonols and tannins are able to reduce the risk of certain chronic diseases, including cancer. A particular anthocyanin, delphinidin, inhibits the formation of new blood vessels that feed growing tumours, demonstrating an additional mechanism that reduces cancer risk. Consumption of the fruit has been associated with increased cognitive function, reduced risk of Alzheimer's disease and

WARNING
Blueberry leaves contain moderately high concentrations of tannins, so they should not be used continually for extended periods of time.

other conditions related to ageing. Animal studies show that regular long-term consumption of blueberries improves motor control, memory and learning new tasks, lowers "bad" cholesterol and blood lipid levels, increases "good" cholesterol levels, attenuates inflammation, deters the development of obesity and suppresses insulin resistance. This evidence points to the possibility of blueberry anthocyanins as a foundation for treating people with obesity, diabetes and cardiovascular disease. Given the plethora of medical benefits provided by these super berries, any health-conscious individual would do well to include them regularly in his or her diet.

OTHER USES: Blueberry leaves were sometimes dried and smoked. The berries were used to dye clothing navy blue.

DESCRIPTION: Deciduous shrubs with thin, oval leaves 1–3 cm long, whitish to pink, nodding, urn-shaped flowers 4–6 mm long, and round, 5–8 mm wide, bluish berries, sometimes with a greyish bloom.

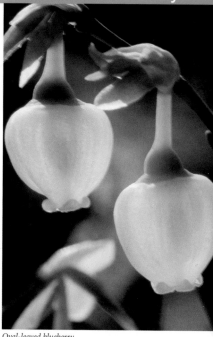
Oval-leaved blueberry

Velvet-leaved blueberry (*V. myrtilloides*) is a low shrub, to 40 cm tall, with densely hairy (velvety) branches, especially when young. Produces dark bluish black to dark red fruits, from August to October. Grows at montane elevations in dry to moist forests and openings and bogs throughout Canada.

Dwarf blueberry (*V. caespitosum*) is a low, usually matted shrub, 10–30 cm tall, with rounded, yellowish to reddish branches and finely toothed, light green leaves. Its 5-lobed flowers produce berries singly in leaf axils, from August to September. Grows at all elevations in dry to wet forests, bogs, meadows, rocky ridges and tundra throughout Canada. See p. 424 for conservation status.

Bog blueberry (*V. uliginosum*) is a low, spreading shrub, 10–30 cm tall, with rounded, brownish branches, but it has toothless, dull green leaves and clustered (1–4), 4- or 5-lobed flowers. Grows in bogs, boggy forests and on alpine slopes at all elevations throughout Canada. See p. 424 for conservation status.

Lowbush blueberry (*V. angustifolium*) is a low shrub, to 60 cm tall, but usually less than 35 cm, with white, bell-shaped flowers 5 mm long, from May to June, and small, dark blue or black berries, 1.2 cm across. Grows in abundance in dry, open barrens, peats and rock from MB to NL and is the main source of wild harvested blueberries in eastern Canada. See p. 424 for conservation status.

Oval-leaved blueberry (*V. ovalifolium*) is a tall shrub, to 2 m tall, with hairless, angled branches. Its leaves are entire or only sparsely toothed. Produces purple berries with a whitish bloom from early July to September. Grows at low to subalpine elevations in dry to moist forests, openings and bogs in BC and AB and from ON to NL. See p. 424 for conservation status.

Alaska blueberry (*V. alaskaense*) is very similar to oval-leaved blueberry, but has flowers appearing before the leaves (versus with the leaves in oval-leaved), flowers that are usually wider than long (versus longer than wide in oval-leaved), and leaves with coarse, stiff hairs along the underside midrib (versus not in oval-leaved). Flowers from April to May. Grows at low to subalpine elevations in mesic to moist forests and openings in BC, mainly coastal.

Highbush blueberry (*V. corymbosum*) is a multi-stemmed shrub, 1.5–4.5 m tall, with green or often red twigs and 5-toothed, white flowers, 6–13 mm long, from May to June. Grows in swamps or dry, upland woods from ON to NS. This is the cultivated blueberry that produces large, sweet berries sold commercially.

Cranberries

Vaccinium and *Oxycoccus* spp.

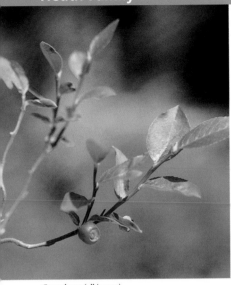

Grouseberry (all images)

Note: Common names can be confusing here. Species of *Vaccinium* with blue fruits are usually called blueberries (p. 114), and taller shrubs with fruits that **aren't** blue are usually called huckleberries (p. 113). Shorter *Vaccinium* species with tart, red berries are commonly called cranberries.

FOOD: Cranberries can be very tart, but they make a refreshing trail nibble, and they are also added to fruit salads or cooked in pies and cobblers (usually mixed with other fruits). They make delicious jams and jellies, and they can be crushed or chopped to make tea, juice or wine and to flavour cold drinks. Cranberry sauce is still a favourite with meat or fowl. It is easily made by boiling berries with sugar and water or, more traditionally, by mixing cranberries with maple sugar and cider. Cranberries are a delicious addition to pancakes, muffins, breads, cakes and puddings. Firm, washed berries keep for several months when stored in a cool place. They can also be frozen or canned. First Nations sometimes dried cranberries for use in pemmican, soups, sauces and stews. Some tribes stored boiled cranberries mixed with oil and later whipped this mixture with snow and fish oil to make a dessert. Freezing makes cranberries sweeter, so they were traditionally collected after the first heavy frost. Because they remain on the shrubs all year, cranberries can be a valuable survival food. These low-growing berries are difficult to collect, so some people combed them from their branches with a salmon backbone or wooden comb.

MEDICINE: Cranberry juice has long been used to treat bladder infections. Research shows that these berries contain arbutin, which prevents some bacteria from adhering to the walls of the bladder and urinary tract and causing an infection. Cranberry juice also increases the acidity of the urine, thereby inhibiting bacterial activity, which can relieve infections. Increased acidity also lessens the urinary odour of people suffering from incontinence. The tannins in cranberry have anticlotting properties and are able to reduce the amount of dental plaque–causing bacteria in the mouth, thus are helpful against gingivitis. Another chemical component, a high molecular weight non-dializable material (NDM), has demonstrated the ability to reverse plaque formation and prevent tooth decay.

> **WARNING**
> Large quantities of cranberries can cause diarrhea.

Cranberries also contain antioxidant polyphenols that may be beneficial in maintaining cardiovascular health and immune function, and in preventing tumour formation. Although some of these compounds have proved extraordinarily powerful in killing certain types of human cancer cells in the laboratory, their effectiveness when ingested is unknown. There is evidence that cranberry juice may be effective against the formation of kidney stones. Cranberries were also taken to relieve nausea, to ease cramps in childbirth and to quiet hysteria and convulsions. Crushed cranberries were used as poultices on wounds, including poison-arrow wounds.

OTHER USES: The red pulp (left after the berries have been crushed to make juice) contains red dyes. Hunters often looked for grouse-berry when seeking grouse because it is a favourite food of these game birds.

DESCRIPTION: Dwarf, deciduous shrubs, mostly less than 20 cm tall, with small, nodding, pinkish flowers producing sour, bright red (sometimes purplish) cranberries.

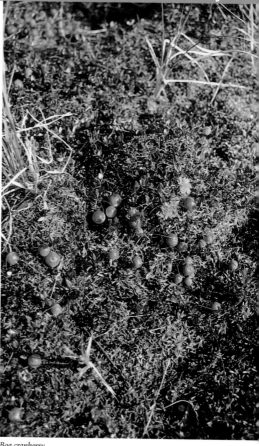

Bog cranberry

Cranberry (*O. macrocarpus*) has 4 petals separated almost to the base, the petals spreading or curved backward, in clusters arising from the leaf axils. Fruit a dark red, globose berry, 10–20 mm wide, appearing from July to August. Grows at low elevations in open bogs, swamps and lake shores from ON to NS, and as a rare escapee from cultivation in other provinces.

Bog cranberry (*O. oxycoccos*) has 4 petals separated almost to the base, the petals curved strongly backward (like little shooting stars), flowers appearing terminal on stems. Fruit a deep red, globose cranberry, about 5–12 mm wide, from July to August. Grows in bogs throughout Canada. See p. 424 for conservation status.

Grouseberry (*V. scoparium*) is a low, broom-like shrub with many slender, green, angled branches. Has thin, finely toothed, deciduous leaves, 6–12 mm long. Has 4 petals fused into urn-shaped flowers, singly from leaf axils. Small (3–5 mm wide), single, bright red berries appear from July to August. Grows on foothill, montane and subalpine slopes in southern BC and southwestern AB.

Lingonberry (*V. vitis-idaea*) is a low, spreading shrub with rounded or slightly angled branches. Has blunt, leathery, evergreen leaves, 6–25 mm long, with dark dots (hairs) on a pale lower surface. Has 4 petals fused into urn-shaped flowers, 1 to several in terminal clusters, which produce bright red cranberries, 6–10 mm wide, from July to August. Grows in sunny mountain meadows, peat moors and dry woods throughout Canada. See p. 424 for conservation status.

False-Wintergreens
Gaultheria spp.

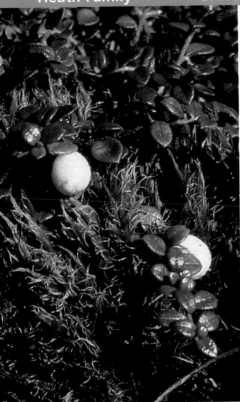

Hairy false-wintergreen

FOOD: The leaves are widely used to make a pleasant tea with a mild wintergreen flavour. The small, sweet berries are eaten fresh, served with cream and sugar or cooked in sauces. Their flavour improves upon freezing, so they are at their best in winter, under the snow, or in spring when they are plump and juicy. The berries were added to teas and were used to add fragrance and flavour to liqueurs. Occasionally, large quantities were picked and dried like raisins for winter use. The young leaves can be a trailside nibble or added to salads. They are often used to make a strong, aromatic tea. The wintergreen flavour can be drawn out if the bright red leaves are first fermented. During the American Revolutionary War, wintergreen tea was a substitute for black tea (*Camellia sinensis*).

MEDICINE: All false-wintergreens contain methyl salicylate, a close relative of aspirin that has been used to relieve aches and pains. These plants were widely used in the treatment of painful, inflamed joints resulting from rheumatism and arthritis. Traditionally, an infusion of the leaves was used to relieve colds, flu, headaches, fevers, kidney complaints, flatulence and colic. Studies suggest that oil of wintergreen is probably an effective painkiller. The berries were soaked in brandy, and the resulting extract was taken to stimulate appetite, as a substitute for bitters. The leaf tea of hairy false-wintergreen was used as a digestive tonic for those who had overeaten. The leaves were chewed to dry the mouth or applied as a poultice on burns, cuts and sores.

WARNING

Oil of wintergreen (most concentrated in the berries and young leaves) contains methyl salicylate, a drug that has caused accidental poisonings. It should be taken internally only in very small amounts. Avoid applying the oil when you are hot because dangerous amounts could be absorbed through your skin. There have been reported cases of fatalities in small children, and in April 2007, a 17-year-old cross-country runner died from having absorbed too much methyl salicylate through excessive use of topical muscle pain relief sports creams. It can cause skin reactions and severe (anaphylactic) allergic reactions. People who are allergic to aspirin should not use false-wintergreen or its relatives.

OTHER USES: The leaves, plants and berries were boiled in water to add to baths for pregnant women. Oil of wintergreen has numerous commercial applications: it provides fragrance to various products such as toothpastes, chewing gum and candy and is used to mask the odours of some organophosphate pesticides. It is a flavouring agent (at no more than 0.04 percent) and an ingredient in deep-heating sports creams (see **Warning**). The oil is also a source of triboluminescence, a phenomenon in which a substance produces light when rubbed, scratched or crushed. The oil, mixed with sugar and dried, builds up an electrical charge that releases sparks when ground, producing the Wint-O-Green Lifesavers phenomenon. To observe this, look in a mirror in a dark room and chew the candy with your mouth open.

DESCRIPTION: Delicate, creeping shrublets with leathery, evergreen leaves, small, white to greenish or pinkish flowers, mealy to pulpy, fleshy, berry-like capsules and a mild, wintergreen flavour.

Hairy false-wintergreen or **creeping snowberry** (*G. hispidula*) has stiff, flat-lying, brown hairs on its stems and lower leaf surfaces. Leaves very small (4–10 mm long). Tiny (2 mm wide), 4-lobed flowers, from May to June, and small (generally less than 5 mm in diameter), white berries. Grows in cold, wet bogs and coniferous forests in montane and subalpine zones throughout Canada. See p. 424 for conservation status.

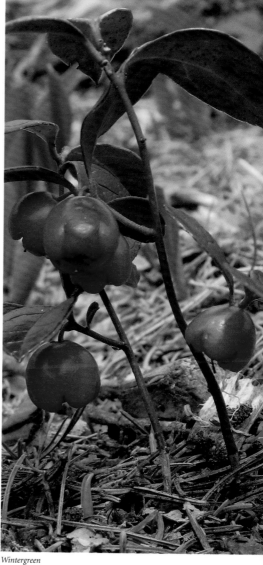

Wintergreen

Alpine false-wintergreen (*G. humifusa*) has 1–2 cm long, glossy leaves, rounded to blunt at tips with pinkish or greenish white, 5-lobed, 3–4 mm wide flowers and scarlet, pulpy, 5–6 mm wide berries. Grows in moist to wet, subalpine to alpine meadows in southern BC and southwestern AB. See p. 424 for conservation status.

Slender false-wintergreen (*G. ovatifolia*) is similar to alpine false-wintergreen, but it has reddish, hairy (rather than hairless) calyxes and 2–5 cm long leaves that are pointy-tipped. Grows in moist to wet forests, heaths and bogs in montane and subalpine sites in southern BC.

Wintergreen (*G. procumbens*) has thick, shiny, oval, 2.5–5 cm long leaves, small, oval flowers from April to May and dry, red berries that dangle beneath the leaves. Grows in poor or sandy soils under evergreens or in oak woods from southeastern MB east. See p. 424 for conservation status.

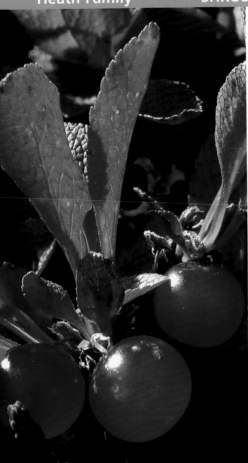

Bearberries or Kinnikinnick

Arctostaphylos spp.

FOOD: Bearberries are rather mealy and tasteless, but they are often abundant and remain on branches all year, so they can provide an important survival food. Many tribes used them for food. To reduce the dryness, bearberries were usually cooked with salmon oil, bear fat or fish eggs, or they were added to soups or stews. Sometimes, boiled berries were preserved in oil and served whipped with snow during winter. Boiled bearberries, sweetened with syrup or sugar and served with cream, make a tasty dessert. They can also be used in jams, jellies, cobblers and pies, dried, ground and cooked in mush or fried in grease over a slow fire until they pop like popcorn. Scalded mashed berries, soaked in water for an hour or so, produced a spicy, cider-like drink, which was sweetened and fermented to make wine. The dried leaves were used to make tea. Although fairly insipid, juicy alpine bearberries are probably among the most palatable fruits in the genus, but because they grow at high elevations and northern latitudes, they have been the least used. Manzanita berries

Red bearberry (above)
Common bearberry (below)

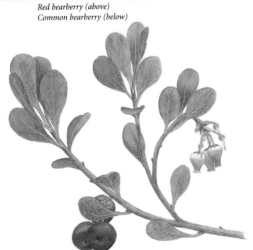

> **WARNING**
> Too many bearberries can cause constipation. Bearberry is rich in tannin and arbutin. Extended use (e.g., for more than 3 days) causes stomach and liver problems (especially in children). Bearberry should not be used by pregnant women. It can stimulate uterine contractions and reduce permeability of the placenta-uterine membrane.

are very similar to the ones of common bearberry, and they were an important food for many tribes.

MEDICINE: The leaves are widely used today in medicinal teas or extracts for treatment of urinary tract infection. Studies show that bearberry has an antiseptic effect on the urinary tract, and it has been shown to inhibit the growth of Gram-positive bacteria. It also has a mild vaso-constricting effect on the uterus and may help to relieve menstrual cramps. The tea was traditionally used to treat kidney and bladder problems, lower back pain, bronchitis, diarrhea, gonorrhea and bleeding. It can be used in sitz baths and washes to reduce inflammation and infection.

OTHER USES: The leaves and bark were widely smoked, often mixed with red-osier dogwood (p. 111) and alder (p. 151) bark, tobacco (p. 240) and other ingredients. Usually, the

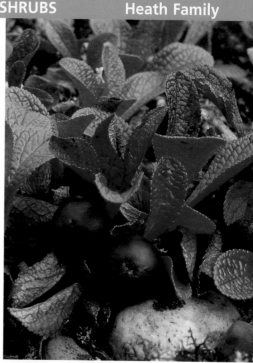

Alpine bearberry

leaves were toasted near a fire until crisp and brown and then crushed and smoked. Some people say that smoking bearberry leaves can cause dizziness and even unconsciousness in the uninitiated. The tannin-rich leaves have been used to tan hides. Hikers sometimes chew the berries and leaves to stimulate saliva flow and relieve thirst.

DESCRIPTION: Evergreen or deciduous shrubs with clusters of nodding, white or pinkish, urn-shaped flowers and juicy to mealy, berry-like drupes containing 5 small nutlets. The genus *Arctostaphylos* contains 2 main groups of species—the bearberries, which are low, trailing to tufted shrubs found most abundantly in arctic and alpine regions, and the manzanitas, which are erect or spreading, taller shrubs of western Canada.

Common bearberry or **kinnikinnick** (*A. uva-ursi*) is a trailing, evergreen shrub, to 15 cm tall, with leathery, evergreen, spoon-shaped leaves, 1–3 cm long. Small (4–6 mm long) flowers appear from May to June and produce bright red, 5–10 mm diameter, mealy fruits by late summer. Grows in well-drained, often gravelly or sandy soils in open woods and rocky, exposed sites at all elevations throughout Canada. See p. 424 for conservation status.

Alpine bearberry (*A. alpina* var. *alpina*) is a trailing, deciduous shrub, to 15 cm tall, with thin, veiny, oval leaves, 1–5 cm long, with hairy margins (at the base) that often turn red in autumn, the previous year's dead leaves usually evident. Small (4–6 mm long) flowers appear from June to July and produce mealy fruits that are purplish black, 5–10 mm in diameter, by late summer. Grows in moderately well-drained, rocky, gravelly and sandy soils on tundra, slopes and ridges in circumpolar Canada, including all territories and northern parts of BC, AB, SK, MB, ON, QC and NL.

Red bearberry (*A. alpina* var. *rubra*) is similar to alpine bearberry, but it has longer leaves (to 9 cm long) with hairless margins, the leaves of the previous year not persistent. Berries bright red. Grows in the same habitats as alpine bearberry and over the same range.

Hairy manzanita (*A. columbiana*) is a much taller shrub, 1–3 m tall. Has 2–5 cm long, oval, evergreen leaves and red fruits. Grows in open, coniferous forests and openings in extreme southwestern BC.

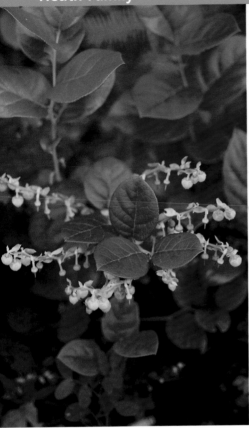

Salal
Gaultheria shallon

FOOD: The dark, juicy berries grow in many places on the Pacific coast and were traditionally the most plentiful and important fruit for Aboriginal people. They were eaten fresh or dried into cakes. The Kwakwaka'wakw ate the ripe berries, dipped in eulachon grease, at large feasts. For trading or selling, ripe salal berries were mixed with currants (p. 104), elderberries (p. 124) or unripe salal berries. The berries were also used to sweeten other foods, and the Haida used salal berries to thicken salmon eggs. In recent times, salal berries have been prepared as jams or preserves, and ripe berries from healthy bushes are hard to beat for flavour and juiciness. They can be used as ingredients in syrups, pancakes, muffins, cookies and fruit cake. The young leaves were chewed as a hunger suppressant by some West Coast bands. The leafy branches were used in pit-cooking and cooked as a flavouring in fish soup.

MEDICINE: The leaf tea of salal was used as a stomach tonic for diarrhea, coughs and tuberculosis.

OTHER USES: A purple dye is obtained from the fruits, and a greenish yellow dye from the infused leaves. The plant is harvested for export and sold to florists worldwide for use in floral arrangements.

DESCRIPTION: Erect to partially creeping, freely branching, evergreen shrub, to 3 m tall, with broadly oval leaves, 3–9 cm long, 1–6 cm wide and finely serrated. Leaf stalks, flower stems and bracts and young branches reddish and hairy. Flowers white to pinkish, urn-shaped, 5-lobed, 7–9 mm long, in 5- to 15-flowered clusters. Fruits purplish black, berry-like, to 1 cm in diameter. Most abundant shrub over much of Canada's Pacific coast, growing in dry to wet forests, bogs and openings to montane elevations in coastal BC and, much less commonly, southern interior BC.

Crowberry

Empetrum nigrum

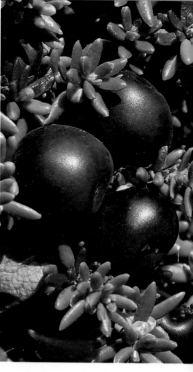

FOOD: Next to cranberries (p. 116) and blueberries (p. 114), crowberries are one of the most abundant edible wild fruits found in northern Canada and were a vital addition to the diets of First Nations. The Inuit call them *paurngait*, meaning "looks like soot," referring to the fruit's black colour, and traditionally dried or froze them for winter use. Because they are almost devoid of natural acids, they taste a little bland and were often mixed with blueberries or lard or oil. Their taste improves after freezing or cooking, and their sweet flavour peaks after a frost. The fruits are high in vitamin C, about twice that of blueberries, and rich in antioxidant anthocyanins (the pigment that gives them their black colour). Their high water content was a blessing to hunters seeking to quench their thirst in the waterless high country. They have a firm, impermeable skin and are not prone to becoming soggy, and are ideal for making muffins, pancakes, pies, preserves and the like. A fine dessert is made by cooking the berries with a little lemon juice and serving them with cream and sugar. Crowberries are usually collected in autumn, but because they often persist on the plant over winter, they can be picked in spring. Approximately 2 cups of berries can be collected per hour. The twigs reportedly make a pleasant tea.

MEDICINE: Consuming too many berries alone may cause constipation, so these berries were especially recommended for patients suffering from diarrhea. People with runny stools were also treated with an infusion or decoction of the stems, as were those with general kidney problems. A decoction of the leaves and stems, mixed with Labrador tea (p. 131) and young spruce tips (p. 30), was taken for colds and chills. A cooled decoction of the root was used as a wash for sore eyes and to remove any growths on the eyes. The leafy branches were recommended as a diuretic, especially in children with fever.

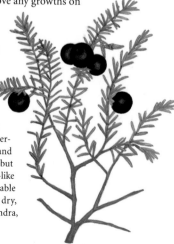

OTHER USES: The berries provide a black dye. The branches were used to make a loosely woven summer mattress, and the stem used like a pipe cleaner to clean gun barrels.

DESCRIPTION: Dwarf or low shrub, 5–10 cm tall, prostrate and mat-forming, to 30 cm long. Leaves alternate but grow so closely together as to appear whorled, needle-like, evergreen, 2–6 mm long. Flowers 1–3, pink, in leaf axils, 3 petals and sepals, petals 3 mm long, with male and female flowers separate but on the same plant, from July to August. Fruit a juicy, black, berry-like drupe, 3–6 mm in diameter, containing 2–9 brown seeds, available from July to November, sometimes overwintering. Grows in dry, acidic, rocky or gravelly soil on slopes, ridges and seashores in tundra, muskeg and spruce forests at all elevations throughout Canada.

Elderberries

Sambucus spp.

FOOD: Generally, raw elderberries are considered inedible and cooked berries edible (see **Warning**), but some tribes are said to have eaten large quantities fresh from the bush. Cooking or drying destroys the rank-smelling, toxic compounds. Most elderberries were steamed or boiled or were dried for winter use. Sometimes clusters were spread on beds of pine needles in late autumn and covered with more needles and eventually with an insulating layer of snow. These caches were easily located by their bluish pink stain in the snow. Only small amounts were eaten at a time—just enough to get a taste. Sometimes elderberries were steamed with black hair lichens for flavouring. Today, they are used in jams, jellies, syrups, preserves, pies and wine. Because they contain no pectin, they are often mixed with tart, pectin-rich fruits such as crab apples. Elderberries are also used to make teas or cold drinks and to flavour some wines (e.g., Liebfraumilch) and liqueurs (e.g., Sambuca). Red elderberry juice was sometimes used to marinate salmon prior to baking. The flowers can be used to make tea

Red elderberry (all images)

WARNING

The stems, bark, leaves and roots contain poisonous cyanide-producing glycosides (especially when fresh), which cause nausea, vomiting and diarrhea, but the ripe fruits and flowers are edible. The seeds, however, contain toxins that are most concentrated in red-fruited species. Many sources classify red-fruited elderberries as poisonous and black- or blue-fruited species as edible.

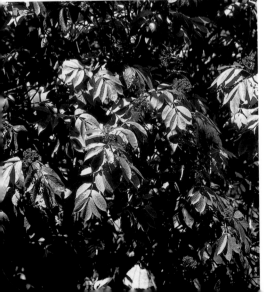

or wine, and in some areas, flower clusters were popular dipped in batter and fried as fritters or stripped from their relatively bitter stalks and mixed into pancake batter.

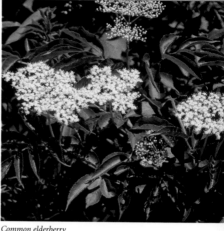
Common elderberry

MEDICINE: Teas made from the bark and leaves were used in washes for healing eczema, sores and rashes and were drunk to treat a wide range of ailments, but ingestion is not recommended (see **Warning**). In Europe, black elderberry tea made from the flowers is used to alleviate cold and flu symptoms and to reduce fevers. Elderberry flowers also stimulate urination and bowel movements, so they have been used in diet pills and laxatives. Dried elderberry flowers have been used to make washes for treating sores, blisters, hemorrhoids, rheumatism and arthritis. The inner bark tea has been used to treat epilepsy, induce vomiting, empty the bowels and stimulate sweating and urination. Some species are included in herbal purges. Elderberries are rich in vitamin A, vitamin C, calcium, potassium and iron. They have also been shown to contain antiviral compounds that could be useful in treating influenza.

OTHER USES: The pithy branches were hollowed out to fashion whistles, flutes, drinking straws, blowguns, pipe stems and spigots for tapping sap from trees, but see **Warning**. The berries produce crimson or violet dyes. Elderberry wine, elderberries soaked in buttermilk and elderflower water have all been used in cosmetic washes and skin creams. The leaves were crushed to make mosquito repellent or boiled to make a caterpillar repellent for spraying on garden plants.

DESCRIPTION: Unpleasant-smelling, 1–3 m tall, deciduous shrubs with pithy, opposite branches often sprouting from the base. Leaves pinnately divided into 5–9 sharply toothed leaflets about 5–15 cm long. Flowers white, 4–6 mm wide, forming crowded, branched clusters, from April to July. Fruits juicy, berry-like drupes, 4–6 mm across, in dense, showy clusters.

Blue elderberry (*S. caerulea*) has flat-topped flower clusters and dull blue fruits with a whitish bloom. Grows in gravelly, dry soils on streambanks, field edges and woodlands in BC and AB.

Common elderberry (*S. canadensis*) bears large corymbs (20–30 cm across) of white flowers and dark purple to black berries. Grows in rich, moist soils along streams and rivers in eastern Canada from MB to NS.

Red elderberry (*S. racemosa*) has pyramid-shaped flower clusters and shiny fruits, the tastiest of the genus. Includes 2 common varieties: **black elderberry** (var. *melanocarpa*), with purplish black fruit, and **red elderberry** (var. *pubens*), with red fruit. Both grow in open woods, forest edges and roadsides on montane and subalpine sites throughout Canada.

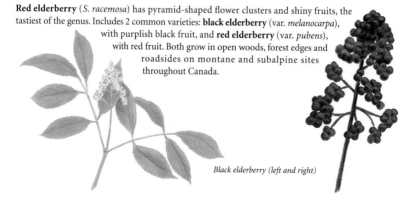
Black elderberry (left and right)

Bush-Cranberries

Viburnum spp.

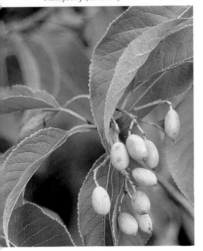

High bush-cranberry (above)
Nannyberry (all below)

FOOD: These berries are best picked in autumn, after they have been softened and sweetened by freezing. Some people compare their fragrance to that of dirty socks, but the flavour is good. The addition of lemon or orange peel is said to eliminate the odour. Raw bush-cranberries can be very sour and acidic (much like true cranberries, p. 116), but many native peoples ate them, chewing the fruit, swallowing the juice and spitting out the tough skins and seeds. They were also eaten with bear grease, or, in an early year, they could be mixed with sweeter berries such as saskatoons (p. 109). Bush-cranberries are an excellent winter-survival food because they remain on branches all winter and are much sweeter after freezing. Some tribes ate the boiled berries mixed with oil, and occasionally this mixture was whipped with fresh snow to make a frothy dessert. Today, bush-cranberries are usually boiled, strained (to remove the seeds and skins) and used in jams and jellies, or as a cranberry sauce. These preserves usually require additional pectin, especially after the berries have been frozen. Early settlers found that berries that were not fully ripe (not yet red) jelled without pectin. Bush-cranberry juice can be used in cold drinks or fermented to make wine, and the berries can be steeped in hot water to make tea. Their large stones and tough skins limit use in muffins, pancakes and pies.

MEDICINE: Bush-cranberries are rich in vitamin C. The bark is said to have a sedative effect and to relieve muscle spasms, so it has been widely used to treat menstrual pains, stomach cramps and sore muscles. Bush-cranberry bark has also been used to relieve asthma, hysteria and convulsions, and it was sometimes given to women threatened with miscarriage (to stop contractions). There is

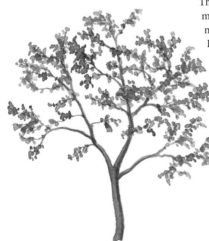

> ### WARNING
> Some sources classify raw bush-cranberries as poisonous, while others report that they were commonly eaten raw by native peoples. A few berries may be harmless, but large quantities cause vomiting and cramps, so it is probably best to cook them before eating. One source reports that the bark tea caused nausea and vomiting.

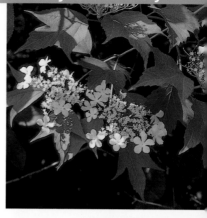

some controversy over bush-cranberry's ability to relieve cramps, but some sources report that pharmacological research supports this use. Commercial "crampbark" was sometimes really the bark of mountain maple (*Acer spicatum*) because of mistakes made by collectors.

OTHER USES: A few people smoked bush-cranberry bark. The berries give a lovely reddish pink dye. The acidic juice was also used as a mordant to set some dyes. American bush-cranberry is used as a garden ornamental.

DESCRIPTION: Deciduous shrubs with opposite, 3-lobed leaves, 3–12 cm long. Flowers white, small, 5-petalled, forming flat-topped clusters, from May to July. Fruits juicy, strong-smelling, red to orange, berry-like drupes, 1–1.5 cm long, with a single flat stone.

Mapleleaf viburnum (*V. acerifolium*) is a 90 cm–1.8 m tall shrub with maple-like leaves and small, white flowers in flat-topped clusters. Flowers 6 mm wide in clusters 5–7.5 cm wide. Grows in moist, upland, hardwood forests in ON, QC and NB. See p. 424 for conservation status.

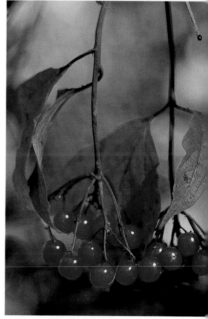

Hobbleberry (*V. alnifolium*) is a 90 cm–3 m tall shrub. Leaves heart-shaped, 7.5–20 cm long, with prominent veins, finely saw-toothed margins and star-like, rusty hairs beneath. Fragrant, flat-topped clusters (5–15 cm wide) of small, white flowers, the outer flowers larger (2.5 cm wide) than the inner ones. Grows in moist woods and shady ravines from ON to the Maritimes. See p. 424 for conservation status.

High bush-cranberry, mooseberry or **squashberry** (*V. edule*), which is sometimes called low bush-cranberry, is a 50 cm–2 m tall shrub whose small, relatively inconspicuous flower clusters lack showy, sterile blooms. Distinctive, musty smell. Grows in shady woods, thickets and cool mountain slopes throughout Canada. See p. 424 for conservation status.

Nannyberry (*V. lentago*) is a shrub, to 9 m tall, with long, tapering leaf tips and winged petioles. Heartwood has an unpleasant, goat-like smell. Fruit raisin-like. Grows in rich soils along woodland edges, streams and rocky hillsides from SK to NB. See p. 424 for conservation status.

American bush-cranberry (all above)
Marsh cranberry (below)

American bush-cranberry or **pembina** (*V. opulus*), which is sometimes called high bush-cranberry, is a 1–4 m tall shrub with relatively deeply cut leaves. Flower clusters have a showy outer ring of large (12–25 mm wide), sterile flowers. Grows in damp soils, hedges, scrubs and woodlands throughout Canada.

Marsh cranberry (*V. trilobum*) is a 3–4.5 m tall shrub with large, showy, white, sterile outer flowers in each cluster, and bright red, translucent berries in late summer and autumn. Grows in low, moist sites and along streambanks throughout Canada. See p. 424 for conservation status.

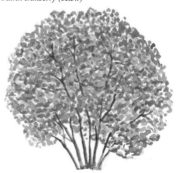

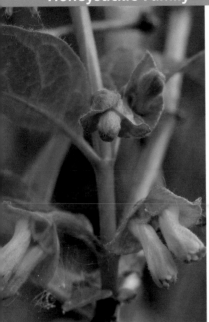

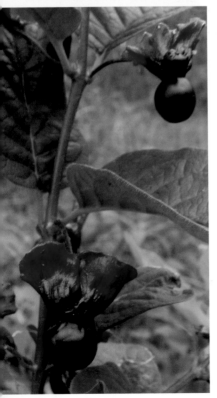

Black Twinberry
Lonicera involucrata

FOOD: The shiny, black, bitter berries were not eaten and were considered poisonous by many. On the Pacific coast, they acquired names such as "raven's food" and "monster food," and there were some taboos against eating them. The Kwakwaka'wakw, for example, believed that eating black twinberries would render a person unable to speak.

MEDICINE: Twinberry bark was taken for coughs and its leaves chewed and applied externally to itchy skin, boils and gonorrheal sores. Berry tea was used as a cathartic and emetic as a means to purify the body and cleanse the stomach and chest. A decoction of twinberry leaves or inner bark was used as daily eyewash to bathe sore eyes. It was used alone or mixed with other plants, most often yellow-cedar (p. 48), on painful areas of the body, most often the shoulders, feet and legs. A tea made from the bark was rubbed on a mother's breast to stimulate milk flow. Boiled leaves and sticks were applied externally to swellings, sores, scabs and broken bones. Boiled bark was applied to burns, infection and wounds.

OTHER USES: The stems were used by First Nations as building materials and to make fibres for mats, baskets, bags, blankets and toys. The hollow stems were used by children as straws. A black dye was obtained from the crushed berries of twinberry and used for basketry materials. It was also rubbed onto the scalp as a tonic to prevent greyness. The tiny berries were crushed and rubbed in the hair for dandruff. Historically, a decoction of twinberry bark was eaten by whalers to relieve the effects of sexual abstinence. Twinberry is resistant to air pollution and sometimes planted as an ornamental.

DESCRIPTION: Deciduous, erect shrub, to 5 m tall, with 4-angled twigs that are greenish when young, greyish with shreddy bark when older. Leaves oval, to 16 cm long and 8 cm wide, sharp-pointed at tip. Flowers bell-shaped, yellow, 1–2 cm long, from May to July, in pairs surrounded by fused bracts (an "involucre," hence the scientific name *involucrata*). Fruits shiny, black berries, to 1.2 cm across. Grows in moist or wet soil in forests, clearings, riverbanks, swamps and thickets across Canada from YT and BC to QC. See p. 424 for conservation status.

Buffaloberry & Soapberry

Shepherdia spp.

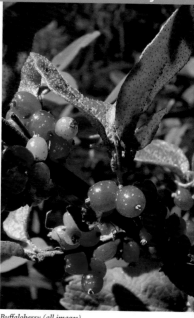

Buffaloberry (all images)

FOOD: Soapberries were collected by beating the branches over a canvas or hide and then rolling the berries into a container to separate leaves and other debris. Soapberries were eaten fresh, or they were boiled, formed into cakes and dried over a small fire for future use. Blackfoot ate buffaloberries fresh or dried for winter, preserved in jellies or cooked with sugar to make pudding. More recently, the berries have been preserved by canning or freezing. Because their juice is rich in saponin, soapberries become foamy when beaten. They were mixed about 4:1 with water and whipped like egg whites to make a white to salmon-coloured, foamy dessert called "Indian ice cream." Traditionally, this dessert was beaten by hand or with a special stick with grass or strands of bark tied to one end, but these tools were eventually replaced by egg-beaters and mixers. Like egg whites, soapberries will not foam in plastic or greasy containers. The foam is rather bitter, so it was usually sweetened with sugar or with other berries. Soapberries were also added to stews or cooked to make syrup, jelly or a sauce for buffalo steaks. Canned soapberry juice, mixed with sugar and water, makes a refreshing "lemonade." Although they are bitter, soapberries are often abundant and can be used in moderation as an emergency food (see **Warning**).

MEDICINE: Soapberries are rich in vitamin C and iron. They have been taken to treat flu and indigestion and have been made into a medicinal tea for relieving constipation. Buffaloberries were used to treat stomachaches. Canned soapberry juice, mixed with sugar and water, was said to cure acne, boils, digestive problems and gallstones. Soapberry bark tea was a favourite solution for eye troubles. Twigs of soapberry and buffaloberry were boiled to make a laxative tea.

OTHER USES: The soapy berries of soapberry were crushed or boiled and used as soap.

DESCRIPTION: Deciduous shrubs with opposite leaves. Flowers yellowish to greenish, male and female flowers on separate plants, single or forming small clusters. Fruits berries.

Soapberry or **soopolallie** (*S. canadensis*) is a shrub, to 2 m tall, with young twigs covered in a rusty "scurf." Leaves rusty underneath (at least when young). Grows in open woods and on streambanks throughout Canada (except PEI). See p. 424 for conservation status.

Silver buffaloberry (*S. argentea*) is a tall shrub, to 6 m tall, with young twigs covered in a silvery "scurf." Leaves silvery underneath (at least when young). Grows in open woods and hillsides from southern AB to southern MB.

> **WARNING**
> Both species contain saponin, a bitter, soapy substance that can irritate the stomach and cause diarrhea, vomiting and cramps if consumed in large amounts.

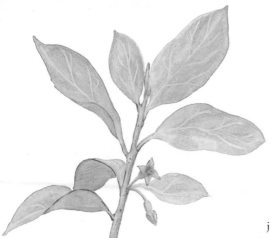

Wolfwillow
Elaeagnus commutata

FOOD: The berries (known as "silverberries") are very dry and astringent, but some northern tribes gathered them for food. Most groups considered the mealy berries famine food. Silverberries were eaten raw or cooked in soup. They were also cooked with blood, mixed with lard and eaten raw, fried in moose fat or frozen. They make good jams and jellies. The berries are much sweeter after exposure to freezing temperatures.

MEDICINE: The bark was used by some First Nations as a medicine. A strong decoction would be mixed with grease or lotion to take away the sting of frostbite or sunburn. When western meadow rue (*Thalictrum occidentalis*) was added to the mix, it was used to treat hemorrhoids. When sumac roots (p. 90) were added, the decoction was used to treat syphilis. A weak tea was taken as a remedy for chest colds.

OTHER USES: The bark was used to make cord, and several tribes used the nutlets inside the berries as decorative beads. The fruits were boiled to remove the flesh, and while the seeds were still soft, a hole was made through each. They were then threaded, dried, oiled and polished. These flowers can be detected from metres away by their sweet, heavy perfume. Some people enjoy this fragrance, but others find it overwhelming and nauseating. If green wolfwillow wood is burned in a fire, it gives off a strong smell of human excrement. Some practical jokers enjoy sneaking branches into the fire and watching the reactions of fellow campers.

DESCRIPTION: Thicket-forming, rhizomatous shrub with 2–6 cm long, alternate, lance-shaped, deciduous, silvery leaves covered in dense, tiny, star-shaped hairs (appearing silvery). Flowers strongly sweet-scented, yellow inside and silvery outside, 6–16 mm long, borne in twos or threes from leaf axils, from June to July. Fruits silvery, mealy, about 1 cm long, drupe-like, with a single large nutlet. Grows on well-drained, often calcareous slopes, gravel bars and forest edges at low to montane elevations from BC to QC and in YT. See p. 424 for conservation status.

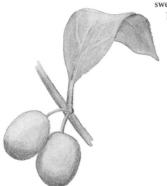

Labrador Teas

Ledum spp.

FOOD: These aromatic leaves, and occasionally their flowers, have been widely used for making tea. Fresh or dried leaves were steeped in boiling water, but some people prepared a stronger, darker brew by boiling them for hours or even days (see **Warning**). The fragrant, steeped brew was served hot, cooled or chilled, either alone or sweetened with sugar. All species have been used for teas, but glandular Labrador tea is relatively toxic (see **Warning**).

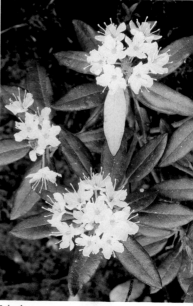

Labrador tea

MEDICINE: Labrador tea was one of the most commonly used medicines of First Nations in Canada. It has been used to treat colds, sore throats and allergies. Although it is slightly laxative, the tea was said to soothe diarrhea and stomach upset. Some people recommended glandular Labrador tea as a relaxant, and Labrador tea was considered a mild narcotic, taken by some Aboriginal women 3 times daily prior to giving birth. Scandinavians let a handful of crushed leaves soak in an alcoholic drink and then used the liquor as a sedative nightcap. Alcohol extracts of the leaves have been used to treat scabies, lice, chiggers and fungal skin diseases. An ointment made from the dried, powdered leaves or roots was applied to ulcers, cracked nipples, burns and scalds. Strong decoctions were applied to inflamed, itchy or oozing skin conditions.

OTHER USES: Dried leaves were sometimes stored in grain to repel mice and rats, and in clothes cupboards to repel insects. They were also added to smoking mixtures, in moderation, for their mild euphoric effect and their flavour. Alcohol extracts of the leaves provided insect repellent and a remedy for insect bites. The plant also provides a brown dye.

DESCRIPTION: Evergreen shrubs, 50 cm–1.5 m tall. Leaves alternate, leathery, elliptic to oblong. Flowers white, about 1–1.5 cm across, 5-petalled, forming flat-topped clusters, from June to August. Fruits round, nodding capsules, 3–7 mm long on 1–2 cm long stalks.

See p. 424 for conservation status. / See p. 398 / Do not confuse Labrador tea with the poisonous bog-laurels (p. 398).

WARNING

Large amounts of Labrador tea can cause drowsiness, increased urination and intestinal disturbance. All species contain narcotic compounds and toxins, which can cause cramps, delirium, palpitations, paralysis and even death. Glandular Labrador tea is poisonous to livestock, especially sheep. Some sources suggest boiling for long periods to destroy the alkaloids, but others say that boiling releases ledol, so it is not recommended. Do not confuse Labrador tea with the poisonous bog-laurels (p. 398). Pregnant women should not use Labrador tea.

Labrador tea (*L. groenlandicum*) has leaves 6 cm long, with rusty-woolly undersides. Grows in cold bogs and coniferous forests at low to montane elevations throughout Canada. See p. 424 for conservation status.

Glandular Labrador tea or **trapper's tea** (*L. glandulosum*) has pale lower leaf surfaces, with dense resin glands among short, white scales. Grows in moist meadows and forests at montane to subalpine elevations in BC and AB. See p. 424 for conservation status.

Marsh Labrador tea (*L. palustre*) has leaves to 1.5 cm long and lacks the glands of *L. glandulosum*. Grows in the arctic and subarctic regions in all territories and northern regions from BC to Labrador and was widely used by the Inuit.

Mayflower
Epigaea repens

FOOD: Once plentiful around the region, mayflower has become scarce because of its sensitivity to abrupt environmental changes. The flowers were often picked from trail sides during long walks and eaten raw or added to salads. The sour-sweet flavour was said to quench thirst.

MEDICINE: Named by the early pilgrims after the ship that had brought them to the New World, the mayflower had long been revered by the native Potawatomi tribe, who believed that this special wildflower came directly from their divinity. The plant was used by First Nations to make a leaf tea to treat kidney disorders, stomachaches, abdominal pains and indigestion. The Shakers once produced and sold this remedy under the name of "gravel plant" to treat gravel (kidney stones) and other kidney, bladder and urethra disorders. The responsible compound, arbutin, has been demonstrated to be an effective urinary antiseptic, but it may be toxic (see **Warning**).

OTHER USES: In a poem entitled "The Mayflowers," American Quaker John Greenleaf Whittier (1807–1892) describes the appearance of the first mayflower bloom as a sign that the pilgrims' first terrible winter was over. The perceived ability of this small, delicate flower to endure the harshest winters made it a powerful symbol of resilience through adversity. Consequently, it has become the floral emblem of NS. The mayflower was officially adopted in 1901 by an Act of Legislature stating that it was "hereby declared to be and from time immemorial to have been the emblem of Nova Scotia." Since at least 1825, it was used as the front cover motif for 2 newspapers, it graced the Lieutenant Governor's chain of state and stamps and coins of the province, and it appeared on the buttons and decorative brass of the NS militia. The plant can be grown as groundcover but is difficult to cultivate.

DESCRIPTION: Trailing, evergreen shrub with sweet-scented, pink or white flowers, 1–1.5 cm wide, in terminal and axillary clusters. Flowers tubular with 5 flaring lobes and hairy within, from February to May. Leaves leathery, 2–7.5 cm long, oval with hairy margins. Fruit a capsule splitting into 5 parts, exposing a whitish pulp covered with tiny seeds. Grows in sandy or rocky woods and clearings from SK to the Maritimes.

WARNING

The active principal of mayflower, arbutin, inhibits the enzyme tyrosinase and thus prevents the formation of melanin. It is therefore useful as a skin-lightening agent. When ingested, it is converted to hydroquinone, a potentially cancerous aromatic organic compound.

Pipsissewa or Prince's Pines

Chimaphila spp.

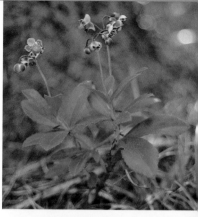

FOOD: Pipsissewa has been used to flavour candy, soft drinks (especially root beer) and traditional beers. The stems and roots were used to make tea, and the leaves and berries have been used as a trail nibble, but they are too tough and astringent to be eaten in large quantities.

MEDICINE: This plant was widely used for a variety of infections. Pipsissewa tea was used as a remedy for kidney and bladder problems, fevers, colds, sore throats, coughs, backaches and stomachaches. It was used as eye drops to relieve irritation from heat, smoke or perspiration. The infusion was also applied externally to heal thrush, sores and skin rashes. Fresh, bruised leaves were applied to the skin to cause redness and blistering as part of the treatment for heart and kidney diseases, tuberculosis of the lymph nodes and chronic rheumatism. A solution made by soaking the leaves in warm water was applied to heal blisters. Pipsissewa was often used to induce sweating and treat fevers. The berries were eaten as a digestive tonic. Recent research has confirmed the potent antimicrobial action of extracts of pipsissewa leaf on a variety of pathogenic fungi. One of the active ingredients has been identified as the anthroquinone chimiphilin.

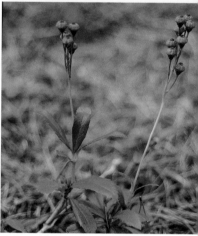

Pipsissewa (all images)

OTHER USES: Some indigenous peoples dried and ground the leaves and used them for smoking.

DESCRIPTION: Semi-woody, low, evergreen shrubs from rhizomes, with whorls of 2–5 glossy, green leaves 2–7 cm long. Flowers light pink or rose-tinged, waxy, about 1 cm across, nodding above the leaves in erect clusters, from June to August. Fruits round capsules, about 5–7 mm wide.

Pipsissewa or **prince's pine** (*C. umbellata*) is 10–30 cm tall, with flowers in clusters of 3–8. Found in dry to mesic mixed woods and coniferous forests all across Canada, except NU. See p. 424 for conservation status.

Little prince's pine (*C. menziesii*) is generally shorter (5–20 cm tall), with 1–3 flowers per stem. Found in dry to mesic coniferous forests in southern BC. See p. 424 for conservation status.

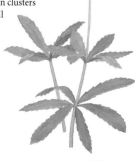

> **WARNING**
> Pipsissewa has shown hypoglycemic activity in experiments. Leaves, bruised and held against the skin, can cause reddening, blistering and peeling.

133

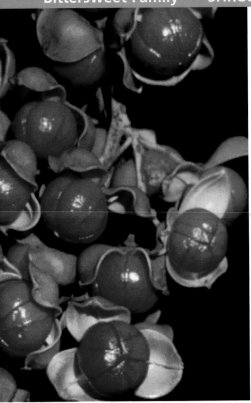

American Bittersweet

Celastrus scandens

FOOD: The showy, berry-like fruits provide winter food for wildlife species such as grouse, pheasant, quail, rabbit and squirrel. To humans, however, they are quite poisonous. First Nations reportedly boiled the bark or inner bark of the stem, said to be sweet and palatable, to make a thick soup. However, this was considered a starvation food and eaten only when other foods were in short supply.

MEDICINE: Although this is a medicinal plant with a history of use by First Nations, it is scarcely used today by modern herbalists. Traditionally, the root bark tea was used to induce sweating, urination and vomiting and considered effective in the treatment of chronic liver and skin disorders, rheumatism, leucorrhea, dysentery and irregular menstruation. It was also given to pregnant women alone or combined with red raspberry leaf (p. 94) to reduce the pain of childbirth. An infusion of leaves and stems would be given to a woman to reduce fever and soreness from pregnancy. An infusion of the bark was taken for upset stomachs, and a decoction for bowel complaints and as a physic, especially for babies. The root was chewed for coughs and tuberculosis. An infusion of the root was prescribed for kidney trouble following childbirth and a leaf tea for diarrhea and dysentery. The bark was applied externally as an ointment on burns, scrapes, tumours and skin eruptions. As a poultice, the boiled root was used to treat obstinate sores and other skin eruptions. Extracts of the bark are reportedly cardioactive.

OTHER USES: The most important use today for bittersweet is as a decorative vine, available in farmers' markets and nurseries from spring to autumn. Historically, First Nations prepared a decoction of the roots and used it as a wash on the lips of bad children. The chewed root was traditionally smeared on the body, believing that the user would be impervious to wounding. Related plants are under study as botanical insecticides.

DESCRIPTION: Twining, woody vine with alternate, oval to lance-shaped, finely serrated leaves, 5–10 cm long. Flowers small, 4 mm wide, green with 4–5 petals, in terminal clusters to 10 cm long, from May to June. Fruits yellow-orange, opening when ripe and exposing the scarlet, berry-like interior. Grows in thickets, woods and on riverbanks from southern SK to NB. See p. 424 for conservation status.

WARNING
All parts of the plant, including the berries, are potentially toxic and should not be consumed, especially by pregnant and nursing women.

Burning Bush

Euonymus atropurpureus

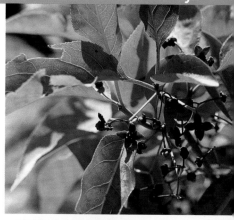

FOOD: Although inedible to humans, the fruit is eaten by several species of birds, such as wild turkey. There have been reports that the fruit was eaten by humans, but it should be avoided considering that the fruit, seeds and bark are poisonous.

MEDICINE: This species was much employed by First Nations and was an extremely popular diuretic drug during the 19th century, especially in England. Historically, the bark was considered a tonic, laxative, stimulant and expectorant, recommended for chest and lung congestion, indigestion and fevers. In small doses, it was said to stimulate the appetite, but larger doses would irritate the intestinal lining. An infusion of the roots was recommended for uterine prolapse, vomiting of blood and painful urination. The bark is employed in modern herbalism as a gallbladder remedy to treat biliousness and chronic liver disease with concurrent fever, and for any skin eruptions associated with it, such as eczema. Some herbal texts describe it as a plant having few equals and no supe-

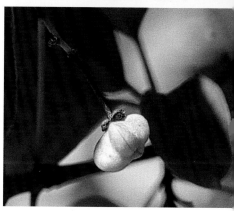

riors in regards to its effect on the liver. Bark tea, syrup or extract was used to treat fevers, upset stomachs, constipation, edema, lung complaints, liver congestion and heart conditions. A 1912 report found that the bark displayed digitalis-like effects on the heart, and this boosted the herb's popularity as a heart medicine. It was dropped as an official drug plant in the US in 1916 but remained on the National Formulary until 1947. First Nations used the plant for a variety of gynecological problems, as an eye lotion and for facial sores. The powdered root was smeared on the scalp as a remedy for dandruff. The seed was used as a strong laxative and emetic.

OTHER USES: The thin, straight stems made ideal hunting arrows.

DESCRIPTION: Fairly nondescript large shrub or small tree, to 2.5 m tall, that can be identified when not in flower by its thin stems, opposite leaves and small, terminal buds. Leaves dark green, simple, elliptic, 4–13 cm long, toothed and pointed with a slightly hairy underside. Buds small, green-tinged red with 5–6 scales. Stems slender, green-brown, smooth and more or less 4-angled. Older stems develop corky striations. Flowers small, deep purple, 4-petalled, in 2–3 branched clusters of 7–15 flowers, from May to July. Fruit a smooth, deeply 4-lobed, purple capsule bearing brown seeds covered with a scarlet aril. Grows in rich woods and thickets in southern ON. See p. 424 for conservation status.

> **WARNING**
> The leaves, bark and berries are potentially poisonous and can cause nausea, cold sweats and prostration. Excess consumption of the bark may result in severe purgative action. This plant should not be consumed.

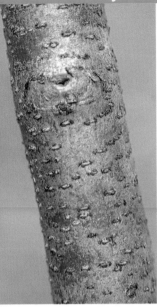

Common Hop Tree
Ptelea trifoliata

FOOD: An infusion of the leaves contains tannic and gallic acids and has a bitter taste resembling that of hops (*Humulus lupus*), hence this plant's use as a hop substitute when brewing beer.

MEDICINE: A tincture of the inner bark is considered to have tonic, antiperiodic and stomachic properties and was recommended as a tonic for convalescents recovering from malaria, to aid digestion, relieve asthma and purify the blood. It is believed to have a soothing influence on mucous membranes and to increase appetite. The bark is known to contain a volatile oil, an oleoresin and the alkaloid berberine. The alkaloid arginine is present in the root. The bark of the hop tree has a strong, medicinal smell akin to that of licorice root, and a disagreeable taste—somewhat resinous, bitter and acrid. The leaves and fruit have also reportedly been used medicinally.

OTHER USES: This relatively small tree makes a striking garden planting either in large containers or directly in the ground. In spring, it provides a mass of young, yellow leaves and orange-scented flowers, the leaves later turning pleasantly aromatic in summer. In autumn, the foliage turns a pretty yellow colour, and the seed wings provide an interesting sight through most of winter.

DESCRIPTION: Deciduous tree, to 6 m tall, forming a broad, rounded canopy and dark grey, almost smooth bark. Leaves consisting of 3 leaflets, elliptic to oval, glossy, dark green above, pale and hairy below, untoothed or sparsely toothed, to 10 cm long and 4 cm wide; glands on leaf surface emit aromatic oil; turn yellow in autumn. Flowers 1 cm wide; green to yellow-green; 4–5 petals, in upright clusters to 7.5 cm across. Fruit pale green ripening to brown, 2 seeds held in the centre of a broad, circular wing to 2.5 cm wide. Inhabits moist woods, alluvial thickets and rocky slopes and gravels in ON; naturalized in southwestern QC. See p. 424 for conservation status.

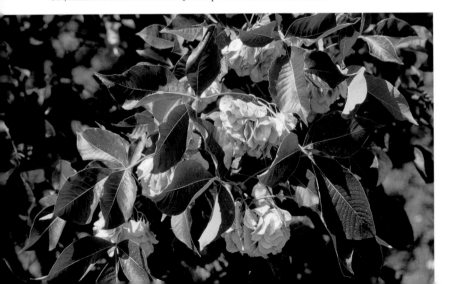

Northern Prickly Ash

Zanthoxylum americanum

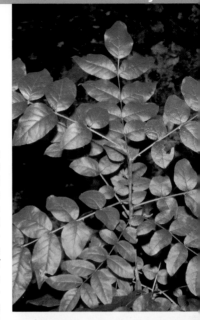

FOOD: This plant was used as a honey plant.

MEDICINE: Prickly ash is used topically by herbalists as a circulatory stimulant and for rheumatism. The Ojibwa made a tea from the bark and berries to treat sore throats and bronchitis and applied the bark to treat toothaches (another common name is toothache-tree). They also made a decoction of the bark and root with the roots of wild ginger (p. 203) and sweet-flag (p. 166) to treat colds and coughs. The Algonquin used a root infusion and a poultice of inner bark to treat rheumatism. Parts of this tree have been used to improve digestion, increase circulation, strengthen the nervous system and treat aching muscles, skin infections and even cholera. Prickly ash is said to have a generally stimulating effect on the body, including the lymph system and mucous membranes, and has been prescribed as a massage lotion for rheumatism and arthritis. It is also recommended for circulatory ailments such as varicose veins and chilblains. Twigs of this tree have been used as toothbrushes. The leaves were used on skin conditions and especially on mouth sores, including both thrush and canker sores. The leaves contain significant quantities of furanocoumarins with potent light-activated antimicrobial properties. Unfortunately, these can photosensitize skin, causing redness and, in extreme cases, blistering in sunlight. The active ingredients in the bark and root are pyranocoumarins and simple phenolics, flavonoids and tannins. Furanocoumarins are not present in these parts, and they are safe to use. Canadian collections of prickly ash contain little in the way of alkaloids, though these compounds are reported from US collections.

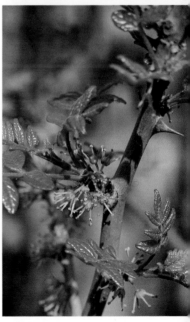

OTHER USES: The wood is considered of little value, but all parts of the plant impart a pleasant, orange-like perfume.

DESCRIPTION: Deciduous shrub or small tree growing to 6 m tall. Leaves alternate, pinnately compound; leaflets 5–11, oval, with pointed tips and toothed edges. Trunk and stems covered in distinctive paired, broad-based prickles. Flowers yellow, small; 4–5 petals, appearing in spring before leaves and forming in clusters on the axils of second-year twigs; male and female flowers on separate plants. Fruits red or reddish brown; pitted surface, opening to expose and eventually drop small, black seeds; fruit smells like oranges when crushed. Found in rich woods and damp thickets in ON and southwestern QC. See p. 424 for conservation status.

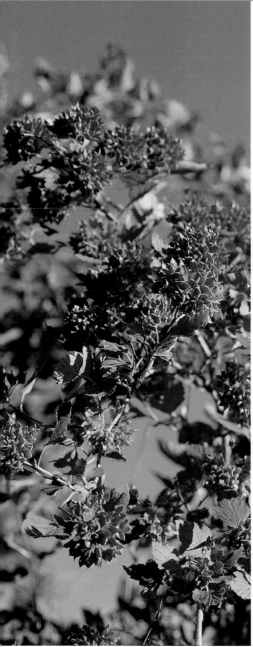

Pacific ninebark

Ninebarks

Physocarpus spp.

FOOD: The roots of mallow ninebark were steam cooked and eaten by the Okanagan-Colville people in BC.

MEDICINE: Pacific ninebark is known for its astringent, diuretic and purgative properties. The roots of Pacific ninebark were boiled and placed as a poultice on sores, burns, swellings and lesions. A decoction of the inner bark was taken as an emetic by people who were "dizzy with pain," as a laxative, to treat gonorrhea and as a wash for scrofulous glands on the neck. The plant contains chemical triterpenes in the stem bark.

OTHER USES: The common name ninebark comes from the exuberant peeling of the bark; it is said that the plant has 9 layers of bark. The flowers are a good nectar source and are eaten by many bird species.

DESCRIPTION: Deciduous shrubs with brown, peeling bark; leaves alternate, simple, 3–10 cm long, palmately lobed with 3–5 lobes; flowers white, 5-petalled, 7–10 mm wide, in terminal rounded clusters, blooming from May to July; fruit egg-shaped, red at maturity, in clusters of 3–5 per flower.

Pacific ninebark (*P. capitatus*) grows to 4 m tall on wet sites; fruits smooth, with 3–5 follicles united only at their base. Found along streams, gravel bars and moist to wet thickets and forests in BC and southwestern AB (Waterton Lakes).

Mallow ninebark (*P. malvaceus*) grows to 2 m tall on dry sites; fruits densely hairy with star-shaped hairs, with 2 follicles united for at least half their length. Found on rocky hillsides, open forests and grasslands in southeastern BC and southwestern AB.

Hardhacks

Spiraea spp.

MEDICINE: Hardhacks have both astringent and diuretic properties, and parts of the plants have been used in the treatment of diarrhea, dysentery, bowel complaints, hemorrhages and ulcers. A compound decoction of shoots or vines was used as a wash for babies with diarrhea. A compound decoction of the bark was taken to induce vomiting and also to treat initial stages of consumption. An infusion of the bark was used as a bodywash to make children stronger in order to walk. An infusion of leaves and flowers of eastern hardhack was taken for morning sickness during pregnancy and to help ease childbirth. A poultice made from hardhack leaves was applied to tumours and ulcers.

OTHER USES: Western hardhack branches were used to make brooms to collect marine dentalia shells, and also to hang salmon for drying and smoking. The dried flower spikes of hardhack are eaten by grouse.

DESCRIPTION: Deciduous shrubs with leaves alternate, simple, irregularly toothed, dark green above, whitish hairy beneath. Flowers deep pink, about 5 mm across, crowded into 5–30 cm long clusters. Fruits follicles. Found in streambanks, wet meadows, swamps or marsh edges.

Western hardhack (*S. douglasii*) is a tall shrub, to 2.5 m tall, with leaves 4–10 cm long, and a shiny fruit that is hairless or nearly so. Found in BC.

Eastern hardhack or **steeplebush** (*S. tomentosa*) is a smaller shrub, to 1 m tall, with smaller leaves (3–5 cm long) and a densely hairy fruit. Found from MB to the Maritimes.

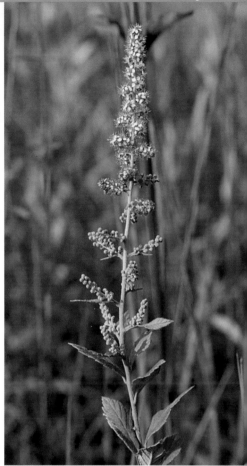

Eastern hardhack (above)
Western hardhack (below)

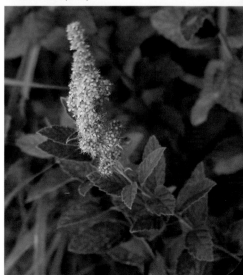

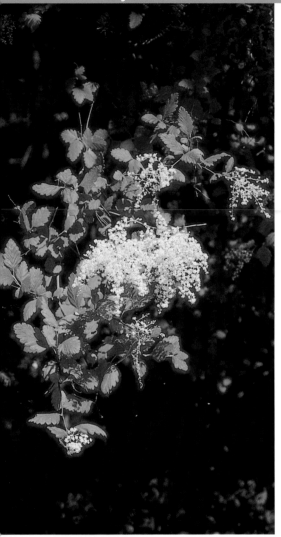

Oceanspray
Holodiscus discolor

FOOD: The small, dry, flattened fruits of this species can be eaten raw or cooked.

MEDICINE: The leaves or dried seeds were boiled to make medicinal teas for treating influenza, and inner bark tea was used as an eyewash. The bark tea was used as a tonic for convalescents and athletes, and it was taken to treat internal bleeding, diarrhea, stomach upset, flu and colds. The bark was dried, powdered, mixed with petroleum jelly and applied to burns. Some indigenous peoples used the flowers to relieve diarrhea, measles and chickenpox and as a blood tonic.

OTHER USES: The wood is extremely hard—other common names included arrow-wood and ironwood—and straight young shoots were used to make arrow, spear and harpoon shafts. It could be made harder by heating over a fire and polishing with horsetail stems. Larger branches were fashioned into a variety of tools and utensils, including digging sticks, cambium scrapers, barbeque sticks, octopus spears, bows, arrows, knitting needles, baby cradle covers, tepee pins, fish clubs, drum hoops and canoe paddles. The wood was reputed not to burn, and for this reason it was used to make roasting tongs. Pioneers made wooden nails, and the Thompson tribe made breast-plates and other types of armour from oceanspray wood.

DESCRIPTION: Slender, deciduous shrub, 1–4 m tall, with arching, slightly angled branches. Leaves oval, coarsely toothed to shallowly lobed, the blades 4–7 cm long, with pale, soft-hairy, lower surfaces. Flowers creamy white, 5 mm across, 5-petalled, forming feathery, pyramidal, terminal, branched clusters, from June to August, that often persist for at least 1 year. Fruits hairy, brown, seed-like achenes, about 2 mm long. Found in open woods, thickets, clearings and forest edges in lowland and montane zones in southern BC and the Bella Coola valley.

Shrubby Cinquefoil

Pentaphylloides floribunda

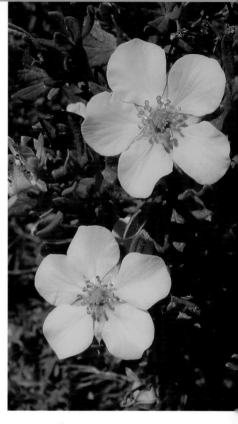

FOOD: The leaves of shrubby cinquefoil were mixed with dried meat to add fragrance and spiciness. The leaves and stems were drunk as a tea that is high in calcium.

MEDICINE: Shrubby cinquefoil leaves, stems and roots were boiled together and drunk to treat fever that is accompanied by body aches. This plant is considered to be a mild astringent, so medicinal teas were also used to treat congestion, including tuberculosis.

OTHER USES: Shrubby cinquefoil used to be known as *Potentilla fruticosa*. Shrubby cinquefoil leaves have been used to fill pillows. The dry, flaky bark was used as tinder when starting a fire with twirling sticks. This species is a common garden ornamental with many cultivars. It has often been used for erosion control, especially along highways.

DESCRIPTION: Multi-branched shrub, to 1.5 m tall, the young branches silky-hairy, older branches hairless with peeling bark. Leaves alternate, deciduous, pinnately compound with 3–7 (usually 5) leaflets to 2 cm long. Flowers yellow, saucer-shaped, single in leaf axils or in small clusters at branch tips. Fruits egg-shaped, hairy achenes to 2 mm long. Widespread; grows in prairies, open forests and wetlands across Canada, including arctic and high altitude, mountainous regions. See p. 424 for conservation status.

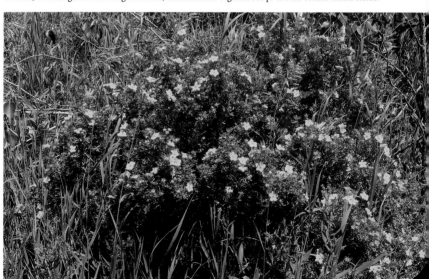

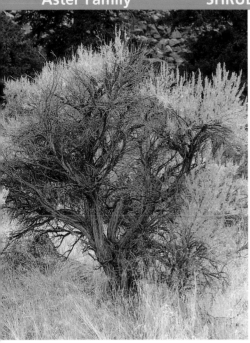

Big Sagebrush
Artemisia tridentata

FOOD: Although sagebrush seeds can be quite bitter, they were used for food by some people, and the seeds of big sagebrush were considered the best. The seeds were eaten raw or dried, but usually they were ground into meal and cooked in pinole, soups and stews. The volatile oils of these plants sometimes added flavour and fragrance to liqueurs.

MEDICINE: Big sagebrush tea was taken to treat colds, fevers, pneumonia and sore eyes and to ease childbirth. It was also used to soak sore feet. Hunters and athletes used it to cleanse the body before long hikes or competitions. The leaves, chewed and swallowed or boiled to make medicinal teas, were taken to relieve stomachaches, coughing, bleeding and postpartum pain and to expel intestinal parasites. Settlers used big sagebrush to treat headaches, diarrhea, vomiting and bullet wounds. Wet leaves were used as poultices to reduce swelling and infection. Sagebrush extracts are believed to kill many types of bacteria and can be applied (with caution; see **Warning**) to cuts, scrapes and other skin problems to combat infection.

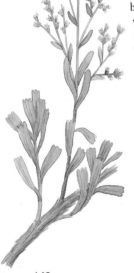

OTHER USES: These shrubs were often burned as firewood, especially if no other wood was available. The aromatic smoke from green, leafy branches provided a ceremonial smudge to cleanse participants of evil spirits and impurities. Leafy branches were used as switches in sweat baths or were tied together with wire to make brooms. Big sagebrush was woven into mats, bags and clothing. The leaf tea was applied to cuts on sheep (from barbed wire, etc.) to speed healing. The aromatic, volatile oils of these plants were used in hair tonics and shampoos and as moth and flea repellents.

DESCRIPTION: Greyish, hairy, fragrant, evergreen shrub, to 2.5 m tall, with greyish brown, peeling bark. Leaves greyish green, 1–2 cm long, narrowly wedge-shaped, 3-toothed at the tip and tapered to the base. Flowerheads 2–3 mm wide, yellow or brownish clusters of 5–8 disc flowers, forming long, narrow (to 7 cm wide) clusters, from July to October. Fruits sparsely hairy seeds (achenes). Covers many acres of dry land in prairies, foothill and montane zones in southern BC and AB. See p. 424 for conservation status.

WARNING
Many people are allergic to big sagebrush, and in rare cases it causes inflammation when applied to the skin. Some classify it as toxic, reporting that it can damage the liver and intestinal tract. It is probably best to use sagebrush for external applications only.

Rabbitbrushes

Chrysothamnus and *Ericameria*

FOOD: The milky sap of these shrubs contains latex (rubbery compounds). The bark of the lower stem and roots of several species of rabbitbrush was widely used as chewing gum. Although the sap also has rubbery properties that make it chewy, it was not extracted for use as gum.

MEDICINE: The roots of common rabbitbrush were boiled to make a strong decoction for treating coughs, fevers, colds and old internal injuries and for easing menstrual cramps. To relieve headaches, the leaves were used to make a medicinal tea that was applied as a lotion. The leaf tea was also taken internally to reduce fevers and relieve constipation, colds and stomach problems. Mashed rabbitbrush leaves were packed onto decayed teeth to relieve toothaches.

OTHER USES: The branches of rabbitbrush were burned slowly to smoke hides. The leafy boughs were used to cover sweat houses and to carpet the floor. Mature flowers were boiled for at least 6 hours to produce a lemon yellow dye. Alum was then added as a mordant, along with the wool or leather to be dyed, and boiling continued for about an hour. When dying baskets, the flowers and buds were boiled overnight and the basket material was then soaked in the dye for about 12 hours. No mordant was used. Immature buds or twigs gave the dye a greenish tinge.

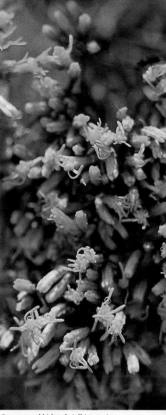

Common rabbitbrush (all images)

DESCRIPTION: Erect, densely branched, perennial shrubs, about 30 cm–1.3 m tall, often flat-topped. Leaves linear, 1–6 cm long, undivided. Flowerheads about 5 mm across, yellow, with about 5 disc flowers and 5 overlapping rows of involucral bracts, forming dense clusters at branch tips, from August to October. Fruits slender, seed-like achenes tipped with a tuft of white hairs (pappus).

Common rabbitbrush (*E. nauseosa*, previously called *Chrysothamnus nauseosus*) is a large shrub, 50 cm–1.3 m tall or more, with felt-covered twigs. Grows on dry prairies, foothill and montane slopes from BC to SK. See p. 424 for conservation status.

Green rabbitbrush (*C. viscidiflorus*) is a much smaller plant, to 35 cm tall, with brittle, minutely hairy twigs. Grows on dry prairies, foothill and montane slopes in extreme south-central BC.

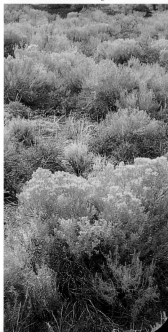

WARNING

Livestock in California are reported to have been poisoned by eating common rabbitbrush. The toxicity of rabbitbrushes is not clear, so these shrubs should not be used in foods or internal medicines.

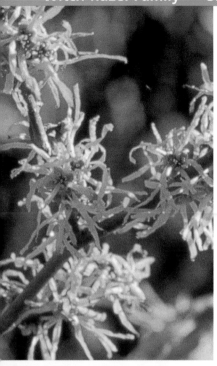

Witch-Hazel

Hamamelis virginiana

FOOD: The plant decoction was sweetened with maple sugar and used as a tea by the Iroquois. The seeds are oily and nutritious and can be eaten.

MEDICINE: Witch-hazel is well known for its astringent and hemostatic (stops bleeding) qualities, and commercial preparations are widely available for topical use. Currently, the leaves and bark of witch-hazel are used in medicinal extracts, skin cosmetics, shaving lotions, mouthwashes, eye lotions, ointments and soaps. Historically, the Iroquois used the inner bark as an emetic, for skin trouble and for sore eyes. First Nations used leaves, twigs and bark to treat skin ulcers, sores, tumours, back problems, dysentery, colds and coughs. It was also used as an astringent and blood purifier. A decoction was rubbed on the legs of participants in games to keep their legs limber.

OTHER USES: The branches, if forked, were often used as divining rods to locate sources of underground water. Branches were also used for bows.

DESCRIPTION: Deciduous shrub or small tree, to 6 m or more tall, with grey or grey-brown bark and several branching stems. Leaves alternate, oval, with wavy edges, to 16 cm long. Flowers 4-petalled, usually yellow (occasionally red), and bloom in autumn. Fruit a woody capsule, 10–14 mm long, that expels the seed explosively (up to 10 m away) in autumn. Most abundant in mesic woods and moist, shaded areas at low to subalpine elevations from southern ON to the Maritimes. See p. 424 for conservation status.

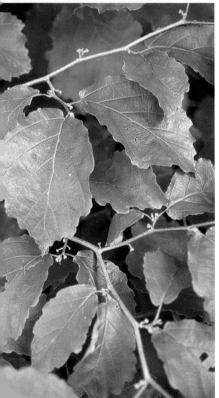

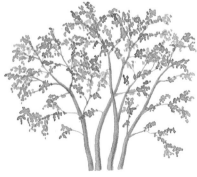

Hazelnuts

Corylus spp.

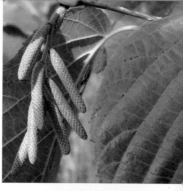

FOOD: One of the more popular and enjoyable wild edibles in North America, hazelnut produces seeds that can be roasted and eaten as is, ground or candied. They can be added to soups, breads, biscuits, sweets and a variety of other foods. They are as good as, but smaller in size than, the cultivated hazelnut (*C. avellana*). Before the seeds ripen in mid- to late autumn, they are softer and sweeter and are especially suited as desserts. Thereafter they are susceptible to being eaten by squirrels. The seeds can be stored for up to 12 months if kept in their shell in a cool, dry place. The seed also provides an edible oil.

MEDICINE: An infusion of the bark of American hazelnut was used by First Nations to treat hives, colds and fevers. The tea is astringent and was used to treat diarrhea, vomiting and cramps. The raw nut was taken for hayfever, childbirth hemorrhage and prenatal strength. A decoction of the roots was mixed with other ingredients and given to teething babies. As a poultice, the bark was used to close wounds and cuts. It was also applied to tumours, old sores and skin cancers. The sharp hairs on the husk were used by First Nations and early physicians to expel worms, although this is a dangerous practice because it causes severe irritation to the intestines. An infusion of the branches and twigs of beaked hazelnut was used by First Nations as a blood purifier to treat heart complaints and gastrointestinal disorders.

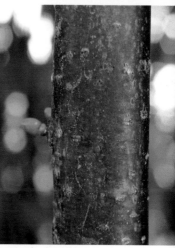

American hazelnut (all images)

OTHER USES: Hazelnut roots are pliable and used to make carrying baskets, baby baskets and other coarse baskets. The twigs were bundled together and made into brushes to serve as brooms. The seed husks were an important component of making a black dye from butternut (p. 63). The two were boiled together, and the tannins in the husks set the dye. The plants grow densely and make good screening hedges.

DESCRIPTION: Tall shrubs, 3–5 m tall, with simple, rounded leaves, 5–12 cm long, somewhat heart-shaped at the base, coarsely double toothed. Male flowers pale yellow, borne in clusters of catkins, 5–12 cm long, on short, lateral shoots on branches, expanding well before leaves, from April to May. Female flowers distal to male, in small clusters largely concealed in the buds, with only the protruding bright red styles visible. Fruit a thin-walled nut, 1–2 cm long, surrounded by a husk that partly to fully encloses the nut.

American hazelnut (*C. americana*) has stem and leafstalks with stiff, glandular hairs. Husk slightly longer than twice the length of the fruit. Grows in moist to dry, open woods and thickets, disturbed sites and on roadsides at low to mid-elevations in southeastern SK and southern MB and ON. See p. 424 for conservation status.

Beaked hazelnut (*C. cornuta*) has glabrous to pubescent branchlets, with or without glandular hairs. Husk soft and bristly, forming a beak 2–5 times longer than the fruit. Grows in moist to dry woodlands, forest edges, disturbed sites and on roadsides throughout southern Canada.

Lewis' Mock-Orange
Philadelphus lewisii

MEDICINE: Historically, mock-orange was used mainly as a topical agent. Fresh mock-orange leaves were bruised and used as poultices to heal infected breasts. Salves were made using either dried leaves or charcoal from burning the wood. Both were ground to a fine powder, which was then mixed with pitch or bear grease. These salves were used for treating sores and swellings. Mock-orange branches, with or without blossoms, were boiled to make medicinal infusions that were used to wash or soak skin affected by eczema and to stop bleeding hemorrhoids.

OTHER USES: Mock-orange wood is stiff and hard. It was used to make a wide variety of items such as combs, knitting needles, basket rims (for birch-bark baskets), pipe stems, fish spears, cradle hoods, arrow and harpoon shafts, snowshoes, digging sticks, clubs, breastplate armour and bows and arrows. The plant was also used as soap, either through soaking the bark, mashing the leaves in water or bruising the leaves and flowers with the hands (to lather into a foam). The blooming bushes also served as an indicator that groundhogs were fat. This attractive shrub, with its dark green foliage and showy, fragrant flowers, makes a lovely addition to sunny or partly shaded gardens. Several cultivars are available from greenhouses and nurseries.

DESCRIPTION: Erect, deciduous shrub, 1.5–3 m tall, with loosely spreading branches and reddish brown bark turning grey and flaking with age. Leaves opposite, oval to rounded, 3–5 cm long, with 3 main veins from the base, slightly roughened. Flowers deliciously fragrant, white, about 3 cm across, with 4 broad, spreading petals, forming showy clusters of 3–15 at the branch tips, from May to July. Fruits woody capsules to 1 cm long. Grows on well-drained sites, along streams, in fields and open forests, in steppe and montane zones from southern BC to southwestern AB.

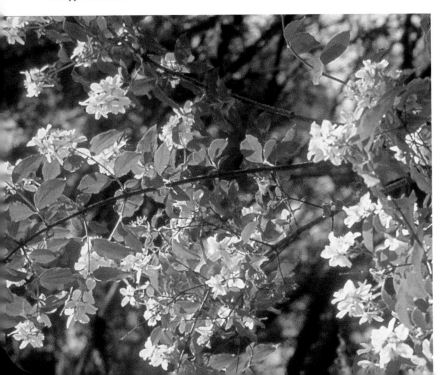

Buttonbush

Cephalanthus occidentalis

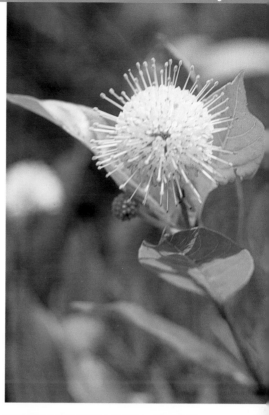

MEDICINE: A tea of buttonbush bark is believed to have astringent, febrifuge, emetic and tonic qualities. A decoction of the bark has been used to treat diarrhea and dysentery as well as stomach ailments and hemorrhages and as a wash for eye inflammations. The inner bark was chewed to treat toothaches, and a decoction of either the roots or fruit has laxative properties. The Ojibwa used tea made with buttonbush stems and leaves to reduce menstrual flow, pain and cramps. Early settlers used the bark as a quinine substitute to treat malaria.

OTHER USES: Buttonbrush flowers are distinctive, pretty, sweet-smelling and attractive to bees and butterflies, making this a good garden plant.

DESCRIPTION: Deciduous shrub, to 8 m tall. Leaves opposite or in whorls, glossy, oblong to elliptic, to 20 cm long and 7 cm wide. Flowers numerous in globular clusters 2.5–3.5 cm in diameter, white to pale yellow, on a 2.5–5 cm long stalk. Individual flowers tubular, 4-lobed, with a long, protruding style. Flowers from June to August. Fruit a hard, spherical ball containing tiny, multiple, 2-seeded nutlets, which usually persist on the plant through winter. Found in swamps and margins of ponds and streams in ON, southwestern QC, NB and NS. See p. 424 for conservation status.

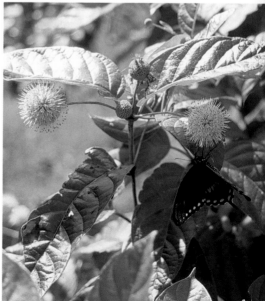

WARNING
Foliage is poisonous to livestock.

Buckbrushes

Ceanothus spp.

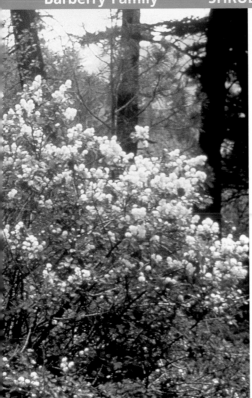

Red-stemmed buckbrush

FOOD: These shrubs are well-known tea substitutes. Dried leaves and flowers were steeped for about 5 minutes to produce a pale, yellowish tea, milder and sweeter than commercial teas. Some people recommend species with resinous leaves, but others prefer less-resinous species.

MEDICINE: Tea made with buckbrush was applied externally and taken internally to relieve alarm or calm nerves. The roots were used to make a medicinal tea for treating inflamed tonsils, enlarged lymph nodes, nonfibrous cysts and enlarged spleens. This tea was also said to be an excellent home remedy for relieving excessive menstrual bleeding, nosebleeds, hemorrhoids, old ulcers and bleeding from vomiting and coughing. It has been recommended for heavy drinkers with inflammation of the stomach, whiskey nose and other symptoms of weak capillaries.

OTHER USES: Buckbrush tea was used as a shampoo and hair tonic. When the flowers are rubbed in water, they produce a soapy foam. The resinous leaves of some species have been used as a substitute for tobacco (p. 240). Buckbrush makes an attractive garden plant. The shrubs are difficult to transplant, so they are best propagated from seed.

DESCRIPTION: Sprawling, spicy-scented shrubs, usually in dense patches. Leaves broadly oval, finely toothed or toothless. Flowers white, tiny, fragrant, forming dense clusters at the tips of side branches, from June to August. Fruits glandular-sticky, 3-lobed capsules, 4–5 mm long, ejecting 3 shiny seeds when mature.

Snowbrush (*C. velutinus*) is a medium-sized shrub, 50 cm–2 m tall, with pyramid-shaped flower clusters. Evergreen leaves sticky and shiny above, with finely toothed blades and 2 tiny (1 mm long) lobes at the stalk base. Found on fairly open sites (shrublands, grasslands, dry, open woodlands) in foothill and montane zones in southern BC and southwestern AB. See p. 424 for conservation status.

Red-stemmed buckbrush (*C. sanguineus*) is a large shrub, 1–3 m tall, also with pyramid-shaped flower clusters. Deciduous leaves neither sticky nor shiny above, and bear 2 slender, 3–8 mm lobes at the base. Found on well-drained slopes and dry, open forests and burns in the foothills of southern BC.

New Jersey tea (*C. americanus*) is a smaller shrub, to 1 m tall, with rounded flower clusters. Deciduous leaves neither sticky nor shiny above, but they are pointy at the tips, which leaves of red-stemmed buckbrush are not. Found in dry, open areas such as roadsides, forest gaps and edges in southern ON and southwestern QC. See p. 424 for conservation status.

WARNING
People with blood disorders or allergies to aspirin should not take buckbrush, and it should be used in moderation during pregnancy.

Sweet Gale
Myrica gale

FOOD: The fruits, leaves and nutlets are edible and can be added to soups and stews. The leaves can be used for tea.

MEDICINE: The Bella Coola would take a decoction of pounded branches alone or with fruits as a diuretic and to treat gonorrhea. The Micmac pounded the roots and soaked them in hot water to treat inflammation. The stem leaf and catkin decoction was drunk to treat tuberculosis.

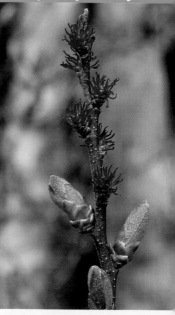

OTHER USES: The Cree used the buds and bark as a yellow dye for porcupine quills, tanning leather and dying wool. The Ojibwa boiled down the branch tips for a brown dye and the seeds to obtain a yellow dye. Woods Cree women gathered female catkins and, once dried, would use them as an ingredient in their lures. Because of its aromatic properties, sweet gale has often been used in households to provide a pleasant scent to linens and cloths and to repel fleas. The essential oil is in demand in the aromatherapy industry. Sweet gale was used to flavour English ale, but fell out of favour after hops became widely available. Although an individual plant will have only male or female catkins, that plant can change sexes from year to year. This may have evolved as a response to preferential feeding on female plants, perhaps by sasquatches. Bacteria growing in root nodules on sweet gale can fix nitrogen, pulling nitrogen gas out of the air and making it available to the plant, which enables it to survive in nitrogen-poor environments such as peat bogs.

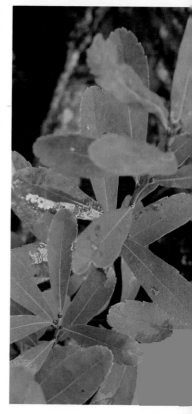

DESCRIPTION: Low, perennial shrub, 50 cm–2 m tall, with loosely branched, brown stems. Leaves fragrant, alternate, to 6 cm long and 3 cm wide, dotted above and below with bright yellow wax glands, whitish underneath, lance-shaped, edges toothed on upper third of leaf. Flowers greenish yellow, waxy catkins, which appear before leaves in spring; male and female on separate plants, male and female catkins to 1.5 cm long. Fruits small, oval nutlets, 2.5–3 mm long, coated with resinous wax, with 2 wing-like scales, in erect brown, cone-like catkins that are 8–10 mm long. Found at low elevations in bogs, swamps, streambanks and thickets in all provinces and territories in Canada. See p. 424 for conservation status.

WARNING
The plant is known to induce abortion, so should not be ingested by pregnant women.

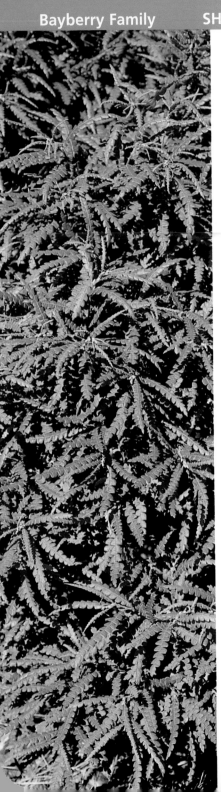

Sweet-Fern
Comptonia peregrina

FOOD: The fruits are edible, and the aromatic leaves are said to make a palatable tea. The Micmac used the berries, bark and leaves as a beverage.

MEDICINE: Sweet-fern was employed medicinally by a number of First Nations living in eastern Canada (Algonquin, Maliseet, Micmac, Ojibwa). The leaves were often made into a poultice to treat wounds such as sprains, swellings, inflammation and poison-ivy (p. 240). Sweet-fern leaves were combined with yarrow (p. 358) to treat swelling and combined with catnip (p. 278) to treat fevers. The leaves were taken internally to treat flu and stomach cramps. The leaves were also used to treat headaches either by ingesting an infusion or inhaling the "perfume" from crushed leaves. The root was also used to treat headaches and inflammation. The plant was smoked as a respiratory aid. One account describes a woman boiling the whole plant and applying it to the outside of her cheek while very hot to treat a toothache. The berries, bark and leaves were ingested as an "exhilarant."

OTHER USES: The Ojibwa lined their buckets with sweet-fern leaves when picking blueberries and covered the berries with leaves to prevent spoiling. The leaves have been used in steam baths and burned as incense. The crushed leaves also repel insects and can be thrown on a campfire to keep mosquitoes away.

DESCRIPTION: Shrub to 1.5 m tall, forming colonies from rhizomes. Stems red-brown to grey, covered in long, white hairs. Leaves sweet-scented, fern-like, alternate, 6–15 cm long, blade cut into 20 or more rounded lobes, tapered at the end, dark green above, pale grey-green and hairy below, with resinous glands covering both surfaces. Flowers small catkins that bloom during April and May; male catkins long (to 5 cm) and narrow, female catkins short (to 5 mm) and rounded; both can be found on an individual plant. Seeds nutlets, 2.5–5.5 mm long, with 4 brown-olive and shiny seeds. Found in open, sandy soils, pinelands, clearings or edges of woodlots at low to montane elevations from ON to NL.

Alders

Alnus spp.

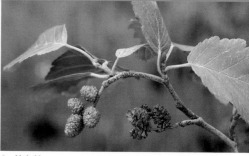
Speckled alder

FOOD: Although the buds and young catkins are not very tasty, they are edible and high in protein and can be eaten in an emergency. Similarly, the inner bark may be eaten raw, cooked or dried and ground into flour.

MEDICINE: Alder bark tea was taken hot to treat tuberculosis of lymph nodes (scrofula) and to regulate menstrual periods and relieve cramping. It was also used as a wash or douche for healing hemorrhoids and vaginal infections. Tea made by boiling the leaves or inner bark has been used as a soothing wash for insect bites, poison-ivy (p. 395) rashes, sores, burns and other skin problems. Bags of heated alder leaves have been used as hot compresses on people suffering from rheumatism. Some tribes chewed the bark and used it as a poultice on cuts, wounds and swellings. The ancient Romans recommended alder leaves for treating tumours. Scientists have discovered 2 tumour-suppressing compounds, betulin and lupeol, in red alder (p. 54).

OTHER USES: Alder was a preferred fuel for smoking fish, meat and hides. It makes excellent fires, with few sparks and little ash. The twigs and inner bark were used to dye hides, feathers, moccasins and fish nets reddish brown or orange. Dyed nets were thought to be harder for fish to see. Boiling produced more brilliant colours, and bark tannin set the colour, so no mordant was needed. Some people even dyed their hair red with alder bark. The bark was sometimes chewed, spat onto hides and rubbed in for colouring. Its high tannin content also helped the tanning process. Alder leaves were used as insoles to ease tired feet. Young boys enjoyed chewing alder buds in spring and spitting jets of dark juice onto the snow—just like real chewing tobacco (p. 240). If someone wanted to appear to be spitting blood, he or she could chew the inner bark and spit red saliva. Moist alder leaves are said to attract fleas, which can then be killed or at least moved outside.

DESCRIPTION: Clumped, deciduous shrubs with scaly, often lichen-covered bark. Leaves alternate, toothed, 4–10 cm long. Flowers tiny, in dense clusters (catkins), with male and female catkins on the same branch. Pollen (male) catkins slender and loosely hanging. Seed (female) catkins woody, cone-like, 1–2 cm long. Fruits tiny nutlets in the seed cones.

Speckled alder (*A. incana* ssp. *rugosa*) is a tall shrub, to 10 m tall, with dull green, thick-textured, double-toothed leaves that are wrinkled above and hoary beneath, veins deeply impressed above. Grows on streambanks, lake shores, in bogs, swamps, wet field edges and roadsides at low to mid-elevations from SK to NL. A closely related species, **mountain alder** (*A. incana* ssp. *tenuifolia*) has thinner and smoother leaves with veins that are not impressed above. Grows on lake shores, wetland margins and in wet forests at montane elevations from YT and BC to SK.

WARNING

Green bark can cause vomiting and sharp pains in the bowels. Bark should be aged for at least a few days prior to use, and bark decoctions were often left to sit until they had changed from yellow to black (2–3 days).

Green and **Sitka alders** (*A. viridis*) are shorter shrubs, to 5 m tall, with dark yellowish green, often shiny leaves with single or double teeth, and seed cones that develop with the leaves on new twigs. **Green alder** (*A. viridis* ssp. *crispa*) grows in sandy or gravelly areas, or on wetland margins, at low to subalpine elevations from eastern AB and eastern NT to NL. **Sitka alder** (*A. viridis* ssp. *sinuata*) grows in similar habitats from YT and northwestern NT to BC and western AB (mostly Rocky Mountains).

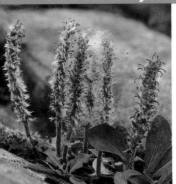

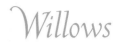

Willows

Salix spp.

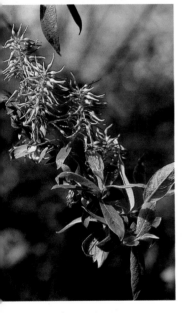

Arctic willow (above)
Bebb's willow (all below)

FOOD: The young shoots and leaves, buds and inner bark of willow are edible, though rather bitter, and they can be used raw or cooked as an emergency food that is rich in vitamin C. These tender plant parts were eaten raw with seal oil by the Inuit and could also be preserved in fish or seal oil for up to a year. The young spring leaves were also dried or canned and used to make tea or soup. The young shoots of some willow species are said to taste somewhat like watermelon or cucumber. The inner bark is considered to be more palatable dried and ground into flour. In the Arctic, half-digested willow twigs from the stomachs of slaughtered caribou were considered a special treat.

MEDICINE: Willow bark has been used for centuries to relieve pain, inflammation and fever. It contains salicin, which is related to acetylsalicylic acid (aspirin). Willow bark was chewed or made into medicinal teas for treating diarrhea and other digestive problems, headaches, arthritis, rheumatism and urinary tract irritations. Aspirin has been shown to delay the formation of cataracts and reduce the risk of heart disease in men. Willow bark is less potent than aspirin but also has fewer side effects (e.g., less stomach upset, no impact on blood platelet function). Some herbalists recommend taking willow bark to lose weight, but there is no clinical evidence yet to support this use. Bark tea or strips of bark softened by chewing or boiling were used in washes and poultices on minor burns, insect bites, cuts, scrapes, rashes, ulcers, corns and even cancers. In ancient Rome, ash from willow leaves or twigs was believed to remove corns, calluses and facial blemishes, and mashed leaves were taken with drink to check overly lustful behaviour (though overdoses could cause impotence).

OTHER USES: Flexible willow branches are easily found. They were used to make many common articles, including pins, pegs, backrests, mattresses, fish traps, fox traps, cradle boards, snowshoes, gambling wheels, walking sticks, stirrups, hide-scrapers, hoops for catching horses, baskets, drums, meat racks and

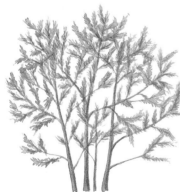

WARNING
People who are sensitive to aspirin should not take willow internally. Large amounts irritate the stomach and contain tannin, which is potentially cancer-causing in high doses.

frames for sweat houses and temporary tepees. Willow bark was stripped and twisted to make twine, baskets and fishing nets that were strong when wet but brittle when dry. Willow bark was chewed to clean teeth and prevent cavities. Dried, crushed willow roots were soaked in water and mixed with grease to make a dandruff tonic. Leaves and twigs were boiled to make a hair rinse for curing dandruff, or the hair rinse was sometimes mixed with wine and used as shampoo. Willow whistles can be made in spring. The prolific male catkins offer an early spring feast for bees. The diamond-shaped patches on some branches of Bebb's willow, much prized by artisans, are caused by fungal infections which produce attractive reddish orange to brown patterns in the pale wood. When peeled and sanded, such "diamond willow" branches are used to make walking sticks, lampposts, furniture and rustic plaques and clock faces.

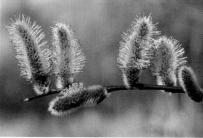

Pussy willow (above)
Sandbar willow (below)

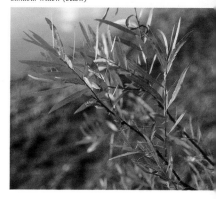

DESCRIPTION: Perennial shrubs or small trees with alternate leaves. Flowers tiny and borne in separate male and female catkins, in most species on separate male and female plants. Fruits capsules containing hair-tufted seeds.

There are more than 65 species of willow in Canada; a handful of the more common and widespread species are described here.

Arctic willow (*S. arctica*) is a prostrate shrub, usually less than 10 cm tall but to 25 cm tall. Found on tundra and in exposed places from far northern Canada south to BC, AB, ON, QC and NL. See p. 424 for conservation status.

Bebb's willow (*S. bebbiana*) is a tree or tall shrub, generally 1–6 m tall (occasionally to 10 m), crown broad and rounded. Trunks clumped, 6–15 cm in diameter; young bark reddish brown to grey; mature bark greyish brown, furrowed. This willow has extremely variable leaf form and twig hairiness among varieties, over one plant at a given time and among plants of different ages. Found in moist to wet forests, thickets and streambanks at low to montane elevations in all provinces and YT.

Pussy willow (*S. discolor*) is a variable, erect shrub, 2–6 m tall, with red-brown to yellowish, hairy or hairless twigs. Leaves elliptic to oval, to 14 cm long, soft-hairy to nearly hairless on both surfaces, the margins entire or toothed. The soft-hairy catkins of many willow species are called pussy willows; those of this species are commonly collected. Found in moist areas (wetlands, streambanks, open forests) in all provinces.

Sandbar willow (*S. exigua*) is a spreading shrub, to 3 m tall. Stems long and smooth with pinkish brown bark. Leaves greyish green, long and narrow and slightly toothed at the margins. Found on streambanks and in alluvial soils, often a pioneer species on sandy shores in YT and NT, interior BC, MB, northernmost ON, QC and NB.

Scouler's willow (*S. scouleriana*) is a tall, spindly shrub or multi-stemmed, small tree, 2–12 m tall (occasionally to 20 m); branches dark brown to yellowish brown, often velvety; twigs densely velvety. Young leaves also densely velvety, especially below, older leaves dark green above, the lower side sparsely hairy with some rust-coloured hairs. Found in moist to dry woodlands, rocky slopes and floodplains in central YT, northern BC, AB, SK and MB.

False Virginia Creeper

Parthenocissus vitacea

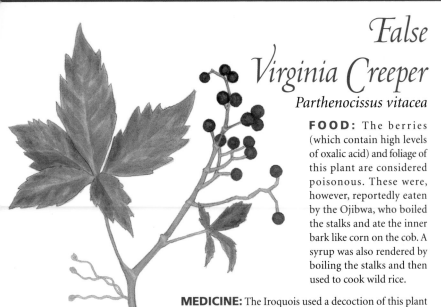

FOOD: The berries (which contain high levels of oxalic acid) and foliage of this plant are considered poisonous. These were, however, reportedly eaten by the Ojibwa, who boiled the stalks and ate the inner bark like corn on the cob. A syrup was also rendered by boiling the stalks and then used to cook wild rice.

MEDICINE: The Iroquois used a decoction of this plant to treat urinary problems and skin ailments.

OTHER USES: This plant is attractive as a garden climber or groundcover, particularly for its showy autumn foliage, which provides a vibrant display of fiery red, purple and scarlet leaves after the first frosts. It is also notable for its purplish black berries and red stems, which remain on the plant after the leaves have fallen, providing an interesting winter display. False Virginia creeper is useful as a wildlife attractant. The berries are a popular food for winter birds, in particular many species of songbirds, and deer and livestock browse its foliage. Because of its perennial root system and ground-covering habit, this plant has been used in slope stabilization, and it can also provide valuable cover for small mammals and birds.

DESCRIPTION: Woody, scrambling or climbing, deciduous vine reaching 20–30 m in length or height; tendrils sparsely branched. Leaves alternate, long-stalked, palmately compound with 5 leaflets; leaflets elliptic to oval, long-tapered at tips, wedge-shaped at base, 5–12 cm long, dark green and shiny above, paler beneath, short-stalked; margins coarsely and sharply toothed above middle; becoming brilliant scarlet in autumn. Flowers greenish, small, about 5 mm across; 25–200 or more in forked, branching clusters, from June to July. Fruits round, purplish black berries, 8–10 mm in diameter, with a thin layer of flesh around 3–4 seeds; stalks often bright red, from August to September. Found in moist soils in woods and thickets and open ground along roadsides in southern MB and ON, and also in NB and NS (where perhaps introduced). It has been introduced and is naturalized in some parts of PEI and southern BC.

This plant is almost indistinguishable from true Virginia creeper (*V. quinquefolia*), the only major difference being that false Virginia creeper lacks the adhesive, sticky discs on its tendrils that allow the true Virginia creeper to climb smooth surfaces. The result of this is that false Virginia creeper rambles through trees and along the ground, attaching itself with twining tendrils similar to those of a grape, rather than vertically adhering itself to walls, trellises and bare tree trunks. The foliage (including showy autumn colouring) of these 2 species is identical.

Grapes
Vitis spp.

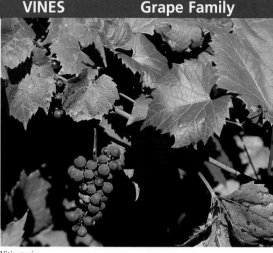

Vitis *species*

FOOD: The fruit of wild grapes (from which the concord grape is derived) is small and tart, but juicy and flavourful. The Iroquois, Maliseet, Huron, Ojibwa and probably other First Nations valued the berries (eaten fresh or preserved for winter) as a food source. They are said to be best when harvested after the first frost, which makes them taste sweeter, but they are often consumed rapidly by birds. More recently, the berries have been made into jelly and wine. The wine of our native grapes has a musky, "foxy" flavour. The Iroquois also ate the fresh shoots.

MEDICINE: The Ojibwa used a tea made of grape roots and branches to treat pulmonary troubles. They made a tea of boiled twigs to clear up afterbirth, and they drank the sap to treat bowel and stomach troubles. The Iroquois made an infusion of the vines together with American bittersweet (p. 134) to remedy anemia. Wine and grapeseed extract contain the compound resveratrol, which has beneficial cardiovascular and antidiabetic properties.

OTHER USES: The winter vines, when twisted together, make a solid and decorative base for Christmas wreaths. The leaves can be pickled to use in making *dolmades*, a Greek delicacy of rice and meat wrapped in vine leaves. Did your grandmother insist on stuffing a grape leaf in each jar of pickles she made? The leaves contain varying amounts of a natural inhibitor that reduces the effects of a softening enzyme present on mouldy cucumber blossoms. Adding a grape leaf to each jar of homemade pickles is a traditional practice that really does result in pickles that are less likely to go soft. Riverbank grape is a key parent species in breeding modern grape varieties for fruit and wine that are disease- and cold-resistant.

DESCRIPTION: Woody, deciduous vines either climbing by means of tendrils or trailing on the ground. Leaves alternate, 3-lobed, 7–20 cm long, toothed. Flowers greenish, inconspicuous; compact in pyramidal clusters. Fruits black, spherical, with a waxy coating giving them a bluish caste; small, 10–12 mm across.

WARNING

Do not confuse wild grapes with Canadian moonseed (*Menispermum canadense*), a vine that is related, but with only a superficially similar appearance. The dark blue, berry-like fruits of moonseed are highly poisonous and may be mistaken for edible grapes, particularly by children. The leaves of moonseed are smooth rather than toothed, and the seed is a single, crescent-shaped body in each fruit rather than the many seeds found in wild grapes.

Summer grape or **pigeon grape** (*V. aestivalis*) has leaves unlobed to deeply 3- to 5-lobed; green above, densely hairy below (at least when young), shallowly toothed. Flowers in a dense panicle, 5–15 cm across. Found in dry woods and thickets in southern ON.

Riverbank grape or **frost grape** (*V. riparia*) has leaves mostly 3-lobed (some unlobed), hairless or slightly hairy below, coarsely toothed. Quite variable; individual plants may vary considerably from the above species description. Inhabits moist thickets from southern SK to the Maritimes. See p. 424 for conservation status.

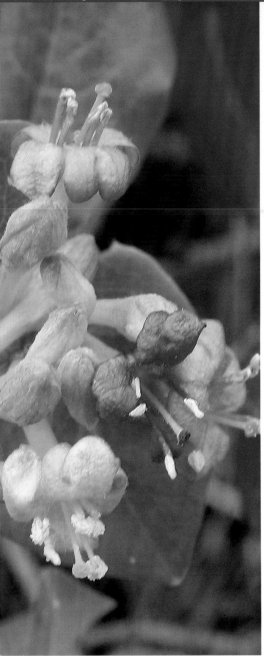

Twining honeysuckle

Honeysuckles
Lonicera spp.

FOOD: Although some honeysuckle berries are nauseously bitter, those listed here are mildly pleasant, though not tasty enough to go out of your way to find them. Their small size, almost always less than 1 cm wide, is also a disadvantage. The flowers produce sweet nectar at their base that can be sucked out.

MEDICINE: Honeysuckle has been employed by a number of First Nations for a diverse range of ailments. The leaves of orange honeysuckle were prepared as an infusion and used as a contraceptive and tonic and for any problems of the womb. In the form of a decoction, it was used to treat colds and tuberculosis. An infusion of the twigs was ingested as a tonic, for colds and sore throats and in small amounts for epilepsy. Sufferers of epilepsy also took baths in a decoction of the woody parts of the vine and sucked the nectar from the flowers. Chewed leaves were applied as a poultice to heal bruises, as a bodywash to strengthen the body and as a hair wash to encourage hair growth. Leaf tea was used in steam baths to promote milk flow. An infusion of the bark of twining honeysuckle was used by First Nations as a cathartic and diuretic to treat kidney stones, menstrual difficulties and dysuria. A tea made from its peeled, internodal stems was used for urine retention, flu and blood clotting after childbirth. A decoction of the root was mixed with other ingredients to treat gonorrhea. A tea from the berries and bark was ingested by pregnant women to expel worms. A decoction of the whole plant was given to children for fevers and general sickness. In spite of the myriad traditional medical uses of honeysuckle, the plant is rarely used today in modern herbalism.

OTHER USES: The stems were used by First Nations as building materials and to make fibres for mats, baskets, bags, blankets and toys. The hollow stems were used by children as straws. The plant was used in a number of love potions, charms and medicines to either form or destroy a relationship. During Victorian times, teenage girls were not allowed to bring honeysuckle home in the belief that it induced erotic dreams. Pieces of orange honeysuckle vines were sometimes placed under pillows to ensure sound sleep.

DESCRIPTION: Twining, woody vines, climbing to 5 m or more tall, with opposite, simple, oval leaves, to 10 cm long. Flowers sweet-scented, bell-shaped, 2–4 cm long, with a sweet, edible nectar from May to July. Fruit an orange or red berry about 1 cm across containing several seeds.

Orange honeysuckle (*L. ciliosa*) has orange-yellow to red flowers and leaves that are long-hairy on the margins. Grows in mesic to dry forests and thickets at low to montane elevations in southern BC.

Twining honeysuckle (*L. dioica*) has yellow to orange flowers (sometimes dark reddish with age) and leaves that are not hairy on the margins. Grows in dry woods, thickets and rocky slopes from BC to QC, and in YT and NT. See p. 424 for conservation status.

Twining honeysuckle

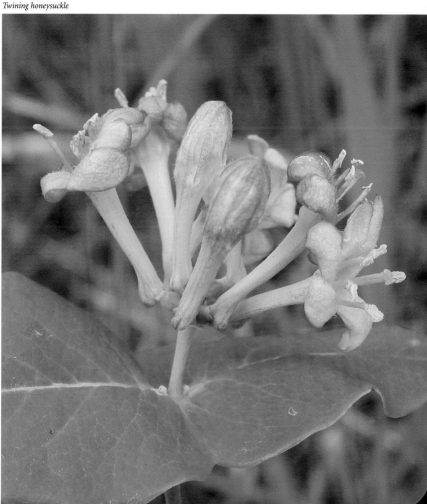

Manroot
Marah oreganus

FOOD: The generic name is derived from Hebrew, meaning bitter, which alludes to the very bitter, and potentially poisonous, quality of the plant (see **Warning**). Despite this, the leaves were reportedly used as a vegetable. A tea was made by one First Nation, who used the young shoots combined with licorice fern rhizomes (p. 381). Seeds of the genus are said to be hallucinogenic (see **Warning**).

MEDICINE: Manroot was used medicinally by a number of First Nations. The seeds were consumed as a treatment for kidney problems, and a decoction of the plant drunk for venereal disease. It was also applied externally as a poultice on scrofula sores (a tuberculous skin disease). This condition was also treated by burning the root and mixing the resulting powder with bear grease and smearing it on the sores. The upper stalk of the plant was mashed in water and used as a bath to soak aching hands. Bruises, boils, rheumatic joints and swellings were treated with a poultice of the crushed roots, as were sores that appeared on horses. A tea made from the peeled, sliced and dried roots was used as an eyewash for sore eyes.

OTHER USES: The bitter root was crushed and placed in streams to stupefy fish. Because it is rich in tannins, the plant has been used for tanning. The fruits were used as toys by Aboriginal children, who either threw them at each other or constructed representations of animals by inserting twigs in them.

DESCRIPTION: Perennial vine borne from a large, woody root. Stems trailing or climbing, herbaceous, nearly hairless, leafy, bearing tendrils. Leaves glossy, alternate, to 20 cm long, shallowly palmately lobed. Flowers whitish, 6–12 mm wide, with 5 flaring lobes, deeply bell-shaped, from April to June. Male flowers in racemes, while female flowers borne singly in axil at base of racemes. Fruit green, weakly spiny, inflated, gourd-like, 3–8 cm long, with several (3–6) large seeds inside. Seeds disc-shaped to flat, 16–22 mm long. Rare but distinctive (and suggestively named) species found in shrubby thickets, moist fields and forest edges at low elevations in extreme southwestern BC. See p. 424 for conservation status.

WARNING
The seeds are poisonous if ingested. They contain bitter principles called cucurbitacins, which are compounds produced by saponic glycosides. In 1986, an Oregon man drank a homemade tea from the seeds in the hopes of obtaining a hallucinogenic effect, went into shock, lost consciousness and died 24 hours later. Death was attributed to heart failure and internal bleeding.

Wild Cucumber
Echinocystis lobata

FOOD: Despite what the name suggests, the cucumber-like fruit is inedible.

MEDICINE: Wild cucumber was once considered to be "the greatest of all medicines and always useful" by one First Nation. An extremely bitter tea was brewed from the roots and used as a tonic and analgesic to treat stomach problems. An infusion of the plant was taken for rheumatism, chills, fevers and kidney complaints and to stimulate the flow of obstructed menses. The pulverized root was applied topically as a poultice for headaches.

OTHER USES: The seeds make excellent beads for jewellery. The roots were sometimes used as an ingredient in traditional love potions.

DESCRIPTION: Climbing, perennial vine, to 8 m or more tall, with an angular stem. Leaves palmately lobed, maple-like, to 8 cm long, with 3–7 mostly triangular lobes. Flower stalks and 3-forked tendrils arise in leaf axils. Flowers small (1.3–1.6 cm wide), greenish white, 6-petalled, with male flowers in racemes and female flowers solitary or in small clusters below, from June to October. Fruit a single, 4-seeded, fleshy berry, to 5 cm long, covered with weak spines, dry when mature. Grows in moist woods and streambanks at low elevations from SK to NS, and introduced to southern BC and AB.

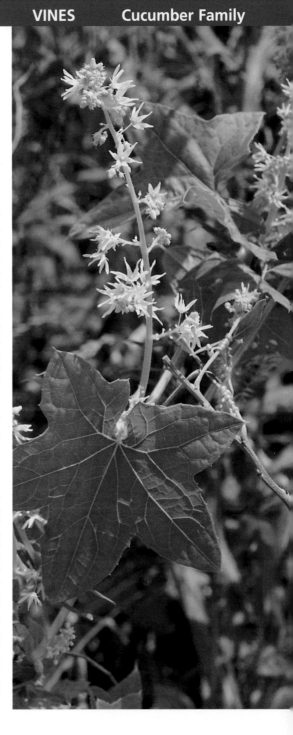

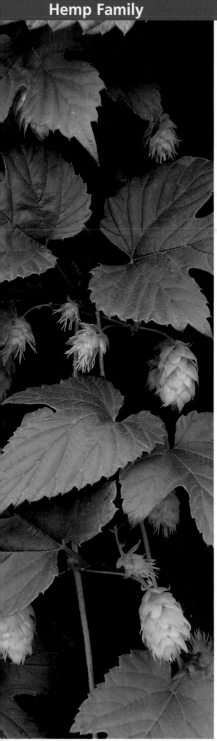

Hops
Humulus lupulus

FOOD: Hops have been used in beer for their preservative action and bitter taste for over 1000 years. They were originally used to prevent the growth of Gram-negative bacteria in the brew but were later noted to impart a pleasant aroma and bitter flavour. The first documented instance of hops cultivation was in Germany in 736. England did not start adding hops to their beers until almost 2 centuries later. Prior to this, malt was brewed alone or from a mixture of honey and a variety of bitter and/or aromatic herbs such as heath, ground ivy and wormwood. This liquor was called "ale" after the Old English drink *ealu*, but once hops were added, the brew adopted the German name *bier*, or "beer." Today, Germany and the United States supply hops for more than half the world's beer production. First Nations boiled hops and used them to flavour drinks, wheat flour and potatoes. In Rome and during medieval times, the tender new shoots were prepared like asparagus. They have recently been rediscovered as a delicacy in parts of Germany, Belgium and England, where they are served raw with vinaigrette, boiled or fried in batter. They are also used to prepare *risotto* (a rice dish) and *frittata* (an omelette dish) in Veneto, Italy. The young leaves contain rutin, a powerful antioxidant, and make a fine addition to green salads.

MEDICINE: It was observed that hoppers (hop pickers) tired more quickly than other labourers, apparently from the accidental hand-to-mouth transfer of the resinous powder of the hops. They were first thought to engender melancholy, but soon gained a reputation as a popular sedative. Pillows were filled with hops to help with sleeplessness and nervous tension. As a bitter tonic, usually prepared as an infusion or tincture, hops were traditionally used to improve appetite, digestion, jaundice and other afflictions of the stomach and liver. Research confirms that hops improve sleep disturbances when given in

WARNING
Contact dermatitis can occur in sensitive people.

combination with common valerian (p. 329). The sedative principle in the resin was found to be 2-methyl-3-buten-2-ol (dimethylvinyl carbinol), present in very small amounts, but it may be formed *in vivo* by metabolism of the α-bitter acids. In combination with chicory (p. 330) and peppermint (p. 287), hops have been found to be effective in relieving pain in patients with chronic cholecystitis. The antibacterial activity toward Gram-negative bacteria is attributed to the unstable polyphenolics humulone and lupulone, which vary enormously in concentration with hop variety. First Nations used hops for breast and uterus problems, and even though the plant was reported to possess estrogenic activity, none could be found in an experiment using immature female mice. However, research has demonstrated that lupulin, an alkaloid that has sedative and hypnotic effects, increases milk flow in nursing mothers. The fruit is applied externally as a poultice to relieve toothaches, fevers, ulcers, boils, painful swellings, tumours, pneumonia and wounds. Because hops are in the same family as marijuana (p. 314), some herbalists have advocated smoking the plant as a mild euphoric. This practice is strongly discouraged because of unpleasant side effects and unknown toxicity.

OTHER USES: The stems are a source of fibre and have been suggested for pulp or biomass production. It is very durable, but not as strong as hemp fibre and is difficult to separate, requiring several months of soaking. Paper can also be made from the fibre by cooking it for 2 hours with lye and hand pounding it with mallets or ball milling it for another 2. The leaves and flowerheads produce a fine brown dye. The essential oil from hops is used in perfumery and as an ingredient in some European skin creams and lotions.

DESCRIPTION: Prickly, twining perennial, 2–15 m tall, growing from a stout, horizontal, cold-hardy rhizome. Leaves opposite, heart-shaped, 3- to 5-lobed, margins serrate, sinuses rounded, yellow, resinous granules beneath, 12–25 cm long and broad. Male and female flowers on separate plants. Female flowers green to pale yellow, in racemes, 1–2 cm long, forming an inflated cone, with yellow glands on the bracteoles, from July to August. Fruit a yellowish, compressed, glandular achene. Both a native North American variety (var. *neomexicanus;* from SK to the Maritimes) and the escaped, cultivated European variety (var. *lupuloides*) grow in waste places, moist thickets, roadsides and edges of woods throughout southern Canada.

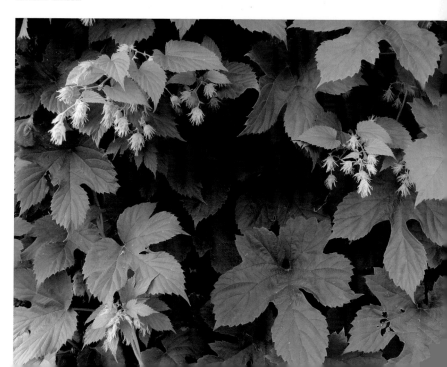

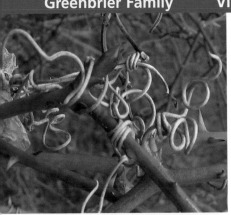

Carrion-Flower & Greenbrier

Smilax spp.

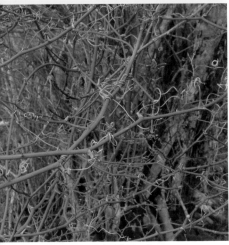

Common greenbrier (all images)

FOOD: The fruits, rootstocks and shoots of a number of *Smilax* species were used as food by First Nations in the southeastern US, but no existing records could be found for similar uses of the related species we have here in Canada. In the US, carrion-flower was used by First Nations and early settlers. The tubers can be roasted and ground into a flour used in breads and for thickening stews. The small berries are edible and can be eaten raw (they should be fully ripe, however) or made into jam. The young leaves and shoots reportedly taste similar to asparagus and can be eaten raw or cooked.

MEDICINE: The dried and powdered leaves of carrion-flower have been used as a healing dressing on burns, and the wilted green leaves as a dressing on boils. The rhizome has analgesic qualities, and a decoction can be prescribed to treat back pain, stomach complaints and kidney problems. The beverage and medicinal sarsaparilla is brewed from the rhizomes of *S. regelii* and related species.

OTHER USES: The flowers of these species smell like rotting carrion, thereby attracting the flies relied on for pollination. These plants can be used as garden ornamentals (but far away from open windows where a breeze could blow into the house during flowering!) and wildlife attractants, particularly for bird species that are fond of the berries as winter food. The dried and powdered root can be used as a gelatin substitute.

DESCRIPTION: Deciduous to semi-evergreen, male or female vines from tuberous rhizomes; either climbing or forming a tangled bush. Bark green, turning brown on old stems. Leaves green, glossy. Tendrils paired, emerging from the leaf axils. Flowers green-yellow, 2.5 cm wide, with a pervasive rotting-flesh smell; borne in small, round clusters in late spring. Fruit dark bluish black berries, often with a powdery bloom, 5–8 mm in diameter, borne in clusters, persisting over winter; 1–3 seeds.

Carrion-flower (*S. herbacea*) is a thornless, smooth, annual vine growing to 2.5 m long. Inhabits alluvial thickets, low, moist woods and meadows, often in calcareous soils, in ON, QC and NB. See p. 424 for conservation status.

Common greenbrier (*S. rotundifolia*) is a woody, deciduous or partly evergreen, perennial vine or tangled bush with wiry, prickly stems to 10 m long. Inhabits moist to dryish woods and thickets from southern ON to southwestern NS. See p. 424 for conservation status.

Jack-in-the-Pulpit

Arisaema triphyllum

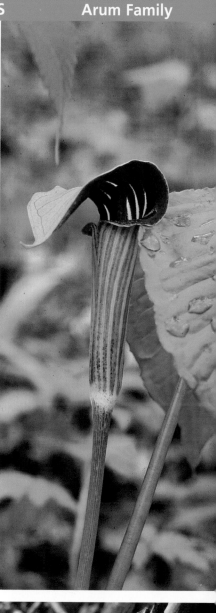

FOOD: To make this poisonous plant (see **Warning**) edible, Jack-in-the-pulpit root was thinly sliced and carefully cooked in a pit oven for 3 days to release its poisonous compounds.

MEDICINE: Jack-in-the-pulpit root and rhizome were used mostly for medicinal purposes by First Nations and European settlers, but the whole plant and the corm were also used. Root decoctions were used as an eyewash for sore eyes and taken internally for relief of general pain. Root infusions were gargled to help heal a sore throat. Roots were pounded, boiled and mixed with meal into a poultice and applied directly to boils. Simple poultices of pulverized roots were applied to sore eyes. Roots were also allegedly used to reduce swelling from rattlesnakebites. Whole plants were prepared into hot poultices and applied to face sores and bruises, or dried whole plants were ground and prepared into poultices for abscesses and boils. The corm was crushed and sprinkled on the head and temples to help with headaches, or it was prepared into a poultice and applied as a counter-irritant for rheumatism.

OTHER USES: Seeds were considered to have divinatory properties and were used to help predict recovery or death. They were also placed in gourd shells to make rattles.

DESCRIPTION: Perennial herb, to 60 cm tall, from an underground stem. It has 1–2 green, veined leaves composed of 3 leaflets each. Flowers tiny, yellow, arranged on a yellowish, club-shaped structure (spadix). Spadix enveloped in an upright, green to purplish brown, ridged or sometimes striped, cup-like bract (spathe) with a curved flap. Found in moist woods from MB to PEI and NS. See p. 424 for conservation status.

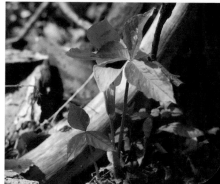

> **WARNING**
> Jack-in-the-pulpit is a poisonous plant, including its roots and corm. It is not recommended as a food or medicinal plant.

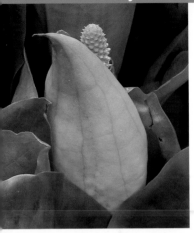

American Skunk-Cabbage

Lysichiton americanus

FOOD: Despite being a poisonous plant (see **Warning**), parts of American skunk-cabbage were cooked and eaten by some First Nations. American skunk-cabbage blossoms were cooked overnight before being served, and a person could eat no more than 2 or 3 blossoms without becoming ill. Young leaves were steamed and eaten or placed over roasting camas (p. 199), wild onion (p. 192) and garlic (p. 192) to add flavour. Root centres were boiled at least 8 times before being eaten.

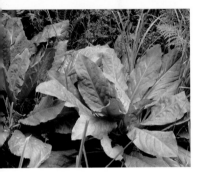

MEDICINE: American skunk-cabbage roots and leaves were used mostly for medicinal purposes (see **Warning**). Roots were chewed for nausea, and decoctions of root were taken for stomach discomforts, to "clean out the bladder" and to ease childbirth; a cold infusion of the roots was considered a panacea. Simple or compound poultices of pounded roots were applied to sores, "blood poisoning," boils, burns, carbuncles and swellings. Charred and ground rhizome was mixed with bear grease and used to help heal animal bites and infections. Pulverized roots were thought to increase hair growth when directly applied. American skunk-cabbage root was used in steam baths for strokes and to ease arthritis and lumbago. Smoking the root was also thought to help with influenza, rheumatism and bad dreams. Leaves were used in sweat baths for general weakness and sickness (including rheumatism), and warm leaves were applied directly to the chest to relieve pain and to help draw out thorns and splinters. Poultices were prepared with leaves for rheumatism, burns and joint pain and to help heal boils, carbuncles and sores. Poultices of heated blossoms were also applied to the body for rheumatism.

OTHER USES: Leaves were popular as tools for cooking, baking, steaming, drying, drinking and storing. Large leaves could be folded into drinking cups or large containers to hold berries or leftover food. Fish, meat, vegetables, berries or cakes were wrapped in leaves and baked, cooked, steamed or boiled. Native peoples lined cooking pits and steaming boxes with American skunk-cabbage leaves and also used the leaves to dry various berries and cakes. Spadices were placed on sticks and used in distance throwing contests by children. Charcoal from the plant was thought to protect against "witchcraft."

DESCRIPTION: Fragrant (some say foul-smelling), perennial, semi-aquatic or terrestrial herb, to 70 cm tall. Large leaves 50 cm–1.3 m long and 30–80 cm wide when mature. Yellowish green flowers arranged in a 4–14 cm long spadix. Spadix enclosed within a large, bright yellow or yellowish green, 30–40 cm tall spathe. Found in swamps and wet areas in woods and along streams in southern BC.

WARNING
Roots and possibly the whole plant are poisonous. Roots may contain abortifacient properties. Caution is advised.

Skunk-Cabbage
Symplocarpus foetidus

FOOD: Young leaves and shoots were cooked and served with salt, pepper and butter (see **Warning**).

MEDICINE: Skunk-cabbage leaves and roots were used as medicines (see **Warning**). Small pieces of fresh leaves were eaten or rolled and chewed for epileptic seizures. Infusions made with leaves were taken for colds, and poultices of crushed leaves were applied to the skin to help reduce pain and swelling. Skunk-cabbage roots were infused and taken as cough medicine, and ground root was used on the skin as a deodorant. Dried root made into poultices was applied to wounds, and steam from compound decoctions of roots was inhaled for rheumatism.

OTHER USES: Skunk-cabbage root was used as a tattoo image because it was believed to protect the bearer from disease.

DESCRIPTION: Perennial herb, to 60 cm tall, with a strong, skunky odour. Leaves 30–40 cm wide and 30 cm–1.2 m long, veined, green. Flowers greenish yellow with a 5–10 cm long, knob-like, yellow to dark red-purple spadix contained in a 10–15 cm tall, brownish purple and green, shell-like spathe. Flowers from February to May. Found in moist soils in MB, ON, QC, NB and NS. See p. 424 for conservation status.

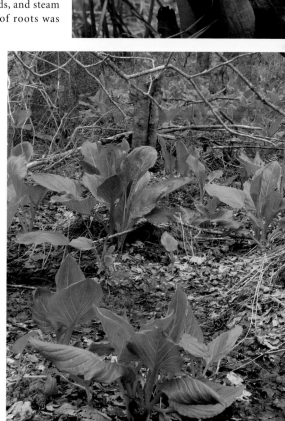

WARNING
The roots are considered toxic, and eating the leaves causes inflammation and burning sensations.

Sweetflags
Acorus spp.

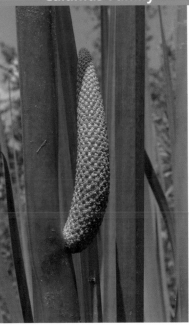
American sweetflag

FOOD: Sweetflag has been an item of trade for centuries and was propagated in North America by settlers for its edible and medicinal properties. The rhizome was sometimes eaten raw after being washed and peeled to remove the bitterness. More often, it was candied by first peeling and cutting the rhizome into 1 cm slices, boiling the pieces for about an hour in 4 or 5 changes of water until tender, and then simmering them in a rich sugar syrup for about 20 minutes before setting them out to dry. The rhizome is also quite palatable when roasted and can be powdered and used as a flavouring substitute for ginger, cinnamon or nutmeg. In Europe, it was often added to wine and is an ingredient in some absinthes. The somewhat sweet, young, tender spadix was sometimes eaten by children as a snack. The tender interior of the spring shoots, when about 30 cm tall, can be eaten cooked or raw or added to salads.

MEDICINE: Long considered a powerful stimulant and aphrodisiac in the Orient and ancient Egypt, sweetflag has been used medicinally by First Nations for a variety of ailments. The rhizome was nibbled fresh or used dried in a tea as a tonic for stomachaches, gas, indigestion or any other digestive complaint. Small doses are said to reduce stomach acidity, while larger doses stimulate stomach secretions, thereby stimulating or normalizing the appetite. For this reason, sweetflag is considered useful for treating appetite disorders such as anorexia nervosa. The chewed rhizome was also useful for alleviating toothaches and sore throats and removing the craving for tobacco. An infusion of the rhizomes was taken for heartburn, headaches, bronchitis, sinusitis, fevers, colds and coughs. In Ayurvedic and traditional Chinese medicine, sweetflag was highly valued for its effects on the central nervous system (CNS). Pharmacological research supports this use: the rhizome has demonstrated sedative, CNS-depressant, anticonvulsant, antispasmodic and memory-enhancing activity in various *in vitro* and animal experiments. In addition, the rhizome displays strong anti-inflammatory, antioxidant, antidiarrheal, antihelmenthic and hypolipidemic activity, all of which have been attributed to the essential oil compounds α- and β-asarone. These are only produced, however, in sweetflag varieties that contain 3 (triploid) or 4 (tetraploid) sets of chromosomes, which grow in Central Europe, India and East Asia. Those in North America contain only 2 (haploid) sets of chromosomes and are devoid of these compounds. Perhaps this is just as well because asarones are genotoxic and mutagenic, thereby limiting their therapeutic use.

OTHER USES: All parts of the plant can be used as an insecticide against fleas, bedbugs, moths, lice and so forth.

Sweetflag was added to rice stored in granaries as an effective means to reduce loss caused by insect damage. The rhizome was used as an incense stick, reminiscent of patchouli. Leaves were used in thatching for roofs, basket making and mat-weaving. The plant's common name refers to its sweet scent and the flag-like appearance of its wavy-edged leaves. Because of the phallic appearance of its flower, sweetflag is considered a symbol of male love, and its species name, *calamus*, is associated with Kalamos, the mythological son of a Greek river god who transformed himself into a reed after his male lover, Karpos, drowned. The rustling sound of the plant in the wind was interpreted as a sigh of lamentation.

DESCRIPTION: Erect, perennial, 30 cm–1.2 m tall, semi-aquatic herb from a thick rhizome; gives off a sweet, tangerine-like fragrance when bruised. Leaves stiff, sword-like and light green. The 2-edged stalk is topped by an outward-jutting, club-like spadix, 5–9 cm long, bearing tiny, greenish yellow flowers clustered in diamond-shaped patterns from May to August. Fruits small, gelatinous berries that eventually dry.

American sweetflag (*A. americanus*) has leaves with numerous veins prominently raised. Mature fruits produced; fertile species. Native to North America ; grows in wet, open areas, marshes and along edges of quiet water, in all provinces and NT. Decreased range coincides with the gradual disappearance and degradation of eastern Canada's wetlands. See p. 424 for conservation status.

Sweetflag (*A. calamus*) has leaves with the mid-vein prominently raised, but other veins not evidently raised. Mature fruits never produced; this sterile species spreads vegetatively by rhizomes. This European species was introduced to North America by early settlers for its medicinal value; grows in wet, open areas, marshes and along edges of quiet water from ON to NS.

American sweetflag

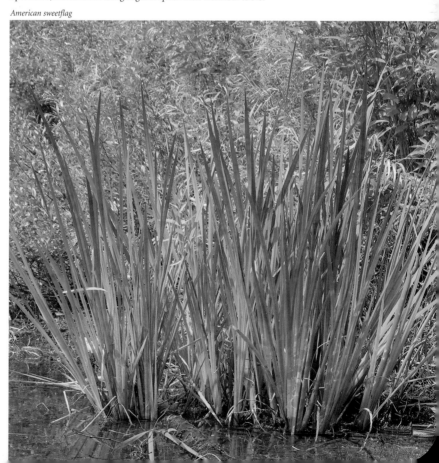

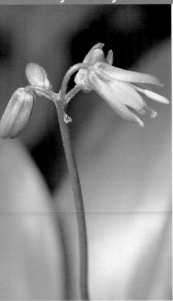

Clintonia & Queen's Cup

Clintonia spp.

FOOD: Young leaves can be eaten raw or cooked and are said to taste slightly sweetish, like cucumber. The berries of both species are mildly toxic to humans and were considered inedible by local indigenous groups.

MEDICINE: A poultice of yellow clintonia leaves was applied to open wounds, infections, ulcers and bruises. A decoction of the plant was taken for the heart and to treat diabetes and was also used as a wash for the body. An infusion of yellow clintonia roots was used to aid childbirth. The toasted leaves of queen's cup were prepared into a poultice and used as a medicine for eyes and wounds.

Yellow clintonia (all images)

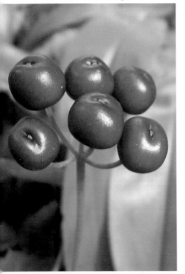

OTHER USES: Dogs were believed to chew the roots of yellow clintonia to poison their teeth and kill the animals they bit. If a person was bitten by a dog suspected of having the poison on its teeth, a poultice of the roots was used to draw out the poison and treat the wound. The crushed leaves of yellow clintonia were rubbed on the face and hands as a protection from mosquitoes. The Nuxalk in BC called the berry of queen's cup wolf's berry because it was considered inedible to humans and edible only to wolves. The berries of queen's cup were used as a dye by the Thompson people in BC.

DESCRIPTION: Perennial herb arising from rhizomes, to 50 cm tall. Basal leaves 2–5 cm wide, shiny, narrowed at both ends, to 30 cm long. Flowering stem 14–40 cm tall, usually hairy at the top. Flowers large and cup-shaped, 1–3 cm long, blooming from May to June. Berries bright metallic blue, 6–12 mm thick. Found in shaded, moist to mesic forests. See p. 424 for conservation status.

Yellow clintonia or **yellow bluebead lily** (*C. borealis*) bears 3–8 yellow flowers. Found in eastern Canada from MB to NL.

Queen's cup (*C. uniflora*) bears 1 or, rarely, 2 white flowers. Found in BC and western AB (Rocky Mountains).

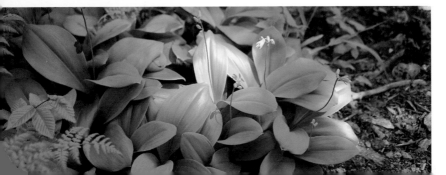

Twisted-Stalks

Streptopus spp.

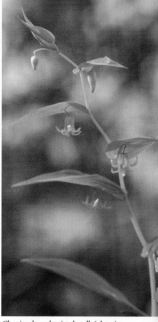

FOOD: Most native peoples regarded twisted-stalks as poisonous, but some ate young plants and/or berries, either raw or cooked in soups and stews. Okanagan First Nations used the bright-coloured berries for food. Clasping-leaved twisted-stalk berries were eaten in large quantities by the Thompson people.

MEDICINE: Twisted-stalks were highly regarded for their general restorative qualities and were taken as a tonic or physic and to treat general sickness. The whole plant was taken by some First Nations to treat coughs, loss of appetite, stomach-aches, spitting up blood, kidney trouble and gonorrhea. The roots were made into a poultice to treat a sty, internal pains and fallen wombs. A poultice was made from the stems to treat cuts. The blossoms were ingested to induce sweating.

OTHER USES: First Nations' names for the berries included owl berries, witch berries, black bear berries and frog berries; the berries were also believed to be eaten by snakes, deer and wolves. Hesquiat children would play with the berries. The plant was sometimes tied to, and used to scent, the body, clothes or hair.

Clasping-leaved twisted-stalk (above)
Rosy twisted-stalk (below)

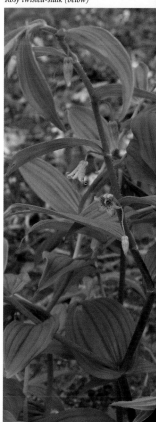

DESCRIPTION: Slender, herbaceous perennial, tall, from thick, short rhizomes. Leaves smooth-edged, elliptical/oval-shaped, alternate, markedly parallel-veined. Flowers small, white, bell-shaped, 8–12 mm long, with 6 petals that flare backward, each hanging on lower side of each stalk, 1 per leaf; flowering late spring to midsummer. Berries hanging, red-orange or yellowish, egg-shaped and somewhat translucent; seeds small, whitish, somewhat visible. Found in shaded forests, clearings, meadows and on streambanks.

Clasping-leaved twisted-stalk (*S. amplexifolius*) grows 50 cm–1 m tall, with loosely branched stems often bent at the nodes (zig-zag), leaves clasping at base; greenish white flowers; yellow to red berries. Found across Canada from BC to NL. See p. 424 for conservation status.

Rosy twisted-stalk (*S. lanceolatus*, also known as *S. roseus*) grows to 30 cm tall, with stems usually unbranched, curved (not zig-zagged), leaves not clasping; rose-purple or pink flowers with white tips; red berries. Found in BC, AB and from MB to NL. See p. 424 for conservation status.

WARNING
Young plants resemble green false-hellebore (p. 401), which is extremely poisonous. Collecting the young shoots of twisted-stalk for consumption is not recommended unless you are absolutely sure of plant identification.

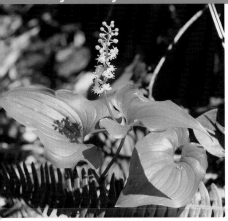

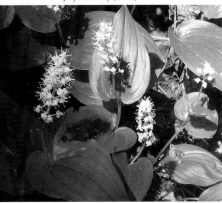

False lily-of-the-valley (above)
Wild lily-of-the-valley (below)

Lilies-of-the-Valley

Maianthemum spp.

FOOD: Berries of both species are edible; however, caution is advised when eating berries of wild lily-of-the-valley. False lily-of-the-valley was eaten by many groups in BC and neighbouring areas, but it was rarely highly regarded. The berries were usually eaten only casually, by children or hunters and berry pickers while out on trips. Some groups, such as the Haida, used the berries to a great extent. They ate berries fresh or picked them when unripe and stored them until they were red and soft. Green berries were sometimes boiled in tall cedar boxes that were lowered into boiling water for a few minutes; the cooked fruit was then mixed with other fruits before being sun-dried into cakes. Sometimes berries were scalded and eaten with animal or fish grease or stored this way. In a Haida myth, a feast for supernatural beings included wild lily-of-the-valley berries. New, "folded" leaves of false lily-of-the-valley were boiled and eaten as greens in spring by the Haida.

MEDICINE: The plant of wild lily-of-the-valley was used to treat headaches and sore throats and "to keep kidneys open during pregnancy." A leaf poultice was used to treat swellings in the limbs. The plant was also used to make smoke for inhaling. False lily-of-the-valley was often made into a poultice to treat boils and cuts, minor burns, sores, wounds and sore eyes. Young leaves were eaten as a spring purge, and the fruit was used as a medicine for tuberculosis. A tea made from the rhizome was drunk to heal internal injuries. The long roots were chewed and the juice swallowed to reverse sterility.

OTHER USES: Wild lily-of-the-valley was given the name "frog berry" by the Slave and Kwakwaka'wakw because the berries were eaten by frogs. The genus name is derived from the Latin word for May, referring to the flowering time of these plants.

DESCRIPTION: Herbaceous perennials arising from rhizomes. Leaves heart-shaped, usually 2 or 3, with prominent parallel veins. Small, white flowers with 4 petals, 4–6 mm wide, borne in distinct terminal clusters, blooming early spring. Berries pea-sized, at first hard and green mottled with brown, then turning soft and red. Found in moist woods and clearings.

Wild lily-of-the-valley (*M. canadense*) is a smaller plant, less than 25 cm tall; leaves stalkless. Found from eastern BC to NL. See p. 424 for conservation status.

False lily-of-the-valley (*M. dilatatum*) is a larger plant, more than 20 cm tall; leaves stalked. Occurs in western BC.

False Solomon's-Seals

Maianthemum spp.

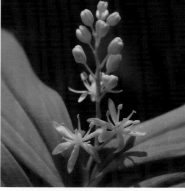

FOOD: Young greens, fleshy rhizomes and ripe berries were eaten by various indigenous peoples across Canada. The Ojibwa soaked the rhizomes in lye "to get rid of their disagreeable taste" and cooked them like potatoes. The Okanagan of BC sometimes chewed the rhizomes raw and used them to flavour black tree lichen and other foods being pit cooked (they were said to resemble onions). The Nlaka'pamux sometimes harvested young shoots in spring, cooked and ate them like asparagus (p. 174), or cooked them as a flavouring in meat. Some BC indigenous peoples believed the berries to be the food of snakes and avoided them. In cases where berries were eaten, it was usually casually (hunters, berry pickers, children). The Gitskan, however, picked them ripe in August, preserved them in eulachon grease and stored them in boxes in a cool place. They were said to be reserved as food for chiefs. The Carrier called the fruits sugar berry. Berries of star-flowered false Solomon's-seal are said to be high in vitamin C.

Star-flowered false Solomon's-seal (above)
False Solomon's-seal (below)

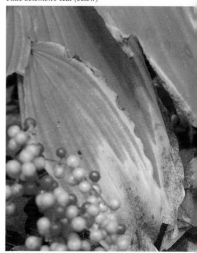

MEDICINE: False Solomon's-seal was often combined with other plants for medicinal purposes. When combined with dogbane (p. 257), it was used to keep the kidneys open during pregnancy, to cure sore throats and headaches and as a reviver. When mixed with black ash the plant was used to loosen the bowels. When mixed with sweetflag (p. 166), false Solomon's-seal was used as a conjurer's root to perform tricks or cast spells. Both the leaf and root were used to reduce bleeding. The rhizome was burned and inhaled to treat a number of ailments: to treat headaches, to quiet a crying child and to return someone to normal after temporary insanity. Leaf decoctions were applied to assist in childbirth and to treat itchy rashes. A rhizome decoction was used to treat back pain and overexertion.

OTHER USES: Some BC groups noted false Solomon's-seal as a favourite food of grizzly bears, as well as being eaten by deer (hence the name "deer berries") and other animals.

DESCRIPTION: Tall, herbaceous perennials growing from thick, whitish, branching rhizomes, often found in dense clusters. Leaves smooth-edged, broad, elliptical, alternate along stems in 2 rows, 5–15 cm long, distinctly parallel-veined, often clasping. Flowers small, cream-coloured, 6-parted, in dense, terminal clusters. Berries small and densely clustered, initially green and mottled or striped, ripening to bright red. Grows in rich woods, thickets and moist clearings from BC to NL. See p. 424 for conservation status.

False Solomon's-seal (*M. racemosum,* previously *Smilacina racemosa*) grows to 1.2 m tall, flowers in clusters of 70–250, berries at first green with copper spots.

Star-flowered false Solomon's-seal (*M. stellatum,* previously *Smilacina stellata*) grows to 50 cm tall, flowers in clusters of 6–15, berries at first green with blue-purple stripes.

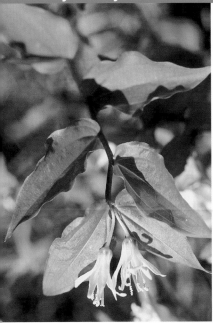

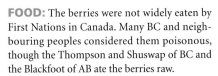

Fairybells

Prosartes spp.

FOOD: The berries were not widely eaten by First Nations in Canada. Many BC and neighbouring peoples considered them poisonous, though the Thompson and Shuswap of BC and the Blackfoot of AB ate the berries raw.

MEDICINE: A compound decoction of roots was taken for internal pains. The whole plant can be boiled and the water drunk as a spring tonic.

OTHER USES: Many BC and neighbouring peoples associated fairybells with ghosts or snakes. Some groups called them snake berries, while another group called them grizzly bear's favourite food. Rough-fruited fairybells were called false raspberries in the Shuswap language. Rodents and grouse are known to feed on the berries.

Rough-fruited fairybells (all images)

DESCRIPTION: Perennial herbs, 30–60 cm tall, with few branches, from thick-spreading rhizomes. Leaves alternate, broadly oval, 3–9 cm long, pointed at tips, rounded to a heart-shaped base, fringed with short, spreading hairs, prominently parallel-veined. Flowers creamy to greenish white, narrowly bell-shaped, 10–20 mm long, drooping, 1–3 at branch tips, blooming from April to July. Berries orange to bright red, ripening in July. Grow in moist woods and thickets throughout southern forest and parklands.

Rough-fruited fairybells (*P. trachycarpa*, previously *Disporum trachycarpum*) has conspicuously rough-skinned, velvety-surfaced berries with 6–12 seeds. Found from BC to ON.

Hooker's fairybells (*P. hookeri*, previously *Disporum hookeri*) has smooth berries with 4–6 seeds. Found in BC and southwestern AB.

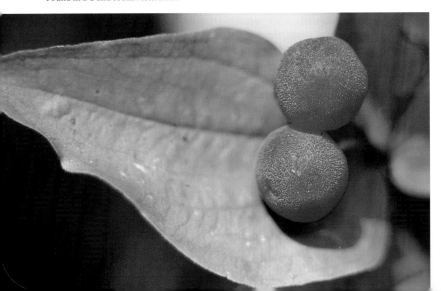

Trilliums

Trillium spp.

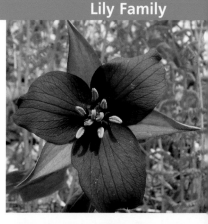

FOOD: There are no records of Aboriginal consumption of trillium for food, but the new leaves are said to be edible and to taste like sunflower seeds.

MEDICINE: Trillium rhizome was commonly taken for female ailments—for example, to lessen the pain and difficulty at time of delivery, to induce labour (blossoms used for this), as an astringent for uterine organs and as "food for woman in the womb." One of its common names is birth root. Red trillium has been used for all forms of hemorrhages, such as bleeding from the nose, mouth, stomach, bowels and bladder. This may be an example of the "doctrine of signatures," in which like treats like. The rhizome was also made into a poultice that was applied to tumours, ulcers, insect stings and stiff muscles and also to treat rheumatism. An infusion of rhizomes from red trillium and flowers from another (unknown) plant were used to treat pimples and sunburn. A snuff for headaches, catarrh and colds was made from a compound of dried roots. Trilliums have

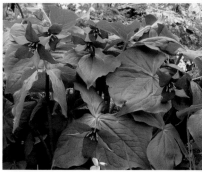

Red trillium (all images)

also been used as a wash to treat itchy skin. Juice extracted from the Pacific trillium plant and rhizomes was used as eye drops or as a wash to relieve sore eyes. White trillium extracts were used as ear drops. The crushed plant was used as a liniment for chapped hands and as a suntan oil.

OTHER USES: An infusion of 1 smashed rhizome was used as a soak for fishing line to help catch fish. The dried rhizome would be carried for luck and for the protection of teeth. Pacific trillium was used in love potions. White trillium is ON's provincial flower.

DESCRIPTION: Hairless, perennial herbs, to 40 cm tall, from short, stout, fleshy rhizomes. Leaves in whorls of 3–5 (usually 3), unstalked, prominently net-veined. Flowers single, on end of stalk, with 3 petals, 3 sepals, blooming from May to June. See p. 424 for conservation status.

Red trillium (*T. erectum*) has flowers with purple or purple-brown petals and purple anthers. Found in cool, rich, dry-to-moist, deciduous and coniferous forests in southern ON, QC, NB and NS.

White trillium (*T. grandiflorum*) has white petals that ascend at the base and then spread, often turning pink as they mature, and prominent yellow anthers. Leaves to 30 cm long. Found in rich, moist soils and floodplains at low to middle elevations of southern ON and southern QC along the St. Lawrence Seaway.

Trilliums are beautiful wildflowers, but they don't transplant well and can be quickly wiped out in an area. Red trillium, for example, was recorded in PEI in the 1950s but has apparently been extirpated there. Enjoy trilliums where they grow!

Pacific trillium (*T. ovatum*) has white petals that spread from the base, often turning maroon as they mature, and prominent yellow anthers. Leaves rarely more than 15 cm long. Found in moist, open to dense forests and moist, mossy, rocky openings at low to middle elevations in southern BC and southwestern AB.

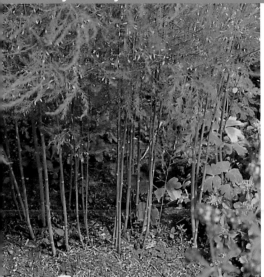

Asparagus
Asparagus officinalis

FOOD: Asparagus has been widely cultivated for over 2000 years as a vegetable and medicinal herb; the Greeks and Romans used it for food and medicine. Young shoots are eaten raw or cooked, and it is often considered a gourmet food. The shoots are a good source of protein and dietary fibre. Roasted seeds are sometimes used as a coffee substitute. The Iroquois ate the stalks, harvesting them in spring.

MEDICINE: The plant reduces muscle spasms, can soothe irritated mucous membranes, promotes sweating and acts as a sedative and tonic. Roots are strongly diuretic and laxative, are said to lower blood pressure and have been used in the treatment of cancer. Roots and shoots have been used to treat problems with the bowels, kidneys and liver. The Iroquois applied stalks externally to treat rheumatism. A decoction of the plant with bark (from an unknown source) was taken before meals for the blood.

DESCRIPTION: Erect perennial herb, to 2 m tall, with fibrous rhizomes. Leaves scale-like, 3–4 mm long. Flowers yellow or yellowish green, 6-parted, 3–7 mm long, bell-shaped, in pairs, stalked, growing along stems, blooming from May to June. Berries red, 6–8 mm long. Found in fields, fencerows, disturbed sites and on roadsides. Introduced to Canada; found from BC to NL.

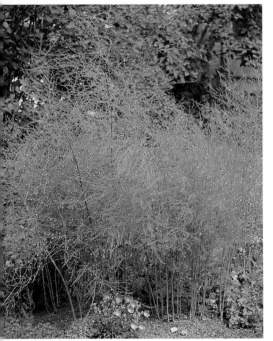

WARNING
Mature plants have poisoned cattle, young plants can cause dermatitis and the berries are suspected of poisoning humans. Compounds produced as asparagus is digested contain sulphur that, when combined with the ammonia in urine, produces a distinctive odour that is detectable by the noses of only some people.

Pokeweed

Phytolacca americana

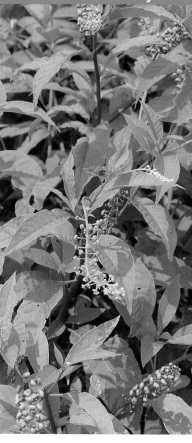

FOOD: The young leaves, according to some accounts, are edible (and quite tasty) only after being boiled in 2 changes of water to remove the toxins (see **Warning**). The berries are said to be poisonous, though some accounts say that cooking inactivates the toxins or that the seed is the only poisonous part of the fruit. Both the Iroquois and the Maliseet gathered the shoots in spring and ate them as greens.

MEDICINE: Pokeweed is known for its immune-stimulating, antiviral, anti-inflammatory and antifungal properties. It has been used traditionally for medicine by the Iroquois and Maliseet. The plant was used as an emetic, purgative, laxative and expectorant; it was also used to treat chest colds and "bewitchment." A poultice of the crushed roots was often applied to bruises, sprains, swollen joints and bunions. A poultice was made from the stalks to treat rheumatism and from the leaves to treat bleeding wounds. Raw berries were rubbed on skin lumps. The toxic/medicinal compounds in pokeweed are phytolaccatoxin, other triterpene saponins, the alkaloid phytolaccin, various histamines and oxalic acid. Pokeweed is currently being investigated as a potential treatment for AIDS.

OTHER USES: A red dye from the ripe berries has been used to colour wine and other foods. The fruits and seeds are said to be an important source of food for mourning doves and other songbirds. The term "poke" could come from the word "pocan" or "puccoon," which resembles an Algonquin term for a plant that contains dye. A close relative of poke-weed, endod (*P. dodecandra*), has been developed in Ethiopia as a botanical molluscicide to control water snails that carry the tropical disease schistosomiasis.

DESCRIPTION: Perennial shrub, to 3 m tall, with large, white taproot; stems green, red or purple. Leaves alternate, large (to 30 cm long), lance-shaped to oval, rounded at base; have unpleasant odour when bruised. Flowers in terminal cluster 6–30 cm long; white or greenish white to pinkish or purplish, 5 sepals (no true petals), 2.5–3.3 mm long, upright or drooping. Fruit purple-black berries, 6–11 mm in diameter with black seeds. Found in damp, rich soils in clearings, roadsides, pastures and thickets in ON, QC and NB. See p. 424 for conservation status..

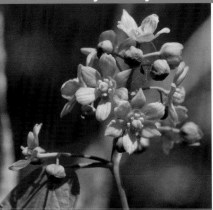

Yellow-flowered blue cohosh

Blue Cohoshes
Caulophyllum spp.

FOOD: Historically, the roasted seeds have been used as a caffeine-free coffee substitute. The attractive, berry-like fruits remain on the plant until autumn, but they should not be eaten, especially by children, because they are potentially poisonous.

MEDICINE: Blue cohosh, also known as "papoose root" or "squaw root," is one of the most important indigenous eastern North American plant medicines. The plant was used extensively by First Nations to facilitate labour, treat irregular menstruation, stimulate the uterus and, with correct dose and timing, induce abortions. It has been labelled "a powerful women's ally" by modern herbalists because of its historical use to treat various gynecological conditions. It is used alone or in combination with other herbs to treat endometriosis, chlamydia and cervical dysplasia. As a homeopathic uterine tonic, it is mixed in a 1:1 ratio with black cohosh (*Cimicifuga racemosa*) and used as a tincture in the last 2–4 weeks of pregnancy to tone the uterus to facilitate childbirth, jumpstart a stalled labour and ease labour pains. If used during early pregnancy, the induced uterine contractions can cause a miscarriage or early delivery. The root contains a number of alkaloids and glycosides, of which the alkaloid methylcytisine and the glycoside caulosaponin seem to be the responsible bioactive constituents. Caulosaponin exerts its oxytocic (childbirth hastening) effects by causing muscle spasms resulting in contraction of the uterus. It also constricts heart blood vessels and has demonstrated cardiac muscle toxicity in animals. For this reason, blue cohosh should not be taken by people with hypertension and heart disease. Methylcytisine displays activity similar to nicotine in animals in that it elevates blood pressure and stimulates respiration and intestinal motility, but it is much less toxic. Other ailments for which blue cohosh root was prescribed include rheumatism, pelvic inflammatory disease, gout, dropsy, colic, sore throat, abdominal cramps, hiccoughs, epilepsy, hysterics, inflammation, urinary tract infections, lung ailments and fevers. It has been used as a diuretic and to expel intestinal worms.

OTHER USES: The bright blue seeds have been used to make seed jewellery. These plants are occasionally grown as woodland garden ornamentals.

DESCRIPTION: Perennial, deciduous herbs from rhizomes, 30–90 cm tall, with large, triple-compound leaves on a single stem; larger stems have 2 leaves, each leaflet ending in 3–5 distinct tips. Flowers borne on spikes, each having 6 greenish yellow to purple, petal-like sepals, with 6 fleshy nectar glands at the base of each sepal. No true fruits, but seed coat develops into a deep blue, berry-like covering for the 2 seeds. See p. 424 for conservation status.

Purple-flowered blue cohosh (*C. giganteum*) has 4–18 purple, red, brown or yellow flowers, 1–4 cm wide, in early spring before *C. thalictroides* flowers. Grows in low elevation, moist woods in southern ON and QC.

Yellow-flowered blue cohosh (*C. thalictroides*) has 5–70 inconspicuous, purplish brown to yellow-green flowers, 1–2 cm wide, borne on a loosely branched cluster, from April to June. Grows in low elevation, moist woods from southeastern MB to NB and in Labrador.

WARNING
Handling powdered root can cause irritation to mucous membranes, and possibly also dermatitis. The plant should be taken with careful medical supervision and should be avoided during early pregnancy.

Mayapple
Podophyllum peltatum

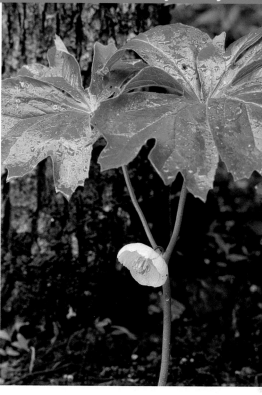

FOOD: The pulp surrounding the seed is sweet and acidic and can be eaten raw or cooked and made into jelly, jams, marmalades and pies. The juice can be added to lemonade. The fruit should be eaten when fully ripe, about the time that the rest of the plant begins to wither and die. If eaten any sooner, it is strongly laxative. If too much is ingested, it may cause colic. The rind should be removed, and no other part of the plant, including the seeds, should be eaten because they are strongly cathartic.

MEDICINE: Unquestionably one of North America's more powerful and useful medicinal plants, mayapple has been used to treat a wide array of diseases but is most noted for its effects on the liver and digestive system. First Nations and early settlers used the plant as a "liver cleanser" to cure jaundice and hepatitis, to expel worms, to relieve constipation and to treat fevers and syphilis. The highly allergenic resin from the root, called podophyllin, contains podophyllotoxin, which is the pharmacological base for the important anticancer drug Etoposide used to treat testicular and small-cell lung cancers. It is also in commercial gels or solutions to treat genital and uterine warts. Podophyllin interferes with the cell replication cycle and inhibits new cell growth. It has been investigated as a potential treatment for ovarian cancer. One of the more common side effects of podophyllin treatment is alopecia, the loss of hair. Because of its cytotoxic effects, mayapple should not be ingested during pregnancy or without the supervision of a qualified professional. The plant has been used by First Nations to commit suicide. Homeopathically, a tincture of the root, gathered after the fruit has ripened, is used for a variety of complaints, most particularly diseases of the gallbladder and intestines.

OTHER USES: An insecticide can be made from an infusion of the leaves and sprayed on potato plants. Corn seeds were once soaked in root resin prior to planting to discourage birds or insects from eating them. Mayapple is sometimes cultivated in woodland gardens.

WARNING
Ingestion of even tiny amounts of the root or leaves is poisonous. The powdered root and resin can cause skin and eye irritation.

DESCRIPTION: Perennial, deciduous herb from rhizomes, 30–60 cm high, with solitary, nodding flower borne in the crotch between a pair of large, deeply lobed leaves, to 30 cm wide. Fragrant flowers to 5 cm wide, have 6–9 waxy, white petals, from April to June. Fruit large, fleshy, lemon-like berry, 3.5–5.5 cm long, containing 30–50 seeds. Grows in mixed deciduous forests and moist, open areas at lower elevations in southeastern ON and southwestern QC. See p. 424 for conservation status.

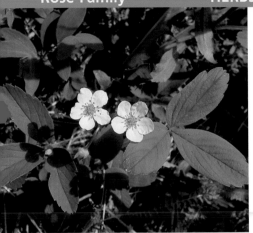

Strawberries

Fragaria spp.

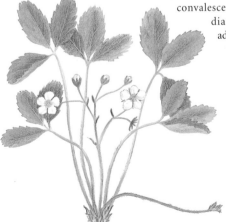

FOOD: These delicious little berries seem much more flavourful than a typical large, domestic strawberry. Wild strawberries are probably best enjoyed as a nibble along the trail, but they can also be collected for use in desserts and beverages. A handful of bruised berries or leaves, steeped in hot water, makes a delicious tea, served either hot or cold. Today, strawberries are preserved by freezing, canning or making jam, but traditionally, they

Wild strawberry (all images)

were sun-dried. The berries were mashed and spread over grass or mats to dry in cakes, which were later eaten dry or re-hydrated, either alone or mixed with other foods as a sweetener. Strawberry flowers, leaves and stems were sometimes mixed with roots in cooking pits as a flavouring. Wild strawberry and coastal strawberry are the original parents of 90 percent of cultivated strawberries.

MEDICINE: A vitamin C supplement can be made by covering fresh strawberry leaves with cold water, blending them to a pulp and simmering the mixture for 15 minutes. Strain the following day and store in the refrigerator or freeze for later use. The leaf tea was used as a tonic and stomach cleanser, as a medicine for fevers, dysentery, diarrhea and kidney problems and as a wash for eczema, sores and other skin problems. It is said to be one of the best home remedies for diarrhea. Dried, ground leaves were used as a gentle disinfectant on open sores, applied as a powder or mixed with fat and used as a salve. Strawberries contain many quickly assimilated minerals (e.g., sodium, calcium, potassium, iron, sulphur and silicon), as well as citric and malic acids, and they were often taken to enrich the bloodstream. Strawberry leaf tea, accompanied by fresh strawberries, was used as a remedy for gout, rheumatism, inflamed mucous membranes and liver, kidney and gallbladder problems. Stems and roots, collected late in the season, were boiled to make medicinal teas for healing sore throats and mouth sores and for strengthening convalescents. The root tea was used to treat diarrhea and infant cholera. With the addition of yarrow root (p. 357), this tea was believed to cure insanity. Cooked strawberry plants were eaten to strengthen gums, "fasten" teeth,

> **WARNING**
> Partially wilted leaves can contain toxins. Always use fresh or completely dried leaves. Some people develop a rash or hives after eating large quantities of strawberries.

soothe inflamed eyes and relieve hayfever. A chemical, D-catechin, found in the leaves is said to inhibit histamine production. Although the leaf tea has little effect on its own, it seems to enhance the action of antihistamine drugs. Strawberries are a good source of ellagic acid, a chemical that is believed to prevent cancer.

OTHER USES: To remove tartar and whiten discoloured teeth, strawberry juice was held in the mouth for a few minutes and then rinsed off with warm water. This treatment is most effective with a pinch of baking soda in the water. Large amounts of fruit in the diet can slow dental plaque formation. Strawberry juice, rubbed into the skin and later rinsed off with warm water, was used to soothe and heal sunburn.

DESCRIPTION: Low perennials with long, slender stolons. Leaves 5–10 cm across, with 3 sharply toothed leaflets. Flowers white, 1.5–2 cm across, forming small, loose clusters, from May to August. Fruit tiny, seed-like achenes embedded in a red, fleshy receptacle.

Coastal strawberry (*F. chiloensis*) has green, thick, leathery leaflets, with the end tooth shorter than its adjacent teeth. Found only on dunes and sea bluffs in coastal BC.

Wood strawberry (*F. vesca*) has yellowish green leaflets, with the end tooth projecting beyond its adjacent teeth. Found in dry to moist, open woods and meadows and on streambanks all across Canada except YT.

Wild strawberry (*F. virginiana*) has bluish green leaflets, with the end tooth narrower and shorter than its adjacent teeth. Found in dry to moist, open woodlands and clearings, often in disturbed areas on well-drained sites in prairie to subalpine zones all across Canada.

Wood strawberry

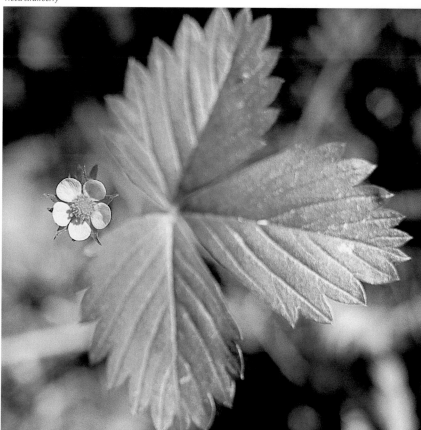

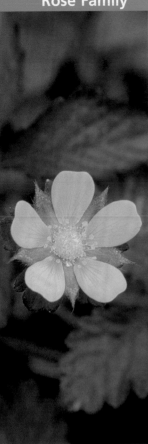

Indian Strawberry

Duchesnea indica

FOOD: The fruit is edible, though it is tasteless.

MEDICINE: Fresh leaves were crushed and applied as a poultice to treat external injuries such as boils, abscesses, swellings, weeping eczema, ringworm, snakebites, insect bites and traumatic injuries. Indian strawberry was also taken as a decoction to treat laryngitis, ulcers of the mouth and acute tonsillitis. An infusion made from the flowers was used to activate blood circulation, and the fruit was used to cure skin diseases.

OTHER USES: This plant is often mistaken for wild strawberry, but there are a few distinguishing features. Indian strawberry has yellow flowers and red seeds in the fruit, whereas wild strawberry has white flowers and yellow seeds in the fruit. The fruits of wild strawberries are also very tasty fruits compared to the bland, tasteless fruits of Indian strawberry. This plant will produce flowers and fruit sporadically throughout the growing season.

DESCRIPTION: Perennial, strawberry-like herb, with trailing, hairy stems to 30 cm long. Leaves alternate, in threes with oval to elliptical, toothed lobes, roughly veined beneath. Flowers solitary, yellow, with 5 petals and 5 leaf-like, 3-toothed bracts, blooming from April to June. Fruit pulpy red, like a strawberry, surrounded by 5 large bracts. This introduced Asian species is found in open forests and disturbed places (fields, lawns) in a few locales in southwestern BC and southern ON.

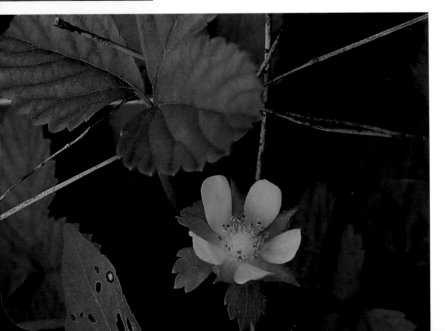

Prickly-Pear Cacti
Opuntia spp.

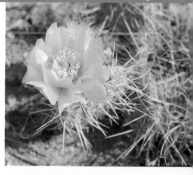

FOOD: Prickly-pear cacti were widely used for food in western Canada, though the fruits of Canadian cacti are smaller and less fleshy than those of their southern relatives. The flavour ranges from bland to sweet to sour and has been likened (at best) to sweet pomegranates or cucumber. Spines were peeled off, burned off, picked off (with fingers protected by deerskin tips) or removed by sweeping piles of fruit with big sagebrush (p. 142) branches. The fruits were then split to remove the seeds and eaten raw (alone or with other fruits), cooked into stews and soups as a thickener or dried for later use. More recently, the sweet flesh has been added to fruit cakes or canned as fruit juice. Berries can also be boiled whole and strained to make jellies or syrups. Dried seeds were added to soups and stews or ground into flour and used as a thickener. Raw cactus stems were usually eaten only when there was a shortage of food. Young segments were boiled and peeled to remove their spines, and the pulpy flesh was fried. Alternately, roasted or pit-cooked stems were simply squeezed until the edible inner part popped out. Cactus stems have also been pickled or candied.

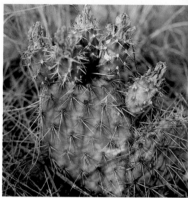

Plains prickly-pear cactus (all images)

MEDICINE: The peeled, mucilaginous stems were used for dressing wounds or were mashed and placed on aching backs. Stems were also boiled to make a medicinal drink for relieving diarrhea and lung problems and for treating people who could not urinate. More recently, studies have suggested that the juice may be effective in lowering blood sugar levels in diabetics, especially those with chronic hyperglycemia.

OTHER USES: When forage was limited, the spines were singed off and cactus stems were fed to livestock. Split stems were placed in containers of muddy water, where they exuded large amounts of mucilage, which cleared the water and made it drinkable. Freshly peeled stems were sometimes rubbed over painted hides to fix the colours. The fruit provides a pink to red dye. The gum from the stem was sometimes used as an adhesive.

DESCRIPTION: Spiny, perennial herbs from fibrous roots, 5–40 cm tall, with thick, fleshy, segmented stems. Leaves reduced to spirally arranged, starburst clusters of short bristles and rigid, barbed, 1–5 cm long spines. Flowers yellow (sometimes pinkish when older), broadly bell-shaped, with many paper-thin, overlapping petals, solitary at branch tips, from May to June. Fruits fleshy (though often rather dry), seedy, somewhat spiny, oval berries 1.5–2.5 cm long.

Brittle prickly-pear cactus (*O. fragilis*) has strongly barbed spines in white-woolly tufts on small (less than 5 cm long), rounded stem segments that detach easily. Grows in dry, open ground in prairie to foothills from southern BC to southwestern ON. See p. 424 for conservation status.

See p. 424 for conservation status.

WARNING

Always protect your hands with gloves when collecting these spiny plants.

Plains prickly-pear cactus (*O. polyacantha*) has slightly barbed spines in brown-woolly or hairless tufts on large (often 5–12 cm long), flattened stem segments that do not break apart easily. Grows in dry, open prairie and on sandhills and rocks from extreme southeastern BC to SK.

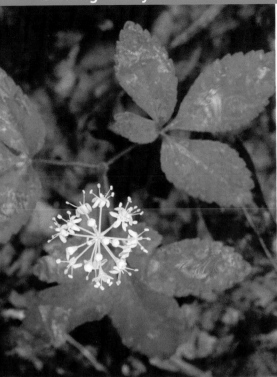

American ginseng

Ginsengs
Panax spp.

FOOD: The aromatic roots can be eaten raw, cooked or candied and chewed. The berries are also edible and taste much like the root. The leaves can be used to make a pleasant tea.

MEDICINE: The most popular and best documented use of ginseng root is as an adaptogen, a substance with the ability to boost the immune system, increase mental efficiency and physical performance and aid in adapting to high or low temperatures and stress. The North American species are considered to have similar medicinal properties to the Asian species, *P. ginseng*, though they are milder in their potency and are thus prescribed primarily to younger patients. The root has a rich 5000 year history of herbal use and plays a crucial role in regulating the balance between yin and yang according to traditional Chinese medical theory. In China, the root is highly prized as an aphrodisiac and as a panacea to promote health, vigour and long life. In the West, ginseng is considered a general health tonic useful for promoting appetite and digestion. Considered a virtual cure-all, the plant is prescribed for a wide array of disorders, including stomachaches, neuralgia, rheumatism, gout, irritation of the respiratory tract, gastrointestinal illness, weak circulation and a variety of nervous disorders. Research has shown that ginseng both stimulates and relaxes the nervous system, promotes hormone secretion and improves stamina and disease resistance. Its ability to lower blood sugar and cholesterol levels is being studied, and the herb may one day provide a therapeutic benefit to diabetic patients. Isolated ginseng saponins have demonstrated a strong radio-protective effect in cancer patients prior to gamma-irradiation. In Canada, First Nations used a decoction of ginseng root for a variety of ailments including fevers, coughs, headaches, nausea and vomiting. Although the herb was not normally prescribed to pregnant women according to Chinese practice, in North America, women regularly consumed a decoction of the root for everything from normalizing menstruation to easing childbirth. The age of the root is believed to correspond to its potency, and older roots should theoretically be given in smaller doses. If using 6–7-year-old root, approximately 3 oz. of the dried, powdered root in 1 cup of near-boiling water is recommended before each meal.

WARNING
Large doses have been reported to increase blood pressure and cause headaches and a variety of other side effects, especially when taken with caffeine, alcohol, turnips and bitter or spicy foods.

OTHER USES: Some First Nations have used it as an ingredient in love potions and charms.

DESCRIPTION: Perennial herb from a fleshy, often forked taproot. Tiny flowers with 5 petals grow in round clusters atop a slender stalk. Fruits berries. See p. 424 for conservation status.

American ginseng (*P. quinquefolius*) is 30–50 cm tall, with whorls of 3 long-stalked leaves, 12–30 cm long, each leaf divided palmately into usually 5 sharp-toothed leaflets. Flowers whitish or yellow-green, 2 mm wide, appear from July to August. Fruit a 2-seeded, white berry, growing in clusters. Grows in moist, rich woods from southern ON to southwestern QC.

Dwarf ginseng (*P. trifolius*) is smaller, 10–20 cm tall, with whorls of 3 sessile (stalkless) leaves, to 8 cm long, each leaf palmately divided into 3–5 coarsely-toothed leaflets. White flowers appear from May to June. Fruit a yellow, 2- to 3-seeded berry. Grows in rich woodlands from southern ON to the Maritimes.

Commercial exploitation in Canada during the 1700s has significantly decimated the ginseng population such that it is now illegal to export wild plants and roots. Canada has since become the world's largest commercial grower of cultivated American ginseng, and it is Ontario's fifth most valuable cash crop. Throughout its growing range in Canada, the species is considered threatened, and a fine is imposed for collection between January and September.

Dwarf ginseng

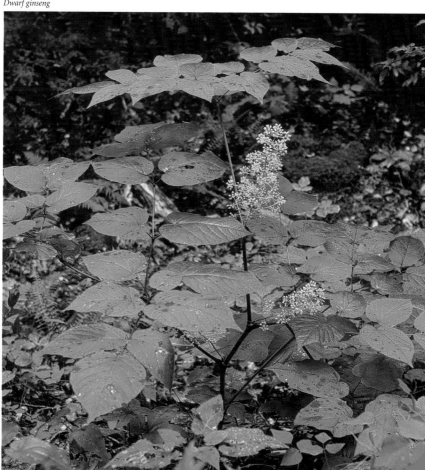

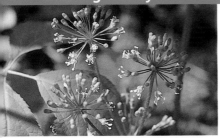

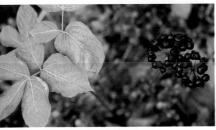

Wild sarsaparilla (all images)

Sarsaparillas
Aralia spp.

FOOD: These rhizomes were generally considered emergency food only, but some indigenous hunters and warriors are said to have subsisted on them during long trips. The fragrant plants have a warm, aromatic, sweetish taste that is most intense in the rhizomes and berries. The rhizomes were used to make tea, root beer and mead. The berries were used to flavour beer and to make wine (similar to elderberry [p. 124] wine), and a tea was sometimes made from the seeds. The berries are generally considered inedible. Some sources report that they have been used to make jelly, but it is not recommended (see **Warning**). Young shoots were sometimes cooked as a potherb.

MEDICINE: The rhizomes (and occasionally the leaves) were pulverized by pounding or chewing and were used in poultices to soothe and heal wounds, burns, sores, boils and other skin problems and to relieve swelling and rheumatism. Mashed rhizomes were also stuffed into noses to stop bleeding and into ears to stop aching. The rhizomes and berries were boiled to make medicinal teas and syrups or soaked in alcohol to make tinctures. These medicines were used to treat many different problems, ranging from stomachaches to rheumatism and syphilis. The pleasant-tasting rhizome tea was valued as a blood-purifier, tonic and stimulant and as a medicine for stimulating sweating. It was widely used for treating lethargy, general weakness, stomachaches, fevers and coughs. Wild sarsaparilla was widely used in patent medicines in the late 1800s.

OTHER USES: Wild sarsaparilla rhizomes were boiled with sweetflag (p. 166) rhizomes to make a solution for soaking nets to be used for fishing at night. This practice was said to increase the catch.

DESCRIPTION: Perennial shrubs or herbs with rhizomes. Leaves large and compound. Flowers whitish and grow in terminal clusters. Fruits dark berries. See p. 424 for conservation status.

Hairy sarsaparilla (*A. hispida*) is a perennial shrub, to 1 m tall, with sharp, stiff bristles at the base. Leaves twice compound with oval, toothed leaflets. Flowers small, greenish white and growing in globe-shaped clusters, from June to August. Fruits dark, foul-smelling berries. Grows in sandy, open woods from SK to NL.

Wild sarsaparilla (*A. nudicaulis*) is a perennial herb, to 70 cm tall, with a long, horizontal rhizome. Leaf blades horizontal, with 3 major divisions, each of these divided into 3–5 oval leaflets 3–12 cm long. Flowers greenish white, 5–6 mm long, forming 2–7 (usually 3) round, 2–5 cm wide clusters, from May to June, usually hidden under the leaf. Fruits dark purple berries, 6–8 mm long. Grows in moist, shaded forests from YT and BC to NL.

Spikenard (*A. racemosa*) is a perennial herb, to 2 m tall, with dark green or reddish stems. Leaves 3 times compound with 6–21 toothed, heart-shaped leaflets. Flowers small, whitish, growing in small clusters along a branching raceme, from June to August. Grows in rich, moist woods from southern MB to the Maritimes.

WARNING
Some people have reported being very sick after eating wild sarsaparilla berries.

Bunchberry
Cornus canadensis

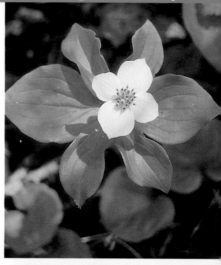

FOOD: The scarlet fruits are edible, but opinions of their flavour range from insipid to good. They were eaten raw as a trail nibble and were said to be good cooked in puddings. Bunchberries (often mixed with other fruits) have been used whole to make sauces and preserves or cooked and strained to make syrups and jellies. Some people enjoy the crunchy little poppy-like seeds.

MEDICINE: Bunchberry is said to have anti-inflammatory, fever-reducing and pain-killing properties (rather like mild aspirin), without the stomach irritation and potential allergic effects of salicylates. It has been used to treat headaches, fevers, diarrhea, dysentery and inflammation of the stomach or large intestine. The berries were eaten and/or applied in poultices to reduce the potency of poisons. They were also chewed and applied to burns. Bunchberries were steeped in hot water to make a medicinal tea for treating paralysis, or they were boiled with tannin-rich plants (such as common bearberry, p. 120, or commercial tea) to make a wash for relieving bee stings and poison-ivy (p. 395) rash. Native peoples used tea made with the entire plant to treat aches and pains, lung and kidney problems, coughs, fevers and fits. The root tea was given to colicky babies. Bunchberry has been studied as a potential anti-cancer agent.

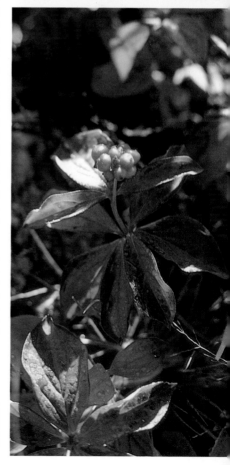

DESCRIPTION: Perennial, rhizomatous herb, 5–20 cm tall, with a whorl of 4–7 wintergreen, 2–8 cm long leaves. Flowers tiny, in a dense clump at the centre of 4 white to purple-tinged, petal-like bracts, forming single, flower-like clusters about 3 cm across, from May to August. Fruits bright red, berry-like drupes, 6–8 mm wide, in dense clusters at the stem tips. Grows in cool woods and damp clearings at low to subalpine elevations in all provinces and territories. See p. 424 for conservation status.

> **WARNING**
> Unripe berries may cause stomachaches, and large quantities have a strong laxative effect.

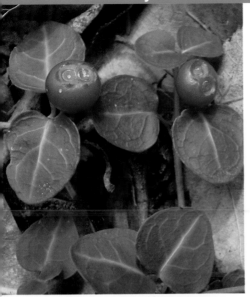

Partridge Berry

Mitchella repens

FOOD: The Mi'kmaq, Iroquois, Montagnais and Maliseet ate partridge berries fresh or preserved and sometimes cooked into a jam. The Mi'kmaq also reportedly used this plant to make a beverage. The berries are considered edible, though not very tasty.

MEDICINE: Historically, the whole plant, or more often the vine, was used medicinally. First Nations reportedly used partridge berry to ease childbirth. The Montagnais used a jelly made from the cooked berries to treat fevers, and the Abenaki reduced swelling with a salve of partridge berry mixed with plantain (p. 256).

OTHER USES: Its trailing stems and pretty red berries make this plant a good Christmas decoration. Partridge berry was also combined with other plants and used for smoking. Wildlife such as ruffed grouse and wild turkey, and presumably partridge, enjoy the bud, leaf, flower and fruit of this plant.

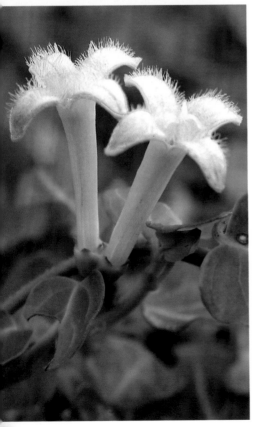

DESCRIPTION: Small, trailing, perennial, evergreen vine less than 50 cm long. Stems slender, wiry. Leaves dark green, opposite, stalked, blades blunt at tip, rounded at base, 1–2.5 cm long and as wide, smooth, with a pale midrib, often variegated with white lines above; margins toothless. Flowers white (occasionally purple-tinged), tubular with coarse hairs inside, with usually 4 spreading lobes, 10–15 mm long, fragrant, in pairs, from June to July. Fruits scarlet, double berries (ovaries of 2 flowers united) with indentation and 2 star-shaped marks, containing 8 seeds; ripen from August to September, persist all winter. Roots easily, often forms large mats. Found in dry or moist woods, sandy to coarse, loamy, upland sites, in hardwood, mixed wood and pine stands from ON to NL. See p. 424 for conservation status.

Horse-Gentian & Feverwort

Triosteum spp.

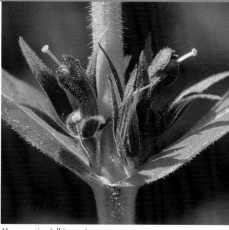

FOOD: Horse-gentian has another common name, wild coffee, that provides a hint of what it was used for. The ripe berries can be dried and ground, and 1–2 teaspoons added to a cup of cold water and heated. When the coffee comes to a boil, remove it from the heat and let it steep for a few minutes. Opinions vary greatly on the taste.

Horse-gentian (all images)

MEDICINE: The plants are a valuable homeopathic remedy for diarrhea with colic pains and nausea. It is useful for patients who experience numbness of the lower limbs after passing stool. First Nations used a decoction of the leaves to induce perspiration and urination in the treatment of fever and malaria. The roots, about 15 mm long, have an unpleasant odour and a bitter, nauseating taste. When given in large doses, they are emetic and cathartic. As an infusion, the plants have been used to treat severe colds, pneumonia, irregular or profuse menstruation, painful urination, stomachaches and constipation. A cold tea was used for bad colds, dry throats and coughs. A decoction was taken for venereal disease. Early physicians used the root tea for headaches, colic, vomiting, diarrhea and indigestion. It was said to be useful for adults and children who needed to put on weight. Externally, the roots were applied as a poultice on snakebites and sores and on the heads of newborn infants with sore heads. The plants secrete an ooze that has been used as a wash to soak sore feet and rub swollen legs.

DESCRIPTION: Perennial plants, 30 cm–1.2 m tall, with erect, round, hairy, hollow stems. Leaves entire, oval to lance-shaped with few-flowered clusters in the axils of the upper leaves. Flowers red to greenish, 2 cm long, with 5-lobed corolla and 5 long sepals, from May to July. Fruit a hairy, yellow-orange berry with persistent, 5-lobed calyx and 3 seeds. Grow in open, rocky woods and thickets. See p. 424 for conservation status.

Horse-gentian (*T. aurantiacum*) has leaves tapering to bases, a smooth or slightly hairy stem, reddish purple flowers and a bright orange-red berry. Found in southern ON, QC, NB and Labrador.

Feverwort (*T. perfoliatum*) has bases of paired leaves united as to appear to be pierced by the stem, a densely hairy, glandular stem, greenish yellow to purplish flowers and a dull orange-yellow berry. Found in southern ON and QC.

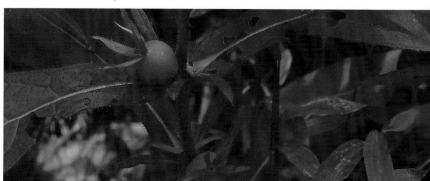

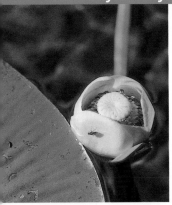

Cow-Lilies
Nuphar spp.

FOOD: The seeds of these aquatic plants were an important food for some tribes. Dried capsules were broken open and winnowed to separate the seeds, which were then popped and eaten like popcorn or fried in bear fat. Dried, fried or popped kernels were also ground into flour. Some people consider cow-lily rhizomes extremely bitter and unpleasant, even after prolonged boiling in several changes of water, but others have described them as sweet, excellent eating. The rhizomes are probably best in late autumn or early spring. They were usually roasted or boiled and then peeled, sliced and eaten with meat in soups and stews. Thin, cooked slices were dried and then stored or ground into flour for making gruel and for thickening soups.

MEDICINE: Cow-lily rhizomes were used in medicinal teas to treat sore throats, inflamed gums, diarrhea, gallstones, stomach inflammation, sexual irritability, venereal disease, blood diseases, chills with fever, heart problems and impotence. Some present-day herbalists have recommended the seeds or dried rhizomes as a cooling astringent and anti-inflammatory for treating irritated digestive tracts, urinary tracts and reproductive organs. Mashed rhizomes have been used as poultices on wounds, bruises, boils, swellings and inflamed and swollen joints. They contain mucilage, tannin and steroids, and some of their alkaloids are reported to stimulate the heart, constrict blood vessels and relieve or prevent spasms. They also contain antagonistic alkaloids: for example, one reduces blood pressure and one increases blood pressure.

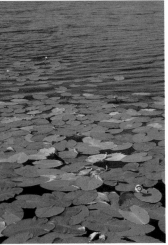

Western cow-lily (all images)

OTHER USES: Bruised rhizomes, steeped in milk, produced an insecticide for killing beetles and cockroaches. Smoke from burned rhizomes was said to drive away crickets.

DESCRIPTION: Aquatic, perennial herbs with fleshy stems to 2 m long from massive rhizomes (to 5 m long and 15 cm in diameter). Leaves floating, long-stalked (stalks 1–2 m long), leathery, round to heart-shaped, 10–40 cm across. Flowers yellow, often tinged green or red, 6–10 cm across, with about 6–9 waxy, petal-like sepals and 10–20 tiny true petals, partially hidden below the stamens; a large, yellow, disc-like stigma is borne singly, on or above the water surface, from May to August. Fruits leathery, oval capsules.

NOTE: The 2 species described here are called subspecies of *Nuphar lutea* in many earlier books.

Yellow cow-lily (*N. variegata*) has slightly flattened, winged leaf stalks and purple fruits. Grows in standing water (ponds, lakes, meandering streams) at low to montane elevations in all provinces and territories from eastern BC and YT eastward.

Western cow-lily (*N. polysepala*) has rounded leaf stalks with no wings, and green to yellow fruits. Grows in the same habitats as yellow cow-lily, but only in western BC and YT and the north-western corner of NT.

WARNING
Large amounts of these rhizomes are potentially poisonous.

Fragrant Water-Lily

Nymphaea odorata

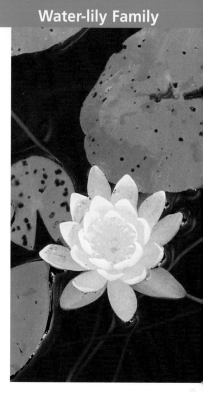

FOOD: The flowers, leaves, rhizomes and seeds are edible. One Ojibwa group ate the flower buds. The flower buds can be cooked as a vegetable or pickled, the flowers eaten raw, the leaves eaten raw or cooked and used in soups and stews, the rhizome boiled or roasted and the ripe seed cooked or ground into a meal.

MEDICINE: The plant was used medicinally by First Nations living in eastern Canada (Mi'kmaq, Ojibwa, Montagnais) and, to a lesser degree, in BC (Okanagan-Colville); it was often taken to treat colds or respiratory ailments. The rhizomes were the part of the plant most often used; they were taken to treat coughs, suppurating glands, tuberculosis and swellings and to inhibit the sexual drives of men for 2 months at a time. However, the rhizomes were considered poisonous by the Okanagan-Colville (they are said to be strongly astringent). The leaves were used for colds and grippe. The stem was placed directly on the tooth to treat a toothache.

OTHER USES: Water-lilies are beautiful water plants with fragrant blossoms and are popular ornamental plants with numerous cultivars. The genus name comes from Greek "nymphs," female nature creatures often associated with, appropriately, springs and mountain streams. The starchy rhizomes are eaten by wildlife.

DESCRIPTION: Aquatic, perennial herb from thick, frequently branched, creeping rhizomes. Leaves simple, nearly circular, floating, to 40 cm in diameter. Underside of leaves often red or purple with many veins. Long stem attached to centre of leaf. Fragrant flowers, opening in the morning and closing by late afternoon, either on the surface of the water or elevated slightly above it, large (10–23 cm in diameter), showy, white or (rarely) pink with yellow centres, 8 to many petals, 4 sepals mostly greenish, blooming from May to September. Fruit leathery, oval-shaped, berry-like capsule, 1–2 cm in diameter, containing many seeds. Found in standing or slow-moving water (lakes, ponds, sluggish streams, sloughs) at low to montane elevations from SK to NL, and introduced in southern BC. See p. 424 for conservation status.

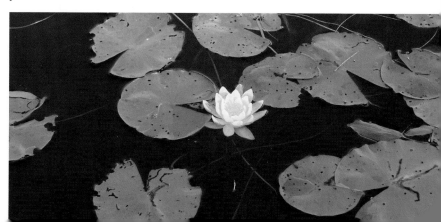

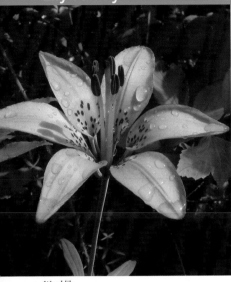
Wood lily

Lilies
Lilium spp.

FOOD: The flowers, seeds and bulbs of lilies have all been used as food. Although the bulbs have a strong, bitter, peppery flavour, they were very popular among native peoples. They were generally cooked and eaten with other foods, such as venison, fish and saskatoons (p. 109) or as a flavouring and thickening agent for stews. Some tribes also ate lily bulbs fresh or dried them for winter storage. Usually, lily bulbs were boiled in 2 changes of water or steamed in fire pits. Cooked bulbs were also dried for winter use, either singly or mashed and formed into thin cakes. The flowers have been used in salads and are delicious as well as beautiful.

MEDICINE: Northern native peoples used wood lily roots to make medicinal teas that were taken to treat stomach disorders, coughs, tuberculosis and fevers and to help women in labour deliver the afterbirth. These teas were also used as a wash for swellings, bruises, wounds and sores. An infusion of the plant combined with sweet viburnum (*Viburnum odoratissimum*) roots was used to treat irregular menstruation. Lily roots combined with roots of blackberries (p. 93), raspberries (p. 94) and staghorn sumac (p. 90) were used to treat coughs, fevers and consumption.

OTHER USES: Bulbs were dried, mashed with stink bugs, powdered and used against "plhax," (i.e. witchcraft). A decoction of the roots was taken by a wife as an emetic and used as wash if her husband was unfaithful. Wood lily is the provincial flower of SK.

DESCRIPTION: Hairless, perennial herbs with single, erect stems from whitish, scaly bulbs. Leaves alternate to (usually) whorled, 5–10 cm long. Flowers showy, usually dark-dotted in the throat, appearing from May to August. Fruits erect, cylindrical capsules, 2–4 cm long.

Canada lily (*L. canadense*) has stems to 1.8 m tall, nodding flowers, spreading or curled backward, colour variable, but most typically yellow with spots on inside of flower. Found in wet meadows, moist, rich woods, marshes, swamps and along wet roadsides and railroads in eastern ON, QC, NB and NS. See p. 424 for conservation status.

Tiger lily or **Columbia lily** (*L. columbianum*) has stems to 1.2 m tall, 2–20 smaller (3–4 cm wide), nodding, orange flowers, with purple-spotted petals that curl back toward the base. Found in coastal scrub and prairies, meadows, conifer or mixed forests and on roadsides in southern BC.

Wood lily (*L. philadelphicum*) has stems to 70 cm tall, whorled upper leaves (usually in sixes) and 1–3 large (about 8 cm wide), erect, goblet-shaped flowers, with orange to brick-red petals and paler, purplish dotted throats. Grows in tall-grass prairies, open woods, thickets, dunes, heathlands and on roadsides from BC (Rocky Mountains) to QC.

Lilies are seldom plentiful, and when they are picked or mowed, all the leaves are removed with the stalk and the plant dies. Digging, mowing and over-picking have caused the near extinction of these beautiful wildflowers in many populated areas. Please leave them for others to enjoy.

Large-Flowered Triteleia

Triteleia grandiflora

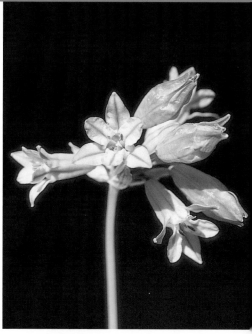

FOOD: Large-flowered triteleia (also called white hyacinth or gophernuts) was one of the first roots to be dug in spring. It was collected in large quantities by both native peoples and settlers, often with the bulbs of yellowbells (p. 196), and was reported to have saved at least one family from starvation. Plants had to be marked the previous year so that their corms could be located the following spring before shoots appeared above ground. Large-flowered triteleia was sometimes eaten fresh, but was said to be rather gluey when raw. The flavour improved with a few minutes of simmering, but the corms were considered best roasted in hot ashes or over a slow fire for about an hour. Cooking breaks down some of the starches and makes the corms much sweeter. Some tribes dried the boiled corms for later use. The young seed pods were also eaten raw as a nibble or cooked as a green vegetable.

MEDICINE: Large-flowered triteleia was believed to have some magical powers and was included in medicine bags to increase their potency.

DESCRIPTION: Slender, perennial herb, 20–60 cm tall, with 1–2 flat, grass-like leaves above a scaly, bulbous stem base (corm) about 2 cm thick. Flowers deep to light blue, about 2 cm long and wide, bell-shaped, with 3 ruffled, inner petals and 3 smooth-edged outer petals, forming flat-topped clusters (umbels), from April to July. Fruits rounded capsules, 6–10 mm long. Found in grasslands, sagebrush, pine forests and hills across southern BC. See p. 424 for conservation status.

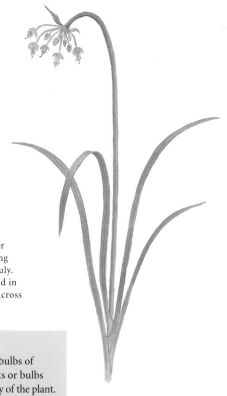

> **WARNING**
> These corms could be confused with the bulbs of death-camas (p. 402). Never eat wild roots or bulbs unless you are absolutely sure of the identity of the plant.

Wild Onions

Allium spp.

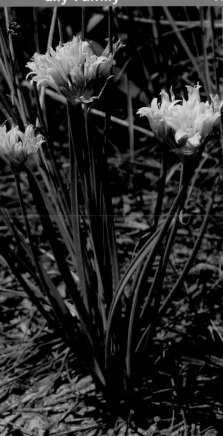

Wild onion

FOOD: All *Allium* species are edible, though some are much stronger than domestic onions. These plants were widely eaten by native peoples and European settlers, either raw or cooked. Wild onions can be served as a hot vegetable but are usually used to flavour other greens and roots or are fried or boiled with meat in casseroles, soups and stews. Cooking removes the strong smell and flavour, converting the sugar inulin to the more digestible fructose, and the bulbs become very sweet. The tender young leaves of most onions (before flowering) have been used raw in sandwiches and salads or cooked with the bulbs. The bulbs were sometimes rubbed in hot ashes to singe off the outer fibres and remove some of the strong taste. They were then eaten immediately or dried and stored for winter. Some tribes layered onions between alder (p. 151) or saskatoon (p. 109) branches in cooking pits and steamed them for several hours, until they were sweet and almost black. Often, onions were steamed with camas bulbs (p. 199) or hair lichen. The sweet, cooked bulbs were usually eaten immediately, but they could also be dried, singly or in cakes, for future use.

MEDICINE: Onions are reported to have antibacterial, antiviral and antifungal qualities, and they have been used for many years in the treatment of cuts, burns and insect bites and stings. *Allium* species contain a complex mix of allyl sulphur compounds, which are the active antimicrobials. The juice from the bulbs was boiled to make a syrup, sometimes sweetened with honey, for treating colds and sore throats. The bulbs have traditionally been used to relieve indigestion, gas and vomiting and were reputed to cure sexual impotency caused by mental stress or illness. They were also dried, ground and used as snuff for opening the sinuses. Frequent doses of onions have been shown to reduce blood lipid (cholesterol) levels and blood pressure and to prevent blood clots from forming.

OTHER USES: Wild onions make an attractive, hardy addition to wildflower gardens and have the added benefit of being edible. Nodding onion was rubbed on the skin to repel insects.

> **WARNING**
> Wild onions resemble and often grow in the same habitats as their poisonous relative, mountain death-camas (p. 402). Some tribes believed that wild onions in the mountains were poisonous, probably because of earlier confusion with death-camas. Mountain death-camas does not smell like an onion. If it doesn't smell like an onion, don't eat it. Some people develop skin reactions after handling onions.

DESCRIPTION: Slender, perennial herbs with oval bulbs, smelling strongly of onions. Flowers bell-shaped, 6-sepalled, clustered at the tips of slender, leafless stems. Fruits capsules.

Canada garlic (*A. canadense*) grows to 50 cm tall. Lower portion of stem has flat, thin, linear leaves 0.5 cm wide and 30 cm long. Flowers often replaced by bulblets; when flowers are present, they're small and white, with a magenta stripe in the centre of each petal. Fruits small, black, triangular-shaped capsules. Found in waste areas and moist woods in southern ON, QC and western NB. See p. 424 for conservation status.

Nodding onion (*A. cernuum*) has bulbs coated with parallel (not netted) fibres, pinkish mauve to white flowers in nodding clusters, and capsules tipped with 6 small crests. Found in dry, open woodlands, prairies and on rocky slopes from BC to ON. See p. 424 for conservation status.

Two common onions have erect flowers and netted, fibrous bulb coats. **Geyer's onion** (*A. geyeri*) has 3 or more leaves and (usually) deep pink flowers, whereas **wild onion** (*A. textile*) usually has 2 leaves and white flowers. Both species grow on prairie, foothill and montane slopes, Geyer's onion from BC to SK and wild onion from AB to southwestern MB. See p. 424 for conservation status.

Prairie onion (*A. stellatum*) grows to 50 cm tall and has narrow, basal leaves. Numerous showy, pink or lavender, star-shaped flowers appear from July to August. Found in rocky prairies or limestone-rich areas from SK to western ON.

Wild leek (*A.tricoccum*) has lance-shaped leaves to 20 cm long and 6 cm wide, with a distinct, slimmer leaf stalk and white flowers. Found in moist areas (rich forests, streamsides) in southern MB, ON, QC, and NS. See p. 424 for conservation status.

Nodding onion

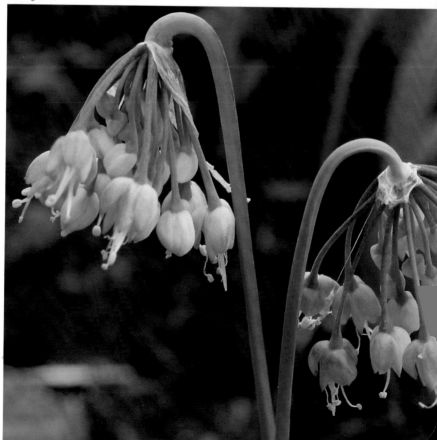

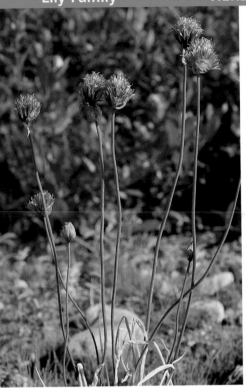

Wild Chives

Allium schoenoprasum

FOOD: Wild chives have been used like domestic varieties—for flavouring soups, salads, sandwiches, vegetables and meat dishes. For example, some Dene peoples of NT ate them raw with moose meat or boiled them in soups; both the Woods Cree and Chipewyans of SK ate the leaves with boiled fish (e.g., trout); and the Inuit used the leaves as a soup condiment, ate the leaves raw with seal oil, meat and fish or fried the leaves with meat, fat, other greens, vinegar, salt and pepper. The leaves, bulbs and flowerheads are all edible and were pickled or used as a cooked vegetable, served hot with butter. Chives contain less sulphur than most onions and are more easily digested. They are a good source of sulphur and iron. Chives were dried or frozen for future use or packed with alternate layers of rock salt and stored in a cool place.

MEDICINE: The most common medicinal use of chives was to treat coughs and colds. The juice was boiled down to a thick syrup, or a sliced bulb was placed in sugar and the resulting syrup was taken. Dried chive bulbs were burned in smudges to fumigate patients, or they were ground and inhaled like snuff to clear the sinuses. Wild chives were also said to stimulate appetite and aid digestion. On the other hand, water in which chives had been crushed and soaked for 12 hours was swallowed on an empty stomach to rid the system of worms. Crushed plants were used to treat insect bites and stings, hives, burns, scalds, sores, blemishes and even snakebites.

OTHER USES: The flower clusters dry well and make a beautiful, purplish addition to dried flower arrangements. Chives are attractive, edible garden plants that flower through-out the growing season. They are easily propagated from seed or by dividing. Some gardeners recommend chives as companion plants for carrots, grapes, roses and tomatoes. They have also been reported to deter Japanese beetles and black spot on roses, scabs on apples and mildew on cucumbers. Chive leaves and bulbs were sometimes rubbed onto skin and clothing as insect repellent.

DESCRIPTION: Slender, perennial herb, 20–50 cm tall, with hollow, cylindrical leaves from elongated bulbs to 1 cm thick, smelling strongly of onions. Flowers deep pink to lilac or white, bell-shaped, 6-tepalled, forming clusters at the tips of hollow, leafless stems, from May to August. Fruits small, membranous capsules, containing shiny, black seeds. Found in moist, open sites (wet meadows, gravelly streambanks and lake shores) across Canada. See p. 424 for conservation status.

WARNING
Without flowers, wild chives might be confused with its poisonous relatives, the death-camases (p. 402), but those plants have flat (not hollow) leaves and no onion-like smell.

Beargrass

Xerophyllum tenax

FOOD: The extensive, stringy rhizomes are edible, but it is recommended that they be roasted or boiled.

MEDICINE: The Blackfoot applied a poultice of chewed rhizomes to wounds and used grated rhizomes to stop bleeding and to treat breaks and sprains.

OTHER USES: Bears eat the fleshy leaf bases in spring, hence the plant's common name. This large, common plant provides an abundant supply of fibre. The tough, fibrous leaves were pounded to separate their fibres, which were then twisted together to make ropes and cord. The plant was also used as twining material for wrapped and twined baskets. The leaves would turn a creamy white colour when dried in the sun and were often used to weave designs in baskets. Some Aboriginal groups wove the long, slender leaves into hats, baskets and capes or used them for trimming the edges of mats, sometimes after shaving and dying the leaves. This plant was known for making baskets that were watertight. Beargrass is difficult to grow, and it does not do well in gardens, so it is best left in its natural habitat. Although beargrass is very showy when in bloom, most plants flower only once every 3–10 years. Often, all the plants in a population bloom together, covering a slope with white and filling the air with a fragrant, lily-like perfume.

DESCRIPTION: Robust, evergreen, perennial herb from rhizomes, with large clumps of tough, wiry, grass-like leaves, 20–60 cm long, edged with sharp, fine teeth. Flowers fragrant, white, about 1.5 cm cross, with 6 spreading tepals, forming showy, club- or bottlebrush-like clusters to 70 cm long, from May to August. Fruits dry, oval, 3-lobed capsules 5–7 mm long. Grows on dry slopes, open coniferous woods, dry ridges and clearings in southeastern BC and southwestern AB. See p. 424 for conservation status.

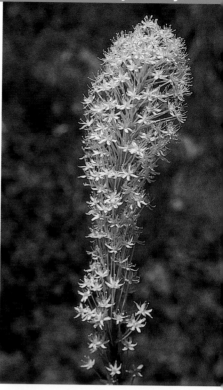

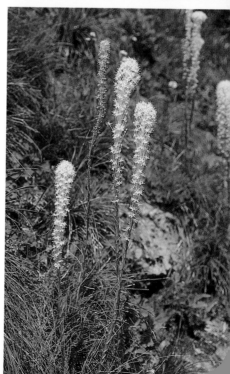

Fritillaries
Fritillaria spp.

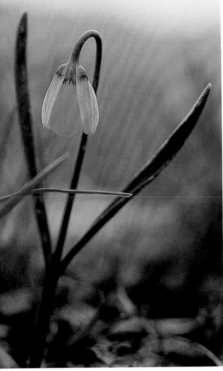
Yellowbells

FOOD: The fleshy bulbs of northern riceroot produce tiny bulblets about the size of rice grains, which give that species its common name. Both rice root bulbs and bulblets are edible, either raw or cooked. Several tribes gathered these roots in early spring, before flowering, or in summer or autumn, using a digging stick, a digging spade or their fingers. The roots would be either cooked immediately or dried for storage and eaten over winter. The bulbs and bulblets would be steamed in cedarwood boxes, mashed into a paste after being boiled or sometimes baked in ashes. They would sometimes be combined with bitterroot (p. 204), which was collected at the same time. They were combined with oil (e.g., eulachon grease) or cooked in stews and soups with fish and eggs or eaten raw with fish eggs. Chocolate lily and yellowbells bulbs were also popular root foods of BC Aboriginal peoples, and they were either boiled or steamed in pits, or sometimes dried for storage.

OTHER USES: The appearance of the flowers of northern riceroot and yellowbells signalled the New Year to the Hanaksiala and Okanagan-Colville of BC, respectively, and the flowers were put on Hanaksiala costumes for the New Year "flower dance."

DESCRIPTION: Slender, perennial herbs, 20–50 cm tall, from scaly bulbs surrounded by tiny, rice-like bulblets. Leaves alternate to whorled, slender. Flowers bowl- to bell-shaped, nodding, 1–2 cm long, with 6 tepals, single or in loose clusters of 2–4, with a disagreeable odour. Fruits small capsules.

Chocolate lily (*F. affinis*) flowers bell-shaped and usually nodding, brownish purple, either mottled yellow or purple, or unmottled, blooming from March to June. Found in oak or pine woodlands and grasslands in southern BC.

Northern riceroot (*F. camschatcensis*) flowers bowl-shaped and usually nodding, dark greenish brown to brownish purple, sometimes streaked or spotted with yellow, blooming from May to July. Found in moist areas from tide flats to mountain meadows in western YT and BC. See p. 424 for conservation status.

Yellowbells (*F. pudica*) flowers yellow to orange, some lined with brown turning to brick red with age, blooming from March to June. Found in grassy, shrubby or woody slopes in southern interior BC and AB. See p. 424 for conservation status.

WARNING

Many members of the Lily family appear very similar before they flower, and several are poisonous. Some tribes considered yellowbells poisonous, probably because of confusion with other plants. Only plants with flowers or flower remains could be positively identified.

●●●

Harvesting the bulb destroys the plant, and over-collecting can eradicate populations of these beautiful wildflowers.

Trout-Lily, Glacier-Lily & Fawn-Lilies

Erythronium spp.

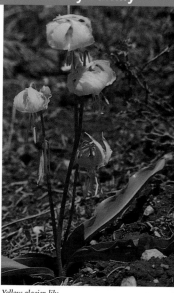

Yellow glacier-lily

FOOD: Slender bulbs of glacier-lily (and to a lesser extent, pink fawn-lily) were collected in large quantities by many Aboriginal peoples in BC and AB, and strings of dried bulbs were a popular trade item. The bulbs can be eaten raw, but like many bulbs and roots, they are made sweeter and more easily digestible by long, slow cooking. Drying also helps this process. Usually they were steamed, roasted or boiled, and many were dried for winter use. A hundred kilograms or more was considered a good winter supply for a family. Dried bulbs were soaked and then boiled or steamed. Once cooked, the bulbs became chocolate brown, soft and sweet. Some First Nations ate the bulbs with soup or stews, or sometimes with meat or fish at feasts. Most tribes used only the bulbs, but the leaves were also eaten occasionally, raw or cooked. Also, the fresh green seed pods were said to taste like string beans when cooked.

MEDICINE: The leaf tea has been shown to inhibit growth of a wide range of bacteria and can be used as an antiseptic wash for cuts, scrapes and sores. Compounds extracted from these plants have also been shown to be slightly antimutagenic and to have tumour-reducing qualities. Bulbs were ingested to treat bad colds. Teas made from other species of *Erythronium* have been used to treat fevers, swelling and infection and to reduce the chances of conception.

OTHER USES: These beautiful wildflowers would make lovely additions to a wildflower garden, but they can be difficult to cultivate.

DESCRIPTION: Perennial herbs, 10–40 cm tall, with 2 basal, lance-shaped to oval or elliptic leaves (10–20 cm long) from deeply buried, elongated, corm-like bulbs (3–5 cm across). Flowers nodding, 3–6 cm across, with 6 tepals curved upward and 6 large stamens projecting downward, usually solitary on leafless stalks from April to August. Fruits erect, 3-sided, club-shaped capsules, 3–4 cm long.

Trout-lily (*E. americanum*) has green leaf blades, irregularly mottled. Flowers yellow, blooming from April to May. Found in shaded areas and moist meadows in ON, QC, NB, PEI and NS.

Yellow glacier-lily (*E. grandiflorum*) has green leaf blades. Flowers bright yellow, blooming from April to July. Abundant in mountain meadows in BC and AB (Rocky Mountains).

White fawn-lily (*E. oregonum*) has leaf blades mottled with streaks of brown or white. Flowers white to creamy white with yellow at base, blooming from March to May. Found in open, coniferous forests, rocky outcrops, oak woodlands and meadows in southwestern BC. See p. 424 for conservation status.

Pink fawn-lily (*E. revolutum*) has leaf blades mottled with streaks of brown or white. Flowers clear violet-pink, blooming from March to April. Found on shaded streambanks, river terraces and in wet places in forests in southwestern BC.

> **WARNING**
>
> The bulbs sometimes cause a burning sensation, and too many can cause vomiting. Large quantities of the leaves and seed pods can cause vomiting and diarrhea.
>
> •••
>
> Over-collecting can eradicate populations of these beautiful wildflowers.

197

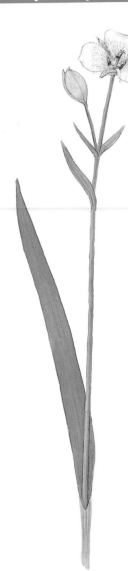

Three-Spotted Mariposa-Lily

Calochortus apiculatus

FOOD: The bulbs of mariposa-lilies are crisp, sweet and nutritious, and they were eaten by many native peoples and settlers. They were sometimes used raw in salads, but usually they were boiled, roasted in ashes or over a smoky fire or steamed in fire pits. Some bulbs were dried for future use. Dried bulbs were boiled in soups and stews or ground into flour for thickening soups and supplementing breads. More recently, these bulbs have been preserved by canning. In 1848, sego-lily (*C. nuttallii*) bulbs, a closely related species that grows in the United States, were reported to have saved the lives of many Mormons when crops were destroyed by crickets, drought and frost. The nectar-rich flower buds of some species were eaten raw as a sweet nibble.

MEDICINE: Juice from the leaves was applied to pimples, and the whole plant was boiled to make a medicinal tea that was given to women in labour to facilitate delivery of the afterbirth.

DESCRIPTION: Slender, perennial herb, 30–45 cm tall, with deep, fleshy, onion-like bulbs. Leaves flat, grass-like and mainly basal. Yellowish white flowers broadly cupped, about 2–4 cm across, with 3 wide, rounded or abruptly pointed petals, each with a distinctive nectar gland and fringe of hairs near the base, borne in loose clusters of 1–5. Flowers have 3 small, round, purplish black dots, and nodding, 3-winged capsules. Grows on foothill and montane slopes in extreme southern BC and AB. See p. 424 for conservation status.

WARNING
Harvesting the bulb destroys the plant. Collecting and overgrazing by cattle and sheep have resulted in the loss of many populations of this beautiful wildflower.

Camases
Camassia spp.

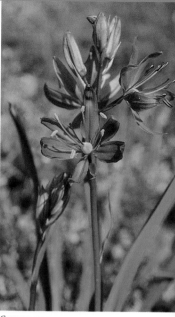

Common camas

FOOD: Camases provided one of the most prized root crops to First Nations in southwestern BC (and US tribes from Montana to California). They were a valued food and trade item, and BC First Nations would often trade camases with neighbouring groups (e.g., First Nations in the BC interior and AB). The bulbs were typically dug in summer, following flowering. The harvest would often take a number of weeks, and the entire family would take part. Large areas of camases were managed by clearing brush and burning. These areas were often owned by individual families and were passed from one generation to the next. The bulbs were harvested with digging sticks, and only large bulbs were taken (smaller bulbs were left for the following year's harvest). They were eaten raw, roasted or stone-boiled, but most were cooked and dried. Usually, bulbs were baked in pits with hot stones for several days until they were dark brown, with a glue-like consistency and a sweet taste, like that of molasses. They were then mashed together and made into cakes, which were sun-dried for storage. During the cooking process, inulin (an indigestible sugar) breaks down to fructose, which is sweet and easily digested. Some cooked, dried bulbs are 43 percent fructose by weight. Camas bulbs were the principal sweetening agent for many tribes prior to the introduction of sugar. Cooked, dried bulbs were sometimes ground and made into small cakes that were eaten with flour, cream and sugar. Concentrated liquid from boiling the bulbs was made into a sweet, hot drink or was mixed with flour to make gravy. The Cowichan served the bulbs at potlatches or winter dances.

MEDICINE: The Blackfoot used a decoction of the roots to induce labour, and they used an infusion of the leaves for vaginal bleeding after birth and to help expel afterbirth.

DESCRIPTION: Slender, perennial herbs, with oval bulbs 1–3 cm thick and grass-like leaves. Flowers pale to deep blue or violet, about 4–5 cm across, with 6 linear, 3- to 9-nerved petals, forming 5–30 cm long clusters, from April to June. Fruits oval capsules, 12–15 mm long. Found in open woods, prairies, fields and on streambanks and roadsides.

WARNING

Harvesting the bulb destroys the plant. Over-collecting has resulted in the loss of many populations of this beautiful wildflower, so leave it untouched in the wild.

●●●

Camases can cause gas and indigestion in the uninitiated; large quantities can result in vomiting and diarrhea. These bulbs could be confused with those of the death-camases (p. 402), so eat at your own risk.

Great camas (*C. leichtlinii*) grows to 60 cm tall and blooms 2–3 weeks later than common camas. Flower segments twist together in a spiral when they wither. Found in southwestern BC.

Common camas (*C. quamash*) is generally smaller and shorter (usually less than 45 cm tall) than great camas and blooms from April to May. Flower segments remain spreading as they wither. Found in southern BC and AB. See p. 424 for conservation status.

Eastern camas (*C. scilloides*) grows to 50 cm tall and has much paler (whitish with a lilac tinge) flowers from April to May. Found in extreme southern ON. See p. 424 for conservation status.

Lady's-Slippers
Cypripedium spp.

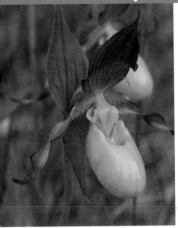

Yellow lady's-slipper (above)
Sparrow-egg lady's-slipper (below)

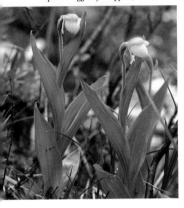

MEDICINE: Lady's-slipper is known widely for its sedative, antispasmodic and tonic properties. Scientific research on yellow lady's-slipper rhizome supports these properties. The rhizomes (the part most commonly used) contain an active compound called cypripedin. Rhizomes were used for menstrual disorders, headaches, insomnia, venereal disease, stomachaches, kidney troubles in children, urinary tract problems and nervousness. Pink lady's-slipper was used medicinally by Algonquin, Iroquois, Mi'kmaq and Cree. A decoction was taken for pains all over the skin and body resulting from "bad blood." A poultice was made from smashed leaves and applied to bites from rabid dogs. As a folk medicine, pink lady's-slipper has been used as a substitute for the European valerian. It has been commonly used for any nervous irritability, hysteria, epilepsy, restlessness and as a sleeping aid; it was sometimes combined with other plants, such as skullcap (p. 273), to make the medicine "more powerful."

OTHER USES: Lady's-slippers have no nectar and attract pollinators by deceit, through the bright colour and the sweet scent of the flower. Bumblebees quickly learn to avoid these plants because they offer no rewards; as a result, lady's-slippers generally have low pollination rates. Like other orchids, lady's-slippers require a fungus for survival. Pink lady's-slipper is PEI's provincial flower.

DESCRIPTION: Herbaceous perennials from slender rhizomes. Oval to lance-shaped leaves, to 20 cm long, have parallel veins and sparse hairs. Solitary flower at end of stalk. Fruits capsules with thousands of tiny seeds.

Pink lady's-slipper (*C. acaule*) grows to 55 cm tall, has 2 basal leaves and no stem leaves. Flower subtended by green bract, with 2 purplish brown to brown, often green-striped sepals, with similar petals. Lip is pouch-shaped, inflated, drooping, magenta to whitish pink. Flowers bloom from May to July. Found in dry, acidic, open woods, on slopes or steep hillsides, edges of swamps, sphagnum bogs and sand dunes in all provinces and territories in Canada except BC and YT. See p. 424 for conservation status.

Yellow lady's-slipper (*C. parviflorum*) grows to 70 cm tall, has alternate stem leaves. Flowers have yellow, sac-like lower lip with purple veins and twisted, spreading, purple-brown lateral petals, 3 petal-like sepals. Flowers bloom from May to June. Grows in moist, calcareous sites, hardwood and mixed woods stands in all provinces.

Sparrow-egg lady's-slipper (*C. passerinum*) grows to 30 cm tall, has 3–5 leaves on lower stem. Small, nodding flowers have a white (occasionally pinkish) pouch and white petals. This sub-arctic plant is found on moist, acidic forest floors, calcareous sites or sandy riversides from northeastern BC to northwestern QC, including much of the Rocky Mountains, YT and NT.

WARNING
The gland-tipped hairs on the stem and leaves cause rashes on some people. These rare and beautiful flowers depend upon an association with a mycorrhizal fungus to grow and will not usually survive harvesting or transplanting.

Rattlesnake-Plantain

Goodyera oblongifolia

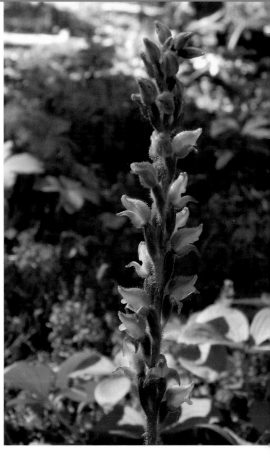

FOOD: An exudation from the plant can be used as a chewing gum.

MEDICINE: Rattlesnake-plantain was used medicinally by Aboriginal peoples on the northwest coast. It was taken for many pregnancy-related issues: the plant was chewed by a woman before and at the time of childbirth; the leaves were chewed prenatally to ensure an easy delivery; and the leaves were split open and blown on several times by women wishing to become pregnant. The leaves, prepared either as a poultice or infusion, were applied to cuts and sores and used in the bathwater of sprinters and canoers as a liniment for stiff muscles. Early settlers believed that the plant could be used to cure rattlesnakebites because of the resemblance of the leaf pattern to snakeskin markings.

OTHER USES: The leaves were chewed to determine the sex of the baby. Some people used the plants as a good luck charm. Children would make balloons from the leaves by rubbing the plants until the leaves separated into 2 layers, then inflating them by blowing through the stem. The plant is named after a 17th-century botanist, John Goodyer. The plant acquired the "plantain" part of its common name likely because it has flattened basal leaf rosettes, similar to real plantain (p. 256).

DESCRIPTION: Evergreen, herbaceous perennial, to 40 cm tall, from rhizome. Leaves 3–7, forming basal rosette, oblong to elliptical, 3–8 cm long and 2–4 cm wide, dark green or blue-green, mottled or with a prominent white stripe along midrib. Flowers dull white to greenish, downy, in terminal spikes of 10–40 flowers, often borne on 1 side, sometimes spiralled; petals and 1 sepal form hood over the lip. Sepals oval, 5–10 mm long and 3–4 mm wide, smooth and white inside, outer surfaces hairy and greenish. Petals spatula-shaped, 5–10 mm long and 3–4 mm wide. Bloom from late July to late August. Fruits erect, hairy capsules, to 1 cm long, with many small seeds. Found in dry to moist, shady, coniferous or hardwood forests at low to montane elevations in all provinces except MB and NL (though most widespread by far in BC). See p. 424 for conservation status.

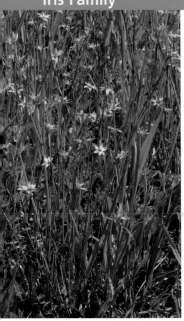

Mountain blue-eyed grass (all images)

Blue-Eyed Grasses
Sisyrinchium spp.

FOOD: Some sources consider these plants poisonous, but leaves were occasionally cooked or mixed with other greens.

MEDICINE: Blue-eyed grass was not widely used but is best known for treating stomach ailments. Some native groups took a decoction of roots and stalks before morning meals for constipation. Other groups made a tea from the roots (an astringent) that was used to treat diarrhea. A compound was made with the plant for "summer complaint," stomach complaints and stomach worms. Herbalists have used the plant to treat menstrual disorders and prescribed leaf tea as a form of birth control. Some native groups used decoctions of mountain blue-eyed grass to treat malaria and typhoid fever, but other groups considered the plant poisonous. Needle-tip blue-eyed grass was used medicinally to treat nose troubles and sore throats.

DESCRIPTION: Despite its common name, this plant belongs to the Iris family. If you feel the stems of blue-eyed grass, you'll discover they are flat or 2-sided, not round like the stems of grasses. Clumped, perennial herbs, to 50 cm tall, stems flattened and ridged. Narrow, basal, grass-like leaves 1–4 mm wide. Flowers pale blue to violet, with 6 pointed tepals and a yellow eye, 8–10 mm long, forming clusters of 3–6 at stem tip. Fruits small, dark brown or black capsules.

Narrow-leaf blue-eyed grass (*S. angustifolium*) has stalked spathes (the bract surrounding the flowers). Flowers from spring to early summer. Found in moist meadows, moist, open woods and on streambanks and swamp edges at low to montane elevations in southern ON, QC, NB, NS and NL. See p. 424 for conservation status.

Mountain blue-eyed grass (*S. montanum*) has stalkless spathes, and stems with wings 1–3.5 mm wide. Flowers from late May to July. Found in moist, open sites in all provinces and territories except NU.

Needle-tip blue-eyed grass (*S. mucronatum*) is similar to mountain blue-eyed grass but has narrower leaves (1–2 mm wide, versus to 3 mm wide in *S. montanum*) and smaller capsules (3–4 mm long, versus 4.5–6 mm long in *S. montanum*). Flowers in early spring. Found in open sites including fields, roadsides, rocky or sandy shores from eastern SK to southern QC.

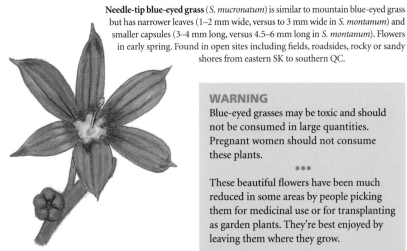

WARNING
Blue-eyed grasses may be toxic and should not be consumed in large quantities. Pregnant women should not consume these plants.

• • •

These beautiful flowers have been much reduced in some areas by people picking them for medicinal use or for transplanting as garden plants. They're best enjoyed by leaving them where they grow.

Wild Gingers

Asarum spp.

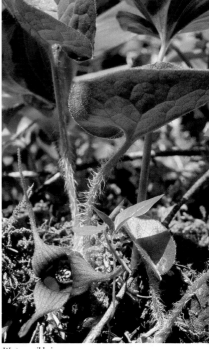
Western wild ginger

FOOD: Wild ginger smells and tastes like commercial ginger (*Zingibar officinale*) and has been used in much the same way, but these two plants are not even distantly related. The leaves of wild gingers are more strongly flavoured than the rhizomes, and they are generally milder than commercial ginger. The rhizomes of wild ginger have been eaten fresh or dried and ground as a ginger substitute, and the leaves have been used to make a fragrant tea. Rhizomes, boiled until tender and then simmered in syrup for 20–30 minutes, are said to make excellent candy. They have also been pickled in brandy.

MEDICINE: Candied rhizomes were used to relieve coughing and stomach problems. The leaves have antifungal and antibacterial properties, and they were used as poultices on cuts and sprains. Rhizomes were boiled to make medicinal teas for treating indigestion and colic. A stronger decoction was taken by women as a contraceptive and was used as drops for curing earaches. The leaf tea is said to stimulate sweating and increase secretions from the tear ducts, sinuses, mouth, stomach lining and uterus. It has been taken to relieve fevers, gas, stomach upset and slow, crampy menstrual periods, and to cleanse the skin when treating measles, chicken pox, rashes and acne. Wild ginger contains aristolochic acid, an antitumour compound.

OTHER USES: Wild ginger in the bedding of ill or restless babies was believed to have a quieting, healing effect. Dried, powdered leaves were used as a deodorant. Some wild ginger plants contain a potential slug repellent: plants growing in areas with slugs produce chemicals that kill or repel these pests, whereas plants in slug-free habitats do not.

DESCRIPTION: Trailing, 15–30 cm tall, often matted, perennial herbs from extensive rhizomes, with 2 shiny, dark green leaves, 5–10 cm wide, smelling strongly of lemon-ginger when crushed. Flowers purplish brown to greenish yellow, bell-shaped, with 3 slender-tailed, petal-like sepals, single, at ground level (often hidden beneath the leaves), from April to July. Fruits inconspicuous, fleshy capsules.

WARNING

Wild ginger should not be used by pregnant women. Large doses can cause nausea. People with sensitive skin may develop rashes from handling the fuzzy leaves. This unusual little plant is becoming less and less common as its habitat disappears. Please leave it in its natural environment. Commercial ginger is readily available to use in its place.

Canada wild ginger (*A. canadense*) has more kidney-shaped leaves and erect flowers with sepals generally less than 2.5 cm long. Grows in moist, rich, usually deciduous woods from MB to NB. See p. 424 for conservation status.

Western wild ginger (*A. caudatum*) has heart-shaped leaves and horizontal flowers with sepals generally longer than 3 cm. Grows in moist, shaded lowland and montane forests in southern BC.

Bitterroot

Lewisia rediviva

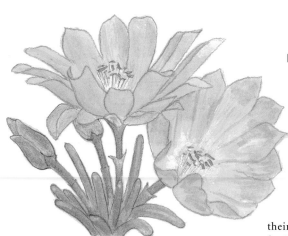

FOOD: Bitterroot was an important staple food for many indigenous peoples in the west, but Europeans usually found it too bitter to enjoy. It was described by Thompson during his expeditions for the NorthWest Company in southern BC and adjacent US, and by Lewis and Clark when their US expedition reached present day Montana. The starchy roots were collected just before the plants flowered, when the bitter, brownish black outer layer could be easily peeled off by rubbing between the hands. Removal of the extremely bitter orange-red heart and storage for 1–2 years was said to reduce bitterness (though some people say that stored roots become increasingly bitter). Peeled, cored and washed roots were pit cooked, steamed or boiled in watertight baskets using red-hot stones; they were sometimes eaten plain, but more often they were mixed with berries or powdered camas roots (p. 199), added to soups (e.g., fish-head soup) and stews, used to thicken gravy or used as an ingredient in fruit cake. They were also cooked with black tree lichen, dough and fresh salmon and made into a pudding. Extra roots were dried for a few days, either loose or on strings if they were large roots, and stored for future use. A 23 kg bag of roots was considered enough to sustain a person through winter, and it took a woman 3–4 days to gather this amount. The brittle, white, dried roots were reconstituted by soaking and boiling, during which they would swell 5–6 times in volume and develop a jelly-like consistency.

MEDICINE: The roots were ingested to treat diabetes and poison-ivy (p. 395) rashes. A poultice of raw roots was applied to sores, and the pounded dried root was a remedy for sore throats.

OTHER USES: The dried roots were an important trade item—a bag of bitterroot could be traded for a good horse. The roots were often traded for dried salmon and other items.

DESCRIPTION: Low, perennial herb, 15–20 cm tall, with fleshy, club-shaped basal leaves 1–5 cm long, from deep, fleshy taproots. Flowers deep to light rose-pink (sometimes whitish), with yellow to orange centres, 4–6 cm across, with 12–18 lance-shaped petals and 6–9 pinkish, oval sepals, borne singly on 1–3 cm tall stalks above a whorl of slender bracts, from April to July. Fruits oval capsules, with 6–20 dark, shiny seeds. Grows in dry grasslands and open forests at foothill and montane elevations in extreme southern BC and AB. See p. 424 for conservation status.

WARNING
Dried bitterroot swells in the stomach, so it should not be eaten in large quantities.

•••

This beautiful wildflower is becoming increasingly rare as a result of overgrazing and human development. It should be harvested only in an emergency.

Spring-Beauties
Claytonia spp.

FOOD: The nutritious corms of many *Claytonia* species have been a valued food source for First Nations in Canada and served as a staple food for some. In Chilcotin territory in BC, the mountain range known as the Potato Mountains was named after western spring-beauty. Entire families would camp in subalpine meadows for 2 or more weeks in late May or June and dig large quantities of corms. The corms were collected using digging sticks or were sometimes taken from the caches of small rodents. They were eaten raw or cooked; they would be rubbed clean, cooked in pits or steamed and eaten. They were sometimes buried fresh in underground caches or cooked for winter storage. If cooked, they were sometimes dried singly or in strings or made into cakes (sometimes combined with mashed saskatoons, p. 109). In eastern Canada, the corms of Carolina spring-beauty were appreciated as a food, especially in spring. Siberian miner's-lettuce leaves are edible and are a good source of vitamin C and pro-vitamin A. The leaves can be added raw to mixed salads or cooked as a green vegetable. Eastern spring-beauty leaves are edible as well.

MEDICINE: Spring-beauties were applied to cuts and sores and eaten to treat constipation and to relieve headaches; they were also mixed with pitch and mountain hemlock (p. 41) bark to treat syphilis. The whole plant was chewed and swallowed as a contraceptive or during pregnancy so the baby would be "soft" when born and to hasten or induce labour. A plant infusion was taken as a general tonic for sore throats. Stem juice was squeezed into the eye for sore, red eyes, and a decoction of powdered roots was given to children with convulsions.

OTHER USES: As the common name suggests, the flowers of spring-beauties are very attractive and emerge in spring. Western spring-beauty was said to fatten hogs, and the flowers of Siberian miner's-lettuce were used by children to play a game.

DESCRIPTION: Perennial herbs, from deep, bulb-like, marble-sized corm or (in Siberian miner's-lettuce) from rhizomes. Basal leaves, usually 1–2, 7–15 cm long. Stem leaves opposite. Flowers white or pale pink (sometimes yellow), with deep pink veins, 5 petals, 5–15 mm long, stalked, few to several in loose clusters. Fruits oval capsules with 3–6 black, shining seeds.

Western spring-beauty (*C. lanceolata*) has stems to 25 cm tall, 1–6 basal, lance-shaped leaves. Flowers 8–14 mm in diameter. Found in sagebrush shrublands and grasslands and moist meadows, from steppe to alpine in BC, AB and SK. See p. 424 for conservation status.

Carolina spring-beauty (*C. caroliniana*) has stems to 25 cm tall. Flowers 8–12 mm in diameter. Grows in moist, often rich forests and wetlands at low to montane elevations from southern ON to NL.

Alpine spring-beauty (*C. megarhiza*) has stems to 10 cm tall. Flowers 12–20 mm in diameter. Thick (succulent), oval-shaped leaves change from red to green as they age. Found on talus, scree and gravelly slopes in the alpine in YT, NT, BC and AB. See p. 424 for conservation status.

Siberian miner's-lettuce (*C. sibirica*) has stems to 50 cm tall. Leaves lance-shaped with long stalks. Flowers 8–20 mm in diameter. Grows in wet sites near streams and ponds, and moist, shaded, coniferous forests in BC.

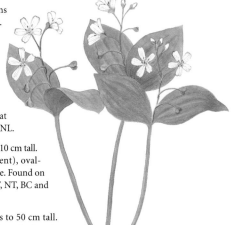

Western spring-beauty

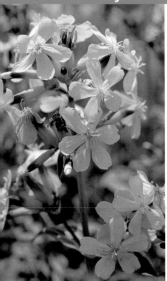

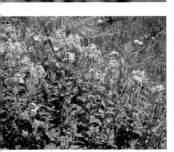

Bouncing Bet
Saponaria officinalis

FOOD: In spite of the toxic potential of bouncing bet, it is used as an emulsifier in the commercial preparation of tahini halva, a sweet confection popular in the Mediterranean and Balkan regions. It is also used in brewing to create beer with a good "head."

MEDICINE: The primary medicinal application of bouncing bet was as an expectorant. The plant contains poisonous saponins that caused the patient to cough and increase the production of a more fluid mucous in the bronchial tubes. The root was taken as a tea for lung disease, asthma, gall disease and jaundice; however, it is rarely used internally today because the saponins irritate the digestive tract. The herb is traditionally used as a poultice to treat spleen pain and boils. The juice from the root was used by some First Nations as a hair tonic. In Europe, the poultice was applied to acne, boils, eczema, psoriasis and poison-ivy (p. 395) rash. A decoction of the entire plant was used as a wash for itchy skin. One of the saponins in this plant, saporin, is useful in biological research applications and is being studied as an anticancer agent. Saporin is a ribosome-inactivating protein, which shuts down protein synthesis inside a cell, essentially causing cell death and, ultimately, the death of the victim. However, saporin and other saponins do not have the molecular means to enter cells on their own and, consequently, are difficult to absorb through the digestive tract. If a method of cellular entry is given to saporin, it becomes an extremely potent toxin. Laboratory experiments have demonstrated that if saporin is directed toward specific target cells, it may be useful in the treatment of cancer.

OTHER USES: The saponins make a soapy lather when mixed with water. This property inspired its genus name (*sapo* means "soap") and its other common name, soapwort. The name bouncing bet is said to originate in England where barmaids, often called "Bets," cleaned ale bottles by filling them with water and a sprig of this plant and shook them violently so as to cause them to bounce. When infusing the plant, especially the root, in warm water, a fine soap is obtained that can be used as an effective cleaner. The soap was said to be especially effective on delicate fabrics. It was used to clean the Bayeaux tapestry, the famous 50 cm by 70 m cloth depicting the 1066 Norman invasion of England. First Nations also used it as a soap and as a shampoo, taking care not to get any lather in the eyes because this caused intense irritation.

DESCRIPTION: Attractive, 30–80 cm tall, perennial herb, from rhizomes and stolons, with stem swollen at nodes. Leaves opposite, oval to lance-shaped, 5–8 cm long, lower ones short-stalked, upper ones unstalked. Flowers 2–3 cm wide, often double, fragrant, with 5 delicate, white to pink petals notched at the tip and with small appendages at their throats, in terminal clusters, from July to September. This introduced Eurasian species grows on roadsides and other disturbed sites throughout Canada.

WARNING
Saponins cause severe irritation to the digestive tract and may cause a skin rash in some people.

Sea Sandwort
Honckenya peploides

FOOD: Sea sandwort, also known as "beach greens" by the Inuit, provides an important source of vitamins A and C to the traditional meat-laden diet of the North. The plants are first rinsed to get rid of the sand and then eaten raw or cooked. The sour leaves and shoots were once more commonly eaten with seal oil and sugar or boiled in several changes of water and stored in large wooden barrels for winter use. In Alaska, the Inuit made "Eskimo ice cream" by souring the boiled, chopped leaves with reindeer fat and berries. The plant was used as a potherb, eaten mixed with other greens or as a side dish to dried fish. The young stems and leaves could also be pickled to make a dish similar to sauerkraut. In Iceland, a liquor that tastes a little like olive oil is obtained from the plant by steeping it in sour whey and allowing it to ferment. The fiddly, small seeds can be used as a garnish or ground into a powder and added to flour.

MEDICINE: According to an Inuit elder, sea sandworts, named *maliksuagait*, were known to have excellent medicinal properties, but the report did not elaborate any further on the subject. Perhaps the plant's nutrient composition was important in preventing deficiencies.

OTHER USES: The plant has been used as fodder for pigs and sheep. On some of the more popular beaches, sea sandwort makes an attractive patch to sit or spread your towel on, but this diminishes the local population.

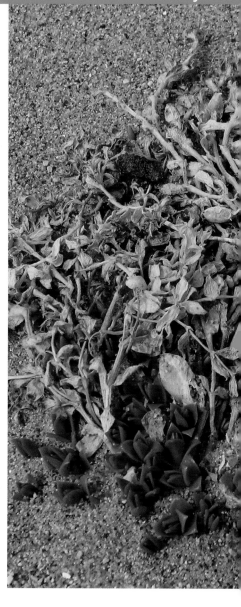

DESCRIPTION: Semi-prostrate, perennial herb, 10–15 cm tall, forming large mat, with alternate, pointed, succulent leaves, 1–4 cm long and 3–20 mm wide. Flowers strongly honey-scented, star-shaped with 5 white petals, 2.5–6 mm long in male flowers, 1– 2 mm long in female flowers, abruptly constricted toward the base, appearing from May to August. Fruit a fleshy capsule, 5–12 mm in diameter. Grows on the top of beaches in fairly stable sand or shingles on the Pacific, James Bay, Arctic and Atlantic coasts.

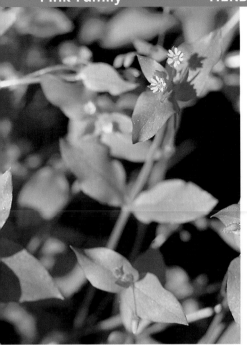

Chickweed
Stellaria media

FOOD: This native of Eurasia has rapidly spread across the Americas and is now a cosmopolitan weed. It is a favourite food of chickens and wild birds. If winter is not too severe, this plant can be eaten year round. The young leaves can be added to salads raw, but they contain some toxic saponins, so not many should be consumed. They are much tastier and safer boiled for 5 minutes and served as greens. Some say that the taste closely resembles that of spring spinach. They are very nutritious and a relatively good source of vitamins A and C. The tiny seeds are also edible, but they are produced in such small quantities throughout the year that gathering a meaningful amount would be a laborious undertaking.

MEDICINE: No herbal is complete without including chickweed in its catalogue. With a long history of use for a wide variety of ailments, it is described by many writers as a valuable herb. However, in spite of extensive scientific investigations of the herb, there is no indication that any of its traditional uses are therapeutic. Modern herbal advocates recommend chickweed for serious constipation, liver ailments, bronchitis, pleurisy, coughs, colds, sore throats, rheumatism, inflammation or weakness of the bowels, stomach, lungs and bronchial tubes, scurvy, kidney complaints, hemorrhoids and cramps. A decoction of the whole herb was taken as a postpartum tonic and to stimulate milk production and menstruation. It was used externally for roseola and other skin diseases, to soothe itchiness and to treat rheumatic pains, wounds and ulcers. The fresh or dried herb was added to bath water to reduce inflammation and promote tissue repair. The juice expressed from the crushed herb was used as an eyewash. The bruised, fresh leaves were used to treat acute ophthalmia, and as an ointment made with fresh lard, were applied to erysipelas (St. Anthony's fire) and other forms of ulcerations. Some of the constituents that occur in chickweed include the flavonoid glycoside rutin and various plant acids, esters and alcohols, none of which possess pronounced pharmacological activity to support its herbal use.

DESCRIPTION: Weak-stemmed, rhizomatous, cool-season, annual herb, 7.5–20 cm tall, with a trailing stem to 40 cm long that is much branched and low to the ground. Leaves relatively smooth, opposite, oval, 1.3–2.5 cm long, with lower leaves stalked, the upper ones sessile. Flowers small, white, to 6 mm wide, with 5 petals cleft so deeply as to appear to be 10, in terminal clusters or solitary in leaf axils, from February to December. Perhaps the most distinguishing feature is the single lengthwise line of fine, white hair on 1 side of the stem that switches sides above and below every node. Found at low to montane elevations in lawns, fields and other disturbed sites throughout Canada.

WARNING
Because the plant contains saponins, excess consumption can cause diarrhea and vomiting. Pregnant women should not consume the plant.

Bloodroot

Sanguinaria canadensis

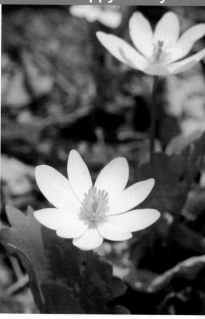

MEDICINE: Bloodroot releases a brilliant red sap when the rhizome is cut. It is well known for its antimicrobial, anti-inflammatory and antioxidant properties and was used extensively by First Nations in eastern Canada (Algonquin, Iroquois, Maliseet, Mi'kmaq). Bloodroot rhizomes were often applied as a poultice or taken as an infusion to threat wounds, growths, sores, swellings and boils, lump hemorrhages, poison-ivy (p. 395) and to draw out thorns or slivers. The plant has also been used for a number of stomach and intestinal ailments: vomiting, stomachaches (cramps), ulcers, intestinal trouble, diarrhea, gas, to "clean" the stomach and to loosen the bowels. Respiratory-related illnesses treated with bloodroot include asthma, bleeding lungs, consumption cough, tuberculosis and inflammation of the mucous membrane in the lungs. Another common use of bloodroot was as a fortifier of blood and internal organs: to make blood redder or purify it, for heart trouble, for internal pain and to treat the kidneys and gallbladder. Other illnesses treated with bloodroot were headcolds, sore throats, earaches, hiccups, sore eyes, fevers, gonorrhea, syphilis and tapeworms. Bloodroot was taken for female-related issues: to induce abortion, for prenatal strength, to help menstruation and "for sickness caught from a menstruating girl." All these blood-related uses are a type of "doctrine of signatures," in which like treats like. Bloodroot was also taken as a medicinal tonic, a panacea and a spring emetic. The active compound in the rhizome of bloodroot is sanguinarine, a potentially poisonous alkaloid at high doses (see **Warning**). At low doses, sanguinarine is a good antimicrobial and was used in commercial toothpaste and mouthwash to fight plaque and gingivitis, but it was withdrawn because of problems with mouth sores in some patients. Research has shown that bloodroot may potentially assist in treating cancer, cardiovascular diseases and other illnesses such as diabetic eye disease and arthritis.

OTHER USES: Bloodroot was often used as a dye, owing to the blood red juice that can be extracted from the rhizome (hence the name bloodroot). A red dye was applied to the skin, clothing and weapons, and sheets were coloured with a yellow-orange dye. It was also used as a love charm and an aphrodisiac. Smoke from bloodroot was used as a wash for a person who had seen a dead person. Bloodroot was also given to horses to induce abortion.

WARNING

This plant contains many alkaloids and is poisonous in large doses. The liquid can cause intense irritation to mucous membranes. Pregnant or breastfeeding women should not use this herb.

DESCRIPTION: Herbaceous perennial, to 40 cm tall, from a reddish orange rhizome. Leaves, typically 1, basal, to 20 cm, mostly palmately 5- to 9-lobed. Flowers white with a yellow centre, to 5 cm wide, often 8 petals (4 large, 4 small) but can have 12 (rarely 16); bloom from March to April. Fruit a 2-part capsule pointed on both ends with a row of seeds on each half. Found in rich woods and thickets, often on floodplains and shores or near streams on slopes at low to montane elevations in MB, ON, QC, NB and NS. See p. 424 for conservation status.

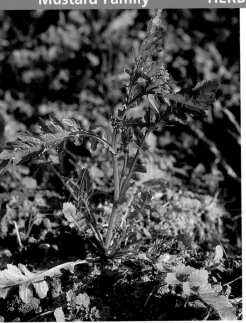

Marsh yellowcress

Watercress & Yellowcress

Rorippa spp.

FOOD: These plants have usually been eaten raw in salads and sandwiches, but they can also be steamed, boiled or stir-fried, like spinach. Common watercress is considered superior, but both are edible. The flavour is similar to peppery lettuce or radishes. Watercress fresh or dried is excellent in casseroles and stews and has also been used in gourmet soups and sauces. Sprigs of flowers can make a pretty, peppery addition to salads. The seeds have been sprouted for use in salads or dried, ground and mixed with salt and vinegar to make "water mustard."

MEDICINE: Carrot and watercress soup has been recommended for treating canker sores and blisters in the mouth. Watercress has also been used to treat a wide range of ailments, including boils, tumours, warts, baldness, eczema, scabies, fevers, flu, rheumatism, asthma, bronchitis, tuberculosis, goiter, nervousness and liver, heart and kidney problems. It was sometimes given to women during labour and was used as a contraceptive and as a cure for impotence. Watercress is rich in vitamins A, B2, C, D and E and in iodine. It was used for many years to prevent and cure scurvy. Watercress is currently under study as a plant that may help to protect smokers from developing lung cancer. The Romans used a mixture of watercress and vinegar to treat people with mental illnesses. From this use came the proverb, "Eat cress and learn more wit." The juice was said to clear the complexion of spots and pimples, and the plants were eaten to improve appetite.

DESCRIPTION: Annual, biennial or perennial herbs of wet places with alternate, pinnately divided leaves, with the largest leaflet at the tip. Flowers small, 4-petalled, forming elongating clusters, from March to October. Fruits sausage-shaped to rounded pods on spreading stalks.

Common watercress (*R. nasturtium-aquaticum*) is a usually prostrate, less than 40 cm tall, sprawling, white-flowered species that roots at its stem joints, producing bright green, tangled masses of shoots. Its relatively short-stalked pods are 1–25 mm long. This European plant has spread to quiet waters across temperate North America.

Marsh yellowcress (*R. palustris*) is an erect, 45 cm–1 m tall, yellow-flowered, fibrous-rooted species, with oblong or oval, 3–12 mm long pods on equally long stalks. Grows on muddy sites in prairies, foothills and montane zones throughout Canada. See p. 424 for conservation status.

WARNING
Never eat raw plants from sites with polluted water. If you would not drink the water, either disinfect the watercress (e.g., soak it in water with water-purification tablets) or serve it cooked. Watercress should not be used medicinally by pregnant women, children or people with kidney inflammation, stomach ulcers or duodenal ulcers. Mustard oil glycosides in watercress can cause intestinal and stomach upset if eaten in large quantities or over long periods.

Shepherd's-Purse
Capsella bursa-pastoris

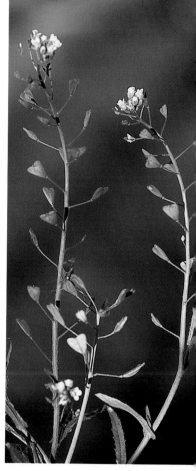

FOOD: All parts of shepherd's-purse are edible, and these plants were once cultivated for greens. Young, crisp leaves have been used in salads, but usually plants were cooked in soups and stews. Shepherd's-purse is said to taste like a delicate cross between turnips and cabbages, and it has been recommended as a substitute for spinach. A pinch of baking soda in the cooking water helps to tenderize older plants. The slightly peppery pods and/or seeds can be used like mustard in cooked dishes, or they can be germinated to produce sprouts for salads and sandwiches. Some tribes crushed the dried pods, removed the chaff by winnowing, parched the seeds and ground them into a nutritious flour used in breads or mush. The roots, fresh and dried, have been used as a substitute for ginger. The fine, grey ash left by burned plants is high in sodium, potassium and other salts. It has been used as a salt substitute and tenderizer in cooked dishes.

MEDICINE: These plants are rich in vitamin C and have been reported to stimulate urination and stop bleeding. A strong decoction was used as drops for relieving earaches. Stems and leaves were steeped in hot water to make a tea for relieving headaches, stomach cramps, hemorrhoids and internal bleeding (especially of the uterus or kidneys). Shepherd's-purse was traditionally used during childbirth, to stop bleeding and aid delivery of the afterbirth by causing the muscles of the uterus to contract (an effect similar to that of oxytocin). As with other members of the Mustard family, shepherd's-purse may have some cancer preventative activity. In animal experiments, shepherd's-purse extracts have been shown to speed healing of stress-induced ulcers, fight chemically induced inflammation, increase urination, lower blood pressure, inhibit quivering contractions of the heart (ventricular fibrillation) and stimulate smooth muscles (especially in the intestines and uterus).

OTHER USES: The seed was used to attract and kill mosquitoes. Submerged in water, it produces a gummy substance that binds insect mouth parts to the seed. It also releases compounds toxic to larvae.

DESCRIPTION: Slender, annual herb, growing 10–60 cm tall from a taproot, with toothed or lobed basal leaves in rosettes and smaller, clasping stem leaves. Flowers white, 4-petalled, the petals to 4 mm long, forming dense, rounded clusters, from March to July. Flower clusters elongate and bear flattened, triangular to heart-shaped pods 4–8 mm long. This introduced Eurasian species is found in disturbed, waste or cultivated ground throughout Canada.

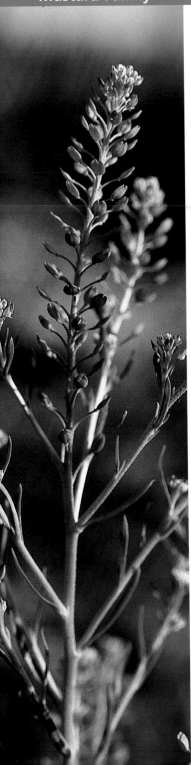

Peppergrass
Lepidium virginicum

FOOD: Aptly named for its pepper-like flavour, the young leaves make a pleasantly pungent addition to any salad or can be used as a garnish. They can also be boiled for 10 minutes and served like spinach. They are a nutritious source of vitamins A and C, iron and protein. The unripe, green seed pods can be eaten raw or added to soups or stews. The seeds can be used as a black pepper substitute, hence its other common name, poor-man's pepper.

MEDICINE: Sometimes used by First Nations as a substitute for shepherd's-purse (p. 211), pepper-grass was traditionally used for a variety of health problems. Its vitamin C content helped to treat scurvy. The plant was also used to treat diabetes, to expel intestinal worms and, when mixed with other ingredients and added to whiskey, as a remedy for tuberculosis. The fresh bruised plant or an infusion of the leaf was applied topically on poison-ivy (p. 395) rashes and as a poultice on the chest to treat croup. A poultice of the bruised root was used to speed the healing of blisters. As a diuretic, it was helpful in the treatment of rheumatic pain. The seeds have been used to treat coughs and asthma with excessive phlegm, to reduce water retention (edema), to decrease urine production (oliguria) and to reduce accumulation of liquid in the chest cavity. The root is used similarly to expel excess mucous from bronchial tubes.

OTHER USES: An infusion of the fresh herb was given to sick chickens as part of their feed to encourage egg laying.

DESCRIPTION: Usually annual herb, 15–60 cm tall, from a slender taproot. Basal leaves, 2–15 cm long, toothed, with large terminal lobe and several small lateral lobes. Stem leaves lance-shaped and unstalked. Tiny, white flowers with 4 petals, 1–3 mm long, in a cross form. Flowers arranged in elongated clusters from June to November. Fruits dry, rounded, flattened pods, slightly notched at the top. Grows in disturbed sites and roadsides in southwestern BC (where native) and ON to the Maritimes and NL (where apparently introduced). See p. 424 for conservation status.

WARNING
Topical application may cause skin irritations and blisters.

Field Pennycress

Thlaspi arvense

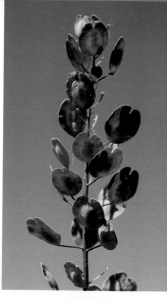

FOOD: The young, tender leaves have been eaten raw in salads, sandwiches and hors d'oeuvres, but they tend to have the characteristic bite of a mustard. Pennycress is too bitter and aromatic for most tastes, but it can be cooked in 1–2 changes of water and mixed with blander herbs or used for flavouring casseroles, soups and sauces. Mature plants are tough and strong-tasting. The seed pods have a peppery flavour and have been used as a mustard-like flavouring in soups and stews.

MEDICINE: Pennycress was historically used as an ingredient in the Mithridate confection (an elaborate preparation that was used as an antidote to poison), but by the early 1900s, it was no longer used in medicine. The plants are high in vitamins C and B2 and also contain relatively large amounts of sulphur. Some reports have suggested that they may have healthful effects similar to those of sulphur and molasses. In some countries, the young plants were eaten to harmonize the internal organs and brighten the eyes. The seeds have been used to treat ophthalmia (inflammation of the eyeball) and lumbago (rheumatic pain in the lower back). Pennycress plants have a broad antimicrobial activity (against *candida*, *eschscherichia*, *mycobacterium*, *proteus*, *pseudomonas*, *staphylococcus* and *streptococcus*), but their high mustard oil content can be very irritating. In Eurasia, pennycress was considered an astringent, purifier, diuretic, stimulant and tonic, and it was also used to treat rheumatism.

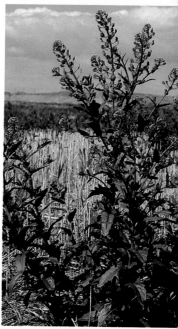

DESCRIPTION: Hairless, yellow-green, annual herb growing to 50 cm tall from a taproot. Basal leaves few, most leaves lance-shaped, reduced upward and clasping the stem. Flowers white, 4-petalled, about 6 mm across, forming dense, rounded clusters, from April to August. These clusters greatly elongate and bear large (9–18 mm long), flat, round, heart-shaped pods that are broadly winged and notched at their tips. Found in disturbed, waste or cultivated ground throughout Canada. It was one of the first weeds introduced to North America from Europe and has since spread across the continent.

WARNING

Pennycress seeds contain the irritating substance mustard oil (isothiocyanate). Cattle have been poisoned by eating hay with 25 percent or more pennycress. Even small amounts of field pennycress can taint the flavour of a cow's milk. People with sensitive skin may react to these plants when contact is accompanied by exposure to sunlight.

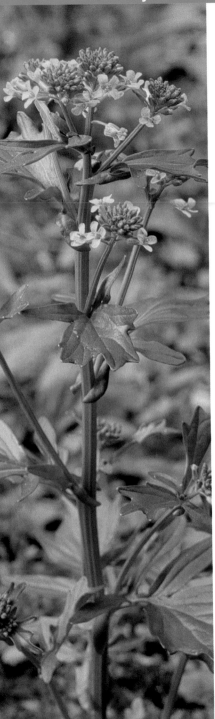

Wintercress
Barbarea vulgaris

FOOD: The bright and abundant yellow flowers are hard to miss on roadsides and other disturbed sites in the middle of spring. The young leaves form dense rosettes that are available year round, even in winter. They can be picked while the nights are still frosty, chopped finely and added to salads or cooked like spinach. They become strongly bitter as they age and as the weather warms up, so they should be cooked in 1 or 2 changes of water. Once the leaves become too bitter, the tight clusters of flowerheads can be harvested, boiled for 5 minutes in 2 changes of water and served like broccoli. Removing the flowering stems as they appear or picking off the outer leaves as they grow increases the growth of younger leaves. However, the plant is yet another aggressive, introduced species, and care should be taken not to encourage its spread.

MEDICINE: A cooked salad was eaten by some First Nations in the belief that it purified the blood. An infusion of the leaves was taken every 30 minutes to suppress coughs. It was also used to stimulate appetite, increase urination and treat scurvy. The herb was used topically as a poultice by Europeans to heal wounds.

OTHER USES: At least one variety of wintercress, called "Variegeta," has ornamental value. Bees are attracted to the plant.

DESCRIPTION: Tufted, biennial herb, 30–60 cm tall, from a slender taproot. Lower leaves to 12 cm long, with 1–2 pairs of lateral leaves, the terminal one large and rounded, upper stem leaves generally lobed. Flowers usually in clusters from leaf axils, sometimes in terminal clusters, the petals to 8 mm wide, bright yellow, with 4 petals forming a cross, from April to August. Fruit an erect seed pod, 1–3 cm long, with a short beak. This introduced Eurasian species grows on road edges, brooksides and in moist fields at low to montane elevations in all provinces.

WARNING
The plant contains an irritant oil that may cause enteritis, diarrhea and kidney malfunction.

Wild Mustards

Brassica spp.

FOOD: Most species have been used for food, though their intensity varies with species, habitat and season. Tender young shoots provide a zesty addition to salads and sandwiches, whereas mature plants are best used as flavouring in soups, salads and casseroles. Wild mustard plants were steamed in fire pits or boiled, sometimes with 2 changes of water, to reduce bitterness. The pods and seeds have a stronger taste than the rest of the plant and were used as peppery additions to meats and salads. The seeds have long been ground to powder and mixed with salt and vinegar to make sharp, peppery sauces (prepared mustards). The cluster of unopened flowerbuds can be boiled for 3–5 minutes and served like broccoli. Make sure not to overcook them or include any of the extremely bitter, upper-stem leaves.

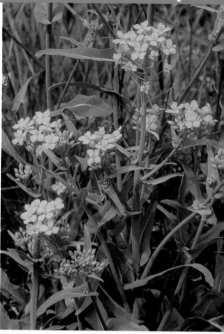

Field mustard

MEDICINE: These plants are rich in vitamins A, B and C and also contain considerable amounts of trace minerals. The seeds, which are said to stimulate the production of digestive juices, have been used for many years to aid digestion. Mustards have also been used as a tonic for fevers, croup, asthma and as a snuff for headaches. Traditionally, mustard seed was used to relieve bronchial congestion by applying it to the chest in the form of a "plaster" (a paste of ground mustard and water sandwiched between 2 sheets of soft cloth). Such remedies should be used with caution (see **Warning**). Mustard seed was used in poultices for healing wounds, burns, rheumatism, chilblains, toothaches and headaches, and it was sometimes taken in large quantities as a laxative (see **Warning**). Plants in the Mustard family contain isothiocyanate derivatives and are considered to have some cancer-prevention properties.

WARNING

Mustard plants are generally not poisonous, but their powdered seeds can be irritating, and mustard oil is one of the most toxic plant oils known. Ingestion of large quantities of mustard plants has caused poisoning of livestock. Mustard plasters redden the skin, and prolonged contact (more than 10 or 15 minutes) raises blisters. Large quantities of mustard seed irritate the digestive tract and cause vomiting. The thyroid is affected by isothiocyanates, which can lead to hyperthyroidism and goiter.

DESCRIPTION: Tall, annual herbs with broad, pinnately divided leaves, conspicuous terminal cluster of 4-petalled, yellow flowers, and erect to ascending, slender pods ending in a beak, containing a single row of seeds. These introduced European species grow in disturbed sites and fields throughout Canada.

Black mustard (*B. nigra*) grows to 1.5 m tall. Upper stem leaves stalked or stalkless, not much broadened at the base and never clasping the stem. Petals to 11 mm or more long. Seed pods to 25 mm long. Flowers from June to October.

Field mustard (*B. rapa*) grows to 60 cm tall. Stalkless upper stem leaves broadened at the base and often clasping the stem. Petals to 8 mm long. Seed pods to 7 cm long. Flowers from April to November.

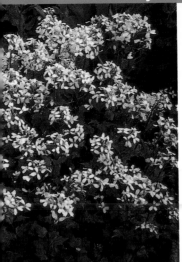

Bittercresses
Cardamine spp.

FOOD: All bittercresses are edible. They can be eaten raw, but some people say they are better cooked in soups, stews and casseroles or served as a puree, like spinach. The delicate, slightly succulent plants add a refreshing, peppery flavour to sauces, salads and sandwiches. The pods of some species have been ground and mixed with vinegar to make a substitute for horseradish.

MEDICINE: Various bittercresses were used by native peoples as medicines. The pungent plants were used to treat fevers, colds, sore throats, headaches, heart palpitations, chest pains, gas, stomach upset and lack of appetite. Europeans used bittercress plants to prevent scurvy and to treat cramps, nervous hysteria, spasmodic asthma, urinary tract problems (especially kidney stones) and tumours. Dried flower clusters were believed to cure epilepsy in children. These plants are rich in vitamin C (and in the salts of iron and calcium), which would explain their effectiveness against scurvy, and, like many members of the Mustard family, they contain compounds that are believed to combat cancer.

Heart-leaved bittercress (above)
Pennsylvania bittercress (below)

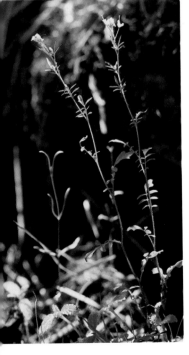

OTHER USES: Bittercresses are easily propagated by root division in autumn or from seed sown in spring. Some of the showier species are cultivated as ornamentals in Europe.

DESCRIPTION: Hairless herbs with basal and alternate leaves, usually pinnately divided, with a large leaflet at the tip. Flowers small, white, 4-petalled, forming elongate clusters, from April to July. Fruits slender, ascending pods, 1–3 cm long. Three common perennial species arise from long, slender rhizomes: Brewer's and heart-leaved bittercress and toothwort.

Brewer's bittercress (*C. breweri*) grows to 50 cm tall and has lower leaves mostly compound but some simple, and petals 3–6 mm long. Grows on wet foothill and montane sites in southern BC.

Heart-leaved bittercress (*C. cordifolia*) grows to 45 cm tall and has mostly simple, broadly heart-shaped lower leaves, with all leaves stalked, and petals 7–12 mm long. Grows in moist streambanks and meadows at montane and subalpine sites in southern BC.

Toothwort (*C. diphylla*) grows 20–40 cm tall, with a prominently toothed rhizome and mostly compound lower leaves, with a pair of toothed stem leaves, each divided into 3 broad leaflets. Grows in rich, damp woods and meadows from southern ON to the Maritimes. See p. 424 for conservation status.

Pennsylvania bittercress (*C. pensylvanica*) is an annual or biennial that grows to 45 cm tall from a taproot, with 3–4 mm long petals and 5–11 linear, lance-shaped leaflets. Grows in moist or wet soils throughout Canada. See p. 424 for conservation status.

Sundews

Drosera spp.

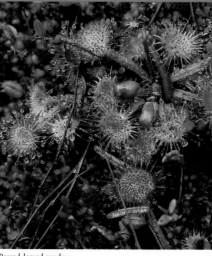

Round-leaved sundew

FOOD: Sundews are not normally used as a food, though in Sweden, a cheese is obtained by adding leaves to milk and heating the mixture until it curdles.

MEDICINE: Sundews have a long history of herbal use as early as the 12th century. They were primarily recommended for all kinds of respiratory disorders. The "dew-drops" were considered quenching to dry, tickly throats and were effective against coughs, laryngitis, pertussis, tracheitis, catarrh, tuberculosis and specifically for asthma and chronic bronchitis with peptic ulceration or gastritis. Research supports some of these herbal uses. Sundew prevented coughing induced by excitation of the larynx nerve in rabbits and prevented hormone-induced bronchial spasms. This action had originally been attributed to the plant's naphthaquinone constituents but is actually a result of the flavonoids hyperoside, quercetin and isoquercetin. These are believed to affect the M_3 muscarinic receptors in smooth muscle, exerting an antispasmodic and anti-inflammatory effect. Today, sundew is an ingredient in some 200–300 registered medicines, mostly cough preparations manufactured in Germany and elsewhere in Europe. These plants also have a reputation as aphrodisiacs. The ellagic acid contained within has been shown to have anti-angiogenic effects, thus benefiting the heart and cardiovascular system. Potent antimicrobial activity against a broad spectrum of bacteria, influenza viruses, pathogenic fungi and parasitic protozoa has been demonstrated in various scientific studies. Traditionally, the leaf juice (with its protein-digesting enzyme) was applied to warts and corns. The plant is usually collected in summer and dried for later use. However, because it has become quite rare in certain areas, it should not be harvested from the wild. Commercial extracts are usually prepared using cultivated, fast-growing species, the most common being round-leaved sundew.

OTHER USES: Round-leaved sundew was traditionally used by the Kwakwaka'wakw of BC as a love charm. The common name sundew comes from the early belief that the "dew" on the leaves persisted through even the hottest sun and possessed the property to endow longevity and youthfulness to those who drank it. We now know that the sticky secretions are not dew, but are in fact a clever trapping and digestion mechanism designed to ensnare and digest insects as a means to obtain nutrients that are lacking in its boggy environment.

DESCRIPTION: Insectivorous, perennial herb, 5–25 cm tall. Leaves arranged in a basal rosette, covered with reddish, glandular-tipped hairs exuding sticky "dewdrops." Flowers with 5 white petals, each 6–10 mm long, in an elongated, 1-sided raceme, opening 1 at a time, from June to August. Fruits many-seeded capsules. Grows in bogs, marshes and fens throughout Canada.

Great sundew (*D. anglica*) has oblong leaves, 1–4 cm long and 3–7 mm wide, with hairless leaf stalks.

Internal use of sundew may cause colouration of the urine, a neat and harmless side effect.

Round-leaved sundew (*D. rotundifolia*) has, as its name suggests, round leaves, usually broader than long, 6–12 mm in diameter, with hairy leaf stalks. See p. 424 for conservation status.

217

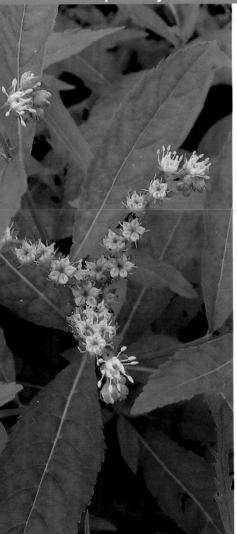

Ditch-Stonecrop
Penthorum sedoides

FOOD: Fresh leaves have an astringent, slightly acid taste that some people enjoy as a potherb or to spice up salads.

MEDICINE: This plant contains tannic acid and a volatile oil most effectively extracted by alcohol. Ditch-stonecrop is considered to have astringent, tonic and laxative properties and has been used to treat conditions such as diarrhea, dysentery and hemorrhoids. The seeds were traditionally used in the formulation of a cough syrup, which appears to have soothed diseased and inflamed mucous membranes and was prescribed to treat tonisillitis, bronchitis and other throat maladies.

DESCRIPTION: Herbaceous perennial growing to 1 m tall from slender, fibrous roots. Stems erect, branched or unbranched; smooth except for some hairs near the flowering parts; sometimes red, especially at the nodes. Leaves usually smooth, alternate, lance-shaped, simple, toothed, 3.5 cm wide and 12 cm long, pointed at the tip, tapering at the base. Flowers to 2 mm long, typically without petals; several, in terminal clusters; 5 green sepals to 1 mm long; 10 stamens, 5 pistils. Blooms from late summer to early autumn. Seeds in clusters of 5 spreading follicles, to 1 cm long, becoming reddish at maturity. Inhabits wet, low grounds such as floodplains and ditches from southeastern MB to ON, QC and NB. See p. 424 for conservation status.

Alumroots

Heuchera spp.

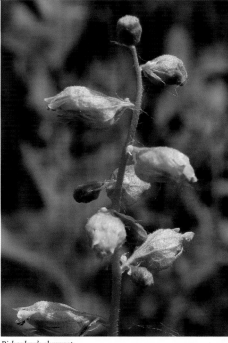

Richardson's alumroot

FOOD: All members of the Saxifrage family, to which the alumroots belong, are edible to some degree. Although the leaves and roots of alumroot are sour and astringent-tasting because of the high level of tannins in the plant, some people consider them a pleasant addition to bland salads.

MEDICINE: Alumroots have as much as 20 percent tannin per dry weight, making this herb highly astringent. Tannins are acidic and are valued medicinally for their ability to shrink swollen, moist tissues. Northwest First Nations used dried and powdered alumroot as a digestive tonic, as a topical agent for sores and for sore throats and arthritis. It is also prescribed by herbalists to reduce inflammation and to stop minor bleeding.

OTHER USES: The Skagit people of BC pounded small-flowered alumroot and rubbed it on little girls' heads to make their hair grow thick.. They also used a poultice of the plant on cuts to stop bleeding and promote healing. Our native alumroots are closely related to the cultivated Mexican coral bells (*H. sanguinea*), which is a popular garden ornamental. Alumroots are tough, persistent plants with striking foliage and delicate flower stems that do well in a variety of garden conditions. They make a striking border and groundcover, especially in cold climates. The plants naturalize easily, and the flowers attract bees and hummingbirds.

DESCRIPTION: Evergreen or semi-evergreen, perennial herbs growing from rhizomes, 30 cm–1.2 m tall. Leaves long-stalked, in clumps 30–60 cm across; individual leaves oval to heart-shaped, sometimes boldly veined, 2.5–7.5 cm across, mainly basal. Flowering stems 1 to several, to 60 cm tall, clothed at base with persistent brown leaf bases and stipules. Flowers generally white to green, small, 5-petalled, saucer- to urn-shaped calyx tubes in narrow, loose panicles or racemes. Fruits many-seeded, beaked capsules; seeds small, black, egg-shaped, covered in rows of tiny spines.

American alumroot (*H. americana*) is also known as rock-geranium. Leaves grow in rosettes, slightly ruffled, 5- to 9-lobed, broadly oval to heart-shaped, glossy, leathery, leaf colour purple, brown or green, with silvery shades between veins, turning reddish in cooler weather; tiny, insignificant, pinkish green to cream flowers borne on broad, open flower clusters in May. Plant forms small mounds to 60 cm across. Grows in rich woods and rocky slopes in southern ON. See p. 424 for conservation status.

Small-flowered alumroot (*H. micrantha*) has flowering stems long-hairy below to glandulary-hairy in the inflorescence, 15–60 cm tall. Leaves kidney- or heart-shaped to oblong, 5- to 7-lobed, sharp- to round-toothed, usually hairy on the leaf stalk and lower surface, often lacking stem leaves. Flowers white, small, numerous, in broad, open clusters. Grows in gravelly banks and rock crevices at low to subalpine elevations in coastal BC, most commonly Vancouver Island and the adjacent mainland.

Richardson's alumroot (*H. richardsonii*) has a narrow flower cluster, the petals purplish. Grows in open areas (grasslands, lakeshores, mountain slopes) from YT and northeastern BC to ON.

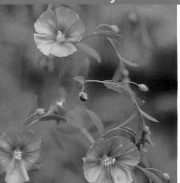

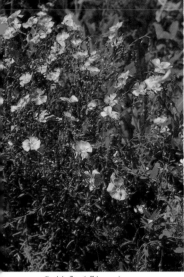

Flaxes

Linum spp.

FOOD: Wild flax seeds are very rich in oil. They were gathered by some tribes, dried, roasted and ground into flour or meal. The seeds were also cooked with other foods as an oil-rich supplement. Flax seeds should not be eaten raw (see **Warning**). Common flax is cultivated for its seeds, which are sold commercially as a healthy source of oil. Taken internally, ground seeds are a good source of dietary fibre and also produce a sticky, glue-like substance (mucilage) when soaked in water, which can be used as an egg-substitute.

MEDICINE: Oil from crushed flax seeds has been used for centuries in Europe to treat rashes, burns and boils. Flax leaves were boiled to make a medicinal tea to treat heartburn. Flax seeds contain healthy oils, both alpha-linoleic and cis-linoleic essential fatty acids, which lower blood fat (lipid) and cholesterol levels, increase the local immune function of prostaglandin and reduce clotting. They also contain several lignans, proven to help prevent breast, prostate and colon cancer.

OTHER USES: The stems of prairie and blue flax contain long, tough fibres (similar to those of common flax) used to make fishing lines and nets, snowshoes and some parts of mats and baskets. Common flax is cultivated for its fibre, which is used to make linen. Flowering plants were sometimes boiled to make a wash for the face and head because the wash was believed to produce beautiful skin and hair as well as treat hair loss.

Prairie flax (all images)

DESCRIPTION: Slender, grey-green, annual or perennial herbs with many linear to lance-shaped, 1–3 cm long leaves. Flowers pale blue, about 2–3 cm across, with 5 fragile petals, soon fading, opening singly in few-flowered clusters, from May to August. Fruits round capsules on curved stalks.

Prairie flax (*L. lewisii*) is a native biennial or perennial herb that grows to 75 cm tall from a woody stem base. Leaves linear, and 3-nerved only at the base. Occurs in dry prairie and rocky, open woods at low elevations from BC to QC.

Blue flax (*L. perenne*) is an introduced perennial herb that grows 30–60 cm tall from a woody stem base. Difficult to distinguish from prairie flax, but check the flowers: those of prairie flax are all the same, while those of this species are of 2 sorts (1 with styles longer than stamens, and 1 with styles shorter than the stamens). Found in similar habitats over a similar range as prairie flax.

Common flax (*L. usitatissimum*) is an introduced annual herb that grows to 1 m tall from a taproot. Leaves more lance-shaped than those of the other species, and 3-veined at least half their length. Found in old fields and disturbed sites across Canada.

WARNING
Eating immature seed pods or large amounts of mature seeds can cause toxic reactions. Although livestock have been poisoned by eating flax, no cases of human poisoning have been reported.

Stork's-Bill
Erodium cicutarium

FOOD: Stork's-bill leaves are edible and considered quite palatable when picked young. The taste is reported to be somewhat sharp, with a parsley-like flavour, and the leaves are suggested as an addition to salads.

MEDICINE: This herb is considered to have diuretic, astringent and anti-inflammatory properties and has been prescribed to prevent postpartum infections and to control afterbirth hemorrhage. It has also traditionally been used to control urinary tract bleeding and as a kidney tonic.

DESCRIPTION: Taprooted, spreading, hairy, annual herb, with ascending stems 3–40 cm tall, sparingly branching from the base, and usually somewhat reddish. Leaves mostly basal (often hugging the ground), stalked, much-divided and fern-like, with very narrow ultimate segments; stem leaves opposite at swollen nodes. Flowers pink, 8–15 mm wide; 5 sepals, bristle-tipped; 5 petals; 10 stamens, 5 short and sterile, 5 longer and fertile; few in umbrella-like clusters on long stalks from leaf axils. Fruits capsules, 3–5 cm long, splitting open into 5 segments each, with 1 or 2 smooth seeds and tipped with a spirally twisting, persistent style. This introduced Eurasian plant is now common in fields, clearings and waste places at low to montane elevations across southern Canada.

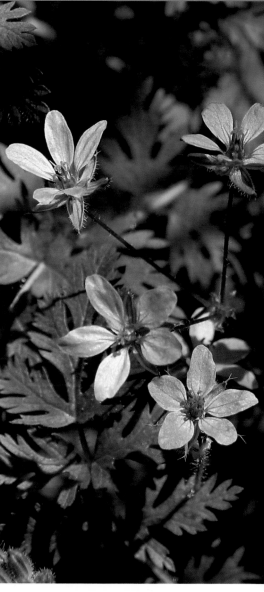

Stork's-bill is a European weed now widespread in North America and on several other continents. Thanks to the long-persistent styles, the fruits resemble stork's bills. As the fruits dry, they split lengthwise into 5 sharp-pointed segments, each attached to its portion of the separated style. The slender style becomes spirally twisted as it dries, but it straightens out again when wet. With alternate moisture and dryness, this uncoiling, squirming action drives the attached seed into the ground. A more correct common name would be heron's-bill because *Erodium* is from *erodios*, the Greek word for "heron."

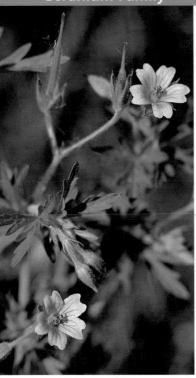

Bicknell's geranium (all images)

Geraniums & Herb-Robert

Geranium spp.

MEDICINE: Herb-Robert has traditionally been prescribed to treat toothaches and nosebleeds. An infusion of the upper plant is said to have diuretic, tonic, antiseptic and styptic (stops bleeding) properties and has also been used to treat dysentery. Geraniums in general are considered astringent and styptic, and Bicknell's geranium has been used as a gargle for sore throats.

OTHER USES: Rubbing the fresh plant, which has a strong smell, on exposed skin and clothes is said to repel mosquitoes. Although invasive if left to their own devices, geraniums make lovely and resilient groundcovers and fillers in ornamental gardens.

DESCRIPTION: Annual, biennial or perennial herbs from a taproot or rhizome; stems branched, bent at the base to upright, spreading, hairy, 10–80 cm tall. Leaves egg-shaped to triangular in outline, palmately or pinnately divided, sparsely hairy on both sides, light green but sometimes reddish. Flowers variable. Fruits 5-parted capsules.

Bicknell's geranium (*G. bicknellii*) is an annual or biennial plant from a taproot. Leaves palmately divided into 5 main segments that are themselves divided or deeply cleft. Flowers pink, borne in terminal and axillary pairs with petals 4–8 mm long. Grows in open forests and recent burns at low to montane elevations across Canada (though apparently not in PEI).

Northern geranium (*G. erianthum*) is a perennial herb from a rhizome. Leaves palmately divided into 3–7 main segments. Flowers blue to pinkish purple (rarely white), borne in terminal clusters of 2–5 with petals 16–20 mm long. Grows in open forests, thickets and moist meadows at higher elevations (montane to alpine) in BC, AB and YT.

Herb-Robert (*G. robertianum*) is an annual plant from a taproot. Leaves pinnately divided into 3–5 main segments that are themselves divided. Flowers pink to reddish purple, borne in terminal and axillary pairs with petals 8–13 mm long. This introduced Eurasian species inhabits open forests, clearings and disturbed sites at low to montane elevations across the country, but is rare northward. See p. 424 for conservation status.

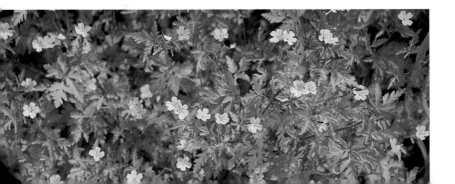

Woodsorrels

Oxalis spp.

FOOD: The woodsorrels are good sources of vitamin C. They can be eaten raw, added to salads or cooked with other milder-flavoured greens. The genus name *Oxalis* is a Greek word meaning "sour," referring to the acidic taste of the leaves. They can be used to give a sour flavour to foods, but see **Warning**. The leaves can be added to soups and stews, made into a sauce, used like rhubarb in pie or pickled to make sauerkraut. Woodsorrels can also be made into a beverage as a lemonade substitute and are said to make a good dry wine. The flowers can be eaten raw.

MEDICINE: As a folk medicine, woodsorrels have been used for a variety of ailments: influenza, fever, urinary tract infections, inflammation of the small intestine, diarrhea, traumatic injuries, sprains and poisonous snakebites. The juice of these plants has been mixed with butter and applied to muscular swellings, boils and pimples, while the juice alone has been applied to insect bites, burns and eruptions. An infusion has been used as a wash to get rid of hookworms in children. Creeping woodsorrel has been found to have antibacterial activity because of the presence of phenolic compounds.

OTHER USES: The flowers can be used to obtain yellow, orange and red to brown dyes.

DESCRIPTION: Low, herbaceous perennials that grow to 30 cm tall from taproots or rhizomes. Stems erect or trailing. Leaves divided into 3 parts, leaflets heart-shaped and folded along their midribs, pointing in toward the centre. Leaves lie flat during the day but fold up at night or in cool weather. Flowers yellow, 5-petalled, 6 mm in diameter, in few-flowered clusters on the end of slender stalks, blooming in May. Fruits narrow capsules with small, brown, wrinkled seeds that are discharged explosively.

Creeping woodsorrel (*O. corniculata*) has main stems creeping and rooting and grows from a taproot. Introduced European species found in greenhouses and waste places (usually near greenhouses) here and there across the country.

Stoloniferous woodsorrel (*O. dillenii*) has at least the main stem erect and grows from a taproot. Range in Canada isn't entirely clear, but it can be expected near gardens and disturbed sites in most provinces.

Upright woodsorrel (*O. stricta*) is an upright, rhizomatous species. Occurs on the same sorts of disturbed sites where the other species do, from SK to NS (and introduced elsewhere).

WARNING

The leaves contain oxalic acid, which gives them their sharp flavour. Oxalic acid binds the body's supply of calcium and could lead to nutritional deficiency if eaten in large amounts; oxalic acid is poisonous in large doses. Oxalic acid amounts are reduced when the leaves are cooked. Caution is advised, especially for people with rheumatism, arthritis, gout, kidney stones or hyperacidity.

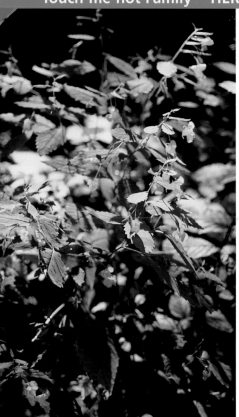

Touch-Me-Nots

Impatiens spp.

FOOD: The seeds are edible and have a walnut-like flavour. The young, succulent stems can be cooked like green beans; however, caution must be exercised. The plant contains calcium oxalate crystals that can cause an intense burning sensation in the mouth and throat, swelling and choking (see **Warning**). The young shoots should be boiled for 10–15 minutes in 2 changes of water, which should destroy most of the calcium oxalate. The cooking water should not be drunk.

MEDICINE: The best known use for touch-me-nots is as an antidote against poison-ivy (p. 395) rashes. How serendipitous that they both share similar habitats, because the remedy is most effective when applied soon after being exposed to poison-ivy. The crushed stems and leaves are rubbed directly on the exposed skin. The mucilaginous fluid that is released is able to neutralize poison-ivy's oily antigen, urushiol. Urushiol induces contact dermatitis by binding to skin cell membrane proteins, which elicits an immune response that results in a rash approximately 24 hours after exposure. It can be transported on clothing and material that has had contact with the plant, which can then contact skin. A study conducted in 1957 found that touch-me-nots were effective in treating urushiol-induced contact dermatitis in 94 percent of patients.

Pale touch-me-not (above)
Spotted touch-me-not (below)

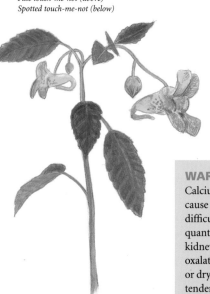

WARNING
Calcium oxalate crystals in touch-me-nots can cause severe digestive upset, breathing difficulties, convulsions, coma and death if large quantities are consumed. Permanent liver and kidney damage can result after recovery from oxalate poisoning. Although thorough cooking or drying destroys the compound, people with a tendency to rheumatism, arthritis, gout, kidney stones and hyperacidity should avoid ingesting the plant.

Touch-me-not mucilage seems effective for countering the irritating toxins of other plants including stinging nettle (p. 312), poison-oak (p. 395) and okra (*Abelmoschus esculentus*) spines, as well as insect bites and razor burn. First Nations used it for a wider range of skin complaints, including wounds, bruises, warts, burns, cuts, acne, eczema, hemorrhoids and fungal dermatitis. A tea can be made from the stem and leaves can be frozen into ice cubes as a method to store touch-me-nots in case there aren't any patches nearby. Some believe that drinking leaf tea acts as a poison-ivy preventative. Touch-me-nots have also been used internally for fevers, difficult urination, measles, stomach cramps and jaundice.

OTHER USES: Touch-me-nots are fun plants to play with in late summer, when the slightest touch to the seed pods causes them to explode open and propel the seeds a fair distance. Their common name reflects this characteristic. Stem mucilage, concentrated through boiling, can be used as an effective fungicide. A yellow dye is obtained from the flower.

DESCRIPTION: Tall, leafy, annual herbs, 50 cm–1.5 m tall, with succulent, smooth stems, often covered with a whitish bloom. Leaves alternate, elliptic to oval, 3–10 cm long, with irregularly toothed margins. Flowers 2.5 cm long, with 3 sepals: the upper 2 small, oval, pale; the third enlarged, petal-like and sac-shaped with 1 end open and the other end tapering onto a narrow, nectar-bearing spur; 3 petals, 2 of them 2-lobed, opened out at the mouth. Fruit a club-shaped capsule, to 2 cm long, smooth, spitting explosively to release its seeds.

Spotted touch-me-not (*I. capensis*) has pendent, golden orange flowers splotched with reddish brown dots, from July to October. Grows in moist, shaded woodlands and lakesides at low to montane elevations in all provinces and NT.

Pale touch-me-not (*I. pallida*) has larger, pale yellow flowers with only occasional brown spots or unspotted, from June to October. Grows in wet woods and meadows, often in limestone sites, from southern SK to the Maritimes and Labrador. See p. 424 for conservation status.

Pale touch-me-not

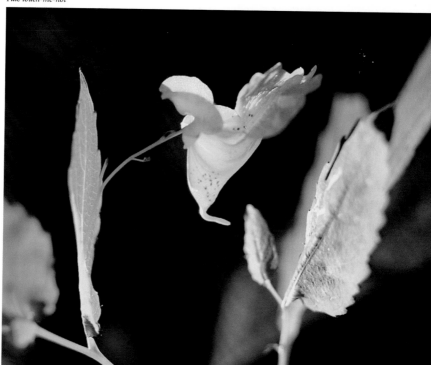

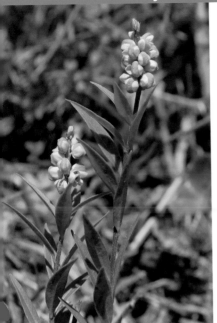

Seneca Snakeroot
Polygala senega

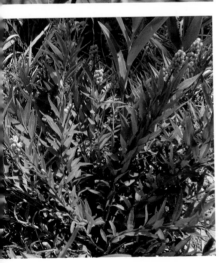

MEDICINE: Seneca snakeroot is one of Canada's most important native medicinal plants. It has long been used as a medicine, and wild populations are still harvested commercially for their medicinal value. Its common name is likely derived from its traditional use in treating snakebites as well as from the snake-like appearance of the root, the medicinal part of the plant. To treat snakebites, the root was chewed and the wound was poulticed with the chewed material. Snakeroot was commonly used for respiratory ailments such as chronic bronchitis, bronchial asthma, laryngitis, whooping cough, sore throats, croup and colds. It was also used to treat earaches, toothaches, heart trouble, bleeding wounds, sore mouths, rheumatism and, in larger doses, as an emetic and cathartic. Snakeroot was valued for its laxative properties and ability to promote sweating and increase urination. The blooms were taken as blood medicine. Snakeroot contains saponins as the active principles (that have been shown to induce bronchial secretions). Europeans learned of the medicinal qualities of snakeroot from indigenous peoples in North America. The increased interest in this plant in Europe, Japan and the US resulted in snakeroot being sold commercially, beginning in the early 1900s. Commercial use of snakeroot is mainly as an expectorant in cough syrups, teas and lozenges or as a gargle for sore throats. In the 1950s, 75 percent of world's supply of snakeroot was harvested by First Nations in the Interlake region of MB. Today, wild populations in MB and SK, along with cultivated plants in Japan, are the major supply source for Seneca snakeroot.

DESCRIPTION: Perennial herb, to 40 cm tall, from yellowish or greyish brown, thick taproot with twisted, snake-like appearance. Stems erect, unbranched. Leaves alternate, simple, lance-shaped, 3–8 cm long, 0.5–3.5 cm wide. Flowers greenish white, less than 4 mm long, crowded into spikes at the tips of branches, blooming from May to July. Fruits hairy capsules, about 4 mm long, with 2 black, hairy seeds. Found in rocky woods, open ground, prairies, roadsides and streambanks in all provinces except PEI, NS and NL. See p. 424 for conservation status.

> **WARNING**
> In large doses, Seneca snakeroot is considered poisonous. It can irritate the lining of the gut, cause diarrhea and vomiting and induce miscarriages.

St. John's-Worts
Hypericum spp.

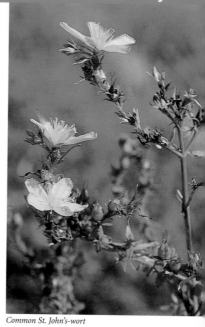

Common St. John's-wort

MEDICINE: St. John's-wort is widely used for treatment of depression. It has proven effective in clinical trials and, like conventional antidepressants, is a selective serotonin re-uptake inhibitor. The main active principle is thought to be the terpene hyperforin, though the light-activated pigments hypericin and pseudohypericin found in black glands in the leaves and flowers also contribute to biological activity through their action on mono-amine oxidase. Although common St. John's-wort has been the most widely used, western St. John's-wort contains similar compounds, but in lower concentrations. St. John's-wort is also rich in tannin, and it was used medicinally by indigenous peoples and Europeans for treating many ailments, including diarrhea, tuberculosis, bladder problems and worms. The fresh flowers were steeped in water, alcohol or oil to make washes and lotions for treating wounds, sores, swellings, tumours, cuts, bruises and ulcers. The tea was taken to treat bladder problems, dysentery, diarrhea, worms, coughs and depression. Experiments have shown St. John's-wort extracts to have sedative, anti-inflammatory and antibacterial effects with efficacy against *Mycobacterium tuberculosis* and *Staphylococcus aureus*. Oil extracts have been taken internally to treat chronic stomach inflammation and stomach ulcers. They have also been applied externally to heal cuts, scrapes and mild burns and to relieve sciatica, back spasms, neck cramps and associated stress headaches. Hypericin and pseudohypericin are potent anti-HIV agents, but the clinical evaluation was abandonded because of side effects.

DESCRIPTION: Hairless, perennial herbs, growing 30 cm–1 m tall, from rhizomes, with opposite, stalkless leaves 1–3 cm long and bright yellow flowers, both usually dotted along their edges with tiny, black glands. Flowers about 2 cm across, 5-petalled, with 75–100 stamens gathered into 3 bundles, borne in leafy, open clusters, from June to September. Fruits small capsules.

WARNING

Cattle, sheep, horses and rabbits have developed severe light-sensitive skin reactions and died from eating large quantities of these plants. In many rangeland areas, common St. John's-wort is a troublesome weed, and efforts are made to control it. Although the human dose for medicine is much lower, some individuals are at risk for photosensitization. St. John's-wort is known to cause adverse drug reactions when combined with conventional pharmaceuticals; in particular, it can reduce the level of the pharma drug in the blood below effective therapeutic levels.

Common St. John's-wort or **klamath weed** (*H. perforatum*) has slender, pointy-tipped sepals (3–5 times longer than wide) and lance-shaped leaves. This European weed now grows on disturbed ground at low to montane elevations across Canada (except for much of the prairies).

Western St. John's-wort (*H. scouleri*) has broader, round-tipped sepals (less than 3 times longer than wide) and oval leaves. Grows in wetlands and on open slopes at low to subalpine elevations in southern BC and AB. See p. 424 for conservation status.

Violets

Viola spp.

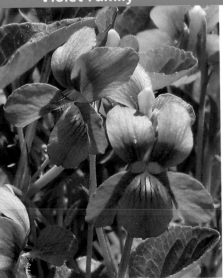

Early blue violet (all images)

FOOD: All upper portions of violets, including garden varieties such as Johnny-jump-ups and pansies, are considered edible. Most leaves are tender and sweet and make an excellent salad green or trail nibble, but they can also be cooked as potherbs or thickeners. Added to soups, the leaves act as a thickening agent. The flowers provide pretty, edible garnishes (fresh or candied) for salads and desserts and delicate flavouring and/or colouring for vinegar, jelly, syrup, jams and preserves. The leaves and flowers have also been steeped in hot water to make tea or even fermented to make wine, and they are delicious added to omelettes and fritters.

MEDICINE: Violet plants are rich in vitamin A (richer than spinach) and vitamin C (½ cup can be equivalent to 4 oranges!), and some contain as much as 4000 ppm salicylic acid (similar to aspirin). The flowers have significant amounts of rutin, a flavonoid that has been shown to strengthen capillary blood vessels. Violet flower tea and syrup have a gentle laxative effect (which is said to be stronger in yellow-flowered species). They have been used to make medicinal teas for treating bronchitis, asthma, heart palpitations and fevers, as well as gargles and syrups for relieving sore throats and coughs. Violets were also traditionally used in the form of poultices, salves or lotions for treating bruises, rashes, boils, skin inflammations, abrasions and eczema. The Cree mixed fresh violet leaves in fresh lard and heated this at a low temperature for an hour. The cooled fat was then used as a salve for skin ailments. Violet leaves, soaked in hot water and drained, were applied directly to sores or wounds as a poultice. They were replaced every 2 hours if the wound was infected. A relaxing tea was made by pouring boiling water over a handful of leaves and letting the mixture cool. This was said to give restful sleep, to moderate anger and to act as a mild laxative. The Ojibwa made a root decoction of Canada violet roots to treat back or bladder pain. Violets are reported to have a mild hormone-regulating action, and early blue violet leaves were used by some women to ease labour. Animal studies have demonstrated that violet plants stimulate urination and that they may be useful in treating rashes. Violet roots, which are not considered edible, were sometimes used to induce vomiting in poison victims.

OTHER USES: Violet flower tea has been used as a substitute for litmus paper; the tea apparently changes colour depending on how acidic or basic a compound added to it is. Mashed violet leaves can also be burned as an incense. Athabascan people placed dried marsh violet roots on top of a hot wood stove, producing a fragrant smoulder that they believed warded off disease. Violet flowers are a popular fragrance for perfumes and have been used in many cosmetics. All parts of the upper plant have emollient properties (softening to the skin) and as such have traditionally been added to skin creams and lotions. The flowers can also be used to produce a dye ranging in shade from yellow to green. Early blue violet's delicate blossoms hold one of the loveliest wildflower fragrances. Enjoy it while you can. The flower's perfume doesn't fade, but your sense of smell is soon dulled by a substance called ionine. In a few moments the perfume returns, only to disappear again just as quickly. Violet seeds have special oily bodies called elaiosomes. These attract ants, which carry them to their nests, thus dispersing the seeds farther. Purple violet (*V. cucullata*) is the provincial flower of NB.

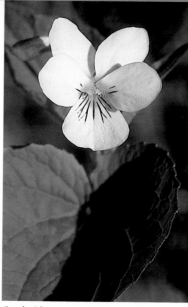
Canada violet

DESCRIPTION: Low, perennial herbs (mostly less than 20 cm tall) with basal or alternate, usually heart-shaped leaves, leaf stalks often with lobes (stipules) at their bases. Flowers with 3 spreading lower petals, 2 backward-bending upper petals and a basal spur, single, from leaf axils, from May to July. Fruits small capsules that shoot out seeds explosively.

Early blue violet (*V. adunca*) is short (2–8 cm tall when flowering) and, as the name suggests, is often one of springtime's earliest flowering plants. Leaves egg- to heart-shaped, 1–2.5 cm wide. Flowers single, blue to deep violet with a white throat; backward-pointing spur, 4–6 mm long; side-petals hairy, 8–15 mm long; from May to June. Inhabits dry to moist meadows, woods, gravelly sites and open ground to near timberline in all provinces and territories. See p. 424 for conservation status.

Canada violet (*V. canadensis*) is a larger (10–40 cm tall) species with broad, heart-shaped stem leaves and purple-lined, pale violet to white flowers. Grows in dry to moist woods, thickets, meadows and on rocky slopes from BC to NS (but apparently not in PEI), and in southwestern YT and NT. See p. 424 for conservation status.

Yellow prairie violet (*V. nuttallii*) has tapered (not heart-shaped) leaves and yellow blossoms. Grows in dry woods, sagebrush areas and prairies at low to moderate elevations from AB to southwestern MB. See p. 424 for conservation status.

Marsh violet (*V. palustris*) grows 5–20 cm tall, with heart- or kidney-shaped basal leaves and white to lavender petals, the lower 3 purple-pencilled and lilac tinged. Grows in moist to wet sites (streambanks, wetlands, moist woods) across Canada.

WARNING

Use violets in moderation. Some leaves contain saponin, which causes digestive upset in large quantities. Only the leaves, stems and flowers should be eaten, and these in moderation. Violet roots, rootstocks, fruits and seeds contain toxins that can cause severe stomach and intestinal upset, as well as nervousness and respiratory and circulatory depression.

Common blue violet (*V. sororia*) grows to 10 cm tall and has densely hairy, heart-shaped leaves and single, fairly large (2 cm or more broad) violet flowers with petals often fading to yellowish at the base. Grows in moist forests and open areas (including lawns) from southern MB to QC.

Johnny-jump-up (*V. tricolor*) is a small plant of creeping habit, reaching at most 15 cm. Leaves deeply cut into rounded lobes, the terminal lobe being considerably larger. Flowers 1.5 cm in diameter and of variable colour (purple, blue, yellow or white, sometimes of one colour but most commonly a combination of all of these in each flower), upper petals generally most showy and of a purple shade, lower petals a shade of yellow. This European native is common in cultivated gardens and naturalized locally across southern Canada.

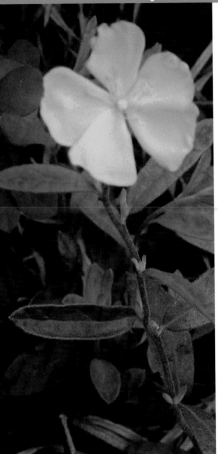

Frostweed
Helianthemum canadense

MEDICINE: The plant has a bitter, astringent, slightly aromatic taste and is said to be astonishingly effective against scrofula, a tuberculous swelling of the lymph nodes. Early physicians treated scrofula with a strong tea made from the entire herb, also recommended for diarrhea, dysentery and syphilis. First Nations used the leaf tea for kidney complaints, sore throats and as a strengthening medicine. Patients were placed inside a tented blanket that held in the steam from the hot tea in which the feet were soaked to treat arthritis, muscular swellings and rheumatism. The tea was used topically as a wash for skin diseases such as prurigo nodularis, itchy nodules that usually appear on the arms and legs, and as an eyewash for infections. Sore throats were treated internally with a tea made from the plant and externally with a poultice of the root to the throat. The oil expressed from the crushed plant was said to be useful in the treatment of cancer. It has been used as a gargle for sore throats, scarlet fever and canker sores. Herbalists use it as a decoction, syrup or fluid extract but recommend that it be used with squirrel-corn (*Dicentra canadensis*) and queen's-delight (*Stillingia sylvatica*) to make it more effective and reduce any side-effects.

OTHER USES: The generic name, derived from the Greek *helio*, meaning "sun," and *anthemum*, meaning "flower," describes the plant's tendency to flower only when exposed to sunlight. The common name refers to ice crystals that form from sap that exudes from cracks near the base of the stem in late autumn. In 1816, professor Amos Eaton, in his work *A Manual of Botany for the Northern States*, observed: "In November and December, I saw hundreds of these plants sending out broad, thin, ice-covered crystals, about an inch in breadth from near the roots. These were melted away by day, and renewed every morning for more than twenty-five days in succession."

DESCRIPTION: Erect perennial, 20–45 cm tall. Leaves to 2.5 cm long, opposite, narrow, simple, dull green and hoary with white hairs underneath. Solitary yellow flower atop a main stem, while later in the season, clusters of inconspicuous, bud-like flowers are produced in the axils of branch leaves. Flowers 2–4 cm wide, with 5 wedge-shaped petals and many stamens, lasting only a single day and producing many seeds, from May to July. Grows in dry, sandy or rocky, open woods and clearings from southern ON to NS. See p. 424 for conservation status.

WARNING
Large doses of the herb tea can cause nausea and vomiting.

Evening Star & Blazing Star

Mentzelia spp.

FOOD: The oily seeds were gathered by some tribes, dried, parched and ground into a nutritious meal for making pinole or mush and for adding to soups and stews. Sometimes seeds were fried, and the water from the fried seeds was used for gravy. The roots were sometimes chewed to relieve thirst.

MEDICINE: Blazing star was one of the oldest and most respected medicines of the Cheyenne. Its roots were gathered early in the year, before the plants had flowered. Because they were considered such a powerful medicine, they were always mixed with other herbs and were never used alone. Blazing star was considered especially good for relieving earaches and pain from rheumatism and arthritis. It was also used to make medicinal teas and salves for treating serious contagious diseases such as mumps, measles and smallpox. A decoction of the leaves was taken for stomach trouble.

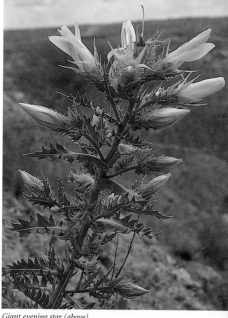

Giant evening star (above)
Blazing star (below)

OTHER USES: These giant, luminous flowers make a wonderful addition to a wildflower garden, especially in dry regions with poor soil, but their beauty remains hidden most of the time. Evening star and blazing star flowers close tightly during the day and open at dusk to attract night-flying pollinators.

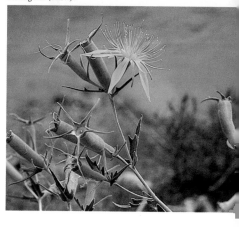

DESCRIPTION: Rough, greyish, perennial (sometimes biennial) herbs, 30–90 cm tall, covered in barbed hairs, with fleshy, brittle leaves that readily catch onto passersby and break off. Flowers large (about 10 cm wide), fragrant, with 5 or 10 spreading, pointed petals around a starburst cluster of stamens, borne singly or in small clusters, from July to September. Fruits oblong capsules, 1.5–4 cm long.

Giant evening star (*M. decapetala*) has creamy to yellowish flowers with 10 "petals" (5 true petals and 5 petal-like stamens); its seeds lack wings. Grows on dry, open slopes and roadsides in prairie, foothills and montane zones in southern AB, SK and southwestern MB. See p. 424 for conservation status.

Blazing star (*M. laevicaulis*) has 5-petalled, lemon yellow flowers and winged seeds. Grows on dry, open sites in prairie, foothills and lower montane zones in southern BC.

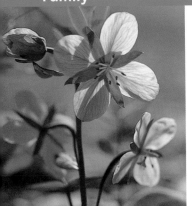

Broad-leaved fireweed (above)
Common fireweed (below)

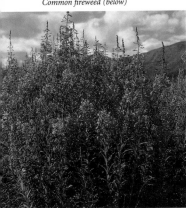

Fireweeds

Epilobium spp.

FOOD: Fireweeds (also called willowherbs) have been widely used as greens, either raw or cooked. The young shoots have been likened to asparagus and the young leaves to spinach. The beautiful pink flowers make a colourful addition to salads, and flower-bud clusters can be cooked as a vegetable. Fireweed tea has been enjoyed around the world, and fireweed honey is popular in some regions. The stem pith was added to soups as a thickener or dried, boiled and fermented to make fireweed ale.

MEDICINE: In Europe, fireweed is used to treat prostate problems, and oenothein B has been isolated as a 5α-reductase inhibitor; common fireweed has also been widely used as a medicine and is under investigation as a possible source for treatments for prostate problems. Common fireweed leaf and flower teas were sometimes used to treat asthma and whooping cough; peeled roots were applied as poultices to burns, swellings, boils, sores and rashes, and the leaves were applied to mouth ulcers. Leaf extracts have been shown to be anti-inflammatory, and the plant has been used to treat yeast infections (candidiasis), hemorrhoids, diarrhea, cramps and general inflammation in the digestive tract (mouth, stomach, intestine), either taken internally in teas or applied externally in washes, enemas and douches.

OTHER USES: Some First Nations used fireweed's stem fibres to make cord and fish nets. The stem pith was dried, powdered and rubbed on the face and hands in winter to protect skin from the cold and to reduce the pain of warming cold hands. Fireweed flowers were sometimes rubbed into rawhide for waterproofing, and the fluffy, down-like substance in mature seed pods provided tinder for fires, padding for quilts and fibres for blankets and clothing. Common fireweed is the territorial flower of YT.

DESCRIPTION: Clumped, perennial herbs with alternate, lance-shaped leaves on erect stems. Flowers pink to rose-purple (rarely white), 4-petalled, with a prominent, 4-pronged style, forming showy clusters, from June to September. Fruits erect, linear pods, splitting lengthwise to release hundreds of fluffy, parachuted seeds.

Common fireweed (*E. angustifolium*) has tall (usually more than 1 m tall) stems, with leaves 10–20 cm long, and produces clusters of 15 or more small (2–4 cm wide) flowers. Grows on open, disturbed, sometimes burned sites at all elevations in all provinces and territories in Canada.

Broad-leaved fireweed (*E. latifolium*) is a smaller (usually less than 40 cm tall) plant, with leaves less than 6 cm long, and with clusters of 1–10 large (2–6 cm wide) flowers. Grows in open sites (river bars, meadows, scree slopes) in montane, subalpine and alpine zones across northern Canada from BC to QC and in all 3 territories. See p. 424 for conservation status.

WARNING
Some people find fireweed has a slightly laxative effect, so start with small quantities.

Common Evening-Primrose

Oenothera biennis

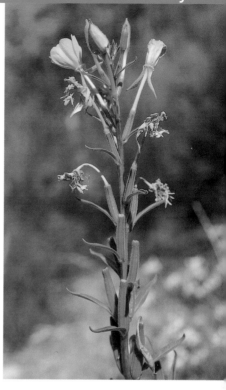

FOOD: The roots of young (first year) plants are said to taste like rutabagas or parsnips, though some people say they are an acquired taste. When gathered in late autumn or early spring, they were sometimes eaten raw, but usually they were boiled for 2 hours and/or in 2 changes of water to reduce their peppery flavour. Cooked roots have been served as a hot vegetable, fried, roasted with meat, sliced and added to soups and stews or boiled in syrup until they were candied. The young leaves, flower buds and green pods have also been cooked as greens, usually in 1–3 changes of water. Flowers and flower buds make a colourful addition to salads. Evening-primrose roots and flower buds have also been suggested for pickling. The oil-rich seeds have been used like poppy seeds, sprinkled on breads and in salads.

MEDICINE: Evening-primrose oil is an important commercial product in Canada. The oil prepared from the seeds is rich in essential fatty acids, such as gamma-linoleic acid and cis-linoleic acid, which the body converts into several important biomolecules. Evening-primrose oil reduces inflammation and imbalances and abnormalities in prostaglandin production and regulates liver functions. Clinical studies have shown evening-primrose oil to be useful for treating asthma, psoriasis, arthritis, weak immune systems, infertility, premenstrual syndrome and heart and vascular diseases. It has also been suggested as a remedy for eczema, rheumatoid arthritis, multiple sclerosis, migraine headaches, inflammations, menopausal and breast problems, diabetes, alcoholism (including liver damage) and cancer. Historically, the roots or shoot tips were steeped in hot water or simmered in honey to make soothing teas and cough syrups, which were said to have antispasmodic, sedative effects. Evening-primrose roots have been used in poultices on swellings, hemorrhoids and boils and rubbed on athletes' muscles to increase strength. Some First Nations used evening-primrose tea to treat obesity and laziness.

DESCRIPTION: Erect, biennial herb with single, hairy stems, to 1.5 m tall, from stout taproot. Leaves in basal rosettes (first year) and alternate (second year), lance-shaped to oblong, 2–15 cm long. Flowers generally open at dusk and close at dawn, bright yellow, about 3–4 cm across, with 4 broad petals and 4 backward-bending sepals, forming long clusters, from June to August. Fruits erect, hairy, spindle-shaped capsules, 2–4 cm long. Grows in moderately dry, open sites, along roadsides and railroad embankments, in waste areas and open woods in all provinces; introduced in BC and NL.

Wintergreens & Pyrolas

Moneses uniflora, Orthilia secunda, Pyrola spp.

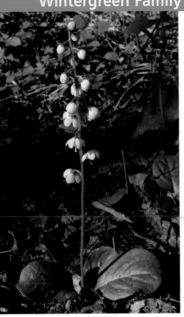

Shinleaf

FOOD: One-flowered wintergreen plants are edible and have been brewed as tea. They are said to be high in vitamin C. The seeds and capsules are edible as well; they can be eaten raw, roasted, parched or ground.

MEDICINE: One-flowered wintergreen tea has been used to treat sore throats, upset stomachs, paralysis, lung troubles (such as tuberculosis), colds, flu, coughs (when mixed with lung lichen [*Lobaria pulmonaria*] and licorice fern [p. 381]), smallpox and cancer; it was also taken for power and good luck. A poultice, tied to the affected area with a cloth bandage, was made to draw pus from boils and abscesses, reduce swellings and treat rashes, bunions, corns and pains. An infusion of the shinleaf plant was taken to treat rheumatism, bad blood, neck sores, indigestion, sore eyes, inflamed lids and styes. The roots of shinleaf were boiled and drunk to treat weakness and "back sickness." The plant was made into a poultice to treat sore legs. The liquid from the steeped plant was used as a gargle for sores or cankers in the mouth. The roots and leaves were given to babies with fits or epileptic seizures. The rhizome of one-sided wintergreen was boiled in water, cooled and used as an eyewash.

OTHER USES: The genus name *Pyrola* comes from the Latin *pyrus*, which means "pear"; not coincidentally, *Pyrola* leaves are often pear-shaped. One-flowered wintergreen has a beautiful flower with a lovely fragrance. Its other common name, single delight, and the genus name *Moneses* derive from the Greek words *monos* ("single") and *hesia* ("delight").

DESCRIPTION: Evergreen perennials from slender rhizomes; leaves often in whorls at stem base. Flowers with spreading petals, single but often close together, nodding on simple leafless stalks, blooming mid-summer. Fruits spherical capsules, 4–12 mm across.

One-flowered wintergreen or **single delight** (*M. uniflora*) has flowering stems 3–10 cm tall. Leaves 1–3 cm long, often basal but sometimes opposite or whorls of 3, egg-shaped, veiny, toothless to finely toothed. Flowers singular, white, waxy, fragrant, 1–2.5 cm across. Found in cool, moist woodlands, often with deep moss, all across Canada except YT. See p. 424 for conservation status.

One-sided wintergreen (*O. secunda*) grows to 15 cm tall. This is the only Canadian wintergreen whose flowers all come off 1 side of the inflorescence (hence the common name). In all others, the flowers are arranged spirally. Fruit a 5-part capsule. Found in coniferous and mixed forests throughout Canada.

Shinleaf (*P. elliptica*) has flowering stems 8–30 cm tall. Leaves basal, broadly elliptic to oblong, blunt-tipped, tapering to base, 3–7 cm long, fine-toothed. Flowers greenish white to pinkish, 3–16 in a cluster at stem tip, nodding, 8–12 mm across, curved style that protrudes from flower. Found in bogs, fens, swamps and moist to wet woods in all provinces. See p. 424 for conservation status.

Round-leaved pyrola (*P. rotundifolia*) has flowering stems 15–30 cm tall, with 1 or 2 scale-like leaves; leaves 2.5–7 cm long, round, shining, firm, often with pale green veins. Flowers white petals and green sepals, 8–10 mm across, in clusters at stem tip. Found in bogs and boreal forests in NU and from MB to NL. See p. 424 for conservation status.

Indian-Pipe
Monotropa uniflora

FOOD: Indian-pipe is said to be edible; it is tasteless if eaten raw, but it tastes similar to asparagus (p. 174) when cooked. However, the plant contains several glycosides and is possibly toxic, so caution is advised.

MEDICINE: The root was used traditionally as a sedative and to treat nervous conditions (convulsions, fits, epilepsy), especially in children. The juice of the plant was commonly used as a remedy for inflamed eyes. A poultice from the whole plant or just the stalk (either dried and powdered or burned) served as a treatment for "sores that would not heal." A medicinal tea was made to relieve aches and pains from colds. The flowers were chewed to treat toothaches.

OTHER USES: This plant could potentially be mistaken for a fungus because of its white colour (it has no chorophyll). It is actually a parasitic plant, obtaining its energy from nearby plants through connections with mycorrhizal fungi. Mycorrhizal fungi form associations with roots of photosynthesizing plants and provide nutrients and water while receiving carbon-rich photosynthates from the plant. Indian-pipe, through its connection with mycorrhiza, gets some of these photosynthates. Because it does not photosynthesize, Indian-pipe can grow in dark environments. Indian-pipe served as an indicator for the Thompson people in BC; if there were many Indian-pipes, this indicated that there were going to be many wood mushrooms in the coming season. For the Straits Salish and Nlaka'pamux of BC, the name for Indian-pipe means "wolf's urine"; it is said to grow wherever a wolf urinates. Other names for this plant, ghost flower and corpse plant, are attributed to its unusual appearance. Indian-pipe is also called "ice plant" because it is said to melt like ice if the plant is rubbed.

DESCRIPTION: Herbaceous, perennial herb, 10–20 cm tall, fleshy, waxy, white or rarely pinkish, in clusters of unbranched stems. Leaves alternate, scale-like, linear to oval, to 1 cm long. Flowers single, nodding at first, white, narrowly bell-shaped, the 5 petals 15–20 mm long, with a hairy inner surface, blooming from June to September. Fruits brown, erect, oval to circular capsules, 5–7 mm wide, containing many seeds; split open when mature. Found in dense, moist forests at low to montane elevations in all provinces. See p. 424 for conservation status.

235

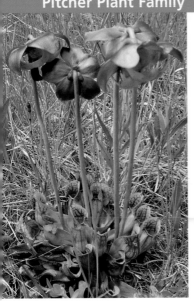

Pitcher Plant
Sarracenia purpurea

FOOD: As a food source for humans, no known use has been recorded, except that the leaves were sometimes used as drinking cups, presumably after the insect corpses inside had been discarded.

MEDICINE: Pitcher plant has a long history of use as a medicine. First Nations made an infusion of the leaves to facilitate childbirth, relieve sickness associated with amenorrhea and treat fevers and chills. A cold infusion of the entire plant was a remedy for whooping cough. A decoction of the roots was used for pulmonary disorders, spitting up of blood, urinary difficulties, venereal disease and liver sickness and was given to mothers to expel afterbirth and to prevent any postpartum sickness. Although an especially virulent form of smallpox was supposedly successfully treated with a strong infusion of pitcher plant root in 1861, modern tests have not confirmed the efficacy of this treatment. Newer studies are exploring the plant's anti-cancer and insecticidal activities. One traditional use supported by Western medicine has been for lower back pain treatments. Sarapin, a distillate from the plant, has been used for the last 70 years as a regional analgesic to reduce chronic neuromuscular or neuralgic pain. The drug reputedly inhibits pain signals in nerves exiting the spinal column without affecting any other nerve function and without adverse side effects. Although recognized and approved by the FDA and the American Medical Association, sarapin is not commonly used in medical practice, perhaps because plant extracts are not patentable, and thus not profitable.

OTHER USES: Pitcher plant was declared the floral emblem of NL in 1954, chosen to symbolize the province and its people because of its hardiness, resilience, adaptability and natural beauty. A true carnivorous plant, pitcher plant digests not only insects, but also isopods, mites, spiders, newts, salamanders and the occasional frog. Prey are attracted to the leaf's striking red veins, baited with nectar, and lured into a pitfall trap. The inside of the cavity has slippery and grooved edges lined with fine hairs that point downward, minimizing any chance of escape. Animals fall into the pool made up of rain, dew and digestive enzymes that soon dissolves the victim. The plant has evolved this unusual method to obtain nutrients otherwise lacking in its bog environment.

DESCRIPTION: Carnivorous perennial with leaves modified into a reddish green, hollow, inflated, curved "urn," 10–30 cm long, with strong red venation, arranged in a rosette. Terminal lip broad, flaring and covered in downward-pointing, stiff hairs. A "keel" on the leaves provides structural support to ensure that the opening is always upright. Flower solitary, deep purplish red, 5 cm wide, with 5 petals, numerous stamens and a style that is expanded into an umbrella-like structure, from May to August. Fruit a capsule with laterally winged seeds. Grows in sphagnum bogs, savannas and wet meadows throughout most of northern Canada from northeastern BC to NL. Because of poaching and diminishing wetland areas, the plant should be left undisturbed in the wild.

Sea-Milkwort

Glaux maritima ssp. *obtusifolia*

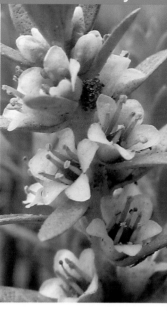

FOOD: Some First Nations in BC ate the fleshy rhizomes of this plant; they were harvested at different times of the year. The Kwakwaka'wakw would mark the plants the previous summer and dig the plants in spring, before they had sprouted. The Sechelt dug them in late summer while also gathering the roots of Pacific silverweed (p. 326). The Comox dug the rhizomes in autumn. After the rhizomes were gathered, they were washed and boiled for a long time in a kettle with a layer of red-hot stones. The rhizomes were typically eaten at family meals, dipped in eulachon grease. Many people would eat the rhizomes of sea-milkwort only before bed because they would cause sleepiness once eaten. They would tend to make a person feel sick if too many were eaten; one of the Kwakwaka'wakw names for sea-milkwort translates into "squeamish." The succulent leaves were used in Europe as a pickle.

OTHER USES: This plant is called milkwort (real milkwort is *Polygala vulgaris*) because nursing mothers drank an infusion of the plant to increase their milk supply. It was thought to increase milk supply in both livestock and humans. The genus name *Glaux* is from the Greek *glaucos*, meaning "bluish green," a good description of the plant colour; the species name *maritima* means "of the sea," its main habitat.

DESCRIPTION: Fleshy, often bluish green, perennial herb from rhizomes, the leafy stems 3–30 cm tall. Leaves opposite low on stem, alternate high on stem, oval to oblong, 5–25 mm long, 1.5–10 mm wide. Flowers white to pinkish, small (4–5 mm long), 5 petals, stalkless in leaf axils around middle of stem, blooming from May to July. Fruit a capsule, 2.5 mm long, with several flattened seeds. Found in moist, saline soil, inland alkaline marshes, wet meadowlands and coastal tidelands across Canada. See p. 424 for conservation status.

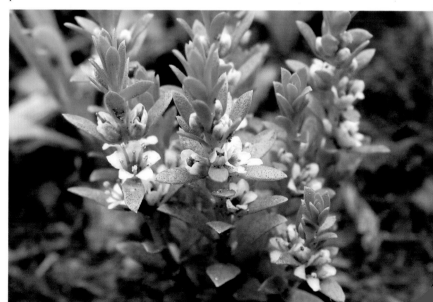

Gentians

Gentiana spp., *Gentianella* and *Gentianopsis*

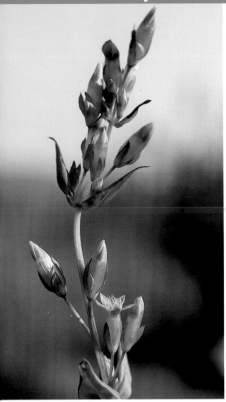

Northern gentian (all images)

FOOD: Before the widespread introduction of hops, gentians were occasionally used in Europe, with other bitter herbs, for brewing beers.

MEDICINE: Gentian roots (and occasionally the flowers) have been used in many forms (powders, teas, syrups and alcohol extracts) to treat many ailments (fever, indigestion, jaundice, fluid accumulation, skin diseases and gout), but usually they have been used in bitter tonics to aid digestion. Grieve (1931) recommends gentian for many purposes: as a general system "strengthener," as a tonic and purgative, to combat jaundice and as an emmenagogue, anthelminthic and antiseptic. His tonic ("60 ml root, 30 ml dried orange peel and 15 ml cardamom seeds in a quart of brandy") apparently restores appetite and promotes digestion. Present-day herbalists still recommend gentian root tea as one of the best vegetable bitters for stimulating appetite, aiding digestion, relieving bloating and flatulence and preventing heartburn. The bitter principles (iridoids and secoiridoids) are also said to normalize the functioning of the thyroid gland. Recent research has confirmed the antimicrobial activity of Canadian species.

OTHER USES: Many gentians are both beautiful and hardy, and they make excellent subjects for wildflower, rock and alpine gardens.

DESCRIPTION: Hairless annual, biennial or perennial herbs with opposite, essentially stalkless

> **WARNING**
> Overdoses cause nausea and vomiting, but only the most grimly resolute could manage to eat large amounts of these extremely bitter plants. Pregnant women and people suffering from stomach or duodenal ulcers or very high blood pressure should not use these plants.

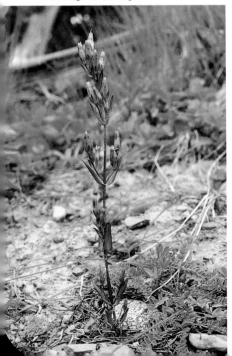

leaves. Flowers usually blue to purple, tubular to bell-shaped, tipped with 4–5 erect to horizontal lobes, borne from June to September. Fruits small capsules. See p. 424 for conservation status.

Mountain bog gentian (*Gentiana calycosa*) grows to 15 cm tall and has solitary, 3–4 cm long, usually deep purplish blue flowers with 5 blunt, spreading lobes and 5 pleated, fringed clefts. Grows in moist, open montane to alpine sites in southeastern BC and southwestern AB.

Stiff gentian (*Gentiana quinquefolia*) is a large plant, to 80 cm tall, with bluish purple, tubular flowers. Grows in moist soils along rocky, wooded banks, ledges, thickets and streams and in moist woodlands in southern ON.

Northern gentian (*Gentianella amarella*) is an annual or biennial herb with branched stems. Purplish blue to pale yellow and blue flowers have fringed throats and form clusters of large and small, 10–15 mm long, tubular flowers. Grows in open woods, thickets, beaches, meadows, clearings and moist areas in general, up to subalpine meadows, in all provinces and territories.

Fringed gentian (*Gentianopsis detonsa*) has 2–5 cm long, purplish blue flowers with 4 broad, widely spreading, fringed lobes, and its calyx lobes have glossy, purple, central ridges. Grows in meadows, bogs and moist ground in YT, northern AB, northern ON, QC and western NL.

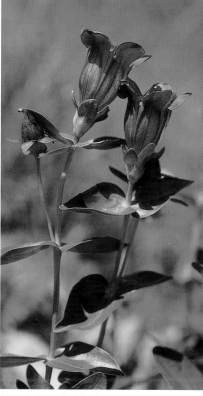

Mountain bog gentian (above)
Fringed gentian (below)

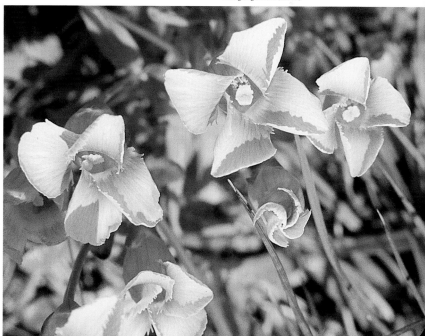

Tobaccos
Nicotiana spp.

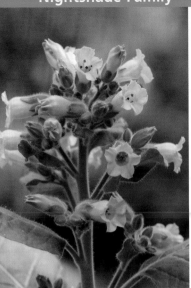
Wild tobacco

MEDICINE: Tobacco has traditionally been valued for its sedative, diuretic, emetic, antispasmodic, antinausea and expectorant properties. Nicotine, a volatile oil that is the main medicinal compound in tobacco, can be absorbed through the skin as well as inhaled, sniffed or ingested. The Algonquin used the leaves to stop bleeding and treated earache by blowing tobacco smoke into the affected ear. A poultice of the leaves applied directly to the skin was also used to reduce swelling and to treat skin ailments. In large doses, however, nicotine produces muscular weakness, vomiting and sweats. Excessive ingestion of nicotine can cause such problems as heart palpitations, cardiac irregularities, arterial degeneration and vascular contraction. Nicotine is now recognized as highly addictive, so its use in modern medicine is limited.

OTHER USES: Tobacco leaves are most commonly processed into forms for smoking (cigarettes, cigars or loose for a pipe or hookah), chewing or inhaling (snuff). In Canada, this plant was historically used by eastern First Nations' shamans and medicine men in large doses as an entheogen (consciousness altering, hallucinogenic). Tobacco was considered a sacred plant and used only on special occasions, such as during rites of passage, to seal a bargain or to make peace. Archaeological evidence suggests that tobacco has been used by First Nations for over 3000 years, and the plant remains religiously and culturally significant. The Metis, Cree and Ojibwa, for example, continue to use tobacco with prayers to the Creator, as part of the sweat lodge tradition, and in pipe and smudging ceremonies. Tobacco is still presented as a gift, especially when asking an elder for information or advice. Because tobacco is considered a sacred plant, its abuse through addiction and thoughtless smoking is frowned upon by many First Nations. Tobacco is also highly regarded as a garden flower: tall and stately with thick foliage and sweetly scented flowers, it attract butterflies, moths, bees and hummingbirds. Nicotine is a powerful neurotoxin, particularly deadly to many insects. Prepared as a diluted infusion, tea or decoction, tobacco produces an effective insecticide against common garden and houseplant pests such as aphids. Other familiar plants of the Nightshade family such as eggplant, tomato, potato and capsicum also contain nicotine, but not in the high concentrations found in tobacco.

DESCRIPTION: Annual, herbaceous plants, 1–2 m tall, from fibrous roots. Stems erect, round, hairy and viscid; branching near the top. Leaves large, numerous, alternate, stalkless, elliptic or oblong-oval, 30–60 cm wide, pointy tipped, hairy. Flowers 3–5 cm long, lobes oval. Seed capsules 1.5–1.7 cm long.

Tobacco (*N. tabacum*) has funnel-shaped flowers that are usually yellowish with purple tips. Native of the tropical Americas, this is the cultivated, commercial species, but it occasionally escapes to waste places in southern ON.

Wild tobacco (*N. rustica*) has yellow flower tubes that are slender, opening abruptly into flat lobes. This Peruvian species has long been cultivated by indigenous peoples of North America and occasionally escapes and natu-ralizes, as in southern ON.

WARNING
All parts of the tobacco plant are poisonous.

Ground-Cherry
Physalis heterophylla

FOOD: While the plant itself is poisonous, the fruit of the ground-cherry is delicious, an orange jewel held in a dry, papery husk and popping like a sweet-sour explosion in the mouth when eaten. Equally tasty fresh, in pies or in jam, it also stores well for months in the fridge or a cool room, providing a welcome burst of summer flavour as late as Christmas. Although this plant is native to eastern Canada, it grows well in warm, sunny gardens across the country. Many eastern First Nations relished the berries as a fresh autumn food source or dried them for winter use.

MEDICINE: The Iroquois used an infusion of dried leaves and rhizomes externally as a healing wash for scalds and burns and to treat sores caused by venereal disease, and internally as an emetic. A poultice of rhizomes and leaves was used to treat wounds and inflammation.

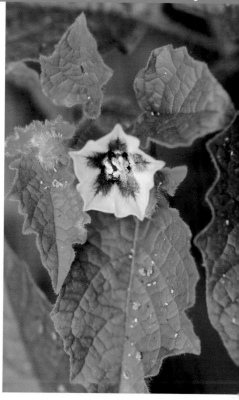

OTHER USES: Ground-cherry does well as an ornamental garden plant.

DESCRIPTION: Perennial plant, to 50 cm tall, growing from stout rhizomes. Stems erect, densely hairy, branching. Leaves glandular-hairy on upper and lower surfaces; 6 cm long, 5 cm wide; alternate, oval, typically heart-shaped with a few coarse, irregular teeth on margins. Single, yellow, funnel-shaped flowers hang from leaf axils, purplish at base, glandular-hairy externally. Seeds many, held in an orange (when ripe) fruit 3 cm long, 2.5 cm in diameter, enclosed in a papery husk. Grows in fields and open woods from MB to NS.

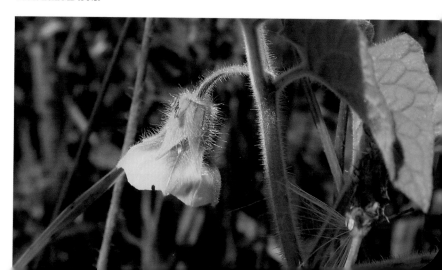

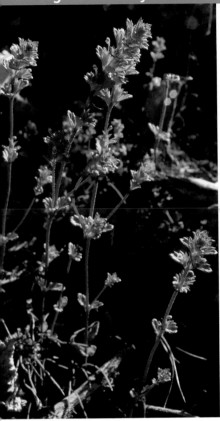

Eyebrights
Euphrasia spp.

FOOD: The leaves are occasionally enjoyed in salads for their slightly bitter flavour.

MEDICINE: As their name suggests, eyebrights have traditionally been used to treat afflictions of the eye, such as conjunctivitis and styes. The herbs were applied mostly as a poultice steeped in a decoction or taken internally as a tea. They are also prescribed to treat related areas of the sinuses, nasal passages and middle ear. Eyebrights are high in iridoid glycosides, flavonoids and tannins. The plants are strongly astringent, hence their use as a topical treatment to reduce inflammation and mucous drainage. Eyebrights are also reported to have anti-inflammatory, digestive and tonic qualities. Eyebrights have been shown to tighten the mucous membranes of the eye and appear to reduce related inflammation. Plants should be harvested when in flower and either prepared fresh or dried for later use. Dried eyebright is an ingredient in herbal smoking mixtures used in the treatment of bronchial colds. Eyebright is grown commercially in Europe for its widespread use in herbal remedies.

Arctic eyebright

DESCRIPTION: Small, herbaceous, annual herbs from taproots, growing 10–40 cm tall. Stems slender, squarish, simple or branched, downy. Leaves opposite, egg-shaped to nearly round, prominently toothed, to 1.5 cm long. Flowers solitary from leaf axils, these 5–10 mm long; strongly 2-lipped, upper lip concave and 2-lobed, lower lip 3-lobed, spreading; clustered in terminal spikes. Partially parasitic on other plants.

Note: Scientific names are very confusing for eyebrights. Eastern eyebright is called *E. americana* and *E. officinalis* in some books, and arctic eyebright has been called called *E. arctica* and *E. disjuncta*.

Eastern eyebright (*E. nemorosa*) has hairy leaves and pale lavender flowers with purple lines and a yellow spot on the lower lip. This introduced European species grows in dry, open areas (usually disturbed sites such as fields, meadows and roadsides) at lower elevations from QC to NL, and in southwestern BC.

Arctic eyebright (*E. subarctica*) has hairless (or nearly so) leaves and white flowers with purple lines and a yellow spot on the lower lip. Grows in wet, open areas (streambanks, mountain meadows, bogs) at higher elevations across northern Canada in all provinces and territories.

WARNING
Eyebrights are sometimes confused with *Euphorbia hypericifolia*, which is also commonly called eyebright but is acrid and poisonous. It is easy to differentiate the two: *Euphorbia hypericifolia* is much larger at 30–60 cm high, has purple, much-branched, prostrate stems to 60 cm long, and yields an acrid, milky juice when broken.

Great Mullein
Verbascum thapsus

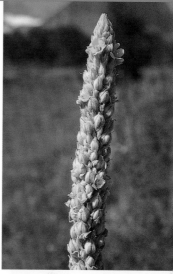

FOOD: Dried leaves have been steeped in hot water to make tea, but this tea should always be strained (see **Warning**).

MEDICINE: The leaves contain large amounts of mucilage, which soothes mucous membranes and has been shown to be anti-inflammatory. Mullein leaves and flowers were traditionally used to make medicinal teas for treating chest colds, asthma, bronchitis, coughs, kidney infections, diarrhea and dysentery. They were also applied as poultices to ulcers, tumours and hemorrhoids, or they were soaked in oil to make ear drops for curing earaches and killing ear mites. Chopped, dried leaves were smoked to relieve asthma, spasmodic coughing and fevers. Tea made with the stalks was used to treat cramps, fevers and migraine headaches. The roots are said to stimulate urination and to have an astringent effect on the urinary tract, so root tea was taken to tone the bladder, thereby reducing bed-wetting and incontinence. The flowers were soaked in oil to make antimicrobial drops for treating ear infections and removing warts. Mullein flower tea was said to have a pain-killing, sedative effect.

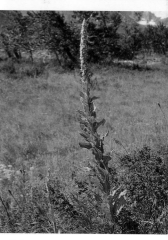

OTHER USES: The large, fuzzy leaves provide soft toilet paper (but see **Warning**). They can also be used as padded insoles for foot-weary travellers. Some native peoples smoked the dried leaves (though too much was said to be poisonous) or used mullein smoke to clear the nostrils of horses with colds. The Iroquois used an infusion of the roots with the flowers of white clover (p. 263) to treat asthma. The stems and leaves provided lamp wicks (before cotton was used), and dried flower stalks dipped in tallow were burned as torches. The seeds were put into ponds and slow streams as a narcotic fish poison, to stun fish. Roman women used the flowers to make yellow hair dye, and soap made with mullein ashes was said to return grey hair to its previous colour.

(p. 263)

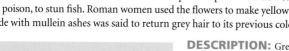

WARNING

This plant is generally considered safe for consumption in reasonable quantities, but it does contain tannin as well as rotenone and coumarin (see sweet-clover, p. 264), which are classified as potentially dangerous by the US Food and Drug Administration. Mullein seeds are toxic. The leaf fuzz may irritate sensitive skin and throat membranes.

DESCRIPTION: Greyish felted, biennial herb with single stems, 40 cm–2 m tall, from a taproot. Leaves many, 10–40 cm long, in basal rosettes (first and sometimes second year) and alternate on the flowering stem (second year). Flowers bright yellow, 1–2 cm wide, 5-lobed, forming dense, spike-like clusters 10–50 cm long, from June to August. Fruits egg-shaped, woolly capsules, 7–10 mm long. This introduced Eurasian weed grows along roadsides and waste places in all provinces.

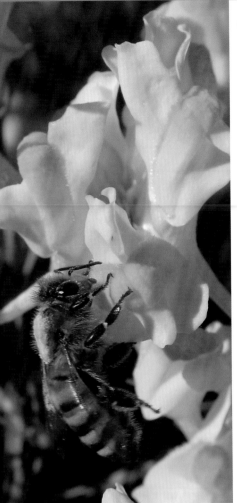

Butter-and-Eggs
Linaria vulgaris

MEDICINE: Butter-and-eggs is reported to have astringent, hepatic, purgative, diuretic and detergent properties. It was traditionally prescribed to treat jaundice and liver problems as well as applied topically to reduce hemorrhoids and to soothe some skin ailments such as ulcers, sores, piles and skin eruptions.

DESCRIPTION: Perennial herb from creeping rhizomes, erect, often branched above, evil-smelling, hairless throughout and somewhat glaucous; 20–80 cm tall, exuding a milky latex when broken. Leaves alternate, stalkless, smooth-margined, numerous, linear to narrowly lance-shaped, 2–10 cm long. Flowers yellow with a central, bearded, orange patch; snapdragon-like with a long, straight spur at the base; in spike-like clusters at first compact, then elongating. Fruits capsules, broadly cylindrical, 2-celled, to 1 cm long; seeds numerous, flattened with tiny bumps, winged. This Eurasian species is a common weed of disturbed sites at low to middle elevations in settled parts of all provinces.

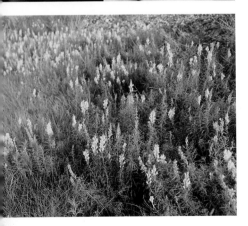

The pretty, yellow flowers tinged with reddish orange are the reason this plant is called butter-and-eggs.

●●●

The plant has been reported as mildly toxic to livestock. It is an aggressive colonizer, spreading by both rhizomes and seeds, and as such outcompetes many native plants and is difficult to eradicate once established. It is listed as a noxious weed in many provinces.

Turtlehead

Chelone glabra

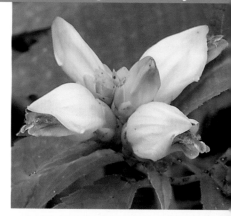

MEDICINE: The whole of this plant is considered medically useful and has tonic and detergent properties. The plant is harvested when in flower and can be processed fresh or dried for later use. Turtlehead has been used as a tonic for the liver and related digestive system problems such as gallstones, to treat consumption and jaundice and as a vermifuge for children. As an ointment it is recommended to soothe ulcers and inflamed tissues. The active compounds in turtlehead can be extracted as an alcohol-based tincture or a decoction. The plant was reportedly used by First Nations as a tonic, laxative and purgative. The Algonquin used turtlehead root with cedar as a medicinal tea, and the Maliseet used it to prevent pregnancy.

OTHER USES: Turtlehead adapts well to an ornamental garden and provides a bushy mound of pleasant-looking foliage with upright stems of large, long-lived, hooded flowers in early summer. It is easily divided from root cuttings or propagated from seed. It does best in moist sites as a border and is excellent as a cut flower and butterfly attractant.

DESCRIPTION: Herbaceous perennial, 60–90 cm tall, from creeping rhizome. Stems slender, erect, smooth, branched or unbranched. Leaves opposite, simple, oblong; 7–15 cm long, to 5 cm wide; narrow, sharply toothed, paired; stalkless or nearly so; pointed at the tip, tapering to the base; with a somewhat tea-like odour and strong bitter taste. Flowers snapdragon-like, 2-lipped, lower lip bearded in the throat, anthers and filaments woolly, colour highly variable (white, purplish, cream or rose); in tight clusters to 10 cm long, crowded onto terminal spikes. Fruits nearly spherical capsules to 1 cm in diameter; many seeds. Inhabits wet, open areas (thickets, streambanks, meadows, wetlands) from MB east. See p. 424 for conservation status.

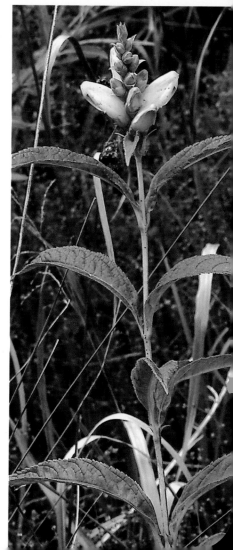

This plant's common and scientific names refer to the shape of the corolla, which resembles a tortoise's head (*Chelone* comes from the Greek word for "tortoise").

Brooklime & Speedwells

Veronica spp.

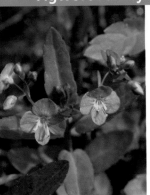

American brooklime

FOOD: All *Veronica* species are edible (but see **Warning**). The young leaves, stems and flowers of common speedwell and American brooklime are eaten raw or cooked and are high in vitamin C. The taste is said to range from bland to peppery or bitter and to be superior to that of watercress. These plants are used widely as a salad vegetable and potherb. The leaves and stems also make a pleasant tea popular in Europe that reportedly tastes like Chinese green tea. Leaves are best if harvested in spring and early summer before flowering.

MEDICINE: American brooklime is the most widely recognized of the plants in this genus for its medicinal properties and has been used for centuries to treat urinary and kidney complaints and as a blood purifier. It is often combined with other herbs, for example with coltsfoot (p. 362) for lung problems, with dandelion root (p. 332) for liver complaints, and with elderberry (p. 124) for eczema and acne. Common speedwell has been used medicinally as a strengthening and wound-healing plant and against coughs. Other uses include as an expectorant for respiratory problems such as bronchitis and asthma and as an ingredient in cough syrups, sore throat gargles and skin salves. The most common methods of preparing these plants are as a tea, tincture or juice.

OTHER USES: Infusions of American brooklime have been used as a conditioning rinse for hair and for pore-cleansing herbal steams. Added to bath water and massage oils, it is soothing to the skin. These plants are also increasingly popular in ornamental gardens for their pretty flowers and love of wet sites. Blue flowers, such as those of common speedwell, were a traditional gift of good luck for departing guests.

DESCRIPTION: Perennial herbs growing from shallow, creeping, branching rhizomes or rooting from trailing stems. Stems erect or trailing. Leaves opposite, usually 3–5, elliptic or lance-shaped to oval, tapered to a short stalk. Flowers generally blue (violet to lilac) or whitish with dark blue lines, 4-lobed, in several many-flowered, narrow, terminal clusters, 5–7 mm wide and 3–6 cm long, from May to July. Fruits round to heart-shaped capsules, finely glandular-hairy; seeds small, few to many.

American brooklime (*V. americana*) grows 10–70 cm tall and has leaves sharply pointed and toothed, saucer-shaped, not strongly lipped, with 2 large, spreading stamens, in long, loose clusters along stem. Found in wet spots and shallow water in all provinces and YT. See p. 424 for conservation status.

Common speedwell (*V. officinalis*) is a hairy, trailing, mat-forming species, 20–30 cm tall or long. Leaves 2–4 cm long and 1–2 cm wide, hairy; margins uniformly toothed, except near base. Fruits capsules 4–5 mm wide and nearly as long. Eurasian weed common across Canada in woodlands and disturbed sites.

Thyme-leaved speedwell (*V. serpyllifolia*) has stems 10–30 cm long, rooting at the nodes, finely hairy. Leaves entire or weakly toothed; lower leaves hairless, 1–2.5 cm long, 4–8 mm wide, saucer-shaped, stalked. Fruits notched capsules. Found in meadows, woodlands, disturbed sites and on streambanks across all provinces. Reportedly 2 types, a native variety with pale blue to dark blue corolla to 8 mm broad, and an introduced variety with whitish to pale blue corolla to 5 mm broad, both widely distributed. See p. 424 for conservation status.

WARNING

Avoid harvesting plants that are growing in or near polluted water. If you are uncertain, add a few drops of bleach to the rinse water when you get home and allow the plants to sit in it for a few minutes to reduce the risk of contamination by water-borne pathogens.

Louseworts
Pedicularis spp.

FOOD: Some First Nations cooked the leaves of these plants in the same way that we cook spinach.

MEDICINE: Historically, the whole plant was used medicinally. The roots of Canadian lousewort were prescribed as a blood tonic and in the form of a tea for sore throats, stomachaches, ulcers, anemia and heart troubles. The Ojibwa steeped the roots in hot water and drank the tea to treat stomach ulcers. They used fresh or dried leaves as a gargle to treat sore throats and took dried root internally to treat anemia. A poultice of the root is said to reduce swelling and sore muscles. An infusion of the leaves is an abortifactant. Elephanthead lousewort leaves and stems were steeped in water, then taken to relieve coughing.

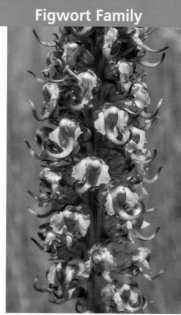

Elephanthead lousewort (above)
Canadian lousewort (below)

OTHER USES: These flowers can be detected from metres away by their sweet, heavy perfume. Some people enjoy this fragrance, but others find it overwhelming and nauseating. Lousewort is reported to have aphrodisiac qualities. The finely grated root was secretly added to the victim's food. The root was also historically included in a feed mixture for ponies. Interestingly, louseworts are semi-parasitic plants relying on grass species. Their presence profoundly alters the structure and composition of grassland communities. Some estimates suggest that louseworts can parasitize at least 80 different grass species in 35 genera.

DESCRIPTION: Perennial herbs from fibrous roots, to 50 cm tall. Leaves basal and alternate, sparsely hairy, lance-shaped to oblong, finely divided. Flowers fairly showy, in dense terminal clusters. Fruits capsules, oblong to lance-shaped, flattened, reddish brown or brown, about 15 mm long; seeds many.

Canadian lousewort (*P. canadensis*) has yellow flowers with an upper lip that is rounded, hood-like, with 2 teeth near tip; blooms from May to June. Found in woodlands and open areas at low to middle elevations in MB, ON, QC and NB. See p. 424 for conservation status.

Elephanthead lousewort (*P. groenlandica*) has reddish purple flowers with an upper lip that extends into a long, cylindrical, upturned beak (resembling a tiny elephant's head and trunk); blooms from June to August. Found in meadows, swamps and wet fields from BC and YT to NL (but not in the Maritimes).

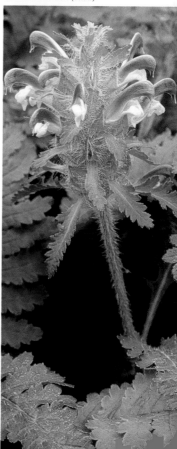

WARNING
Louseworts are considered poisonous to humans and animals if ingested in quantity.

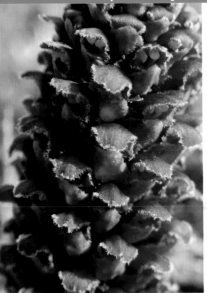

Vancouver groundcone (all images)

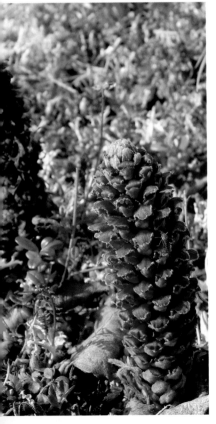

Groundcones

Boschniakia spp.

FOOD: While plants were in fruit, the thickened stem bases of Vancouver groundcone were harvested by some BC coastal First Nations, including the Kwakwaka'wakw. The stem bases were eaten raw. A classic west coast sasquatch tale features Albert Ostman, who was kidnapped and held for nearly a week by a family of sasquatches near Toba Inlet, BC in 1924. Ostman reports that the sasquatch family ate, among other things, "some kind of nuts that grow in the ground. I have seen lots of them on Vancouver Island." These "nuts" may have been the dried stem bases of Vancouver groundcone.

MEDICINE: The roots were used to treat coughs.

OTHER USES: A common name for Vancouver groundcone, poque, is derived from the Kwakwaka'wakw name for the plant, *p'ukw'es.* Some central coastal First Nations considered Vancouver groundcone to be a good luck charm. These plants are root parasites (they obtain their nutrients by attaching to roots of other plants) and do not produce chlorophyll.

DESCRIPTION: Perennial, parasitic herb from corm-like stem base and fleshy roots, resembling an upright Sitka spruce cone (p. 31). Plants solitary or clustered, covered with many scaly, broad bracts. Flowers crowded between bracts, each flower 1–1.5 cm long, blooming from June to July. Fruit capsules 1–1.5 cm long, with numerous tiny seeds.

Vancouver groundcone (*B. hookeri*) is a smaller, yellow to red or purple plant (8–12 cm tall) with yellow to purple flowers and entire bracts. Grows in moist to mesic forests at low elevations in southwestern BC and Haida Gwaii (Queen Charlotte Islands), where it is usually parasitic on salal (p. 122).

Northern groundcone (*B. rossica*) is a larger, brownish plant (10–14 cm tall) with rusty red flowers and fringed bracts (at least the upper ones). Grows in moist to mesic forests at montane elevations in northern BC, YT and NT, where it is parasitic on a number of shrubs, mostly in the Birch family, and most commonly on alders (p. 151).

Beechdrops

Epifagus virginiana

MEDICINE: In modern herbal medicine, beechdrops have been used externally for wounds, bruises, cuts and skin irritations. A tea made from the fresh plant was taken to treat dysentery, mouth sores, cold sores and diarrhea. It is said to have a bitter, astringent taste.

OTHER USES: Beechdrops are parasitic on the roots of the American beech tree (p. 61). (The genus name, *Epifagus*, translates into "upon the beech.") This plant is often overlooked because its brown stems are difficult to see against dead leaves on forest floors. Beechdrops has 2 kinds of flowers, some that open to cross-pollinate and others that don't open and self-pollinate. Another common name for this plant is cancer root because it was thought by settlers to be a remedy for cancer.

DESCRIPTION: Annual, parasitic herb, 15–50 cm tall, stem with many branches, pale brown with thin purple lines; leaves alternate, scale-like. Flowers yellowish white, reddish or brown, on thin stalks, 2 kinds: lower flowers cup-like, ribbed, 5-lobed; upper flowers tubular, 4-lobed, and often with 2 brown stripes 1–1.5 cm long; bloom from August to October. Found in mesic to moist forests, with American beech, in ON, QC, NB, NS and PEI.

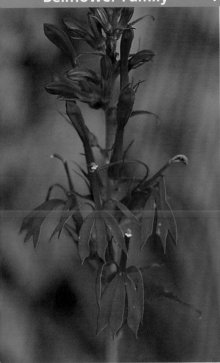

Cardinal flower (all images)

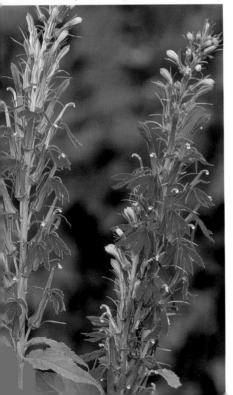

Indian-Tobacco & Cardinal Flower

Lobelia spp.

MEDICINE: Indian-tobacco was one of the more valuable medicinal plants of First Nations, used as a remedy for a wide variety of complaints. Its common names capture some of its traditional uses: wild tobacco, asthmaweed, vomitwort, pukeweed and gagroot. The taste and smell of dried lobelia somewhat resembles tobacco, and the leaves were smoked, paradoxically, as a treatment for asthma, bronchitis, sore throats and coughs. The plant was taken internally to treat the same respiratory conditions, as well as for fevers and to induce sweating and vomiting. Indian-tobacco was added to herbal mixtures to enhance or direct the action of other plants.

In the early 1800s, US herbalist Samuel Thomson, founder of the idiosyncratic form of medicine called Thomsonianism, popularized the herb as an emetic in large doses, and in smaller doses as a nauseant expectorant in cases of asthma and chronic bronchitis. The popularity of Indian-tobacco was renewed in the 1970s as a mild euphoriant, taken as a tea or powdered capsule and said to induce feelings of mental clarity, happiness and well-being.

The principal component of Indian-tobacco is lobeline, an alkaloid with similar pharmacological properties to nicotine, but less potent. Thus, lobeline initially stimulates peripheral and central nerves, followed by respiratory depression. Today it is marketed as

WARNING
Side effects of Indian-tobacco are similar to those of nicotine and include nausea and vomiting, diarrhea, coughing, tremors and dizziness. Overdosing causes convulsions, hypothermia, hypotension, coma and death.

a stop-smoking treatment. Studies have found that lobeline may diminish some of the effects of nicotine, specifically nicotine-induced release of the neurotransmitter dopamine. Because dopamine plays a role in drug addiction, it was theorized that lobeline could be helpful for those seeking to stop smoking. Despite widespread marketing, there is little evidence that the treatment works. There is, however, a potential benefit for addiction to amphetamines. Animals in which lobeline was injected experienced deeper respiration, enhanced memory and reduced pain.

Another constituent of *Lobelia* species, beta-amyrin palmitate, has antidepressant and sedative effects. Use of the plant requires caution (see **Warning**). Excess doses cause nausea, vomiting, drowsiness, respiratory failure and potentially death. The alkaloids can induce muscle paralysis in much the same way as curare so that not even the smallest muscles can be used. This condition was termed "the alarm" and, although uncomfortable, was not considered dangerous by early herbalists.

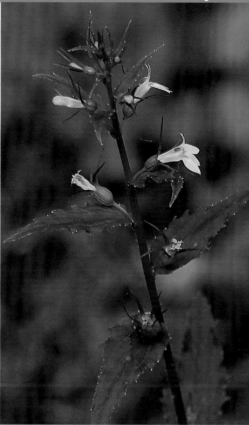

Indian-tobacco

Topically, Indian-tobacco is employed as a salve or tincture for swellings, inflammations, pleurisy, rheumatism, tennis elbow, whiplash injuries, boils and ulcers. Cardinal flower was considered to possess similar activity to Indian-tobacco, but less potent, and so used less often by First Nations. An infusion of the roots was used for the treatment of epilepsy, syphilis, typhoid, stomachaches, cramps and worms. Leaf tea was used for croup, nosebleeds, colds, fevers, headaches and rheumatism.

OTHER USES: Cardinal flower, possibly because of its bright red flowers, was a common ingredient in love charms, potions and spells. Smoke from Indian-tobacco was used to drive away gnats.

DESCRIPTION: Perennial herbs from fibrous roots, with terminal racemes of variously coloured flowers, each flower with 2 narrow lobes above and 3 wider lobes forming a lip below. Fruits capsules. See p. 424 for conservation status.

Indian-tobacco (*L. inflata*) grows 30–60 cm tall, with oval, wavy-toothed leaves to 5 cm long. Tiny, white to pinkish to blue-violet flowers, to 12 mm long, from June to October. Calyx surrounding fruit becomes distinctly inflated and balloon-like, to 8 mm across. Grows in open fields, woods and roadsides from southern ON to NS and PEI, and also in BC's lower Fraser Valley, where introduced.

Cardinal flower (*L. cardinalis*) grows 60 cm–1.2 m tall, with lance-shaped, toothed leaves to 15 cm long. Larger (to 4.5 cm long), brilliant red, tubular flowers, with narrow, leaf-like bracts beneath, from July to September. Grows in damp sites and along streams from southern ON to NB.

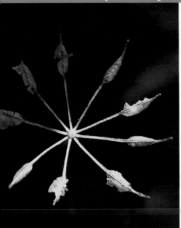

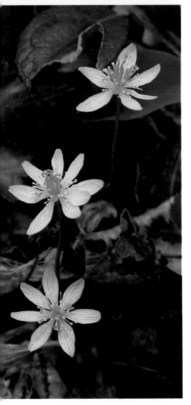

Three-Leaf Goldthread
Coptis trifolia

FOOD: The whole plant of three-leaf goldthread is said to be edible. It has been mixed with sassafras root bark (p. 103) and Irish moss (the seaweed *Chondrus crispus*) and brewed into a kind of herbal root beer.

MEDICINE: Three-leaf goldthread is a very bitter tasting herb that has been used for medicinal purposes by First Nations including the Iroquois, Maliseet, Mi'kmaq, Ojibwa, Abenaki and Algonquin. The root was often used to treat illness in babies and children, such as mouth sores (oral cankers), teething pains, vomiting and sickness caused by "bad blood" from the mother. An infusion of the rhizomes was used to treat stomach cramps, worms, vomiting, jaundice, diarrhea, sore eyes (as an eyewash), earaches, toothaches, dizziness, trench mouth, raw throat, colds, coughs and respiratory troubles and to ease digestion. A compound decoction of the whole plant was taken as blood purifier and blood remedy as well as for venereal disease. The plant was said to relieve cravings for alcohol and was often used in compounds administered to fight alcoholism. The plant contains the alkaloid berberine, which is anti-inflammatory, antibacterial, astringent, anticonvulsant, immunostimulant and mildly sedative. Three-leaf goldthread was listed in the US Pharmacopoeia from 1820–82, and 500 g sold for $1 at turn of the last century.

OTHER USES: The rhizomes of three-leaf goldthread, which are golden-coloured, were boiled to make yellow dye; they were sometimes added to other plant dyes to emphasize the yellow colour. The genus name *Coptis* comes from the Greek word *kopto*, which means "to cut," referring to the dissected leaves. The species name *trifolia* comes from the Latin words *tri* (three) and *foliata* (having leaves), "having three leaves." The common name goldthread comes from the distinctive thread-like rhizomes.

DESCRIPTION: Perennial herb, 5–15 cm tall, from bright yellow to orange thread-like rhizomes, found just below ground. Leaves divided into 3 leaflets, egg-shaped with pointed base, toothed, slightly 3-lobed, 1–2 cm long. Flowers erect, solitary, white, the 5–7 petals, club-shaped and half the length of the sepals, the 5 sepals, 4–11 mm long, white, blooming from May to August. Fruits 3–7 long-stalked pods with beaks, 2–4 mm long; seeds shiny, black, 1–1.5 mm long. Found in coniferous and mixed forests, bogs, willow scrub and tundra in lowland and montane zones across Canada except YT.

Marsh-Marigolds

Caltha spp.

FOOD: The broad, fleshy leaves have been boiled until tender (10–60 minutes depending on the plant) and served with butter or in cream sauce; they were cooked as greens or sometimes with meat or fat by the Iroquois, Ojibwa and Abenaki. White marsh-marigold could be an important emergency food at high elevations because it is often abundant in areas where other edible plants are scarce, but it would probably be wise to cook it if possible and to use it in moderation (see **Warning**). Yellow marsh-marigold is said to make an excellent potherb when cooked in 2 changes of water (see **Warning**). The buds have been used like capers, soaked in salt water and vinegar; however, the pickling juice is said to be poisonous. The fleshy roots have been cooked and eaten; these have been described as resembling sauerkraut. The seeds were used as food by the Abenaki.

MEDICINE: Poultices of yellow marsh-marigold leaves were used as counter-irritants to relieve rheumatic pain and inflamed wounds, and the caustic juice was dropped onto warts. The plant has also been used to treat fits, anemia and colds. A tea made from the leaves has been used as a diuretic and laxative. The plant was considered poisonous by some First Nations. An infusion of the smashed roots was taken to vomit, a measure designed to counter a love charm.

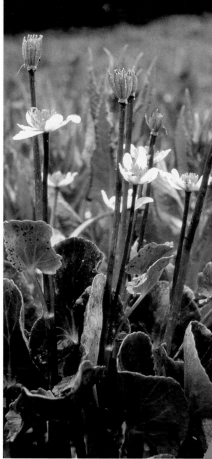

White marsh-marigold

WARNING

Some sources warn against eating marsh-marigolds, but many writers recommend this plant as a potherb, and some say they have used the raw flowers and young leaves in salads with no ill effects. Many marsh-marigolds contain volatile, poisonous glycosides. All parts of yellow marsh-marigold contain protoanemonin and helleborin, poisons that are toxic to the heart and cause inflammation of the stomach. The leaves can cause skin to blister.

DESCRIPTION: Fleshy, perennial herbs, to 60 cm tall, from fibrous roots. Leaves basal, long-stalked. Flowers about 2–4 cm across, with 5–15 oblong to oval, petal-like sepals and no petals, borne singly on leafless stems. Fruits erect clusters of pods (follicles), about 15 mm long. Grows in moist to wet meadows, marshes, fens, swamps, ditches and shallow water. See p. 424 for conservation status.

White marsh-marigold (*C. leptosepala*) has oblong to heart-shaped leaves 2–6 cm long, and white (sometimes bluish-tinged) flowers blooming from June to August. Grows at all elevations in BC, western AB (Rocky Mountains) and southern YT.

Yellow marsh-marigold (*C. palustris*) has kidney-shaped to circular leaves 2–13 cm long, and yellow flowers blooming from April to July. Found at lower elevations across Canada.

253

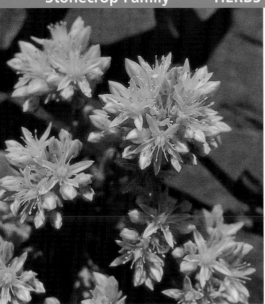

Lance-leaved stonecrop (all images)

Stonecrops
Sedum spp.

FOOD: The leaves of spreading stonecrop are so succulent that they were often referred to as berries by First Nations along Canada's Pacific Coast. For example, the Kwakwaka'wakw referred to spreading stonecrop leaves as crow's-strawberry, though they didn't consider them edible. The Haida and Nisga'a, however, did eat the leaves. Young leaves and shoots have been eaten raw or cooked, but older plants can become bitter. These plants have been eaten raw in salads and as a trail nibble, cooked as a hot vegetable or added to soups and stews. The fleshy rhizomes have also been eaten, either boiled alone or with other vegetables, or pickled in seasoned vinegar. These juicy plants can be a good source of liquid when water is not available.

MEDICINE: The plants are high in vitamins A and C. Because stonecrops are slightly astringent and mucilaginous, their juice or mashed leaves have been applied to wounds, ulcers, minor burns, insect bites and other skin irritations. Stonecrops have also been taken internally to treat lung problems and diarrhea.

DESCRIPTION: Hairless, succulent, perennial herbs with short, thick leaves on erect, 5–20 cm tall stems. Flowers small, 5-petalled, forming dense, flat-topped clusters, from May to August. Fruits compact clusters of 5 pointed capsules that split open along the upper inner edge.

Lance-leaved stonecrop (*S. lanceolatum*) has slender rhizomes and creeping, rooting stems, forming mats. Alternate, lance-shaped, pointy-tipped leaves. Grows on dry, rocky slopes at low to subalpine elevations from BC and YT to SK (Cypress Hills).

Spreading stonecrop (*S. divergens*) is similar to lance-leaved stonecrop, but has mostly opposite, egg-shaped, round-tipped leaves. Grows on rocky cliffs and talus slopes at all elevations along BC's coast.

In addition to these 2 native species, a number of introduced Eurasian species of stonecrop are found escaped from gardens along roadsides and in waste places across southern Canada.

Roseroot & Stonecrop

Rhodiola spp.

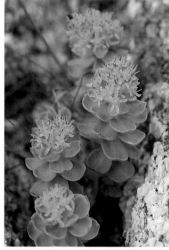

Roseroot

FOOD: Inuit ate the succulent stems and leaves as a green vegetable, harvesting them in early summer when the plants were more tender. Sweetness varies with the species, and roseroot is one of the most popular. A touch of garlic enhances the cucumber-like flavour. Other First Nations fermented rhizomes in water and ate the plants and juice with walrus blubber or oil. The mixture was then stored cold to prevent further fermentation. The herb can be made into a sort of sauerkraut, or cooked and eaten like asparagus (p. 174). The fleshy, tuberous rhizomes were eaten in early spring.

MEDICINE: Roseroot (also called golden root and arctic root) has been used in European and Asian medicine for over 3000 years. The Vikings used roseroot before going into battle. In Middle Asia, roseroot tea was the most effective treatment for cold and flu. Similarly, ledge stonecrop leaves were steeped in hot water or rhizomes were boiled to make medicinal teas for relieving cold symptoms, to soothe sore throats and for washing irritated eyes. In traditional folk medicine, roseroot was used to increase resistance to high altitude sickness and to treat fatigue, depression, anemia, impotence, gastrointestinal ailments, infections and nervous system disorders. More recently, it has been studied as an "adaptogen." These are medicinal herbs that make stress responses less damaging and regulate adaptive reactions when the body is under stress. The plant increases the body's resistance to stress, improves mood, alleviates depression, reduces fatigue, ameliorates mental and physical performance and prevents high altitude sickness. Its unique medicinal activity is attributed to phytochemicals such as the phenylethanol derivative salidroside (rhodioloside) and the rosavins, including phenylpropanoids rosarin, rosavin and rosin.

DESCRIPTION: Fleshy, perennial, rhizomatous herbs, sometimes mat-forming, the stems erect, 5–30 cm tall, numerous, leafy. Leaves alternate, 10–40 mm long, succulent, smooth-margined or coarsely toothed, stalkless. Flower clusters dense and head-like, flowers purple or yellow, from May to August. Fruits erect follicles. See p. 424 for conservation status.

Note: Scientific and common names can be confusing for these species. Both species treated here as *Rhodiola* are sometimes called *Sedum* (p. 254), and both are sometimes treated as subspecies of *Rhodiola* (or *Sedum*) *rosea*. Also, both species described here are also called roseroot in other books!

Roseroot (*R. rosea*) has thick, branched rhizomes and erect to ascending stems (5–10 cm long); not generally mat-forming. Egg-shaped to elliptic leaves to 4 cm long. Found along the east coast of Ungava Bay, in arctic QC; also grows on moist cliffs and alpine ridges, often near the ocean, in NB, NS and NL.

Ledge stonecrop (*R. integrifolium*) is very similar to roseroot, but is generally larger (10 –20 cm), and often mat-forming. Leaves shorter than those of roseroot (generally less than 2.5 cm long), and female flowers purplish black (vs. yellow in roseroot). Grows on cliffs, talus slopes and meadows at low to alpine elevations in BC, AB, YT and NT.

Plantains

Plantago spp.

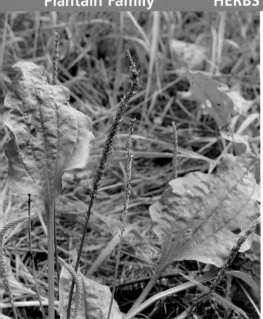

Common plantain

FOOD: It is easy to pull these common weeds from the garden without realizing that they are edible and probably more nutritious than most of the greens we tend to eat. Young leaves have been eaten raw in salads and sandwiches, but as they age they become tough and stringy. Cooking improves palatability and makes it possible to remove some of the tougher fibres. Fine chopping may also make older leaves easier to eat. The flavour has been likened to that of Swiss chard (*Beta vulgaris*). Plantain seeds can be dried and ground into meal or flour for use in bread or pancakes. Plantains are rich in vitamins A, C and K.

MEDICINE: The leaves and leaf juice have been widely used as topical agents in poultices and lotions for treating insect bites and stings, snakebites, sunburn, poison-ivy (p. 395) rashes, sore nipples, blisters, burns and cuts. Plantain leaves have also been heated and applied to swollen joints, sprains, strained muscles and sore feet. In Latin America, common plantain is a prominent folk remedy for treating cancer. Plantain tea has been used for centuries to treat sore throats, laryngitis, coughs, bronchitis, tuberculosis and mouth sores. These plants are said to have anti-inflammatory effects and are rich in the flavonoids allantoin (a nitrogenous compound that promotes healing of injured skin cells) and tannin (whose astringency helps to draw tissues together and stop bleeding). Preliminary studies indicate that plantains may reduce blood pressure, and their seeds have been shown to reduce blood cholesterol levels. Plantain seeds are rich in mucilage, and they were widely used as a source of natural fibre with laxative effects. They were also used in medicinal teas for treating diarrhea, dysentery, intestinal worms and bleeding of mucous membranes. The roots were recommended for relieving toothaches and headaches and for healing poor gums.

OTHER USES: Strong plantain tea was sometimes used as a hair rinse for preventing dandruff. The tough veins of mature leaves are amazingly strong and have been used as a source of fibre for making thread, fishing line and even cloth. Plantain seeds, soaked in water, produce a mucilaginous liquid that was used as a wave-set lotion.

DESCRIPTION: Clumped, perennial herb, to 10 cm tall, with a basal rosette of elliptic to lance-shaped leaves 4–18 cm long and abruptly tapered to winged stalks. Flowers greenish, about 2 mm across, with 4 whitish petals, forming dense, slender, 3–30 cm long spikes, with conspicuous yellow stamens that stick out, blooming from May to September. Fruits membranous capsules 2–4 mm long, opening by a lid-like top to release tiny, dark seeds. These European weeds grow on disturbed, cultivated or waste ground.

Common plantain (*P. major*) has broadly elliptical leaves with strong parallel veins. Found in all provinces and territories except YT.

Narrow-leaved plantain (*P. lanceolata*) has narrower, lance-shaped leaves with several prominent ribs. Found in BC and across Canada from SK to NL.

Dogbanes

Apocynum spp.

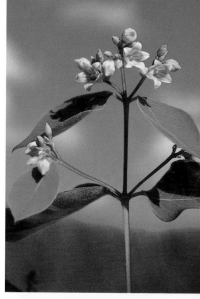

MEDICINE: Dogbane roots were mashed to induce the flow of white latex and applied as poultices or were used to make teas and tinctures that were applied as lotions. These preparations were said to induce sweating, act as a counter-irritant and stimulate blood flow to the skin. They were sometimes applied to the scalp to increase hair growth. Berry and root extracts were taken internally to relieve constipation, induce sweating and vomiting, stimulate the heart, relieve insomnia and expel intestinal worms. However, this use could be very dangerous (see **Warning**). Dogbanes were used to treat headaches, indigestion, rheumatism, liver disease and syphilis. These plants have a powerful action on the heart (similar to digitalis). They also irritate the digestive tract. Some of their glycosides are said to have antitumour properties.

OTHER USES: Mature stems were used to make thread by soaking them in water, removing the tough outer fibres and rolling what remained against the leg into thread. This thread was said to be stronger and finer than cotton thread. Three strands plaited together were used to make bowstrings, and the cord was also made into fishing nets and net bags. Dogbane cord was used to make rabbit nets, up to 1.5 km long, which were used in communal rabbit hunts. These nets were often inherited, and the owner was the recognized leader of the hunt. Indian hemp was preferred because of its longer, tougher fibres. The milky sap (latex) contains rubber.

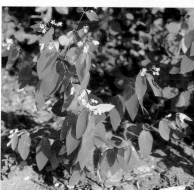

Spreading dogbane (all images)

DESCRIPTION: Erect, perennial herbs, to 1 m tall, with milky sap and opposite, sharp-pointed, short-stalked leaves. Flowers bell-shaped, 5-petalled, sweet-smelling; form showy, branched clusters; bloom from June to September. Fruits hang in pairs of slender pods (follicles), splitting down 1 side to release many small, silky-parachuted seeds.

Spreading dogbane (*A. androsaemifolium*) has oval to oblong, spreading or drooping leaves and 4–8 mm long, pink flowers. Grows in well-drained fields and open forests at low to subalpine elevations throughout Canada, except NU.

Indian hemp (*A. cannabinum*) has narrower, ascending leaves and smaller (2–4 mm long), greenish white to white flowers. Grows in dry to moist, often disturbed sites at low to montane elevations throughout Canada, except NU, Labrador and PEI. See p. 424 for conservation status.

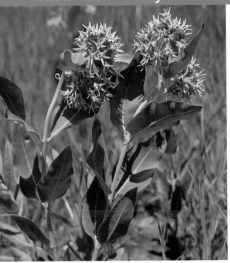
Showy milkweed

Milkweeds
Asclepias spp.

FOOD: Young shoots, unopened flower buds and immature seed pods were eaten raw (see **Warning**) or boiled or fried in oil (with or without batter). Milkweed was often added to soups and stews to thicken broth and tenderize meat. It was usually necessary to boil the plants in 2–3 changes of water to reduce bitterness. Young plants, 10–15 cm tall, could be used like asparagus (p. 174), and young firm pods, 2–3 cm long, like okra. The sweet buds and flowers were boiled down to make a thick syrup. They were also made into preserves. Milkweed seeds were occasionally eaten.

MEDICINE: The milky sap was applied to cuts and burns and to infections and irritations, including warts, moles, ringworm, poison-ivy (p. 395) rash, measles, corns and calluses. The plant tips were boiled to make a wash for treating blindness. The powdered roots were boiled to make medicinal teas for use as a sedative and to treat stomachaches and asthma. Fresh roots were boiled to make teas for treating bowel problems, kidney problems, water retention, rheumatism, intestinal worms, asthma and venereal disease and for use as a temporary contraceptive. Seeds were boiled to make a solution for drawing poison from snakebites, or they were powdered and added to salves for treating sores.

OTHER USES: Dried juice from broken stems provided chewing gum. The milky juice leaves a stain that can persist for days or weeks, and it was sometimes used to temporarily brand livestock. The seed silk was used to stuff pillows, mattresses and comforters and was even woven (with other fibres) into cloth.

DESCRIPTION: Robust, greyish, downy, perennial herbs from rhizomes, with milky sap (latex) and hollow, hairy stems. Leaves opposite, simple and exude a milky sap when bruised. Flowers in umbrella-like clusters, pink or whitish to greenish purple, with 5 backward-bent petals below 5 erect, horn-like appendages, forming rounded clusters, from June to August. Fruits (follicles) single or paired, soft-spiny pods containing flat seeds with parachutes of silky hairs. See p. 424 for conservation status.

Swamp milkweed (*A. incarnata*) is 30 cm–1.2 m tall. Narrow, lance-shaped leaves to 10 cm long. Flowers deep pink and clustered at the top, 6 mm broad. Less milky than the other milkweeds. Grows in swamps, shores and thickets from MB to NS.

Common milkweed (*A. syriaca*) is 60 cm–1.8 m tall. Leaves 10–25 cm long, oval-oblong, light green with grey down underneath. Slightly drooping, purplish to pink flower clusters, 5 cm wide. Grows in old fields, roadsides and waste places from SK to NB.

Showy milkweed (*A. speciosa*) is a western species similar to the more eastern common milkweed, but with branched stems and a more densely hairy appearance. Leaves have a pink-ish midrib and conspicuous side veins. Grows on open ground (roadsides, streamsides, meadows, grasslands) in prairies, foothills and montane zones in southern BC and AB.

WARNING
The milky sap contains poisonous cardiac glycosides. Livestock have been poisoned, but animals usually avoid these plants. The toxins are destroyed by heat, so milkweeds should always be cooked before they are eaten. The rhizomes are considered poisonous.

Lupines
Lupinus spp.

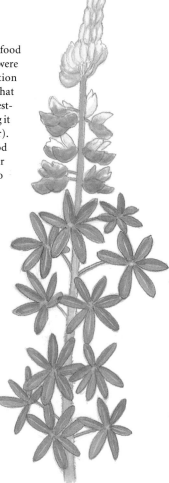

Nootka lupine

FOOD: The fleshy rhizomes of seashore lupine were a food source for a number of coastal BC First Nations. These were harvested in spring before the plant flowered. Preparation was by steaming, roasting, pit-cooking (a slow process that breaks down complex carbohydrates into more easily digestible simple sugars) or simply peeling the rhizome and eating it raw (traditionally with grease and more recently, sugar). The rhizomes were prepared as an important winter food source by cooking, pounding, then moulding into cakes for drying and storage. Nootka lupine rhizomes were also eaten cooked, but not raw unless as a famine food.

MEDICINE: An infusion of crushed seashore lupine seeds was used as a wash for scabby skin conditions.

OTHER USES: Lupine leaves and flowers can be added to provide pretty colour and scent to herbal baths, potpourri, facial steams and body oils. The Okanagan people of BC used the leaves and flowers as a sweet-smelling bedding on the floor of their sweat houses.

DESCRIPTION: Perennial herbs from rhizomes, the stems erect to decumbent, often hairy. Leaves palmately compound. Flowers pea-like, often blue to purple, in stalked, terminal clusters. Fruits pods, often hairy. See p. 424 for conservation status.

Seashore lupine (*L. littoralis*) is prostrate and mat-forming, from bright yellow rhizomes. Blue-green appearance caused by conspicuous covering of silky, white hairs. Shoreline species; restricted to sandy beaches and dunes on Graham Island in the Queen Charlotte Islands, Vancouver Island and the adjacent mainland.

Nootka lupine (*L. nootkatensis*) is erect to ascending, from a branched, woody rhizome. It's generally larger than seashore lupine, with leaflets to 7 cm long (vs. 3 cm long in seashore lupine), flowers 15–21 mm long (vs. 11–13 mm long in seashore lupine) and pods 3–6 cm long (vs. 2–3.5 cm long in seashore lupine). Inhabits moist to wet, open habitats (seashore, streamside, wet meadows, forest openings, gravel bars, rocky slopes) and disturbed sites at all elevations, from southwestern YT to southern BC and the mountains of AB. Nootka lupine has also been naturalized in NL on the Avalon peninsula and Yarmouth County in NS.

WARNING

Like other lupine species (p. 407), rhizomes of these species contain toxic alkaloids, and it is strongly recommended that they not be eaten raw. Because lupines readily hybridize, it may also be difficult to accurately identify edible species. According to ethnobotanical reports, eating lupine rhizomes raw can result in a state resembling a "drunken sleep," dizziness, and even death.

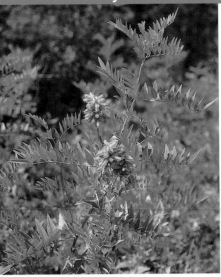

Wild Licorice
Glycyrrhiza lepidota

FOOD: The sweet, young rhizomes were sometimes eaten raw by First Nations, but usually they were roasted in coals, pounded lightly to separate the tough fibres from their centres and then eaten. Lewis and Clark compared them to sweet potatoes. Wild licorice has been used to flavour candy, root beer and chewing tobacco (p. 240). It contains glycyrrhizin, a substance about 50 times sweeter than sugar that quenches (rather than increases) thirst. Wild licorice is very similar to, but less strongly flavoured than, its European relative, licorice (*G. glabra*), from which commercial licorice is obtained.

MEDICINE: Wild licorice tea has been used for treating stomachaches, diarrhea, fevers (especially in children), stomach ulcers, asthma, arthritis and rheumatism. It has also been taken to regulate menstrual flow and aid in the delivery of the afterbirth. The juice from chewing raw rhizomes was held in the mouth to relieve toothaches, and leaves were steeped to make compresses or drops for curing earaches. Wild licorice rhizomes are rich in mucilage, which makes them effective in soothing coughs and sore throats and healing ulcers. Some closely related species act as expectorants and also have proved to be as effective and longer lasting than codeine for suppressing coughs. These rhizomes contain cortisone-like substances that are said to reduce inflammation without the dangerous side effects of steroids. Glycyrrhizin has been suggested as a safe sugar substitute for diabetics and is also believed to be effective as an anti-allergenic, anticonvulsive, antibacterial and antispasmodic medicine. European and Chinese species (*G. glabra* and *G. uralensis*) are among the most widely used medicinal plants in the world. Licorice has been shown to help heal and prevent stomach ulcers, combat bacteria, viruses and yeasts, reduce inflammation, treat bronchitis and urinary disorders and lower levels of complexes that are formed in auto-immune diseases such as lupus.

OTHER USES: Chewed leaves were used as a poultice on horses with sore backs.

DESCRIPTION: Large (30 cm–1 m tall), aromatic, glandular-dotted, perennial herb with leafy stems from deep, spreading rhizomes. Leaves pinnately divided into 7–19 lance-shaped, 2–4 cm long leaflets. Flowers yellowish white to greenish white, pea-like, 10–15 mm long, forming dense, stalked clusters from leaf axils, from May to August. Fruits brown, bur-like pods, 10–15 mm long, covered with hooked bristles; very sticky. Grows in moist, well-drained sites, usually near water, in prairies and foothills zones from BC to ON; thrives in disturbed sites, particularly roadside ditches and along the edges of wet fields. See p. 424 for conservation status.

WARNING

Consumed in large amounts over time, wild licorice can act like a mineral corticoid hormone, raising blood pressure, increasing sodium retention and depleting potassium levels, which can cause water retention, elevated blood pressure, low energy levels, weakness and even death. Pregnant or nursing women, people with heart disease, high blood pressure, glaucoma or kidney or liver disease, and people taking hormones or digitalis should not use this plant.

Alfalfa
Medicago sativa

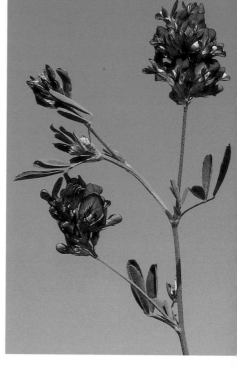

FOOD: Tender young leaves have been added to salads and sandwiches, but usually alfalfa is used to make a rather bland tea. Dried, powdered leaves have been sprinkled on cereal and other food as a nutritional supplement because alfalfa is a mineral-rich herb. The sprouted seeds are a popular addition to salads and sandwiches.

MEDICINE: Alfalfa is rich in vitamins A, B, C, E, K and P, calcium, potassium, phosphorus, iron and protein (about 18–19 percent). Parts used include flowers, leaves and sprouted seeds. Some herbalists have recommended alfalfa tea for use by convalescents, pregnant women and people taking sulfa drugs or antibiotics. It has also been used for treating anemia and celiac disease (in combination with a proper diet), and it is said to stimulate appetite and weight gain, stimulate urination and stop bleeding. Many unproved claims have been made for alfalfa, including treatments for cancer, fungal diseases such as athlete's foot, diabetes, alcoholism, gastritis, eczema, hemorrhoids, constipation and arthritis. It contains the antioxidant tricin, as well as estrogenic isoflavones, which may prevent cancer. Alfalfa has been shown to kill some fungi. In experiments with monkeys, it has reduced both blood cholesterol levels and fatty deposits (plaque) on artery walls, both of which are risk factors for stroke and heart disease.

OTHER USES: Alfalfa provides excellent forage for livestock, though ingestion of large amounts can cause bloating. It also produces abundant, high-quality nectar for bees. Alfalfa has been used as a commercial source of chlorophyll and carotene. To make a toothbrush, peel the root, cut it into 10 cm pieces, dry slowly and gently tap the end with a hammer to separate the fibres.

WARNING

Alfalfa plants contain saponins. When eaten in large quantities, this substance causes the breakdown of red blood cells in livestock and subsequent bloating. Alfalfa also interferes with vitamin E metabolism, and large amounts of alfalfa seed can cause a blood-clotting disorder in humans called "pancytopenia." Alfalfa sprouts contain the non-protein amino acid canavanine, which is potentially toxic and may cause the recurrence of lupus in patients in whom the disease has become dormant.

DESCRIPTION: Sweet-smelling, extremely deep-rooted perennial with weak, reclining stems. Grows to 60 cm tall. Leaves divided into 3 oblong leaflets that are sharply toothed on the upper half. Flowers deep purple to bluish (rarely white), slender, pea-like, 7–10 mm long, borne in dense, 2–4 cm long heads, throughout summer. Fruits small, dark, net-veined pods tightly coiled in 1–3 spirals. Introduced from Eurasia as a forage plant and is now naturalized across Canada, often along roadsides and in disturbed sites.

Clovers
Trifolium spp.

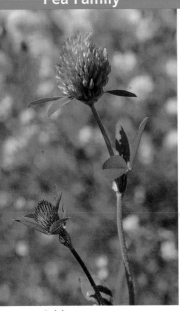
Red clover

FOOD: Clovers are high in protein and are eaten either raw or cooked. However, these plants are difficult to digest and can cause bloating in man and beast, so they should be used in moderation. Cooking helps to counteract this effect, with some native tribes also dipping the leaves in salt water to reduce indigestion. The flowerheads, fresh or dried, have been used in teas, salads, soups and stews, and even made into a flour. Clover sprouts are said to be nutritionally superior to alfalfa sprouts. For many First Nations, the rhizomes and roots of some species of clover were a highly valued food source said to have a sweet flavour similar to young peas. These parts were cooked and served during feasts, with the thicker and longer straight taproots reserved for dignitaries and the shorter, thinner and gnarled horizontal rhizomes eaten by the common folk. In BC, patches of springbank clover were actively tended by many First Nations, who weeded, aerated and removed debris such as rocks and sticks that could negatively affect that clover's growth. Indeed, tribes such as the Kwakwaka'wakw, Nootka and Haida marked good springbank clover patches using stakes and other methods to show ownership and stewardship rights and responsibilities that were passed as a valuable hereditary right from generation to generation. Roots were stored in large quantities for both trade and winter use. These were enjoyed either plain or dipped in grease, sometimes eaten raw but most commonly prepared by boiling, steaming or wrapping in American skunk-cabbage (p. 164) leaves to cook in fire embers or pit-cook.

MEDICINE: Red clover is a major herbal treatment for symptoms of menopause and contains 4 phytoestrogenic isoflavonoids in significant amounts. Clinical evidence for efficacy against some symptoms is available, but there is continuing controversy over whether or not they act as estrogens (potentially promoting cancer) or anti-estrogens (preventing cancer) in breast tissue. Clover tea has been taken to treat coughs, fevers, sore throats, rheumatism and gout and applied topically to treat skin diseases. Its high tannin content makes it rather astringent, which may explain some of these uses. In ancient Rome, clover seeds soaked in wine or clover plants boiled in water were used as antidotes for the poisonous bites and stings of snakes and scorpions. Red clover has long been used as a blood purifier (called "queen of the blood purifiers" by some herbalists) and is reputed to stimulate the liver and to remove toxins from the blood. It has been shown to contain blood-thinning compounds related to coumarin (see **Warning**). Tea made from red clover flowers is recommended by herbalists as a mild sedative and as

WARNING

Although generally considered a nutritious food and medicinally useful plant, ingesting excess amounts of clover can be harmful. Cattle that eat too much clover have been known to die of bloat and to bleed to death if injured due to the conversion of the substance coumarin to dicoumarol, an anticoagulant (see sweet-clover, p. 264). In autumn, red clover may appear normal but may contain toxic alkaloids. Some cattle have been poisoned by late-cut hay containing clover.

a treatment for asthma, bronchitis, coughing, headaches and arthritic pain. Decoctions, teas and salves made of this plant can be applied externally to treat athlete's foot, mastitis, soft tissue inflammations, sores, burns, ulcers and other skin afflictions. Dried flowers were sometimes smoked to relieve asthma.

OTHER USES: Clovers provide excellent forage for cattle—hence the phrase "living in clover" in reference to a luxurious lifestyle. These plants produce large amounts of high-quality nectar and are commonly planted as a bee crop. Clover is also a soil-enriching crop that adds nitrogen to the soil. And who can resist returning to childhood by nibbling on the sweet, nectar-rich end of clover blossoms? Some people carry a 4-leaf clover (a leaf with 4 leaflets, occasionally caused by a mutation) for good-luck. Clover leaves were also sometimes dried and smoked. The flowers of clover make a pretty and sweet-smelling addition to potpourri.

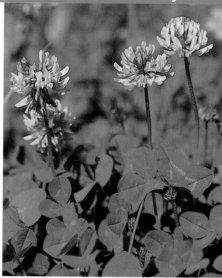

White clover (above)
Alsike clover (below)

DESCRIPTION: Annual or (for the ones described here) perennial herbs from taproots. Stems erect or spreading. Leaves divided into 3 oval leaflets. Flowers slender, pea-like, borne in dense, round heads throughout summer. Fruits pods.

Red clover (*T. pratense*) is the largest of the 3 common and widespread species, with plants 40–80 cm tall and leaflets 2–5 cm long. Large, 12–20 mm long, stalkless, usually red or deep pink flowers in dense, 2–3 cm wide heads with 1–2 short-stalked leaves at the base.

Alsike clover (*T. hybridum*) and **white clover** (*T. repens*) are smaller plants (usually less than 50 cm tall), with smaller leaflets (1–3 cm long) and smaller (7–10 mm long), short-stalked, paler flowers in looser heads on leafless stalks. Alsike clover is relatively erect, with pinkish flowers and leaflets without a notch at the end, whereas white clover is a sprawling plant with rooting joints, mostly white flowers and leaflets usually with a distinct notch at the end. Alsike clover is, as its species name *hybridum* suggests, a hybrid between white and red clover.

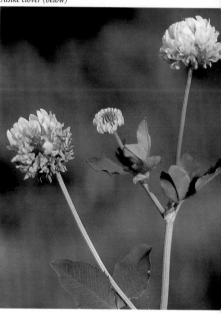

All 3 above species were introduced from Europe and now grow wild on disturbed and cultivated ground across Canada in all provinces and territories.

Springbank clover (*T. wormskjoldii*) has horizontal rhizomes to 75 cm long, often forming dense patches. Leaves longer and narrower than the introduced clovers above and sharply saw-toothed. Flowers pink to reddish purple, often white-tipped, typically clover-like, but with a unique jagged green sheath at the base. This native clover inhabits coastal dunes, tidal marshes, meadows and streambanks along the BC coast, including Haida Gwaii (Queen Charlotte Islands) and, rarely, in southern interior BC.

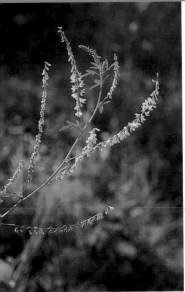

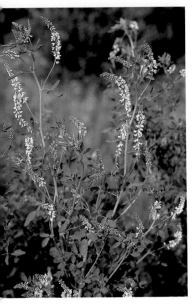

Common Sweet-Clover

Melilotus officinalis

FOOD: These plants are nutritious and rich in protein. The flowers and/or leaves can be used, fresh or dried, to make a pleasant, vanilla-flavoured tea. Young leaves (gathered before flowering has begun) have been used raw in salads or boiled or steamed as a cooked vegetable. In spring, try steaming this nutritious and delicious triad of tender early green shoots, served with butter and lemon: sweet-clover (leaves soaked in salt water for 2–3 hours first), stinging nettle (p. 312) and dandelions (p. 332). The seeds have been added to stews and soups as a flavouring, and crushed, dried leaves are said to give a vanilla-like taste to pastries. These flowers and fruits are used to flavour Gruyère cheese in Switzerland.

MEDICINE: Sweet-clover tea was traditionally used to treat a wide range of maladies, ranging from headaches, gas and nervous stomachs to painful urination, colic, diarrhea, painful menstruation, aching muscles and intestinal worms. People who were chilled from falling in water or being in heavy rain were given cold sweet-clover tea, both as a drink and as a lotion. The plants have also been used in poultices for treating swollen joints, inflammation, ulcers and wounds (especially in tender areas such as around the eyes). Dried leaves of sweet-clover were sometimes smoked to relieve asthma. Sweet-clover contains quercetin, an antioxidant substance that improves vascular health. These plants contain coumarin, which gives them their sweet, vanilla-like smell and flavour. Caution is advised, however; if these plants are allowed to mould, their coumarin becomes dicoumarol, a chemical that can cause uncontrollable bleeding (an anticoagulant). Rat poisons such as warfarin (which prevents blood clotting in rats) have been developed from such coumarins.

OTHER USES: Sweet-clover provides excellent forage for livestock and produces abundant, high-quality nectar for bees. It also increases the soil's nitrogen content.

DESCRIPTION: Sweet-smelling, 50 cm–3 m tall, annual or biennial herb with a strong taproot, sweet-scented when dry. Leaves divided into 3 oblong, 2–4 cm long leaflets edged with fine sharp teeth from near the base to the tip. Flowers yellow or white, pea-like, 4–7 mm long, forming branched clusters of long, slender spikes, from May to September. Fruits small, 3–5 mm long, net-veined, mostly 1- to 2-seeded pods. Introduced from Eurasia and has spread widely to disturbed sites across Canada. Until recently, the white variety was recognized as a separate species, *M. alba.*

Sweet-Vetches

Hedysarum spp.

FOOD: Sweet-vetch roots were an important food for many tribes across Canada and were also enjoyed by trappers, settlers and livestock. Young roots have a sweet, licorice-like taste and were often eaten raw as a sweet treat. They were also boiled, baked or fried as a hot vegetable or added to soups and stews, while some tribes enjoyed them dipped in grease. A hot drink could also be made by frying a small piece of root and then soaking it in hot water. Cooked sweet-vetch roots are said to be delicious, tasting rather like carrots. Alpine sweet-vetch was highly regarded for human use by many First Nations. When quantities permitted, roots were stored in buried caches, preserved in lard or oil or dried for winter use. Alpine sweet-vetch roots were usually collected in spring because they become woody and unpalatable during summer.

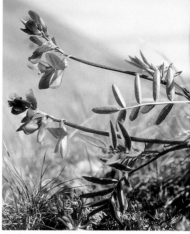

Northern sweet-vetch (above)
Alpine sweet-vetch (below)

MEDICINE: Small pieces of the sun-dried roots of alpine sweet-vetch were burned and the smoke trapped with a blanket over the head as a treatment for sore eyes. The roots of alpine sweet-vetch have also been shown to be a rich source of vitamin C. This species contains mangiferin and isomangiferin, which have anti-inflammatory, liver protecting, antiviral and central nervous system stimulating properties.

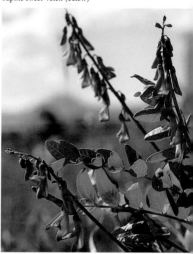

OTHER USES: Pieces of root, softened at one end by chewing, were given to babies as pacifiers, and sweet-vetch roots were softened and fed to infants who lacked mother's milk. Preserved roots were an important trade item among some tribes.

DESCRIPTION: Perennial, taprooted herbs, to 90 cm tall, with alternate leaves divided into 9–21 elliptic to oblong leaflets. Pea-like flowers, usually pink to reddish purple in colour, hanging in 1–2 cm elongating clusters, bloom from June to August. Fruits flattened pods constricted into 1–6 rounded segments.

Northern sweet-vetch (*H. boreale*) has rose to red-purple flowers, very showy and fragrant, and pods that are cross-corrugated and not wing-margined. Grows in fields, thickets, gravel bars, roadsides and open woods; widespread at montane and subalpine elevations across Canada from BC to NL, but missing from the Maritime provinces. See p. 424 for conservation status.

Alpine sweet-vetch (*H. alpinum*) also has rose to red-purple flowers, but its pods are net-veined and wing-margined. Commonly grows in moist, open woods, tundra, lakeshores, meadows and gravelly subalpine and alpine slopes. Widely distributed from BC and YT to NU and NL, but apparently not in NS or PEI. See p. 424 for conservation status.

Yellow sweet-vetch (*H. sulphurescens*) has yellow to whitish flowers. Grows in moderately dry to moist forests and openings from prairies to subalpine elevations in southeastern and northeastern BC and southwestern AB.

Pomme-de-Prairie

Psoralea esculenta

FOOD: Probably the most important food gathered by Great Plains First Nations, the edibility of pomme-de-prairie ("prairie apple") is reflected in the many English names given to it: breadroot, breadroot scurfpea, prairie turnip, Indian turnip and prairie potato. Even the species name is Latin for "edible." The tubers were collected near the end of the growing season when the tops die down and then eaten raw, roasted, boiled or dried for winter storage. Pomme-de-prairie flour made from the dried ground root was added to cakes, porridges, soups, breads and gravies. Made up of 70 percent starch, 9 percent protein and 5 percent sugar, the tubers were nutritious, abundant and palatable, tasting slightly like sweetened turnip. Once a staple of First Nations, early voyagers (Lewis and Clark consumed it on their journeys) and later European immigrants, contemporary use of the plant has declined, but it has always been considered a candidate for commercial domestication.

MEDICINE: Prairie First Nations treated gastroenteritis, constipation, diarrhea, sore throats and chest complaints with an infusion of dried roots. Children with bowel problems chewed raw roots, while colicky babies suffered a more invasive procedure: they had chewed-up roots blown into their rectums. The chewed root was also used as a topical treatment for sprains, fractures and burns, or it was spit into the eyes and ears in cases of local inflammation. Tea made from the lowermost leaves was considered a fever and snakebite remedy.

OTHER USES: So important was this plant to the Blackfoot Nation that they sometimes adorned their garments with dried pieces of root. The Lakota Sioux named the month of June, considered best time to harvest the plant, *tinpsila itkahca wi*, which means "moon when pomme-de-prairie is ripe." The roots were also food for the now extinct plains grizzly, which, according to Lewis and Clark, "dug it from the prairie with passion."

DESCRIPTION: Densely hairy, herbaceous perennial, 30 cm tall, that grows from 1 or more sturdy brown, tuberous roots, each 4–10 cm long. Single or multiple stems bear alternate, palmate leaves with 5 lobes, each leaflet oval, sometimes tapering at the base, 2.5–5 cm long, 1–2 cm wide, with rounded, obtuse or acute tips; upper surface smooth, underside pubescent. Pea-like flowers blue or purple, clustered on a terminal spike 5–10 cm long, terminating on a short peduncle, from May to July. Fruit a flattened, slender-tipped pod. Grows in prairie hillsides and bluffs, stream valleys and open woodlands on the prairies of AB, SK and MB.

WARNING
The plant contains furanocoumarins, which may cause a photosensitive reaction in certain people.

Groundnut

Apios americana

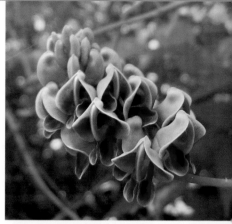

FOOD: Both the beans and tubers of this plant are edible and were an important starch and protein source for First Nations pre-contact. The fruits were eaten fresh in a similar manner to garden peas. Tubers were either dug fresh or parboiled, peeled and dried for winter use. Per dry weight, groundnut tubers have 3 times the starch content of potatoes. However, tubers require 2–3 years of growth before they can be harvested, a trait that has prevented this plant from becoming a common garden or commercial crop. Early settlers and explorers made heavy use of this plant, especially the tubers, which are perennial and can be harvested at any time of the year. They are at their best, however, when dug from late autumn to early spring. Boiled tubers are delicious, tasting somewhat like a cross between a boiled peanut and a potato, with a slightly mealier texture than potatoes. Fresh tubers are eaten boiled, fried or baked, while dried tubers can be ground into a flour substitute for breads or a thickening agent. Eating raw tubers is not recommended and can cause indigestion.

MEDICINE: The boiled and crushed tubers were applied topically to treat ulcers and wounds and to stimulate the growth of healthy tissue.

OTHER USES: Groundnut is an attractive ornamental garden plant.

DESCRIPTION: Perennial, rhizomatous vine growing 3–4 m in length and climbing. Edible tubers, to 5 cm long, form on rhizomes lying 5–8 cm below ground. Leaves pinnate, 8–15 cm long, with 5–7 leaflets. Flowers have 5 parts, the upper one round, white and reddish brown, the 2 side wings curved downward and brown-purple, the lower 2 petals sickle-shaped and brownish red. Fruit shaped like a bean pod, 6–13 cm long, either straight or slightly bent. Seeds oblong or square, dark brown, with a wrinkled surface. Usually found in moist lowlands such as riparian woods and thickets, and commonly found around historic village sites and seasonal camps in ON, QC and the Maritimes. See p. 424 for conservation status.

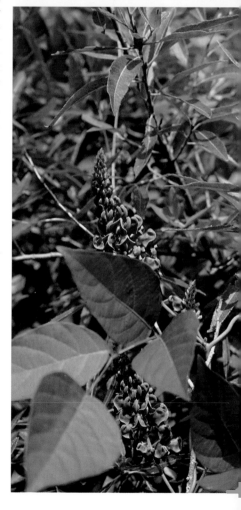

Bedstraws

Galium spp.

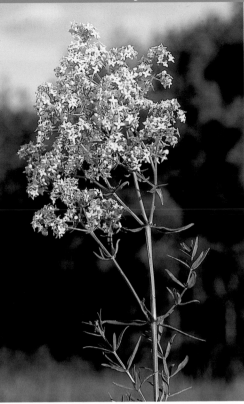

Northern bedstraw

FOOD: Bedstraws are related to coffee, and their nutlets have been dried, roasted until dark brown, ground and used as a good caffeine-free coffee substitute. The dried leaves and roots of all varieties of *Galium* are said to make a pleasant, tasty and sweet-smelling tea. The young plants are edible raw or cooked, but raw plants of rough-barbed species can cause gagging and are best cooked or not consumed at all. The flavour of cooked bedstraw has been likened to that of spinach. Cooked, cooled shoots were sometimes used in salads.

MEDICINE: Bedstraws are rich in vitamin C and have been used in spring tonics and as a cure for scurvy. Of the species described here, cleavers has been used most widely as a medicine. Plants were used in hot compresses to stop bleeding and to soothe sore muscles. They were also dried, ground and sprinkled onto cuts, scrapes and other wounds to stop bleeding and aid healing, or they were made into washes for treating freckles, sunburn, psoriasis, eczema, ulcers and other skin conditions. Crushed plants or fresh plant juice were used to stop nosebleeds and to soothe minor burns and skin irritations. The Ojibwa used a tea made from the whole plant as a diuretic and to treat kidney troubles. They also applied the plant to treat skin problems and bruises, and used a tea of Our Lady's bedstraw (*G. verum*) as a febrifuge for colds and to treat chest congestions. Cleavers tea has been reported to stimulate urination and the drainage of lymph-engorged tissues and to accelerate the metabolism of stored fat. Consequently, it has been used as a treatment for kidney stones and bladder problems and as a weight-loss aid. It was traditionally used in medicinal teas and washes for treating cancer, and it has been found to contain citric acid (reported to have some antitumour activity) and asperuloside (an anti-inflammatory). Cleavers extracts have also been shown to lower blood pressure and combat certain yeasts. Sweet-scented bedstraw contains substances that lower blood pressure.

OTHER USES: The vanilla-scented plants were used to stuff pillows and mattresses, hence the common name bedstraw. They were also used as perfume. The roots of many species produce a red or purple dye. The Blackfoot of AB used the roots of northern bedstraw to make a red

WARNING
People with kidney problems or poor circulation or with a tendency toward diabetes should not use these plants. Continual use of bedstraw will irritate the mouth, and the plant juice can cause rashes on sensitive skin.

dye for their arrow tips. Bristly masses of cleavers make good temporary strainers. The Cowichan people rubbed the plant on their hands to remove pitch and also used the dried plants for starting fires. Belgian lace-makers used the hard fruits as heads for their pins. The juice of Our Lady's bedstraw was historically used to curdle milk (the first step in most cheese making), a result of which was the original sweet flavour and orange colour (from the flowers) of cheddar cheese.

DESCRIPTION: Leafy, perennial or annual herbs, 20 cm–1 m tall or long, with whorled leaves in clusters of 2–8 radiating like wheel spokes on slender, 4-sided, erect to sprawling stems. Flowers small, white to greenish, 4-petalled, forming branched clusters, from June to August. Fruits hairy nutlet pairs (2-lobed burs) covered with hooked bristles, about 2–3 mm long. See p. 424 for conservation status.

Cleavers (*G. aparine*) is a weak, taprooted annual; stems sprawling, leafy, with hooked bristles on the angles, tending to scramble over other vegetation. Leaves usually in whorls of 8. Found in woods, thickets, shores, moist fields, clearings and waste places at low to montane elevations in most provinces and territories.

Northern bedstraw (*G. boreale*) is a perennial from rhizomes, with erect or ascending stems. Stems smooth, numerous, clustered, simple or few-branching, erect. Leaves in whorls of 4. Flowers white or creamy, very fragrant when in full flower. Found in meadows, prairies, open woods and shores, from BC and YT east to the Maritimes.

Sweet-scented bedstraw (*G. triflorum*) is a perennial from rhizomes, sometimes ascending but usually scrambling over other vegetation. Stems leafy, usually hooked-bristly on the angles. Leaves usually in whorls of 6, vanilla-scented. Found in woods and thickets throughout Canada, except NU.

Cleavers (or "clivers") derives from the Anglo-Saxon *clife* and the Dutch *kleefkruid* meaning "cleaving (clinging) herb," and from the Old English *clivers* meaning "claws." Another common name of the annual *G. aparine*, tangleweed, derives from the thousands of tiny, reversed hooks growing on the stem angles, which cause the plant to catch on whatever (or whoever) is brushing past it, thereby spreading its seeds far and wide. The perennial varieties of *Galium*, such as northern bedstraw, do not share this characteristic.

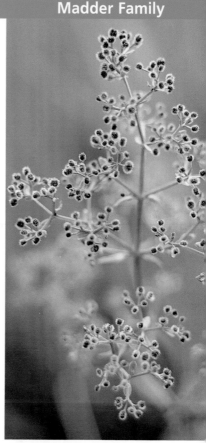

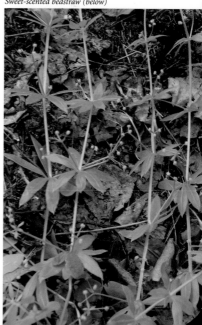

Northern bedstraw (above)
Sweet-scented bedstraw (below)

Common Hound's-Tongue
Cynoglossum officinale

FOOD: The young leaves have been boiled and eaten in small quantities, but this use is not recommended (see **Warning**).

MEDICINE: The plant has been used as medicine but may be dangerous (see **Warning**). Because the fruits and leaves have a rough texture (like a dog's tongue), this plant was beaten with swine grease to make a salve for healing dog bites. Hound's-tongue is said to have soothing and mildly sedative properties, though there is no experimental evidence to substantiate these claims. The roots and leaves have been used in teas and decoctions to treat coughs, colds, shortness of breath, irritated membranes, diarrhea and dysentery. The leaves were boiled in wine to make a cure for dysentery and were applied as poultices to relieve insect bites, burns and hemorrhoids. These plants contain alantoin, a waxy compound that has been used to treat ulcers on the skin and in the intestine.

OTHER USES: Perhaps because they are so hairy, the leaves were used in salves and ointments to cure baldness.

DESCRIPTION: Leafy, softly long-hairy, biennial herb, 30 cm–1 m tall, giving off an unpleasant smell when crushed. Leaves in a large basal rosette (first year), alternate on the stem (second year), lower leaves 10–30 cm long, upper leaves smaller and stalkless. Flowers reddish purple, 5-lobed, about 1 cm across, borne on long, 1-sided, spreading branches, from May to July. Fruits prickly nutlets in 5–8 mm wide clusters of 4. This Eurasian introduction is found in dry, grassy areas and forest edges, disturbed sites and roadsides at low to montane elevations throughout Canada.

WARNING
These plants contain pyrrolizidine alkaloids that may cause severe liver damage. These compounds are most concentrated in roots and young leaves. In cattle and horses, common hound's-tongue causes disorders of the central nervous system, liver failure (in horses) and death. Horses also develop skin reactions following exposure to sunlight. In England, a family who ate these plants suffered vomiting, stupor and sleepiness, which continued for 40 hours, ending with one death. Handling these plants may cause skin reactions. Livestock become distressed when large numbers of nutlets adhere to their faces (wouldn't you?).

Gromwells
Lithospermum spp.

FOOD: Some tribes cooked and ate the large, deep taproots of yellow gromwell. Others gathered wayside gromwell seeds for food.

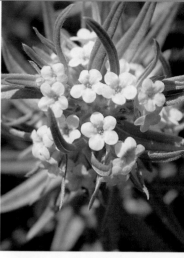

MEDICINE: These species were often used in similar ways as medicines. Teas made from the roots were taken to stop internal bleeding and improve appetite and were used as washes for treating skin and eye problems and rheumatism. Women drank the root tea every day as a contraceptive, and effects are said to have ranged from temporary to permanent sterility. Alcoholic extracts of these plants have been shown to eliminate the estrous cycle in laboratory mice. The leaves of hoary gromwell were also made into a tea to treat fevers and seizures. Powdered yellow gromwell roots were taken by people suffering from chest wounds. If a person had to stay awake, the plant was chewed and blown into his or her face and rubbed over the chest. Roots and seeds were ground together and steeped in hot water to make a medicinal tea that was cooled and used as an eyewash. Some people chewed the roots to relieve coughs and colds.

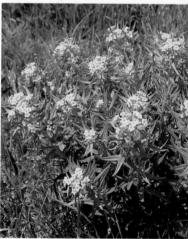

OTHER USES: The hard, shiny nutlets were used as decorative beads. The roots yielded a fast red dye, which was used in face and body paints and for colouring fabrics. Some tribes believed that wayside gromwell had magical powers. It was used by some as a charm to bring rain and by others to stop thunderstorms. Sometimes a plant was prayed over and then placed on an enemy's person, clothing or bedding to inflict sickness or bad luck.

Wayside gromwell (all images)

DESCRIPTION: Clumped, hairy, perennial herbs from woody taproots, with 5–60 cm tall stems bearing dark green, slender leaves 3–8 cm long. Flowers 5-lobed, clustered in the upper leaf axils, from April to July. Fruits 4 shiny, greyish white to brownish nutlets. See p. 424 for conservation status.

Hoary gromwell or **hoary puccoon** (*L. canescens*) grows to 30 cm tall, with bright yellow or orange flowers that appear from March to June. Fruits hard, shiny nutlets that turn yellow with maturity. Grows in dry prairies and open forests from SK to ON.

Yellow gromwell (*L. incisum*) is generally a smaller plant (5–30 cm tall), with larger (15–30 mm long), bright yellow to orange flowers with the lobes ragged-margined, and smaller (3–4 mm) nutlets. Grows on open, dry slopes in prairies and foothills zones from BC to ON.

Wayside gromwell or **lemonweed** (*L. ruderale*) is a larger plant (20–60 cm tall), with small (4–6 mm long), pale yellow to greenish-tinted flowers and large (4–6 mm) nutlets. Grows on warm, dry, open slopes in prairies, foothills and montane zones from southern BC to southwestern SK.

WARNING

Given their effects on hormone levels and glands in the endocrine system, these plants should not be taken internally.

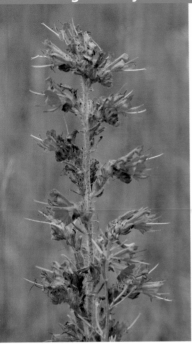

Viper's Bugloss
Echium vulgare

FOOD: The names given to this beautiful wild-flower are undeservedly frightening, leading some people to believe that they are nesting sites for serpents or are associated with vipers in some way. Even the genus name, derived from the Greek word *echis*, means "viper," but refers to nothing more than the nutlet's resemblance to the head of a snake. The young leaves are mucilaginous, hairy and may be irritating to the touch (see **Warning**), but when finely chopped, can be added raw to a mixed salad. They may also be steamed and prepared like spinach. The nectar is used to make commercial monofloral honey. However, the Canadian Honey Council has advised against over-consuming (>2 tbsp per day) honey made from *Echium* because of the presence of naturally occurring pyrrolizidine alkaloids. These compounds are toxic to the liver and may have caused the death of foraging cattle and fighting bulls.

MEDICINE: According to one medieval author, "Viper's bugloss hath its stalks all to be speckled like a snake or viper, and is a most singular remedy against poison and the sting of scorpions." The plant was finely chopped and applied as a poultice to snakebites, or rubbed on exposed skin as a preventative. The treatment would also be used for boils, carbuncles, paronychia (whitlow), inflammation and generally delicate skin. The plant contains allantoin, a compound in several over-the-counter cosmetic and pharmaceutical products said to promote wound healing and protect the skin from irritants by forming complexes with irritant agents, increasing the water content of skin cells and enhancing the exfoliation of the upper dead layers of skin cells. Traditionally, it was used in a similar manner to borage, to which it is related, especially as a medicine to induce sweating and urination. First Nations prepared an herbal infusion to treat fevers, headaches and chest conditions and added it to a compound medicine for milky urine and other kidney disorders. In medieval times, a decoction of the seeds and roots in wine were thought to be mild love potions and aphrodisiacs to "comfort the heart and drive away melancholy." Modern herbalists do not commonly incorporate viper's bugloss in their practice due to the presence of toxins (see **Warning**) and the lack of any interesting medicinal properties.

OTHER USES: First Nations made decorative beads out of the seeds.

DESCRIPTION: Hairy biennial (or occasionally perennial that flowers once and then dies), 30–75 cm tall. Leaves 5–15 cm long, hairy, oblong to lance-shaped. Showy, 5-lobed, tubular, blue flowers, 2 cm long, each with 5 protruding, pinkish red stamens, from June to October. Fruits rough, 1-seeded nutlets. European native introduced as early as 1683; grows in fields, roadsides and waste places, often in alkaline soils, throughout Canada.

WARNING
The sharp hairs on the plant may get lodged in the skin and cause severe dermatitis. Gloves are recommended. The leaves are considered poisonous due to the presence of hepatotoxic pyrrolizidine alkaloids and should not be consumed.

Skullcaps

Scutellaria spp.

MEDICINE: Skullcaps were a widely used treatment for nervous system conditions in the 19th century and have been rediscovered recently as an anxiety-reducing herbal medicine. Skullcaps contain a flavonoid called scutellarin that has been shown to have sedative properties. Some Aboriginal peoples also used skullcaps as a medicine to promote menstruation. The leaves and flowers of marsh skullcap were brewed into a tea to treat ulcers and fever, and the plants were used to treat heart trouble. Powdered roots of blue skullcap were ingested as an infusion to prevent smallpox and to keep the throat clean. Warm tea made from the dried leaves of this plant has been used by herbalists for over 250 years to treat hysteria, neuralgia, epilepsy, multiple sclerosis, Saint Vitus' Dance and convulsions. In the 1700–1800s, blue skullcap was famed for its ability to cure the bites of mad dogs (rabies), which lead to a common name of mad-dog skullcap for *S. lateriflora*, but this ability was later disclaimed. More recently, it has been used to relieve nervous headaches, sciatica, shingles and the tension and irritability of premenstrual syndrome, to prevent epileptic seizures and to help wean addicts from barbituates, Valium and meprobamate. Similarly, skullcaps have been mixed with American ginseng (p. 183) to treat people suffering from the *delirium tremens* of alcoholism.

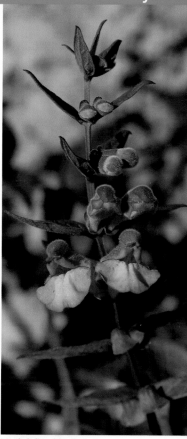

Marsh skullcap (above)
Blue skullcap (below)

DESCRIPTION: Perennial herbs, to 80 cm tall, with weak, 4-sided stems and opposite, 2–8 cm long, blunt-toothed leaves. Flowers blue to bluish purple, trumpet-shaped, with a hooded upper lip, a broad lower lip and a 2-lipped calyx with a small bump on the upper side. Fruits 4 tiny, bumpy nutlets, produced from July to October. Grow in moist prairies, streambanks and wet meadows across Canada. See p. 424 for conservation status.

Marsh skullcap (*S. galericulata*) has relatively few, large (15–20 mm long) flowers in its upper leaf axils (1 per leaf).

Blue skullcap (*S. lateriflora*) has many, smaller (6–8 mm long) flowers in long clusters from the leaf axils.

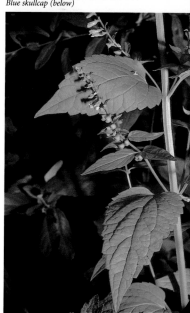

WARNING

Although they are not considered poisonous, skullcaps should be used in moderation. Too much can cause excitability and wakefulness, with giddiness, stupor, confusion and twitching.

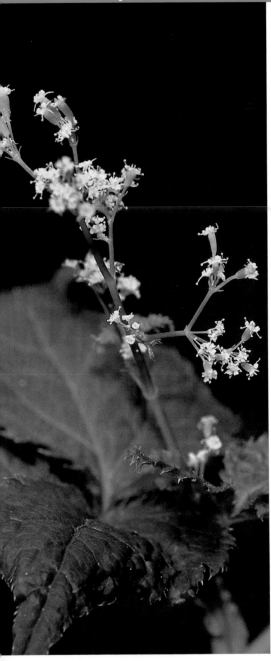

Horehound
Marrubium vulgare

FOOD: The leaves have been used as a seasoning to flavour beer (horehound ale) or liqueurs, which are described as bitter and pungent. Fresh or dried leaves are also used as tea.

MEDICINE: Horehound is a popular herbal medicine used often to treat coughs and colds because it stimulates the removal of mucous from the lungs. The leaves and young stems are the parts most commonly used for medicines, often made into a syrup or candy to disguise horehound's bitter flavour. In addition to being a stimulant and tonic, it relieves muscle spasms or cramps, stimulates the flow of bile and urine, promotes sweating and menstruation, increases the appetite, aids in digestion and liver function and helps to normalize the heart rhythm. The root, combined with plantains (p. 256), has been used as a remedy for rattlesnake-bites.

OTHER USES: Horehound repels flies and has been used to eliminate cankerworm in trees.

DESCRIPTION: Perennial, white-woolly herb from a taproot, the 4-angled stems to 1 m tall. Leaves opposite, roundish to oval, to 5 cm long, deeply veined, blunt toothed, the lower leaves long-stalked. Flowers white, tubular, to 15 mm long, in clusters in leaf axils. Fruits egg-shaped nutlets, in fours. This introduced Eurasian species grows in mesic to dry, disturbed sites across Canada.

Giant-Hyssops

Agastache spp.

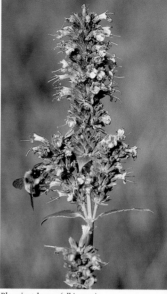

FOOD: The seeds of both nettle-leaved and yellow giant-hyssop can be eaten raw or cooked. The leaves have been used to flavour soups, stews and other hot dishes. They can also be steeped in hot water to make a delicate anise-flavoured tea, best when brewed weakly. The Woods Cree added the leaves to store-bought tea to improve the flavour. The quality of the flavour of these plants can vary greatly from one population to the next.

MEDICINE: Giant-hyssop leaves have been used to make pleasant medicinal teas for treating coughs, colds and fevers and for relieving chest pains (especially those associated with coughing and weak hearts). These plants were said to stimulate sweating, and some tribes took the tea to cure a "dispirited heart." Powdered leaves were rubbed on the body to cool fevers. Blue giant-hyssop flowers were often included in Cree medicine bundles, and an infusion of stem, leaves and other plants was taken for coughing up blood. Blue giant-hyssop leaves were dried, combined with coneflower (p. 350) and goldenrod (p. 342) and applied wet to treat burns. More recently, teas made from the leaves and flowers of giant-hyssops have been used to relieve intestinal gas, to stimulate sweating and as a sedative to relieve tension. A compound infusion of yellow giant-hyssop was used as a wash for poison-ivy (p. 395) and itch.

Blue giant-hyssop (all images)

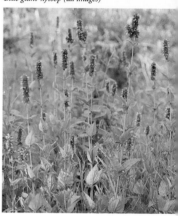

OTHER USES: The flowerhead can be chewed as a breath-freshener. Giant-hyssops make an attractive and useful addition to a wildflower garden; they are easily propagated from seeds, cuttings or root divisions and grow best in limey, well-drained soil, preferably in full sun.

DESCRIPTION: Large, perennial herbs with 4-sided stems, 40 cm–1 m tall, and paired, coarsely toothed leaves 3–10 cm long, smelling of anise. Flowers trumpet-shaped, 2-lipped, with a long stigma and 4 stamens projecting conspicuously from the mouth, whorled in spike-like clusters, from May to August. Fruits 4 small nutlets.

Nettle-leaved giant-hyssop (*A. urticifolia*) has white to pale rose or purplish flowers, 10–15 mm long. Leaves have long (to 5 cm) stalks and green, sparsely hairy to hairless lower surfaces. Found in moist, open foothill, montane and subalpine sites in southern BC.

Blue giant-hyssop (*A. foeniculum*) has blue flowers, about 10 mm long. Leaves have shorter (less than 15 mm) stalks and pale lower surfaces with a whitish bloom and dense, felt-like hairs. Found in meadows, moist thickets and open, deciduous woods from BC to ON.

Yellow giant-hyssop (*A. nepetoides*) has greenish yellow flowers clustered into spikes as long as 1.5 m (much longer than the others). Leaves have long (to 5 cm) stalks and are mostly hairless except for long hairs in the groove of the leaf vein, especially near the base of the leaf. Found in open woods, moist soils and thickets in ON and QC. See p. 424 for conservation status.

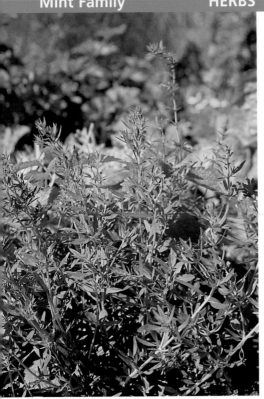

Hyssop
Hyssopus officinalis

FOOD: The leaves, young shoot tips and flowers can be eaten raw or used as a flavouring in soups and salads. Essential oil made from hyssop is used as a food flavouring.

MEDICINE: Hyssop has long been a valued medicine, even considered a cure-all in the past. It has been used as a stimulant, aromatic and tonic, being commonly employed for problems with the respiratory or gastrointestinal tract. It has been used to treat bronchitis, colds, coughs in children, asthma and respiratory infections because it is reputed to remove mucous from the lungs. The plant was gargled with sage for sore throats or tonsillitis. A tea made from the leaves is used in the treatment of flatulence and stomachaches. The plant is also used as a blood regulator because it increases circulation in the blood and reduces blood pressure. Large quantities of this plant can induce a miscarriage. A poultice made from the fresh plant is used to heal wounds and bruises.

OTHER USES: The essential oil from this plant is used in aromatherapy and perfumes. The plant attracts cabbage white butterflies and bees. Hyssop is also used as a potpourri and is useful in controlling bacterial plant diseases. It has been used commercially in wine, food, confectionary and cosmetic industries.

DESCRIPTION: Perennial, shrubby plant with erect, square stem, to 60 cm high. Leaves in pairs, lance-shaped. Blue-purple flowers, stalkless (with stamens protruding), growing in spikes in upper leaf axils in July. This introduced European plant is found on roadsides and in ditches from SK eastward.

Ground-Ivy
Glechoma hederacea

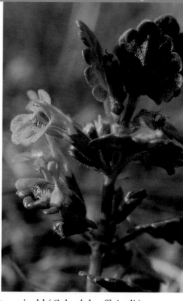

FOOD: The young leaves of ground-ivy can be eaten raw in salads, cooked and added to soups or used as flavouring. A tea can be made from fresh or dried leaves. This plant was commonly used to flavour beer before the use of hops became widespread in the 16th century. The leaves have been added to beer for clarification, preservation and flavour enhancement.

MEDICINE: Ground-ivy has often been used to treat ailments of the mucous membranes (of the ear, nose, throat and digestive system) and as a general tonic for colds and coughs. The plant has been used to treat yellow jaundice, hip gout, sciatica, arthritic hands and knees and to ease grippe pains and gas. The fresh juice of the plant was snuffed up the nose to treat headaches. A poultice can be made from the leaves and applied to wounds. When combined with pot marigold (*Calendula officinalis*), it has been applied externally to treat scabs and other skin irritations. The plant has been shown to have anti-inflammatory properties.

OTHER USES: Ground-ivy was introduced to Canada as a garden ornamental. It is sometimes grown as a potted plant and makes an excellent ground cover. This species has many common names, including cat's-foot, gill-go-by-ground, gill-creep-by-ground, turn-hoof, hay maids, ale-hoof, creeping Charlie and field-balm.

DESCRIPTION: Perennial herb, 5–50 cm tall, from stolons, stem trailing, branches erect. Leaves opposite, heart- to kidney-shaped, with round-toothed edges, 1–3 cm long, 2–3 cm across. Flowers in upper leaf axils in small, loose clusters, bluish purple, 12–24 mm long, petals fused into trumpet shape, opening into an upper 2-lobed lip and lower 3-lobed lip, blooming mid-spring to early summer. Fruits 4 brown nutlets. This introduced Eurasian species is found in thickets, open forests and waste places across Canada. See p. 424 for conservation status.

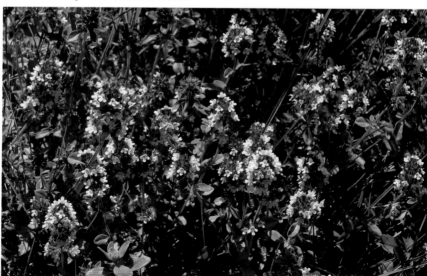

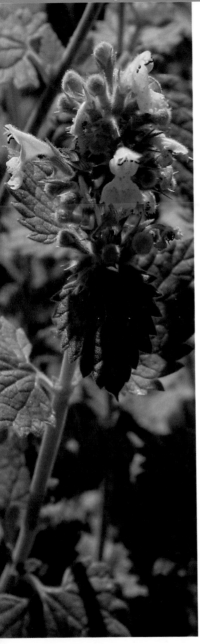

Catnip
Nepeta cataria

FOOD: The young leaves can be eaten raw, in salads. Older leaves are used as flavouring in cooked foods. Fresh or dried leaves can be used in tea.

MEDICINE: Catnip, while most widely known for its effects on cats, has a long history of use as an herbal medicine. It is most commonly used to treat digestive problems and reduce fevers (by stimulating sweating). It is used to treat colds, flus, fevers, and infectious childhood diseases, sometimes being combined with black elderberry (*Sambucus nigra*) flowers. Catnip is calming to the stomach and alleviates flatulence, nausea, diarrhea and colic. Catnip is also considered soothing to the nervous system and is taken for insomnia and hyperactivity. It is reputed to prevent miscarriage and premature birth and to lessen morning sickness. Tea made from the leaves can be used externally on bruises, especially black eyes. Aboriginal peoples in eastern Canada (Iroquois, Ojibwa) used catnip for a wide range of ailments, and it was often provided for illness in children. A plant infusion was taken for headaches, to alleviate vomiting, for "trouble" caused by eating rich foods, for diarrhea, colds, coughs, fevers and chills and for stomachaches due to colds. The flowers and roots were used to treat excess saliva or drooling, and plant tips were given to restless babies who couldn't sleep. An infusion of leaves was taken as a blood purifier. People would be bathed in an infusion of leaves to raise the body temperature.

OTHER USES: Catnip is well known for its pseudo-narcotic affects on some cats. There seems to be a genetic link to whether a cat responds to or is unaffected by catnip. Cats chew, bite and roll in catnip to release the volatile oil trapped in the leaves. The plant deters ants, flea beetles, rats and mice. Leaf extracts or the essential oil contain potent insect repellent ingredients (nepetalactones) and are much longer lasting than citronella. Dried leaves can be used in potpourri.

DESCRIPTION: Perennial herb from a taproot, with upright, 4-angled stems, to 1 m tall, covered in fine, whitish hairs. Leaves 3–6 cm long, hairy, heart-shaped, coarsely toothed, top side green with greyish green underneath. Flowers whitish pink with purple spots, tubular, to 6 mm long, in several clusters toward tips of branches, blooming from June to September. Fruits 4 nutlets. This introduced Eurasian species can be found in mesic to dry, disturbed sites across Canada.

Self-Heal
Prunella vulgaris

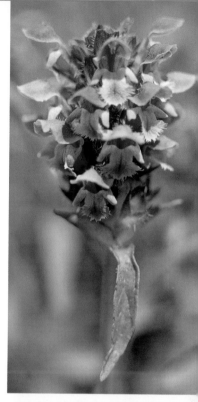

FOOD: The leaves can be eaten raw or cooked and can be used in salads, soups and stews. Tannin in the leaves makes them somewhat bitter, but it can be washed out. A drink is made from a cold-water infusion of fresh or dried and powdered leaves.

MEDICINE: Aboriginal peoples across Canada used this plant for medicine. An infusion of the leaves was used for fevers. A weak decoction of roots, leaves and blossoms was taken for the heart. An infusion of the whole plant was used to wash a burst boil, applied to neck sores, taken for backaches, fed to babies that cry too much, used as an eyewash to keep the eyes moist on cold or windy days, taken for sickness caused by grieving and employed as a tonic for general indisposition. The plant was chewed for sore throats. A decoction of the whole plant was taken for diarrhea and vomiting, as an emetic, for fevers and shortness of breath, in a steam bath for sore legs or stiff knees, to strengthen the womb and for stomach cramps and biliousness. A compound decoction of roots and shoots was taken as a remedy for colds and coughs, as a blood purifier and to treat venereal disease. A compound decoction of roots was used as a wash for piles and taken for shortness of breath and consumption. The leaves were used to treat boils, cuts, bruises and skin inflammations. In addition to Aboriginal use, other people have long made use of the medicinal qualities of self-heal, which gave rise to its common name. It has been used especially in the treatment of external wounds, ulcers and sores but was also taken as a tea in the treatment of fevers, diarrhea, sore mouths and internal bleeding. The whole plant is antibacterial and inhibits the growth of a number of disease-causing bacteria. It was also known to reduce blood pressure, destroy intestinal worms, reduce muscle spasms and act as a general tonic.

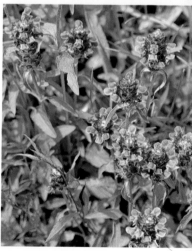

OTHER USES: An infusion of plant was used for saddle and back sores and as an eyewash for horses by the Blackfoot. An olive-green dye can be made from the flowers and stems.

DESCRIPTION: Perennial herb, with upright stems solitary or clustered, 10–50 cm tall. Leaves in pairs, opposite, lance-shaped or oval, entire or obscurely toothed, the lower leaves long-stalked. Violet or purplish flowers, 1–2 cm long, petals fused into 2-lipped tube, with bottom lip divided into 3 lobes, middle lobe fringed; in dense terminal spikes. Produces 4 nutlets. This introduced Eurasian species is a common weed of lawns, fields and roadsides throughout Canada.

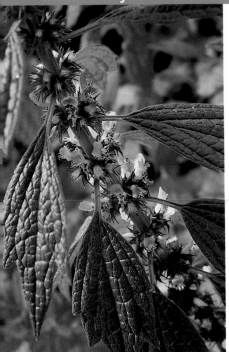

Common Motherwort

Leonurus cardiaca

FOOD: Fresh or dried flowers are used as flavouring in soups, beer and tea.

MEDICINE: The plant was widely used to treat heart problems and female ailments and valued for its calming, sedative qualities. It has been used as a remedy for heart palpitations and is said to strengthen a weak heart (hence the species name *cardiaca*). It will also decrease muscle spasms, temporarily reduce blood pressure, promote sweating and aid in digestion. Motherwort is a uterine stimulant and was taken for problems with menstruation, childbirth and menopause. An infusion of the dried plant was taken to help digestion. It was considered an effective tonic to calm nerves and reduce anxiety and has been used to treat epilepsy. Early Greeks commonly gave motherwort to pregnant women suffering from anxiety, which gave this herb the name motherwort, or "mother's herb." The active compounds are bitter principles known as labdane diterpenes.

OTHER USES: Dark olive-green liquid from the leaves has been used as a dye.

DESCRIPTION: Perennial herb arising from branching rhizomes, with erect, branched stems, to 1.5 m tall. Leaves opposite, palmate, 3- to 7-lobed, to 10 cm long and wide, dark green above, pale below, smaller and less lobed further up the stem. Flowers pale pink to purple, tubular, to 1.2 cm long, with 2-lipped corolla, with long hairs on the upper lip, in whorls of 6–12 in leaf axils, blooming from June to August. Produces 4 nutlets. Common motherwort is an introduced Eurasian species found abundantly in disturbed sites, pastures, fields and roadsides across southern Canada.

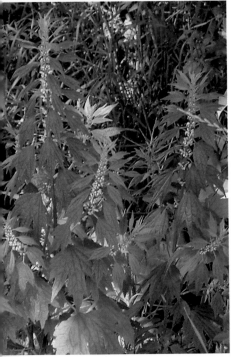

WARNING
Skin contact with motherwort can cause dermatitis in some people. The essential oil can cause photosensitization.

Swamp Hedge-Nettle

Stachys palustris

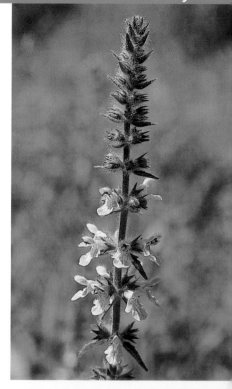

FOOD: The plump, crisp rhizomes, collected in autumn, are said to have a rather agreeable flavour. They have been eaten raw, boiled, baked or pickled. They were also dried, ground and used to make breads in times of food shortage. Young shoots can be cooked as a vegetable (like asparagus, p. 174), but they are said to have a disagreeable smell. The flowers are also edible.

MEDICINE: The leaves were bruised or soaked in water and applied as poultices to stop the bleeding of wounds and open sores (another common name is "woundwort"). The leaves and rhizomes have also been used in poultices to reduce pain and inflammation associated with sprains, gout, cramps, swollen joints and headaches. Fresh rhizomes were chewed alone or were soaked in alcohol that was then gargled to relieve sore throats. Medicinal teas made from these plants have been used to treat inflammation of the bladder and urethra, migraine headaches, headaches from eye strain and hangovers, colic, sprains and inflamed joints.

OTHER USES: Swamp hedge-nettle was used as a yellow dye.

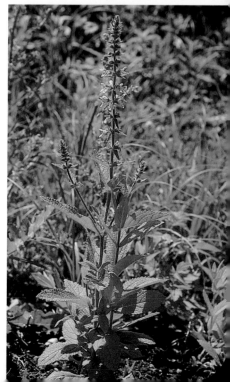

DESCRIPTION: Glandular-hairy, perennial herb, to 90 cm tall, with erect, 4-sided stems bearing opposite, 4–8 cm long, blunt-toothed leaves. Flowers purplish pink to whitish, mottled with darker spots, widely funnel-shaped, with a broad, concave upper lip and a flared, 3-lobed lower lip, 10–15 mm long, borne in spike-like clusters of few-flowered whorls, from July to August. Fruits dark brown nutlets, about 2 mm long, in clusters of 4. Swamp hedge-nettle grows on moist plains, streams, ditches and swamps all across Canada.

These plants are called hedge-nettles because, with their stiff, bristly hairs, they resemble stinging nettle (p. 312). However, unlike true nettles, they do not have stinging hairs, so they are safe to touch.

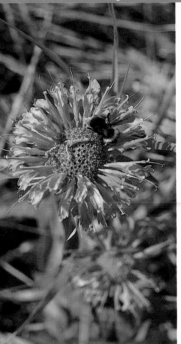

Wild Bergamot
Monarda fistulosa

FOOD: Wild bergamot (also called horsemint) plants have been cooked alone as a potherb or used (like oregano) to flavour meat dishes, soups and stews. They can also make delicious, fragrant teas. This species smells much like oil-of-bergamot (extracted from the tropical tree orange bergamot, *Citrus aurantium*, which gives Earl Grey tea its distinctive flavour. Native peoples sprinkled the dried leaves on meat and drying berries to repel insects.

MEDICINE: The leaf tea has been used to treat coughs, colds, flu, fevers, pneumonia, insomnia, sore eyes, kidney and respiratory problems, nosebleeds, heart trouble, gas, cramps and indigestion and to expel intestinal worms. Studies have shown that wild bergamot stimulates sweating and helps to expel gas, and that it contains the antimicrobial monoterpene thymol. The leaves were packed around aching teeth or applied in poultices to relieve headaches and painful swollen joints and to heal rashes and acne. Dried, powdered plants (sometimes made into a paste) were rubbed on the head, face and limbs and inside the mouth to relieve fevers and headaches, or they were taken internally with water to treat fevers and sore throats. Dried leaves were sometimes wrapped around the neck in a cloth or strip of deerskin to relieve sore throats. Wild bergamot has been used to stimulate menstrual flow and to help expel afterbirth. An infusion of the plant was taken or used as a bath for infant convulsions.

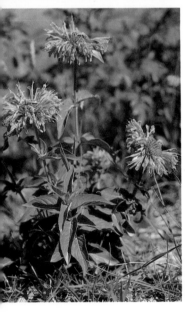

OTHER USES: Some Aboriginal people perfumed favourite horses with the chewed leaves of wild bergamot. Other people mixed bergamot and other sweet-smelling plants with 1–2 drops of beaver castor oil and a bit of water and applied it to their hair, body and clothing as perfume. Today, wild bergamot is used in potpourris and perfumes. Plants were burned on hot rocks in sweat baths as incense. Some native groups used wild bergamot as an insect repellent and burned it in smudges to drive insects away. This beautiful mint attracts many butterflies and hummingbirds, and it deserves a place in wildflower gardens. It is best grown from seed.

DESCRIPTION: Finely hairy, perennial herb, smelling strongly of mint, with square, unbranched stems, 20–70 cm tall, bearing paired leaves 2.5–8 cm long. Flowers bright rose to purplish, 20–35 mm long, tubular, with a long, narrow upper lip and a 3-lobed lower lip, forming short, showy clusters, from June to August. Fruits 4 smooth nutlets. Grows in open, moist to moderately dry prairies, foothill and montane sites from BC to QC. See p. 424 for conservation status.

Mock-Pennyroyals

Hedeoma spp.

FOOD: The leaves of mock-pennyroyals smell and taste mint-like, and can be brewed into tea or used as culinary flavouring. An essential oil from these plants is used as a flavouring in beverages, ice cream and baked goods.

MEDICINE: Mock-pennyroyals have long been used for a variety of medicinal purposes, most commonly to treat digestive disorders and colds and to assist with menstruation and childbirth. An infusion of the plant was taken for cold fevers due to its ability to induce sweating. It was used to treat upset stomachs, intestinal pain and digestive disorders because the plant removes gas from the digestive tract. It was used for a number of female-related conditions, such as promoting menstruation (for suppressed flow), easing painful menstruation and assisting in childbirth. When taken with brewers yeast, mock-pennyroyals can induce an abortion. Mock-pennyroyal is a diuretic and stimulant and also causes irritations and redness when applied to the skin, which promotes circulation. It has also been taken for nervousness and hysteria. The plants can be used fresh or dried after harvesting when flowering.

OTHER USES: The essential oil is used as an ingredient in commercial insect repellents and cleaning products and is reputed to repel ticks when rubbed on the body, but see **Warning**.

DESCRIPTION: Annual, strongly-scented herbs with upright, simple or branching, square stems, to 40 cm high. Leaves lance-shaped to oval, opposite, with few teeth, on short petioles, and hairy on bottom of leaf. Flowers small (3 mm long), blue, 5-parted, a few in each cluster at leaf axils, appearing from June to September. Produces 1-seeded nutlets.

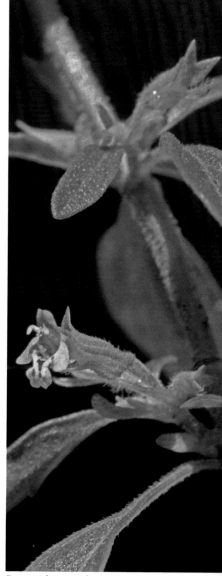

Eastern mock-pennyroyal

WARNING

The essential oil is considered toxic because of the pulegone content, which is associated with hepatotoxicity. Skin contact may cause dermatitis.

Western mock-pennyroyal (*H. hispida*) is a smaller plant, to 20 cm tall, the stems simple or branched, the leaves to 2 cm long. Grows in dry, open places (fields, grasslands) from southeastern BC to QC.

Eastern mock-pennyroyal (*H. pulegioides*) is a larger plant, to 40 cm tall, the stems branched, the leaves to 3 cm long. Found in upland woods, particularly around limestone in ON, QC, NB and NS. See p. 424 for conservation status.

Yerba Buena
Clinopodium douglasii

FOOD: A pleasant scent wafting from the forest floor may alert you to the presence of this elegant plant. Steeping yerba buena leaves in water makes an invigorating tea. Leaves may also be mixed with spearmint, lemon balm or chamomile to make refreshing, aromatic teas, or used to flavour less palatable teas. A refreshing iced tea can be made from a 3:1 mixture of yerba buena and hibiscus, sweetened to taste with honey. Fresh leaves or a few tablespoons of tincture may also be used to flavour lemonade, apple cider or other fruit punches. Runners may be gathered from April to September, dried in a paper bag and stored for up to a year. Typically only the leaves are used, as stems are less aromatic and slightly bitter. Yerba buena tea was used as both a beverage and a tonic, mainly by Saanich peoples, although other Salish groups along Georgia Strait may have occasionally used this plant.

MEDICINE: Teas made from this plant have been drunk to increase perspiration for those suffering from mild fevers. Yerba buena was also used as a skin wash to relieve rashes. Yerba buena contains a monoterpenoid in its volatile oils. Terpenoids contribute to the herb's aroma and are currently being studied for their antibacterial and pharmaceutical properties.

OTHER USES: The name yerba buena stems from the Spanish *hierba buena* or "good herb." Yerba Buena was the original name of San Francisco because the herb was so abundant in the area.

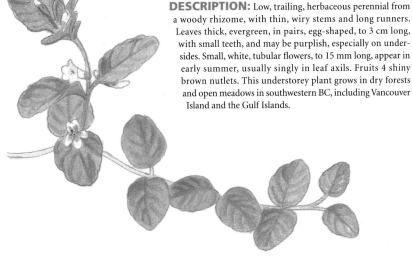

DESCRIPTION: Low, trailing, herbaceous perennial from a woody rhizome, with thin, wiry stems and long runners. Leaves thick, evergreen, in pairs, egg-shaped, to 3 cm long, with small teeth, and may be purplish, especially on undersides. Small, white, tubular flowers, to 15 mm long, appear in early summer, usually singly in leaf axils. Fruits 4 shiny brown nutlets. This understorey plant grows in dry forests and open meadows in southwestern BC, including Vancouver Island and the Gulf Islands.

WARNING
Yerba buena sometimes grows among patches of poison-oak (p. 395). When gathering yerba buena, ensure that it has not come into contact with poison-oak, as traces of the poison-oak oils may cause irritation in sensitive individuals.

Bugleweeds

Lycopus spp.

FOOD: Bugleweed roots were formerly used as a principal food for Interior Salish peoples of BC. The roots would typically be gathered in spring, before they began to sprout. They could be eaten raw, steam-cooked in an underground pit or boiled. First Nations would often mix the roots with meat or fish; some groups ate them as a dessert. They are said to have a sweet taste, similar to a mild radish. They could be stored fresh in a wet sack for a few days and were sometimes dried for long-term storage.

MEDICINE: Bugleweed plants were used in medicines. American bugleweed was used as an astringent, mild narcotic and mild sedative. The plant was said to slow and strengthen heart contractions and be of value in the treatment of

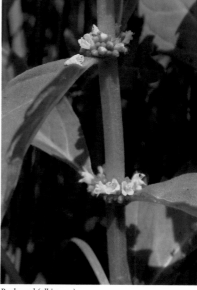

Bugleweed (all images)

hyperthyroidism. American bugleweed was also used in the treatment of coughs, bleeding from the lungs, consumption and excessive menstruation. Bugleweed was used mainly for preventing/relieving coughs and as a sedative. The plant was mixed with other plants to treat children's colds. It contains phenylpropanoid esters which are cyclooxygenase inhibitors.

OTHER USES: Juice from the plant is said to make a good dye.

DESCRIPTION: Herbaceous perennials, about 8–70 cm tall. Stems finely hairy or smooth. Leaves opposite, lance-shaped to elliptic, 2–7 cm long. Flowers white or pinkish, 3 mm long, 4-lobed, hairy within, stalkless, several to many in whorled clusters in leaf nodes, blooming from July to October. Produces 4 hard-ridged, 1-seeded nutlets. Requires moist or wet soil, can grow in partial shade or full sun. Found in streambanks, marshes, lake edges and peat bogs from BC to NL. See p. 424 for conservation status.

Bugleweed (*L. uniflorus*) has irregularly toothed leaves and spreads by stolons, which often produce tubers.

American bugleweed (*L. americanus*) has deeply lobed leaves, the lobes most prominent on lower leaves, and does not produce tubers.

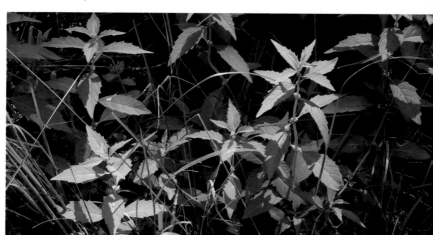

Wild Mints

Mentha spp.

FOOD: These plants can be eaten alone as greens, raw or cooked, but usually they are cooked with soups, stews and meats or used to flavour sauces, jellies and sweets. Mints make delicious, fragrant teas, cold drinks and even wine. Spearmint and peppermint have long been favourite flavours for gums, candies, syrups and liqueurs. All 3 species have been used to improve the flavour of other foods, including fruit juices, sauces and preserves, stout or overly yeasty beer, yogurt and fruit salads. Powdered mint leaves were sprinkled on berries and drying meat to repel insects, and dried mint plants were sometimes layered with stored, dried meat for flavour.

MEDICINE: The active medicinal ingredient, menthol (found in all 3 species), has been shown to expel gas from and relieve spasms of the digestive tract—hence the advent of the after-dinner mint. Menthol calms smooth muscles (e.g., in the digestive tract), facilitates belching and stimulates the liver to produce bile. It can help to prevent retching and vomiting and may also bring some relief from pain, coughing and sinus conjestion. Wild mint tea was used by native peoples to treat colds, coughs, fevers, upset stomachs, gas, vomiting, kidney problems and headaches. Mint plants, menthol and peppermint oil have all been applied in poultices or lotions to relieve arthritis, tendinitis and rheumatism, and leaves were packed into and around aching teeth. Cold wild mint tea was recommended for combating the effects of

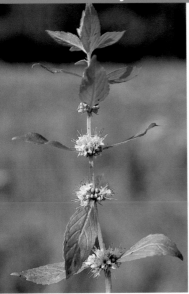

Wild mint (all images)

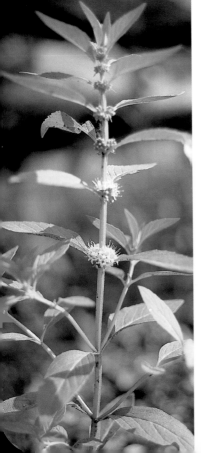

> ### WARNING
>
> Wild mint and spearmint are high in pulegone, which is hepatotoxic and stimulates the uterus, so they should not be used during pregnancy or heavy menstruation. Peppermint oil can cause heartburn and acid regurgitation when injested in large amounts, and it also causes rashes when applied to the skin. These plants should be used in moderation. As little as 1 tsp of pure menthol can be fatal. Also, some people are allergic to menthol or have chemical sensitivities to it. Use caution when giving infants or small children foods or medicines containing menthol or peppermint. They could gag, choke or even collapse from the intense fragrance.

being struck by a whirlwind. In Europe, spearmint was an important medicine for treating diarrhea, stomach and bowel troubles, colic, gas, coughs, toothaches, headaches and hysteria. Peppermint tea may help to relieve morning sickness, but wild mint and spearmint should not be used for this purpose (see **Warning**). Peppermint extracts have been shown to be effective against some bacteria and viruses (including *Herpes simplex*).

OTHER USES: These aromatic plants were hung in dwellings as air-fresheners, and they were also crushed or chewed and rubbed on bodies as perfume (to improve one's love life). Mint was one of the aromatic plants boiled with traps to mask human scent. Mint oils from spearmint and peppermint have been used as a fragrance in toothpaste, soap and perfume and as a flavouring in toothpaste and mouthwash.

DESCRIPTION: Glandular-dotted perennials, to 90 cm tall, smelling strongly of mint, with 4-sided stems bearing paired, sharp-toothed leaves 2–8 cm long. Flowers light purple or pink to whitish, funnel-shaped, with 4 spreading lobes, from June to September. Fruits 4 oval nutlets. Grow in moist areas, streambanks, wet meadows and clearings, springs and lakeshores across Canada.

Wild mint or **field mint** (*M. arvensis*) is a native species that produces whorls of flowers in its leaf axils. See p. 424 for conservation status.

Spearmint (*M. spicata*) and **peppermint** (*M. piperita*) are European introductions with terminal spike-like flower clusters. Spearmint has stalkless leaves and slender flower spikes (5–10 mm wide), whereas peppermint has stalked leaves and thicker flower spikes (10–15 mm wide). If in doubt with these two, taste them!

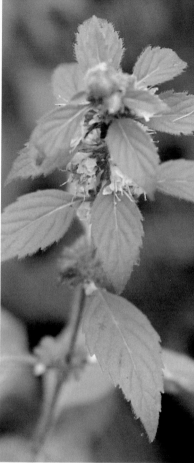

Mint species (all images)

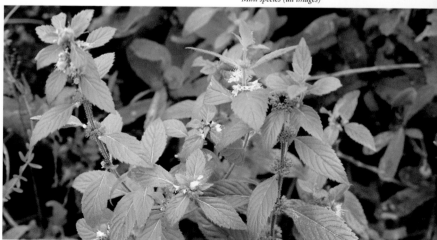

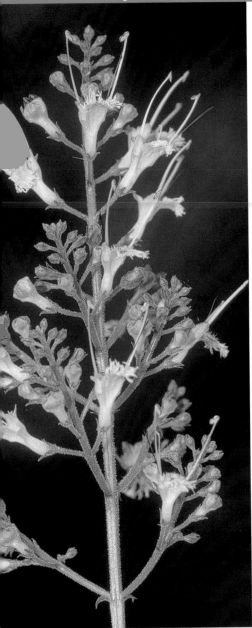

Stoneroot
Collinsonia canadensis

MEDICINE: The root of stoneroot was used extensively as a medicine to treat irritated tissues, heart tonic, urinary tract ailments and hemorrhoids. The Iroquois used a compound decoction of roots for diarrhea with blood and also used stoneroot decoctions as a foot, back, and leg soak for rheumatism. The roots were also used stoneroot decoctions as a blood medicine, for heart trouble, kidney trouble, boils and as a cure-all. An infusion of the smashed roots was given to strengthen listless children and as a wash for babies to give them strength. The Iroquois applied a poultice of the powdered leaves to the forehead for headaches. The plant contains saponins and some novel flavonoids, which may be responsible for its medicinal activity.

OTHER USES: The Cherokee used an infusion of stoneroot as a drench for horses with colic. Flowers were mashed and used as a deodorant.

DESCRIPTION: Perennial herb, 30 cm–1.2 m tall, with square upright stem, with several branches on top. Leaves few, large, opposite, 15–20 cm long and 5–10 cm wide, oval with serrated margins and smell like lemon when crushed. Light yellow flowers, lemon-scented, 1 cm long, with 2 very long, protruding stamens, long lower lip that is fringed at the tip, on stalks, in loose branching clusters; bloom from July to September. Fruit a nutlet containing 4 seeds, which mature in autumn as the plant begins to lose its leaves. Found in moist woodlands in southern ON.

Lopseed

Phryma leptostachya

MEDICINE: The Ojibwa made a tea of lopseed as an analgesic for rheumatism. The root can be dried and then chewed or mixed with water to make a gargle for sore throats. A poultice of the roots is said to soothe insect bites and stings. This plant also grows in southeast Asia, where it is used to treat ringworm, scabies, fevers, ulcers and insect bites.

OTHER USES: The common name lopseed describes how the seeds hang down against the stem.

DESCRIPTION: Erect, herbaceous perennial reaching 1 m in height. Stems simple or branching, hairy, mostly hollow, 4-angled (the angles rounded), purplish, with swollen purple areas above each node. Leaves opposite, stalked, toothed, oval to lance-shaped, to 16 cm in length. Leaf blades near the base of the plant are smaller. Inflorescence with spreading flowers and hanging fruits. Flowers small, purplish white, snapdragon-like, in terminal clusters on very short stalks; bloom from June to September. Fruit a strongly-ribbed achene to 4 mm long, tan when mature. Inhabits rich woods, moist thickets and ravines from southern MB to ON, QC and NB. See p. 424 for conservation status.

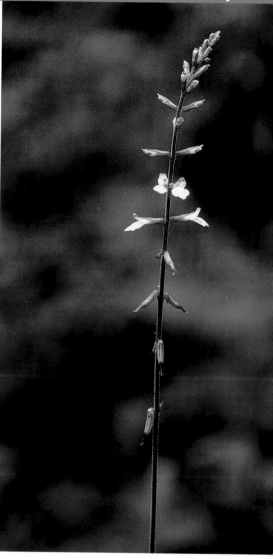

Vervains

Verbena spp.

FOOD: The flowers and leaves of these plants can be used as a tea substitute. The leaves are considered palatable when parboiled, and the flowers make a pretty garnish or addition to salads.

MEDICINE: Vervains are considered to have antibacterial, anticoagulant, antispasmodic, analgesic, diuretic, emmenagogue, stimulant and astringent properties. Plants harvested for medicinal use should be gathered in summer as flowering begins, and dried. Blue vervain was traditionally used to treat convalescents and people suffering from depression, headaches, jaundice, cramps, coughs and fevers. Externally, it has been applied to minor wounds, ulcers, eczema, sores and acne. The root is considered astringent and has been used to treat dysentery. Blue vervain can, however, interfere with blood pressure medication and hormone therapy, and large doses cause vomiting and diarrhea. European vervain (*V. officinalis*), often cultivated in Canadian gardens, has a long history of medicinal use, particularly in the treatment of nervous problems and insomnia.

Blue vervain

OTHER USES: Vervain is pretty as a garden ornamental. Blue vervain's small, deep blue blossoms develop in a ring, starting at the bottom of the flower spike. As the ring approaches the top, the spike often produces more buds at its tip, sometimes extending the flowering period to 3 months. The flowers are pollinated by bees, flies, butterflies and moths and as such attract these species to your garden.

DESCRIPTION: Perennial, roughly hairy herbs from a taproot or fibrous roots. Leaves opposite, coarse-toothed. Flowers violet blue to pinkish (occasionally white), funnel-shaped, 2.5–4.5 mm long, with 5 flaring lobes; in terminal clusters, from July to September. Fruits small (1–2 mm long) nutlets.

Bracted vervain (*V. bracteata*) is a prostrate or decumbent, much-branched plant, 10–60 cm long. Leaves 2–5 cm long, deeply cleft into segments. The common name bracted refers to the long sterile leaves (bracts) below the flower cluster that greatly exceed the cluster in length (bracts of blue vervain are shorter than the flower cluster). Grows in mesic to dry, sandy sites and disturbed areas in steppe and montane zones from southern BC to ON.

Blue vervain (*V. hastata*) is an erect plant, unbranched or sparingly branched, 40 cm–1.5 m tall, with square, grooved, branched stems. Leaves 4–18 cm long, lance-shaped, sharply toothed. Inhabits damp thickets, ditches, wet meadows and shores in lowland to steppe zones from BC to NS (except AB and PEI). See p. 424 for conservation status.

Sweet-Cicelys
Osmorhiza spp.

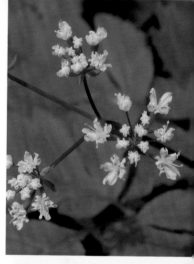

FOOD: Although the southern Kwakwaka'wakw peoples of BC believed that mountain sweet-cicely was sure to kill if eaten, this plant was widely used medicinally. Some native peoples ate the young tops as greens, and the Thompson Indians of BC ate the thick roots.

MEDICINE: Decoctions of the root of Clayton's sweet-cicely were gargled or chewed to relieve a sore throat or were used as an eyewash. Warm infusions prepared with Clayton's sweet-cicely root were taken for coughs and to help ease childbirth. Its roots have an anise-like odour and were also pulverized into poultices that were placed over ulcers and infections. Longstyle sweet-cicely leaves, stems and roots were pulverized and consumed as infusions for stomach discomforts and kidney troubles. Root infusions were also taken for amenorrhea (absence of menses) and for stomach problems. Root decoctions were consumed as an energizing drink, and poultices prepared with longstyle sweet-cicely roots were applied to wounds and boils. One of the active ingredients is falcarindiol, an acetylene. The roots and leaves of mountain sweet-cicely were used in many medicines or medicinal teas to prevent ailments and treat conditions ranging from headaches and colds to stomach sickness.

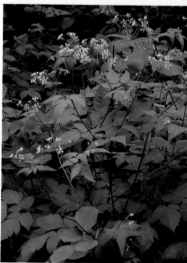

OTHER USES: Some native peoples believed that mountain sweet-cicely was a good luck charm if found growing in an area where it had not been seen before. Other groups considered the roots a powerful love charm. The Blackfoot gave mountain sweet-cicely to mares to prepare them for foaling.

Longstyle sweet-cicely (all images)

DESCRIPTION: Perennial herbs, to 90 cm tall, with small, fern-like leaves (1.5–9 cm long) that are divided into blunt-toothed or lobed leaflets. Small (< 2 mm wide), sparse, compound umbels of white, 5-petalled flowers that occur throughout May and June.

Mountain sweet-cicely (*O. berteroi*, formerly known as *O. chilensis*) has 2 times pinnately divided leaves, white to greenish flowers and a dry, flattened fruit that splits into 2 seeds. Found in cool, moist woodlands across Canada.

Clayton's sweet-cicely (*O. claytonii*) is hairy with thrice-compound leaves and a rank-tasting root. Found from SK to QC, NB, PEI and NS. See p. 424 for conservation status.

WARNING
Poison-hemlock (p. 410) can be mistaken for sweet-cicely species.

Longstyle sweet-cicely (*O. longistylis*) is mostly smooth, and its aromatic root is more sweet-smelling. Found from AB to QC, NB, PEI and NS. See p. 424 for conservation status.

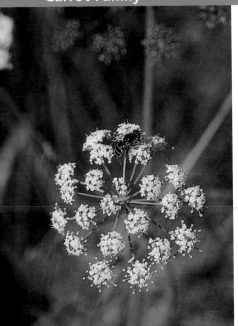

Water-Parsnip
Sium suave

FOOD: Many tribes gathered water-parsnip roots in spring and early summer and ate them raw, roasted or fried. The crisp, fresh roots were said to have a carrot-like flavour. Because the roots were often collected in spring, before the leaves had grown, plants had to be identified using their roots and the remnants of stems from the previous year. Tender young shoots were sometimes eaten, but mature plants were not considered edible.

MEDICINE: The roots were used to treat stomach problems.

OTHER USES: Children sometimes used the hollow stems to make whistles.

DESCRIPTION: Hairless, perennial herb with hollow, ridged stems, 50 cm–1 m tall. Leaves pinnate, divided into 5–17 slender, 5–10 cm long leaflets edged with sharp teeth. Flowers small and white, form twice-divided, flat-topped clusters (umbels) 5–18 cm across; bloom from June to August. Fruits pairs of flattened, ribbed, seed-like schizocarps, 2–3 mm long. Grows in wet sites in prairies, foothills and montane zones throughout most of Canada except NU and Labrador. See p. 424 for conservation status.

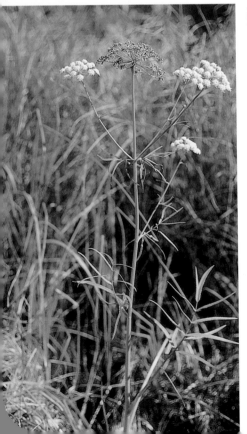

WARNING
Although the stems and roots are edible, the flowerheads may be poisonous. These plants have been confused with the extremely poisonous water-hemlocks (p. 411), with fatal results. Water-hemlocks are recognized by their twice- (rather than once-) divided leaves, their yellowish, strong-smelling (rather than white, sweet-smelling) roots and their smooth (rather than ribbed) stems. If there is any question about the identity of a plant, especially in the Carrot family, consider it poisonous.

Golden Alexander
Zizia aurea

FOOD: One of the earliest blooming prairie plants, the tiny flower clusters (umbels) of golden Alexand er, once removed from their stem, make an excellent contribution to a tossed green salad. As a cooked vegetable, they can be served much like broccoli.

MEDICINE: Some First Nations dried and ground the flower stalks and used them in a compound mixture as a snuff to treat headaches. The root was boiled and taken to alleviate fevers. Historically, the plant was used to heal wounds and induce sleep. Early settlers believed that it was a cure for syphilis.

DESCRIPTION: Erect, branching perennial, 30–90 cm tall, with alternate, twice- or thrice-divided leaves with 3–7 leaflets. Leaflet stalks of terminal leaflet to 4 cm long, those of lateral leaflets to 1.5 cm long, both winged. Leaflets 2.5–5 cm long, toothed, pointed, generally oval to lance-shaped and irregularly divided again. Inflorescences terminal compound umbels with up to 20 rays, each to 4 cm long. Central flower of each smaller umbel (umbellet) stalkless. Flowers yellow, 5-petalled, 2 mm long, glabrous and folding in on themselves, from April to June. Fruit round to oblong, 4 mm long. Grows in prairies, glades, fields, thickets and rich, open woods from SK to NS. See p. 424 for conservation status.

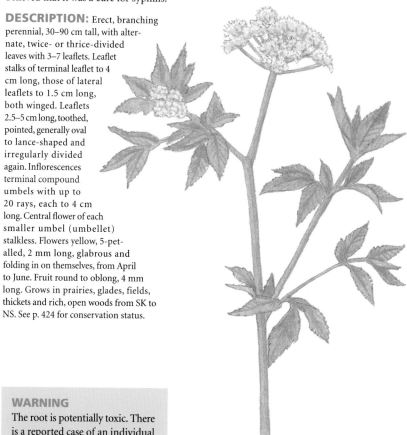

WARNING
The root is potentially toxic. There is a reported case of an individual vomiting violently after eating an entire root. Further adverse reactions are believed to follow. As with other members of this family, the plant should be identified carefully and consumed with extreme caution.

Pacific Water-Parsley

Oenanthe sarmentosa

FOOD: The roots of this plant were highly esteemed by some Pacific First Nations and considered highly toxic by others. They have a sweet, starchy flesh with a cream-like parsley flavour when boiled. The young, tender stem was occasionally eaten raw or boiled and eaten as greens. Some caution is advised, however, because other members of this genus contain the active poison oenanthotoxin.

MEDICINE: Consumption of the roots causes vomiting and has strong laxative effects. Traditionally, they were crushed and swallowed by pregnant women to induce a quick and easy delivery. The purging action of Pacific water-parsley was used by First Nations to purify the body and as a means to seek supernatural powers.

OTHER USES: The hollow stems were fashioned into whistles and played by children. Pacific water-parsley makes a very attractive ornamental for gardens that are seasonally wet.

DESCRIPTION: Perennial herb, 50 cm–1.2 m tall (or long) with green, parsley-like leaves and tall, white flowers. Hairless stems root as they recline to the ground (stoloniferous). Leaves generally 2-pinnate, the leaf stalk 10–35 cm long, blade 10–30 cm long, 6–25 cm wide, with leaflets 1–6 cm long, oval, lobed or toothed. Flowerhead atop a stout stalk, 5–13 cm long, with many bractlets, 4–5 mm long, lance-shaped, rays 10–20. Flower petals 5, 1.5–3 cm long, from May to September. Fruit a reddish schizocarp, round, 2.5–3.5 cm long with wide ribs. Found in marshes, open forests and areas of sluggish water up to an elevation of 1000 m on BC's coast.

Angelicas

Angelica spp.

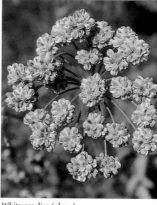

FOOD: Angelica leaves smell like parsley and have a strong but pleasant taste, similar to that of garden lovage. The seeds taste like a cross between celery and cardamom. The leaves have been used as a spice or garnish in soups and stews, and occasionally as a vegetable. Angelica has also been used to flavour gin and liqueurs. Stems of North American species can be candied like those of European species, though generally the roots are not candied because they are too tough. Leaves and stems of kneeling angelica were also considered edible.

White angelica (above)
Kneeling angelica (below)

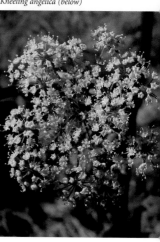

MEDICINE: Teas and extracts made from the seeds and roots of angelica have been used for centuries, the seeds to aid digestion and relieve nausea and cramps, and the roots for their antispasmodic properties. Angelica root tea has been taken to relieve spastic asthma, intestinal cramps, gas and menopausal discomforts, as well as menstrual cramps, constipation and bloating associated with premenstrual syndrome. It is said to relieve spasms without sedating or stimulating the patient. The Chinese medicine *Dong quai*, which is made from cured plants of *A. polymorpha* and/or *A. sinensis*, is widely used to treat problems of the digestive tract and of the female reproductive system. Kneeling angelica root was eaten raw or prepared into a decoction as a purgative medicine.

OTHER USES: Kneeling angelica stems were made into whistles, used as drinking straws and employed as breathing tubes for hiding underwater. They were also used for collecting sap from Sitka spruce (p. 31).

DESCRIPTION: Robust, often ill-smelling, perennial herbs, to 2.5 m tall, with stout stems from taproots. Leaves alternate and compound with 3 major divisions, pinnately divided into sharp-toothed leaflets about 3–10 cm long, with inflated, clasping stalk bases. Flowers small, usually white, borne in large, flat-topped clusters that bloom from June to August. Fruits flat, winged and ribbed, seed-like schizocarps, 3–6 mm long. All 3 species described below have hairless fruits that occur in clusters and don't have bracts at their base. See p. 424 for conservation status.

> **WARNING**
>
> The roots may be toxic when eaten fresh and should be avoided during pregnancy. Because of the presence of photogenotoxic furanocoumarins, *Angelica* species can cause severe skin burn, rash or other skin reactions in some people when skin contact or ingestion is followed by exposure to sunlight. Accurate identification is essential to avoid confusion with the extremely poisonous water-hemlocks (*Cicuta* species, p. 411)

Kneeling angelica (*A. genuflexa*) has the main leaf axis bent, and the leaflets deflexed (bent back). Grows on moist streambanks and open forests at montane elevations in BC and AB.

White angelica (*A. arguta*) has the main leaf axis straight, the leaflets not bent back. Grows mostly in moist sites in montane and subalpine zones in BC and AB.

Purplestem angelica (*A. atropurpurea*) has a smooth, dark purple stem. Found in wet soils as far north as NU, south to ON, and along the coast to NL.

Lovages

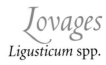

Ligusticum spp.

FOOD: Fresh beach lovage leaves were eaten in salads and considered a good source of vitamins A and C. Stalks were eaten raw like celery or cooked as greens. Beach lovage was also used to flavour soups and season fish or meats. The plant was preserved in seal oil and stored for winter use. Canby's lovage is a very fragrant plant, and all parts are edible. It is usually used in small amounts for flavouring because it tends to be rather overwhelming alone.

MEDICINE: Canby's lovage is a popular medicinal herb still widely gathered and traded by some native peoples. The fragrant dried roots were chewed to soothe a wide range of ailments, including sore throats and colds, toothache, headache, stomachache, fever and heart problems. They have also been used to make medicinal teas for treating colds, coughs, flu and sore throats and for use as eardrops. Some present-day herbalists recommend this plant for treating deep, raspy coughs caused by viral infections. Roots were

Canby's lovage

mashed or cut into fine shavings and used in poultices on abscessed ears. Some said that a piece of root held over a cut would stop bleeding immediately. To calm seizures, lovage roots were chewed and rubbed on the body and were also smoked in cigarettes. Smoking or chewing these roots has been reported to have a relaxing effect. Beach lovage was considered an inferior medicine in BC, but an infusion of the dried root was used to treat coughs or chest colds.

OTHER USES: Some tribes used lovage roots and snowbrush leaves (p. 148) to make a hair rinse. Vocalists chewed lovage roots to give their voices strength and endurance. Root shavings were sprinkled on coals as incense or were used in cigarettes to give a pleasant menthol taste to smoking mixtures of tobacco (p. 240) or common bearberry (p. 120). The roots were also used like chewing tobacco—held in the mouth as a snoose. Washing lovage roots was believed to bring rainstorms.

DESCRIPTION: Perennial herbs from thick taproots. Leaves basal and sometimes stem, finely divided into toothed leaflets. Flowers small, white to pinkish, in compound umbels. Fruits oblong, ribbed schizocarps.

Canby's lovage (*L. canbyi*) grows to 1.2 m tall, with usually basal leaves only, the leaves once divided into threes, then divided in a fern-like fashion. Small fruits (4–5 mm long). Grows on moist sites in open foothills and montane zones in southern BC.

Beach lovage (*L. scothicum*) is a smaller plant (to 80 cm tall), with usually basal and stem leaves, the leaves thick, twice divided into threes, then divided into usually 9 egg-shaped leaflets. Larger fruits (7–8 mm long). Grows on moist to mesic upper beaches and coastal bluffs at or near sea level, along BC's central and north coast and Queen Charlotte Islands, ON and QC (around James Bay), the Maritimes and NL.

WARNING

Lovages could be confused with some of their extremely poisonous Carrot family relatives, including water-hemlock (p. 411) and poison-hemlock (p. 410). Never eat a plant in the Carrot family unless you are positive of its identity.

Common Cow-Parsnip
Heracleum maximum

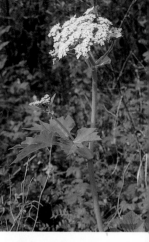

FOOD: Common cow-parsnip was widely used by native peoples. Young stems were gathered before they flowered, were peeled (to remove the strong-smelling outer bark), and the inner stem was eaten raw, steamed or boiled. Cow-parsnip tastes much like celery and has a texture similar to rhubarb. It can replace celery in many recipes, be served as a hot vegetable or used as a tasty snack, raw and dipped in sugar. Unpeeled stems were sometimes roasted in hot coals. More recently, cow-parsnip has been frozen, canned or dried. The roots were used as a cooked vegetable, like parsnips, and are said to taste like rutabagas.

MEDICINE: Cooked roots were eaten to relieve gas, colic and cramps, or were mashed as a poultice for drawing out puss from infected boils. Fresh roots were pounded to a pulp and used as poultices on sores, steeped in hot water to make tea for treating sore throats, coughs, headaches, colds and flu and boiled to make tea for treating epilepsy, asthma and nervous disorders. Some herbalists have recommended alcoholic extracts of fresh roots to stimulate nerve growth after injury. Tinctures of the fruits were applied to gum abscesses and toothaches. These plants contains furanocoumarins, which are light-activated antimicrobials. These compounds have been experimentally tested in treating psoriasis, leukemia and AIDS.

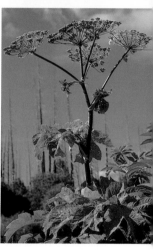

OTHER USES: Common cow-parsnip has previously gone by different scientific names, including *H. lanatum* and *H. sphondylium.* Toy flutes and whistles can be made from the dry, hollow stems, but they may irritate the lips with painful blisters, leading to a medical condition documented mostly with 8–12-year-old boys, known as "pea-shooter syndrome."

DESCRIPTION: Robust, pungent, perennial herb, 1–2.5 m tall, with hollow stems. Leaves divided into 3 large (10–30 cm wide), somewhat maple-like leaflets with inflated, clasping stalk bases. Flowers white, forming large (10–30 cm wide), twice-divided, flat-topped clusters, from late May to early July. Fruits flattened, seed-like schizocarps, 7–12 mm long, with few ribs and 2 broad wings. Grows on moist sites in prairies, foothills, montane and subalpine zones throughout Canada. See p. 424 for conservation status.

WARNING

There is an increasing number of reports of photodermatitis from cow-parsnip in recent years. People with sensitive skin may develop dark blotches, rashes and painful blisters when in contact with this plant, especially with exposure to sunlight. These skin irritations can remain for weeks or even months. Furanocoumarin compounds in cow-parsnip have been shown to damage DNA. When collecting cow-parsnip, protect your skin by wearing gloves and a long sleeved shirt and long pants. Cow-parsnip could be confused with its poisonous relatives, the water-hemlocks (p. 411).

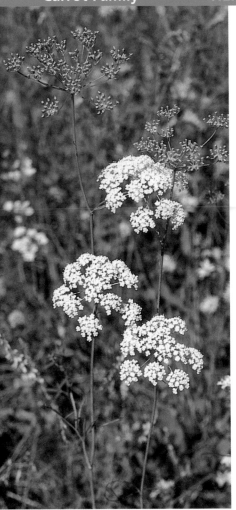

Gairdner's Yampah

Perideridia gairdneri

FOOD: Yampah was an important food for many native peoples and mountain men. Many people considered its roots the best-tasting wild roots in the mountains, with a sweet, nutty flavour, devoid of bitterness. Some people have likened them to carrots and parsnips, while others say they have a sweet, licorice-like flavour. Yampah roots can be eaten raw, but usually they were boiled, steamed or roasted. They were traditionally collected when the plants were in flower, in spring or early summer. Several tribes dried them for winter use, either whole or boiled, mashed and formed into cakes. Yampah was also stored in earth pits lined with pine needles or cottonwood bark, where it was safe from frost and rodents. The dried roots were soaked and boiled alone or with other foods, such as saskatoons (p. 109) and black hair lichen. They were also ground into meal and mixed with hot soup or water to make mush or, more recently, mixed with flour to make a thick pudding. Dried yampah root mixed with powdered deer meat was considered a special treat. The seeds have been used as seasoning and were also parched and added to cooked cereals.

MEDICINE: The root tea was used as a laxative, to stimulate urination, to aid in clearing mucous from the lungs and bronchia and to soothe sore throats. The roots were eaten by travellers, hunters and runners and fed to horses to increase energy and improve endurance. This effect was probably owing to the presence of rapidly assimilated sugars and starches.

DESCRIPTION: Slender, 40 cm–1.2 m tall, perennial herb with a caraway-like fragrance and 2–3 fleshy, tuberous roots. Leaves usually once pinnately divided into slender segments 2.5–15 cm long, but often withered by flowering time. Flowers small and white, and form twice-divided, flat-topped clusters (umbels) 2.5–7 cm across. Bloom in July and August. Fruits brown, rounded, ribbed, seed-like schizocarps about 2 mm long. Grows on open or wooded slopes in prairies, foothills and montane zones from BC to SK. See p. 424 for conservation status.

WARNING
Never eat any plant in the Carrot family unless you are sure of its identity. There are many poisonous species in this family, and experimentation can be deadly.

Pacific Hemlock-Parsley

Conioselinum gmelinii

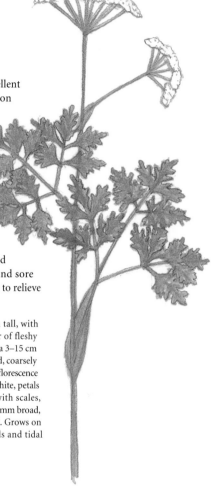

FOOD: The root of this plant is said to be excellent steamed for a few hours and eaten with eulachon grease. Pacific First Nations would mark the herbs in summer and harvest the root the following spring before the new shoots emerged. The root is highly branched and only the larger rootlets are removed, the smaller ones left in the ground to continue growing. Opinions vary on the taste of the steamed root. Some say that it is sweet, while others say it is pungent and causes diarrhea.

MEDICINE: First Nations boiled the leaves and drank the resulting liquid as a tonic for colds and sore throats. The entire plant was used in steam baths to relieve arthritis, rheumatism and general weakness.

DESCRIPTION: Stout, perennial herb, to 1.2 m tall, with a hollow, branched stem from a rhizome and a cluster of fleshy roots. Leaves oval to triangular-oval, 15–30 cm long, on a 3–15 cm long petiole, 2- to 3-times pinnately divided with stalked, coarsely serrate and pinnately-cut leaflets, oval, 1–5 cm long. Inflorescence umbrella-like, with 15–30 rays, to 5 cm wide. Flowers white, petals 2–3 cm long, spreading-ascending, slightly covered with scales, from August to October. Fruit oblong, 6–8 mm long, 3 mm broad, flat on the back with prominent ribs, narrowly winged. Grows on sandy or gravelly beaches, grassy bluffs and headlands and tidal marshes at low elevations along BC's coast.

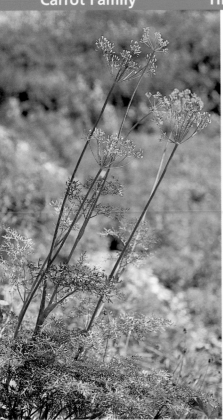

Fern-leaved desert-parsley

Desert-Parsleys & Biscuitroots

Lomatium spp.

FOOD: The leaves have a strong parsley-like flavour and were often used to flavour meat, stews and salads. The starchy, fibrous roots are edible, but some desert-parsleys may have a strong, resinous, balsam-like flavour. Roots of biscuitroot have a mild, rice-like flavour and were very popular. Large roots were roasted or boiled, but more often they were dried and ground into meal or flour for making mush, bread, cakes and biscuits. Large, flat cakes of biscuitroot meal were carried on long journeys for food. Dried roots and meal were also important trade items among some tribes. Barestem biscuitroot was also a popular food plant, and its leaves and tender stems were used as food. Its leaves, stems, flowers and young, green fruits were dried and boiled into tea beverages. Barestem biscuitroot leaves, stems and underdeveloped fruit were eaten raw, and the stalks were used like celery. Leaves could also be frozen or canned for future use or dried and used to flavour soups and stews.

MEDICINE: The roots of fern-leaved desert-parsley were used to make a medicinal tea that was considered a panacea by many native peoples. It was most commonly used for treating coughs, colds, sore throats, hayfever, bronchitis, flu, pneumonia and tuberculosis. Some herbalists still use fern-leaved desert-parsley to treat bacterial and viral respiratory infections and to help bring phlegm up from the lungs and bronchia. Extracts from this species have proved effective in combatting a wide range of bacteria in laboratory studies. Barestem biscuitroot seed, its leaves and decoctions made with the whole plant were medicinally useful. Seeds were eaten for constipation and general internal discomforts, chewed for colds and sore throats and sucked for coughs and to loosen phlegm in the throat. Poultices of chewed seeds were applied to the head for headaches, to the back to relieve muscle aches and itchiness, to the skin for colds, directly to carbuncles to help reduce infection and to the chest to reduce breast swelling in women. Teas prepared with seeds were given to pregnant women to encourage easy childbirth. Compound decoctions of barestem biscuitroot leaves, strawberry leaves (p. 178) and wild ginger root (p. 203) were used as a vitamin supplement for colds. Decoctions of whole barestem biscuitroot or stems and leaves were also taken for colds and fevers.

> **WARNING**
> All *Lomatium* species are edible, but as with all members of the Carrot family, these plants can be confused with poisonous relatives. They should be used only when they are positively identified.

OTHER USES: Long-distance runners sometimes chewed on desert-parsley seeds to prevent side aches. Barestem biscuitroot seed was burned to protect one from illness and evil spirits. Its leaves, seeds and stems were also used as scents or charms, and either the leaves or seeds were used as a lure for devil's club codfish.

DESCRIPTION: Perennial herbs with a parsley-like fragrance and leafy, branched crowns on long, often tuber-like taproots. Leaves usually divided 2–3 times into small or linear segments. Flowers small, borne in open, flat-topped clusters of smaller, round clusters, and bloom from April to July. Fruits flattened, winged, seed-like schizocarps about 5–15 mm long.

Barestem biscuitroot or **naked-stem desert-parsley** (*L. nudicaule*), which grows 20–90 cm tall, and nine-leaved desert-parsley have ultimate leaf segments at least 1 cm long, relatively broad (more than 5 mm). Grows on dry, rocky or grassy slopes at low elevations in southern BC and southwestern AB.

Nine-leaved desert-parsley (*L. triternatum*) grows 15–40 cm tall, has finely hairy, 1–10 cm long, linear (less than 5 mm wide), ultimate leaf segments, plus a whorl of bracts at the base of its yellow flower clusters. Grows on open foothill and montane slopes in southern BC and southwestern AB. See p. 424 for conservation status.

Most other species have small, short (less than 1 cm long) ultimate leaf segments.

Biscuitroot (*L. cous*) is a small plant (usually under 25 cm tall), with yellow flowers above whorls of broadly oval bracts. Grows on dry, open foothill and montane slopes in AB and SK (Cypress Hills). See p. 424 for conservation status.

Fern-leaved desert-parsley (*L. dissectum*) grows to 1.5 m tall, has yellow or purplish flowers, slender bracts and corky-winged fruits. Grows on dry, open foothill and montane slopes in southern BC, AB and SK. See p. 424 for conservation status.

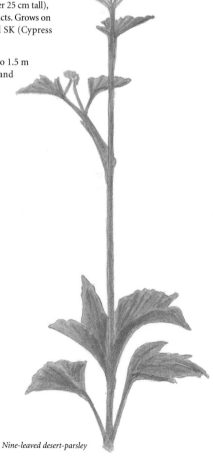

Nine-leaved desert-parsley

301

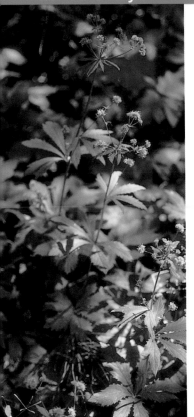

Snakeroot
Sanicula marilandica

MEDICINE: Snakeroot has been reported to have sedative properties, similar to those of valerians (p. 328), for soothing nerves and relieving pain. It was used by native peoples for treating lung, kidney and menstrual problems, rheumatism, syphilis and various skin conditions. It was also said to relieve pain and fever. Herbalists have used snakeroot to cleanse and heal the system, believing that it would stop bleeding, reduce tumours and heal wounds by seeking out the problem area and focusing its effects there. The root tea was used as a gargle for relieving sore throats and as a wash for treating skin problems. Its high tannin content makes it very astringent. The roots were traditionally used as poultices on snakebites, hence the common name snakeroot.

DESCRIPTION: Perennial herb, 40 cm–1.2 m tall, from clustered, fibrous roots. Leaves mainly basal, with long-stalked blades 6–15 cm wide, divided into 5–7 sharply toothed, finger-like leaflets. Flowers greenish white, tiny, forming flat-topped clusters (umbels) of several 1 cm wide, 15- to 25-flowered heads, in June. Fruits oval, seed-like schizocarps, 4–6 mm long, covered with hooked bristles. Grows on moist, rich, wooded sites in prairies and foothills across southern Canada. See p. 424 for conservation status.

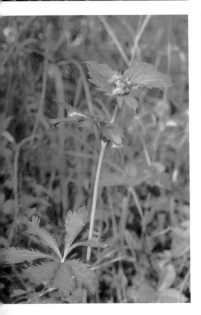

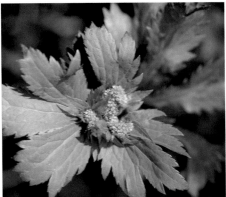

WARNING
Snakeroot roots contain irritating resins and volatile oils. Native peoples believed that snakeroot was a powerful medicine because when its roots were chewed, it could cause blistering on the lining of the mouth.

Wild Carrot

Daucus carota

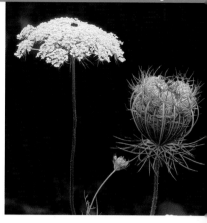

FOOD: Despite its listing as a noxious weed in North America, this introduced species, also known as Queen Anne's lace, is the ancestor of the garden carrot (*D. carota* ssp. *sativus*). Like the carrot, the taproot of Queen Anne's lace is edible when young, but becomes too tough and fibrous in its second year. It can be cooked like carrot or dried and roasted and used as a coffee substitute. The seeds are aromatic and can be used to flavour stews and salads.

MEDICINE: The crushed seeds have long been used as a form of contraceptive or "morning after" pill, its use for this first described by Hippocrates in the 4th century BC, and later by Dioscorides, Scribonius, Largus, Marcellus Empiricus, and Pliney the Elder. Scientific studies in mice confirm that seed extracts possess weak estrogenic activity and inhibit implantation of the fertilized egg. This is believed to be because the seeds block the synthesis of progesterone, a hormone involved in pregnancy. In contrast, another animal study found insignificant antifertility activity in pregnant rats fed oral doses of up to 4.5 g/kg body weight for 100 days. Considering that the plant also has both spasmodic and spasmolytic actions on smooth muscle tissues, the seed should not be consumed by pregnant women. Further research is required to establish the safety and efficacy of this potentially useful natural contraceptive. Traditionally, the root tea was used as a diuretic and prescribed for a number of disorders, including diabetes, edema, kidney and bladder disease, kidney stones, cystitis and expelling worms. This is likely due to the presence of terpinen-4-ol, the diuretic principle that also occurs in juniper. First Nations used an infusion of the plant as a wash to treat swelling, and a decoction of the root was taken by men for lack of appetite, general blood disorders, pimples and baldness.

OTHER USES: The aromatic seed oil has an orris-like scent that is sometimes used in perfumes and cosmetically in creams. The plant was used in rituals and spells to increase fertility in women and libido in men—odd, considering its contraceptive use.

DESCRIPTION: Variable, bristly stemmed, biennial herb, 30–90 cm tall. Leaves 5–20 cm long, finely dissected. Lacy, flat-topped clusters of tiny, cream-white flowers, with 1 dark reddish brown flower at the centre of the umbel, from May to October. Flowers compound umbels, 7.5–12.5 cm wide, with 3-forked bracts below. Fruit bristly, with the umbel contracting inward to become concave, resembling a bird's nest. This introduced Eurasian species grows in dry fields and waste places throughout Canada.

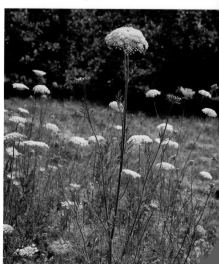

WARNING

Handling of the plant may cause dermatitis and blisters in certain individuals. The plant should not be confused with the deadly water-hemlocks (p. 411) or poison-hemlock (p. 410).

Mallows

Malva spp.

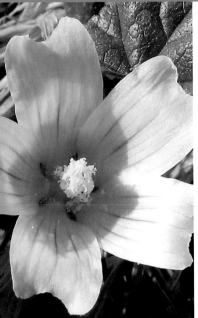

FOOD: Leaves and young shoots of mallow can be eaten raw (in salads) or cooked (as greens); they are said to be highly nutritious. It is better to use young leaves because old leaves become tough and bitter. The leaves are mucilaginous, so they can be used to thicken soups. The immature seeds can be eaten raw or cooked and are said to have a pleasant, nutty flavour. A tea can be made from the dried leaves. Flower buds, flowers and fruits are all edible; the fruits have a crisp texture and have been a common nibble for children in England for centuries.

MEDICINE: Most commonly, the leaves and flowers of the plant are used for medicine. Mallow is known for its anti-inflammatory properties and was often used by the Iroquois as a poultice to treat swellings of all kinds, broken bones and babies with swollen stomachs or sore backs. It was also used to treat fever in infants. The plant also has properties that soothe the skin and has been used as a salve. Due to its mucilaginous qualities, mallow helps soothe irritated tissues and has been used to treat respiratory system diseases or inflammation in digestive or urinary systems. It is said to be an excellent laxative for young children.

OTHER USES: Cream, yellow and green dyes can be made from the plant and the seedhead. The root has been used as a toothbrush.

DESCRIPTION: Annual or biennial, hairy-stemmed herbs, 20–60 cm tall, from taproots. Leaves alternate, long-stalked (several times the length of the blades), bluish green, 2–6 cm wide, short hairs on upper and lower leaf surfaces. Flowers 5-petalled, 1–3 in leaf axils along length of stem, flowering in April. Fruits round and flat, 5–8 mm in diameter, with 12–15 small, hairy, 1-seeded segments. All are introduced European species, often garden escapees, found in waste places, gardens, fields, roadsides and rail-

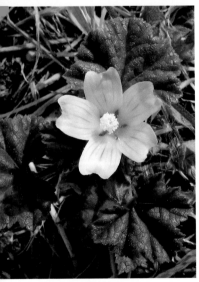

Common mallow (all images)

roads across southern Canada.

Musk mallow (*M. moschata*) has upper stem leaves that are finely dissected, and flowers with white to pink petals.

Common mallow (*M. neglecta*) has upper stem leaves that are 5-lobed and heart- to kidney-shaped, with pale pink or nearly white flowers, the petals 0.5–1.2 cm long.

High mallow (*M. sylvestris*) also has upper stem leaves that are 5-lobed and heart- to kidney-shaped, with bluish purple flowers with pink veins, the petals 1.5–2.5 cm long.

Pickerel Weed

Pontederia cordata

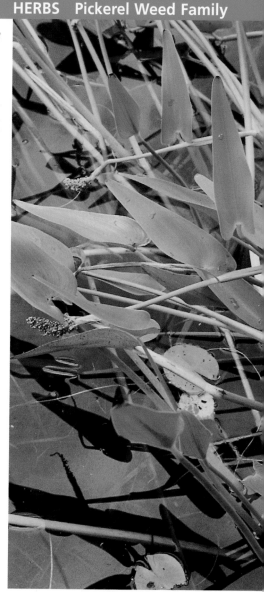

FOOD: The young leaves of pickerel weed can be eaten as a salad green or potherb, cooked like spinach or added to soups. The starchy seeds can be eaten fresh, dried or roasted and ground into a powder. They are said to have a nutty flavour and texture when raw.

MEDICINE: An infusion of the plant was used to prevent pregnancy or to treat illness in general.

OTHER USES: Pickerel weed is an attractive plant with beautiful flowers and is a popular addition to home water gardens. This plant often forms dense stands and protects from erosion. Each blooming flower lasts for only 1 day. The seed is eaten by waterfowl, and the rest of the plant is eaten by geese and muskrats. Fish and sometimes birds and small mammals use the large leaves for cover.

DESCRIPTION: Aquatic perennial arising from creeping rhizomes; grows to 90 cm tall. Leaves basal, arrowhead-shaped to lance-shaped, 10–20 cm long, shiny green, thick-spongy, with parallel veins on fleshy leaf stems. Flowers violet blue with 2 yellow spots, showy, orchid-like, 2.5 cm across, on stalks 60–90 cm tall, blooming from June to October. Fruit corky, oblong, 1-seeded. Found in swamps, lakes, ponds and river bottoms in ON, QC, NB, NS and PEI. See p. 424 for conservation status.

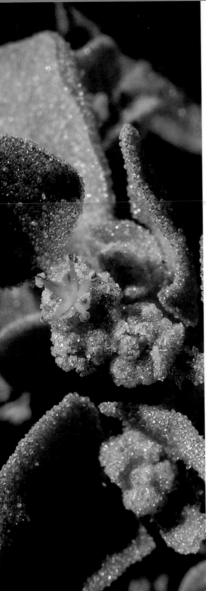

Silvery orache

Oraches
Atriplex spp.

FOOD: Garden orache, also called French spinach, was widely grown as a potherb and has escaped cultivation. The green leaves were once used in Italy to colour pasta. Almost all members of this genus have leaves that can be boiled or steamed for 10–15 minutes and served like spinach. Their bulk tends to reduce substantially, and their taste is slightly salty but mostly bland. They were traditionally served along with other greens such as sorrel to counterbalance sorrel's acidity. The seed is also edible and nutritious, containing a fair amount of vitamin A. Seeds were ground into a meal and used to thicken soups or added to flour when making bread and other baked goods. They are small, so harvesting a reasonable quantity is arduous. The seeds reportedly contain saponins that are potentially toxic (see **Warning**).

MEDICINE: The leaves of garden orache are diuretic, emetic and purgative and have historically been used to treat tiredness, nervous exhaustion and respiratory problems. The plant was considered a spring tonic by some, taken as an infusion to stimulate metabolism. The leaves were applied externally to relieve gout. The seeds, mixed with wine, were recommended as a cure for jaundice. The fruits and seeds were eaten to induce vomiting or as an effective laxative. In western and central Canada, the leaves of silvery orache were used as a fumigant in the treatment of pain. A cold tea of the entire plant was used to treat sickness caused by drinking contaminated water, or added to the water to purify it. A poultice of the leaves was applied externally to spider bites, and that of the chewed roots to sores and rashes. Stomachaches were treated with an infusion of the roots.

WARNING

Although this genus contains no known toxins, the seeds contain saponins that may be potentially poisonous if ingested in large quantities. The leaves are regarded as generally safe, although one report has found that consumption of large quantities caused photosensitivity. The plants tend to concentrate harmful nitrates in their leaves if grown where artificial fertilizers are used. Caution should be exercised.

OTHER USES: Australian researchers found that sheep that grazed on *Atriplex* species had higher than usual levels of vitamin E in their meat. This not only benefits the animal in protecting it from certain diseases, but also extends the shelf life and preserves the red colour of the meat. The seed of orache produces a blue dye. The wood has been used as fuel, and the plant is a potential source of biomass that has applications for fuel conversion.

DESCRIPTION: Small, weedy annuals or perennial herbs or shrubs (those described here are annual herbs) from taproots, 30–90 cm tall, sometimes silvery or mealy. Leaves 5–20 cm long, lower leaves usually opposite, upper leaves alternate, green or grey-green, shape variable. Flowers green, in interrupted spikes in axils, 2–7 mm long, from June to October. Fruiting spikes green becoming black, the fruits containing seeds 2.5–3 mm wide, brown or black. All 3 species described here grow in open, disturbed sites (roadsides, gardens, fields) at low to montane elevations. Many species of this genus are extremely tolerant of salt content in the ground and grow at the seashore and in the desert. See p. 424 for conservation status.

Silvery orache (*A. argentea*) is an erect, greyish green species, 15–80 cm tall, of open, saline sites, with lance-shaped, oval or triangular leaves. Found from southern BC to southern MB.

Garden orache (*A. hortensis*) is a larger, decumbent to erect, green species, (though the young leaves are usually mealy-white), 60 cm–2.5 m tall or long, with lance-shaped to oval leaves. This Asian species has escaped from gardens (where it's grown as a potherb) from BC to QC, and in YT.

Common orache (*A. patula*) is an erect or ascending, green species (though the young leaves are sometimes mealy-white), 5–80 cm tall, with broadly lance-shaped leaves. This introduced Eurasian species grows across Canada.

Silvery orache

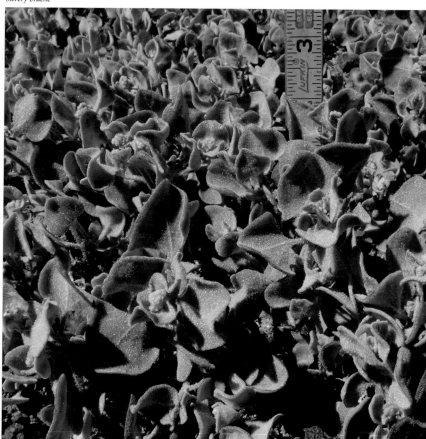

Lamb's-Quarters & Strawberry-Blite

Chenopodium spp.

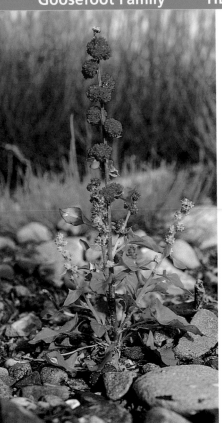

Strawberry-blite

FOOD: This genus includes several plants of minor to moderate importance as food crops, including quinoa (*C. quinoa*), kañiwa (*C. pallidicaule*) and the species included here, lamb's-quarters. The leaves are satisfactory eaten raw, although not too much should be consumed because of possible toxicity (see **Warning**). They are best cooked, boiled or steamed for 10–15 minutes and served like spinach. They are not as tasty as spinach, and lose quite an amount of bulk upon cooking, but they are excellent if stronger flavoured greens are added. If eaten with beans, they reportedly act as a carminative and prevent "wind" and bloating. The leaves are quite nutritious, containing (per 100 g dry weight) 260 calories, 24 g protein, 5 g fat, 45 g carbohydrates, 15 g fibre, plus significant amounts of calcium, phosphorus, iron and vitamin A. They were sometimes dried and stored for later use. The young inflorescences can be prepared in a similar fashion to broccoli. The seed is also edible and highly nutritious and can be boiled to make a breakfast gruel or ground and added to flour for bread. Seeds should be thoroughly washed and soaked overnight in water to remove any saponins. The sprouting seed is a tasty addition to any tossed green salad. The fruits of strawberry-blite are also edible and nutritious, but rather bland. They can be added to salads, eaten raw or cooked.

MEDICINE: The vitamin C content of lamb's-quarters leaves was recognized by First Nations, who ate the leaves to prevent scurvy and to treat stomachaches. A decoction of the entire plant was taken as a spring tonic, to improve circulation and to treat painful limbs and headaches. A decoction of the leaves, alone or with milk, was given to children to expel worms, and an infusion taken for rheumatism. The cold tea was recommended for diarrhea. The root was used for delayed menstrual periods and urethral itching. The leaves were applied topically as a wash or poultice on insect bites, burns, sunburn, rheumatic pain, swollen feet

> **WARNING**
> Saponins in the seeds are potentially toxic and these should not be consumed in excess. The plant also contains some oxalic acid, an antinutrient that can block absorption of certain nutrients, but oxalic acid is mostly removed during cooking. One report states that consumption of very large quantities of raw leaves can cause photosensitivity.

and vitiligo. The juice from the stem was applied to freckles and sunburns, while that of the root used in the treatment of bloody dysentery. Strawberry-blite was traditionally used in lotions for treating black eyes and head bruises. Lung congestion was treated with the juice expressed from the seeds and an infusion of the entire plant.

OTHER USES: Lamb's-quarters was wound into necklaces, stuffed in pillows and made into bags, baskets or tied to clothes as a scent. The stem was fashioned into a snake figurine as a charm for snake infection. A green dye is obtained from the young shoots of lamb's-quarters and a red one from the fruits of strawberry-blite. The crushed roots of lamb's-quarters were used as a mild soap substitute and hair wash.

DESCRIPTION: Succulent, erect, annual herbs from taproots, 30 cm–1 m tall. Leaves alternate, simple, toothed or lobed, sometimes with a greyish, mealy surface. Flowers minute, clustered, greenish, with petals absent and usually 2–5 sepals. Fruit a tiny achene, containing a single seed. See p. 424 for conservation status.

Lamb's-quarters (*C. album*) is a generally greyish, mealy species. Leaf shape variable, from triangular to lance-shaped, oval or diamond-shaped. Clustered spikes of minute flowers, which remain green. Grows in disturbed sites, roadsides and cultivated fields throughout Canada.

Strawberry-blite (*C. capitatum*) is a generally green species. Leaf shape triangular, with an arrowhead-shaped base. Tight, round clusters of tiny flowers, which in fruit become bright red and berry-like, about 12 mm across. Habitat and range are similar to lamb's-quarters.

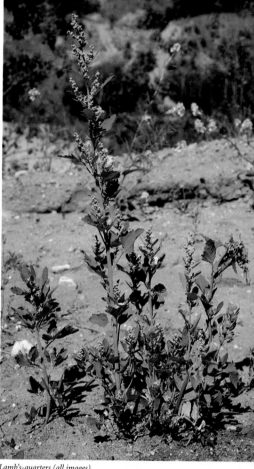

Lamb's-quarters (all images)

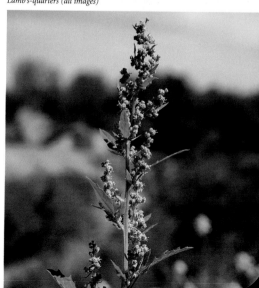

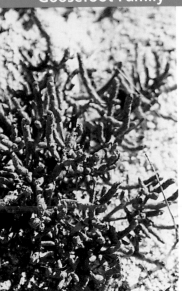

American glasswort (above)
Red glasswort (below)

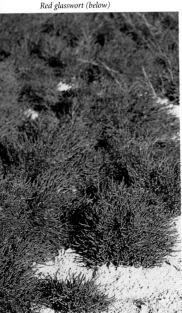

Glassworts

Salicornia spp.

FOOD: Sodium chloride, common table salt, is poisonous to most plants. Glassworts have adapted to saline conditions by integrating salt into their tissues in order to balance the osmotic pressures exerted by environmental concentrations. Consequently, the plants are very salty, and eating them raw without any other foods may irritate the throat. Only small nibbles should be taken. The plant can be added raw to spreads and salads and used as a garnish for cooked vegetable dishes and grains. Glasswort makes a good cooked vegetable dish on is own, sometimes called sea asparagus. It can be cooked for 10–15 minutes in soups, stews or other dishes. The young shoots make excellent pickles after first boiling them in their own salted water. They are available from spring to autumn, but the best time to collect is in late spring when the plant is most tender. The top 10 cm should be collected, leaving the bottom to produce new shoots. Glassworts can be dried, ground into a powder and used as a salt substitute. The seeds are rich in protein and produce a high quality edible oil. They are quite tiny, however, and are difficult to handle.

MEDICINE: American glasswort was used externally by Pacific First Nations to treat arthritic pain, rheumatism, aches, pains and swellings.

OTHER USES: A soap can be made from the ashes.

DESCRIPTION: Fleshy, erect, cylindrical, leafless, opposite-branched annual or perennial herbs, 5–25 cm tall, generally in salt marshes. Flowers minute, 1–2 mm wide, green, sunk into joints with only the stamens visible, from August to November. Fruits membranous bladders surrounded by fleshy flower scales.

Red glasswort (*S. rubra*) is an annual plant, erect, widespread. It's similar to American glasswort, but check the central flowers in each cluster: in this species, they're much longer than the lateral flowers. Grows in salt marshes and alkaline flats at low to montane elevations in all provinces and territories. See p. 424 for conservation status.

American glasswort (*S. virginica*) is a perennial, matted west coast species. Central flowers in each cluster are only a bit longer than the lateral flowers. Grows in marshes and along beaches at sea level along BC's coast.

> **WARNING**
> These plants have a high salt content and excess consumption may induce vomiting. Anyone following a low-sodium diet should avoid them altogether.

Pigweeds
Amaranthus spp.

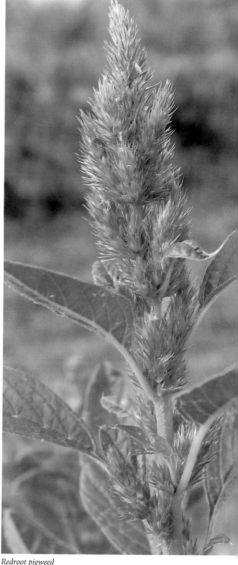

FOOD: Young pigweed plants or leaves were boiled and eaten as greens. Some First Nations boiled smooth pigweed leaves with squash flowers and corn in soup, while others mixed fresh redroot pigweed leaves with wild mustard (p. 215), plantain (p. 256), dock (p. 321) and stinging nettle (p. 312) leaves for salads. Seeds from both species were winnowed, roasted, finely ground and used in soups, breads and dumplings. In Mexico, a related species was domesticated as a cultivated crop and is known as grain amaranth. The grain has a high protein content with balanced amino acid composition.

MEDICINE: Plant infusions prepared with both species were used to help stomach problems, and leaves were used to relieve profuse menstruation. Redroot pigweed leaf infusions were also taken to reduce throat hoarseness.

OTHER USES: Short stem pieces from redroot pigweed were made into snake figurines to help with snakebite infections.

DESCRIPTION: Annual, invasive, introduced herbs, to 2 m tall, with a branched stem and alternate leaves to 15 cm long that are usually flat, with curly or wavy edges).

Smooth pigweed (*A. hybridus*) has a smooth stem that is sometimes reddish purple, but otherwise green. Leaves hairy, flowers borne in erect or ascending, green or reddish spikes. Abundant in waste places, agricultural fields and along railroads, roadsides and riverbanks in BC, MB, ON, QC and NS.

Redroot pigweed

Redroot pigweed (*A. retroflexus*) is a hairier plant with a reddish stem base and flower spikes that are usually erect and sometimes bent back at the tip. Widely distributed across southern Canada in agricultural fields, disturbed sites and wetlands.

Stinging Nettles

Urtica spp.

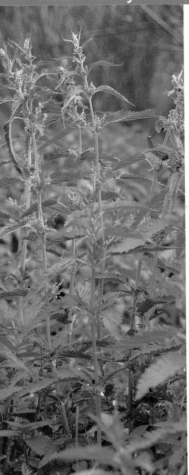

Stinging nettle

FOOD: Tender, young shoots are delicious boiled and eaten like spinach or added to soups and stews. The leaves and shoots can also be eaten raw (they taste rather nutty) if they are rubbed between 2 layers of a tea towel to remove the stinging spines, and they are a great addition to salads. Nettle purée and cream-of-nettle soup are tasty; spanakopita with nettles substituted for spinach is sublime. Nettle cooking water is high in iron and has been flavoured with lemon and sugar as a hot drink or with salt, pepper and vinegar as a soup base. Young plants can also be used to make nettle tea, wine or beer. Older plants become fibrous and gritty from an abundance of small crystals and are not as tasty (and can also cause urinary tract problems). Nettle juice or strong nettle tea produces rennet, which was traditionally used to coagulate milk to make junket or cheese. The roots, gathered in autumn to spring, can be cooked as a starchy vegetable.

MEDICINE: Nettle leaves are rich in protein, minerals, tannins, chlorophyll and vitamins A and C. All parts of the plant may be used, but for medicinal purposes, the leaves are best harvested in May before the flowers begin to form. The leaf tea is rich in iron, and it is also said to aid coagulation and the formation of hemoglobin. Studies suggest that nettle depresses the central nervous system, inhibits the effects of adrenaline, increases urine flow and kills bacteria. It has traditionally been used to treat a wide range of ailments, including gout, anemia, poor circulation, diarrhea and dysentery. Nettle tea was also believed to increase milk production in nursing mothers and to reduce bleeding associated with menstruation, bladder infections and hemorrhoids. Nettle leaf has been recommended for relieving bronchitis, asthma, hives, hayfever, kidney stones, urinary tract

WARNING

Always wear gloves and long sleeves when collecting nettles. The swollen base of each tiny, hollow hair contains a droplet of formic acid, and when the hair tip pierces you, the acid is injected into your skin. The acid can cause itching and/or burning for a few minutes to a couple of days. Rubbing nettle stings with the plant's own roots is supposed to relieve the burning. Dock leaves have also been recommended as an antidote. Nettle should not be used by pregnant women (it has caused uterine contractions in rabbits) or diabetics (it has aggravated the diabetic condition of mice). Most of the stinging compounds in nettles are destroyed by cooking or drying, but eating large quantities may still cause a mild burning sensation.

infections, premenstrual syndrome, gout, sciatica and multiple sclerosis. In mouthwashes, it can combat dental plaque and gingivitis.

The most important therapeutic use of nettle root today is for the enlarged prostate (benign prostatic hypertrophy or BPH). Nettle root has been used internally for difficulty in urination due to BPH, at the rate of 4–6 g/day of the dry cut root for infusions and other preparations (alcoholic tincture, native dry extract, fluid extract) for oral administration. BPH is mediated by hormonal interactions. The lipophilic fractions of the plant (sterols) are inhibitors of aromatase, the enzyme that converts testosterone to estradiol, a major contributing factor in BPH. The phenolics provide an additional benefit in BPH by their affinity to the human sex hormone binding globulin. Several double blind clinical trials with stinging nettle root (alone) have shown statistically signficant improvement in BPH compared to controls. Even better results are obtained in combination therapy with African plum (*Prunus africanum*) bark and saw palmetto (*Serenoa repens*) fruit extract.

Nettles have a long history of association with First Nations, particularly in coastal BC; stinging nettle was not widely eaten for food but rather used in medicine and technology. The Ojibwa used a tea of the roots as a diuretic and to treat urinary ailments. These plants are high in boron, which has been reported to elevate estrogen levels, thereby improving short-term memory and elevating the mood of people suffering from Alzheimer's disease. Urtication (stinging the skin with nettles) has been used around the world for centuries to treat rheumatism, arthritis, paralysis and, more recently, multiple sclerosis. Its effectiveness can vary greatly from one case to the next. The theory is that stinging could act as a counter-irritant, creating minor pain that tricks the nervous system into overlooking the deeper pain. The stingers also inject a mixture of chemicals into the skin including resin, acetylcholine and histamine. Some of these chemicals cause inflammation, which may trigger the body to release more of its own anti-inflammatory chemicals.

OTHER USES: First Nations used the fibrous stems of mature nettles to make important products such as twine, fishing and duck nets, snares, tumplines and even deer nets. Nettle fibres were used traditionally by Europeans to make fishing nets, rope, paper and cloth. When spun together with bird down, nettle fibre was used to make blankets and sleeping bags. The Cowichan people rubbed pigment on nettle thread and ran it under the skin with a fine hardwood needle to make tattoos. To Europeans, the fibres were considered superior to cotton for making velvet or plush, and more durable than linen. The roots can be boiled to make a yellow dye (red if boiled in urine) or a rinse for reducing hair loss. Roman soldiers, chilled with cold, rubbed their feet and hands with nettles to bring back the circulation. Nettles were traditionally dried to feed to livestock during the winter months when nutritional forage was not widely available. An infusion of nettles (dry or fresh) was given to livestock that was ill or anemic.

DESCRIPTION: Erect, annual or perennial herbs, armed with stinging hairs, with 4-sided stems. Leaves opposite, slender-stalked, the blades narrowly lance-shaped to oval, coarsely saw-toothed. Flowers greenish (sometimes pinkish), 0.5–2 mm long, with 4 tiny sepals and no petals, borne in hanging clusters from upper leaf axils, from April to September. Fruits seed-like achenes, 1–2 mm long.

Stinging nettle (*U. dioica*) is a large, rhizomatous perennial, to 3 m tall. Flowers in unisexual (male or female) clusters, on the same or on different plants. This native species grows on moist, rich, sites (alluvial floodplains, streamsides, avalanche tracks) and disturbed ground from low to subalpine elevations across Canada. See p. 424 for conservation status.

Dog nettle (*U. urens*) is a smaller, annual species, to 80 cm tall, from a taproot. Flowers in mixed clusters of male and female flowers. This introduced Eurasian species grows mostly on disturbed sites (roadsides, cultivated fields) from BC to NL, but apparently not in SK.

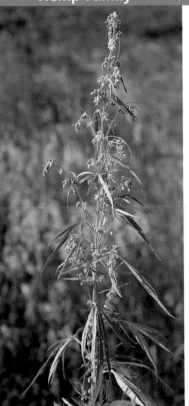

Hemp or Marijuana
Cannabis sativa

FOOD: Although botanically identical, hemp usually refers to the industrial form used for food and fibre, and marijuana to the psychoactive form used as a drug. Cultivated as a food source since the Palaeolithic Age (12,000 years ago), hemp seed is second only to soybeans in having a complete protein profile (containing 8 of the 9 essential amino acids), as well as providing both omega-3 and omega-6 essential fatty acids. The seed imparts a nutty flavour and was often eaten as a condiment or made into cakes and fried. Banned in 1938, the commercial cultivation, processing and sale of the industrial hemp seed was legalized in Canada in 1998, and has since found its way into many new food products, including pasta, tortilla chips, salad dressings, snack products and frozen desserts. It is also used as an ingredient in beer, with many Canadian breweries involved in production. The regulatory system for the commercialization of hemp is strict, ensuring that levels of the psychoactive compound, Δ^9-tetrahydrocannabinol (THC), remain below 0.3 percent of the weight of leaves and flowering parts (marijuana plants often have levels of 5 percent or more). While hemp foods were legalized in the US in 2001, production of the seed remains illegal, thereby stimulating the Canadian market for seed production. Today, about 95 percent of Canada's hemp products are destined for the US, a country whose founding document, the Declaration of Independence, was drafted on hemp paper.

MEDICINE: Marijuana is an ancient drug, used since prehistoric times for the treatment of all manners of disorders ranging from anthrax to whooping cough. The principal active component, THC, belongs to a class of chemicals called cannabinoids that are unique and unlike any other drug molecule, exhibiting features belonging to the stimulant, depressant,

---

WARNING

The production of marijuana for drug use is illegal throughout most of the world, although a 2007 decision in ON provincial court has ruled that criminal possession laws are unconstitutional. Smoking marijuana, like tobacco, is an important risk factor in the development of respiratory disease. Although unusual, dependency on the psychoactive effect of THC can develop, causing distinctive withdrawal symptoms that include restlessness, irritability, mild agitation, insomnia, sleep disturbance, nausea and cramping. The notion of marijuana as a "gateway" drug to harder, more harmful drugs cannot be supported or refuted with existing data. Overdoses of smoking cannabis are unpleasant, but not dangerous medically, causing symptoms of disorientation and delirium.

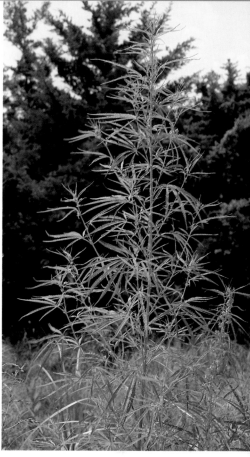

hallucinogen and antipsychotic categories of drugs. Cannabinoids are insoluble in water, thereby rendering medicinal teas ineffective. Rather, they are soluble in alcohol and oil (extraction with solvents results in hashish oil), and when eaten, are absorbed unevenly, causing difficulties in estimating correct dosage. Evidence-based medical science has shown that THC affects the brain (although how this occurs remains unclear), and that humans possess cannabinoid receptors throughout the body, suggesting that cannabinoids play a natural role in pain modulation, control of movement and memory. Accumulated data indicate that cannabinoid drugs have potential therapeutic value for symptoms such as pain relief, control of nausea and vomiting and appetite stimulation, making them well suited for conditions such as chemotherapy-induced nausea and AIDS wasting. Smoked marijuana on the other hand, is a crude THC delivery system that also delivers harmful substances (see **Warning**) and is not recommended for long term medical use. Smoking nevertheless causes a more acute effect that may be useful for certain patients.

Smoking marijuana is useful in the treatment of glaucoma, a condition of increased pressure within the eyeball that potentially leads to blindness, by acting on the cannabinoid receptors of the ciliary body of the eye, resulting in decreased intraocular pressure. The effect, however, is short-lived, and the frequency of smoking needed to sustain lowered pressure can result in systemic toxicity. Marijuana is also reported to reduce muscle spasticity associated with multiple sclerosis (MS). The abundant anecdotal reports that support this therapeutic use are not well-supported by clinical data; nevertheless, a cannabis extract has been approved as a prescription drug in Canada for the treatment of MS. Additional research is needed, rendered difficult by its political and social stigma as a recreational drug.

OTHER USES: A strong, durable fibre is obtained from the stem that has been used to make clothing, rope, coarse fabrics and paper. A drying oil, obtained from the seed, is used for lighting, soap making, paints and varnishes.

DESCRIPTION: Coarse, branching annual, 90 cm–3 m tall, with erect stems. Leaves palmately divided, with 5–7 lobes. Leaflets long (5–15 cm), coarsely toothed, lance-shaped, hairy and tapering. Clusters of small, greenish, unisexual flowers, 3 mm wide, in the leaf axils, from June to October. Grows in well-manured, moist farmyards and in open habitats, waste places and occasionally fallow fields and open woods, cultivated illegally across Canada.

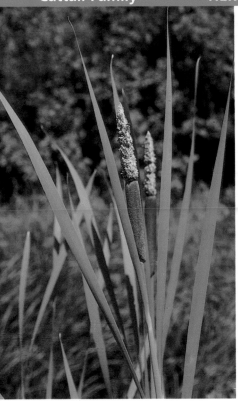

Common cattail

Cattails
Typha spp.

FOOD: The shoots, rhizomes and flower spikes of cattail are all edible but did not enjoy consistently widespread use by First Nations. The tender inner parts of young shoots (with the outer leaves removed) have been likened to celery (*Apium graveolens*) or asparagus (p. 174) and are good raw, steamed or stir-fried. Green flower spikes have been cooked and eaten like corn on the cob. The Ojibwa enjoyed the green flowers boiled or dried and used the pollen to make a flour. Oil- and protein-rich cattail pollen has been used to thicken sauces and gravies or mixed with flour to make muffins, biscuits, pancakes and cookies. It can be gathered by shaking pollen-laden spikes into a bag and sieving the powder. The starchy white core of the rhizomes was eaten raw, boiled, baked or pit-cooked, for example by the Lower Lillooet, Carrier and Chilcotin peoples. It was also dried and ground into flour, boiled to make syrup or fermented to make ethyl alcohol. The starch can be collected by peeling and crushing the rhizomes in water, straining out the fibres and washing the heavy white starch in several changes of water, carefully pouring off the water each time. The seeds were used in breads and porridges. Burning the fluff both separated and parched the seeds. The Woods Cree in SK ate cattails fresh and also dried the rhizomes over a fire to preserve them for winter use. They were consumed by almost all indigenous peoples of Eastern Canada as well. More recently, cattail seed has been suggested as a source of oil, with the by-products providing chicken feed.

MEDICINE: Boiled or raw rhizomes were pounded to a jelly-like paste and applied to sores, boils, wounds, burns, scalds and inflammations. Cattail was once used as a chew for treating coughs, and the rhizomes were recommended for increasing urination and for treating gonorrhea and chronic dysentery. Green flower spikes were eaten to relieve digestive disorders such as diarrhea. Rhizomes were steeped in water or milk to make medicinal teas for treating abdominal cramps, diarrhea and dysentery. Down from the flower spikes was also used, either dry or in salves, to heal burns, scalds and smallpox pustules. The sticky juice was rubbed on gums as a topical anesthetic when extracting teeth.

OTHER USES: Down from flower spikes provided stuffing for bedding and diapers and baby powder for infants. It was also used to stuff mattresses, pillows, sleeping bags and life jackets, and it provided tinder, insulation and soundproofing. Cattail quilts would not let water penetrate, so they were placed over mattresses and used for babies. The down was mixed with ashes and lime to make a cement that was said to be as hard as marble. The leaves were woven into bed mats, chair seats, baskets and water jugs, and they were also fashioned into toy figures of humans and ducks. Cattail mats, often several layers thick, covered tepees, sweat baths and Sundance lodges. Mats were sometimes hung in homes to bring rain and to protect the families and their animals from lightning. Cattail mats also played an important role in food preservation, providing a clean, dry surface for drying berries and root foods as well as serving as plates and dishes. Historically, cattail pollen was widely used in religious ceremonies, but as agriculture developed, it was replaced with corn (*Zea mays*) pollen. It can also be used in pyrotechnics to produce bright flashes of light. Cattail seeds were said to kill mice. Cattail stems have been used to make a type of glue, and the pulp can be made into rayon. Rhizomes and leaves were used for caulking boats and barrels.

DESCRIPTION: Emergent, perennial herbs with pithy stems from coarse rhizomes. Leaves sword-like, rather stiff and spongy. Flowers tiny, lacking petals and sepals, forming dense, cylindrical spikes, with yellow male flowers at the tip (soon disintegrating) and green to brown female flowers below, from June to July. Fruits tiny, seed-like follicles with a tuft of long hairs, borne in brown spikes. See p. 424 for conservation status.

Common cattail (*T. latifolia*) is a large plant (often over 1.5 m tall) with 8–20 mm wide leaves, and the male and female parts of its spikes are contiguous. Grows in calm water, shallow marshes, swamps and lake edges, often forming extensive patches, from BC and YT to the Maritimes and NL.

Narrow-leaved cattail (*T. angustifolia*) is smaller (1–2 m tall), with narrower (5–10 mm wide) leaves, and the male and female parts of its spikes are usually separated by a 1–5 cm gap. Grows in similar habitats but reduced range to common cattail, growing in BC and MB to NS and PEI.

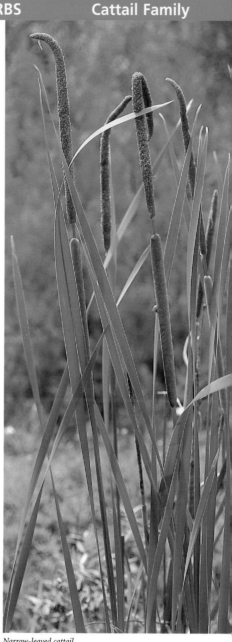

Narrow-leaved cattail

WARNING
Mature cattails are unmistakable, but be careful not to confuse young shoots with poisonous members of the Iris family, such as western blue flag. Plants in salty or stagnant water often have a bad flavour.

Arrowhead & Wapato

Sagittaria spp.

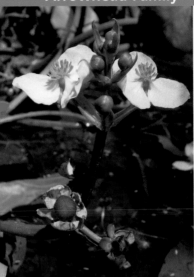

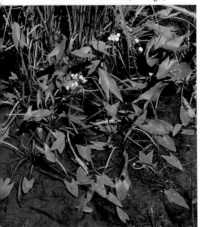

Arum-leaved arrowhead (all images)

FOOD: The entire rhizome of this aquatic plant is edible, but usually only the corms were used. Corms are said to have an unpleasant taste and to be unfit to eat raw, but when cooked, they taste like potatoes (*Solanum* spp.) or chestnuts (*Castanea* spp.). Served like potatoes, freshly harvested corms were roasted in hot ashes or pit-steamed, or dried ones were boiled. They were also made into candies when boiled down with maple syrup. Because the corms are easily separated from the main roots and float to the surface when dislodged, they were traditionally harvested by uprooting them by foot. Muskrats were said to scavenge arrowhead corms and store them in large caches where different tribes would appropriate them. Wapato was preferred over arum-leaved arrowhead because its corm is larger (2.5–5 cm long). Families often owned wapato sites and camped nearby for weeks, harvesting the crop. Raw, unwashed corms can keep for several months, but often they were cooked, sliced and dried for storage. The cooked stems are also said to be tasty.

MEDICINE: Arum-leaved arrowhead was eaten to relieve headaches, and wapato roots were steeped in hot water to make medicinal teas for relieving indigestion. Mashed wapato roots were applied to wounds and sores, and leaves were used as poultices to stop milk production. Wapato leaf tea was used to relieve rheumatism and to wash babies with fevers.

DESCRIPTION: Aquatic, perennial herbs, 20–50 cm tall, with a milky juice and spreading stolons bearing fleshy corms. Leaves all basal; emergent leaves arrowhead-shaped, submerged leaves grass-like; to 1 cm wide. Flowers white, with 3 broad petals, in whorls of 3 (usually), forming elongated clusters from June to September. Fruits flattened, short-beaked, seed-like achenes in round heads.

Arum-leaved arrowhead (*S. cuneata*) has emergent (arrowhead-shaped) leaf blades to 12 cm long on leaf stalks to 50 cm tall, and achene beaks tiny (less than 0.6 mm long) and erect (extending in the same direction as the body).

Wapato (*S. latifolia*) is a larger species with emergent (arrowhead-shaped) leaf blades to 25 cm long on leaf stalks to 90 cm tall, and achene beaks larger (1–2 mm long) and extending at right angles to the body.

Both species are widely distributed in calm waters from coast to coast. See p. 424 for conservation status.

WARNING

Some species of *Sagittaria* cause skin reactions.

•••

Wapato is much less common now because of livestock and development pressures. Cattle enjoy the leaves, and pigs eagerly root out the corms.

Northern Water-Plantain

Alisma triviale

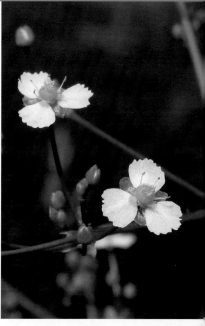

FOOD: The bulbous plant bases are eaten as a starchy vegetable. They can be eaten raw, but they have a very strong flavour and are more palatable thoroughly dried and cooked. The plant was also made into a tea and used by forest runners.

MEDICINE: Native peoples used the roots to make medicinal teas for treating lung and kidney problems and lame backs. They also applied the roots as poultices to bruises, sores, swellings, ulcers and wounds. In China, these plants are used to increase urine flow in the treatment of dysuria (painful urination), edema (water retention), bladder distention, diarrhea, diabetes and many other problems. Studies there have verified the diuretic action of these plants. Laboratory studies have also shown that water-plantain can lower blood pressure, reduce blood glucose levels and inhibit fat storage in the livers of experimental animals. Some Chinese people believe that these plants stimulate female reproductive organs and promote conception, whereas the seeds promote sterility. In Russia, it was believed that northern water-plantain would cure rabies.

DESCRIPTION: Semi-aquatic, perennial herb, with leafless flowering stems, 30 cm–1 m tall, from fleshy, corm-like bases. Leaves basal, oval to lance-shaped or oblong, with rounded or heart-shaped bases, on long, sheathing stalks. Flowers white, about 1 cm across, with 3 broad petals, short-lived, borne in several whorls that form elongated clusters, from June to September. Fruits flattened, grooved, oval, seed-like achenes to 3 mm long. Northern water-plantain grows in marshes and ponds from BC to NL. See p. 424 for conservation status.

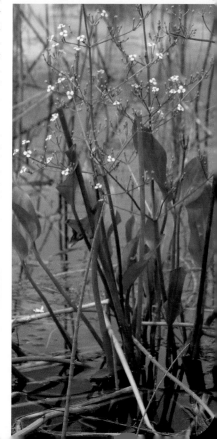

WARNING

Most herbalists consider these plants edible, but some sources describe them as poisonous to people or livestock. Grieve (1931) reported that the leaves of European plants were used as a rubefacient (to redden skin) and could even blister skin, so these plants may cause skin reactions in some people. Never eat aquatic plants from polluted water.

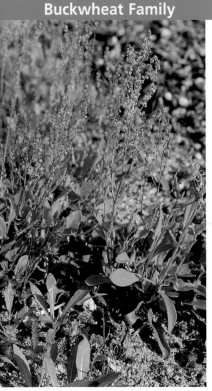

Sheep Sorrel
Rumex acetosella

FOOD: These tart leaves remain fairly tender until the plant flowers. They have been nibbled as a thirst-quenching trail snack or used to add zest to soups, salads and casseroles. They can also be boiled (sometimes requiring 1–2 changes of water, depending on how sour they are) and served as a hot vegetable. Sheep sorrel steeped in hot water and sweetened with honey can make a refreshing tea, and plants have also been simmered, strained and chilled to make a lemonade-like drink. Cucumber pickles, made with brine and large amounts of sheep sorrel, were considered a delicacy in the early 1900s.

MEDICINE: These nutritious plants, rich in vitamins A and C, were used as a spring tonic and a cure for scurvy. Poultices containing the roasted leaves or the plant juice have a long history as a folk-cure for cancer. The leaves were used to make gargles for treating mouth sores and sore throats, and they were sometimes dried, powdered and dusted onto sores. The leaves and roots were also said to lower fevers, stimulate appetite, reduce inflammation and increase urination. The roots were taken to slow menstrual bleeding, and the seeds were used to treat bleeding, diarrhea and dysentery. Some present-day herbalists consider sheep sorrel a blood alterative and liver stimulant, useful for treating skin problems and other metabolic imbalances. The plants contain compounds called anthraquinones, which have laxative, antibacterial and antifungal properties.

DESCRIPTION: Slender, hairless, annual or perennial herb, about 20–30 cm tall, with long-stalked, arrowhead-shaped leaves about 2–4 cm long. Flowers reddish (sometimes yellowish), male and female on separate plants, forming loose, branched clusters, from April to August. Female flowers have 3 scale-like sepals, whereas male flowers have 6 scale-like sepals. Fruits glossy, golden brown, 3-sided, seed-like achenes, closely enveloped in 3 valves. This European introduction grows in fields, grasslands and woodlands across Canada.

WARNING

Sheep sorrel, like its relative spinach (*Spinacia oleracea*), contains oxalates, which irritate the digestive tract and can be toxic, although a large quantity would have to be eaten to cause poisoning. Acid levels can be reduced by parboiling. Also, calcium helps to neutralize oxalates, so the hazard can be further reduced by serving sorrel with calcium-rich foods (e.g., in a cream sauce). Cooled ashes have been suggested as a possible emergency source of neutralizing calcium. Elderly people, small children and people with kidney problems, gout or rheumatism should not use plants with oxalates. People who are allergic to grass, tree or shrub pollen may also be sensitive to sheep sorrel pollen.

Docks

Rumex spp.

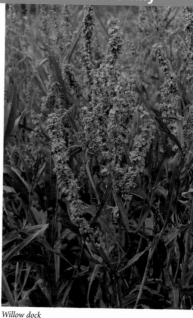

Willow dock

FOOD: All docks are said to be edible, curled dock being one of the best. Young leaves may be too sour to be eaten raw, but these plants remain tender for most of the growing season, providing an excellent cooked vegetable (likened to beet greens). Sometimes they require 1–2 changes of water, depending on how bitter they are. Docks often produce large quantities of fruit, which can be stripped from the plant and then winnowed (with much effort) to separate the outer hulls. The seeds have been boiled into mush or ground into flour or meal for addition to breads, muffins and gravies.

MEDICINE: Docks were often used interchangeably as medicines, but curled dock was one of the most widely recognized and used. The leaves are rich in protein, calcium, iron, potassium and vitamins. Curled dock can contain more vitamin C than oranges and more beta-carotene than carrots. Dried, powdered leaves were sometimes used as dusting powder, added to salves or applied as a paste to heal sores and reduce itching. Dock leaves can be rubbed on nettle (p. 312) stings to relieve the burning; they were also used to make gargles for treating mouth sores. Some present-day herbalists consider curled dock a liver stimulant and blood cleanser, useful for treating liver problems, swollen lymph nodes, sore throats, skin sores, warts and rheumatism. The root tea has been used to treat jaundice and post-hepatitis flare-ups; some believe it helps the body to eliminate heavy metals such as lead and arsenic. Dock plants contain anthraquinones, which have laxative and antibacterial effects and also stop the growth of ringworm and other fungi. Docks have been widely used as mild laxatives and in washes for treating fungal infections.

DESCRIPTION: Robust, often reddish, perennial herbs, 50 cm–1.5 m tall, from taproots. Leaves alternate, narrowly oblong to lance-shaped. Flowers small, reddish, with 3 net-veined, heart-shaped scales (valves), hanging in dense, branched clusters, from June to August. Fruits smooth, seed-like achenes about 2–2.5 mm long, covered by the flower valves.

Curled dock (*R. crispus*), a European introduction, has wavy, curled leaf edges, wedge-shaped to rounded leaf bases, unbranched stems (below the flower cluster), and each valve has a large, oval bump (tubercle).

Western dock (*R. occidentalis*) has wavy to slightly curled leaf edges and notched leaf bases, unbranched stems, and its valves lack tubercles.

<table>
<tr><td>

WARNING

These plants, like sheep sorrel (p. 320), contain oxalates; see Warning for sheep sorrel. Docks produce large amounts of airborne pollen that can cause allergic reactions, such as hayfever and asthma.

</td><td>

Willow dock (*R. triangulivalvis*) has plane or only slightly wavy leaf edges, tapered leaf bases, branched stems, and most valves have a lance-shaped bump (tubercle). See p. 424 for conservation status.

All 3 species grow in waste places, roadsides, cultivated fields, meadows and ditches across Canada. Willow dock and western dock are also found farther north or at slightly higher elevations.

</td></tr>
</table>

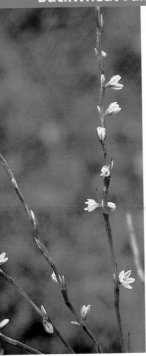

Mountain knotweed

Knotweeds & Smartweed

Polygonum and *Persicaria* spp.

FOOD: Knotweeds and smartweed belong to the Buckwheat family, and, like buckwheat, they have seeds that can be eaten whole or pounded into meal and added to breads and sauces. The plants have also been cooked and eaten, though flavour and texture vary greatly with age, species and habitat. Always test a little for palatability before gathering these plants.

MEDICINE: Common knotweed has a high tannin content and astringency; the juice was used to stop bleeding, especially nosebleeds. Teas made from these plants were applied to hemorrhoids to stop bleeding and as a foot and leg soak for rheumatism; they were taken internally to relieve diarrhea, fever, chills and stomach pain and to treat kidney problems and heart trouble. A decoction of the plant was used as a poultice for pain, headaches and poison-ivy (p. 395). An extract made from oak bark and common knotweed was used as a substitute for quinine. There is a long history of the use of knotweeds, including common knotweed, for treating various forms of cancer.

OTHER USES: Elizabethans believed that if the sprawling plants of common knotweed were eaten, they would stunt growth. The Iroquois rubbed the plant over horses to keep the flies away.

DESCRIPTION: Slender, usually annual herbs with sheathing leaf bases (at least when young) and swollen joints. Leaves alternate, lance-shaped. Flowers inconspicuous, green to white to pinkish, with 5 sepals and no petals, borne in small clusters of 1–4 at leaf axils and in loose, slender spikes, blooming from May to October. Fruits small, brown to black, smooth achenes.

Common smartweed (*Persicaria hydropiper*) grows to 1 m tall, has greenish white flowers on a nodding spike, and petals covered with small, yellow glands.

Spotted knotweed (*Persicaria maculosa*) grows to 1 m tall, has pink to rose flowers, and typically has a purple splotch near middle of leaf blade.

Common knotweed (*Polygonum aviculare*) has spreading stems, to 1 m long, that lie on the ground, small, blue-green, oblong leaves, white flowers and erect fruits.

All three of these species were introduced from Europe and are found in moist meadows, fields, swamps and disturbed areas across Canada. The names are a bit confusing: *Persicaria hydropiper* used to be known as *Polygonum hydropiper*, and *Persicaria maculosa* as *Polygonum persicaria*.

Mountain knotweed (*Polygonum douglasii*) is a native species with erect, 10–40 cm tall stems, oval lower leaves, lance-shaped upper bracts and downward-pointing fruits. Grows on dry slopes in prairies to subalpine zones from BC to QC. See p. 424 for conservation status.

WARNING

Although none of these species is considered poisonous, their sap is often quite acidic, and raw plants can cause intestinal disturbance and diarrhea when eaten in large quantities. Some plants contain the toxin hydrocyanic acid. People with sensitive skin should avoid knotweed.

Bistorts

Bistorta spp.

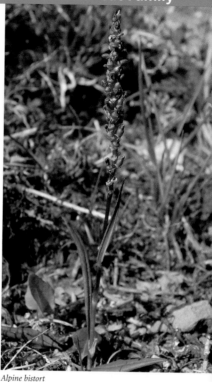

Alpine bistort

FOOD: Indigenous peoples ate these starchy rhizomes raw, boiled in stews and soups or steeped in water and then roasted or dried and ground into flour for bread. The rhizomes can have a pleasant taste, similar to that of almonds or water chestnuts, but occasionally they contain large amounts of tannic acid (as much as 20 percent), making them quite bitter. Mild rhizomes have been suggested as a substitute for raisins or nuts in baking. The leaves and shoots are also edible, with a pleasing tart taste, though flavour and texture vary with age, species and habitat. They have been eaten raw or cooked as a potherb, but the mature stems are usually tough. Like their relative rhubarb, bistorts can be sweetened with sugar and cooked as a dessert or made into jam. The seeds are also edible. They have been roasted whole or ground into meal or flour for adding to breads or thickening stews. The tiny bulblets produced by alpine bistort have a pleasant nutty flavour and can be eaten raw, as a trail nibble or cooked in soups and stews.

MEDICINE: Dried, powdered roots or alcohol or water extracts from the roots are very astringent. They have been used as washes, gargles, douches and enemas to stop bleeding, reduce inflammation and combat infection. These preparations have been used to treat cuts, abrasions and other minor skin problems, infected gums and mouth sores, pimples, measles, insect stings and snakebites. They were also taken internally to treat jaundice and intestinal worms. Bistorts are rich in vitamin C, and the shoots and/or roots were eaten to prevent and cure scurvy.

DESCRIPTION: Erect, perennial herbs with thick rhizomes, usually growing at higher elevations. Leaves alternate, mainly basal, elliptic to lance-shaped, with a sheath (fused stipules) at the base of each stalk, stem leaves generally smaller and fewer and unstalked. Flowers small, with 5 oblong, white or pinkish sepals and no petals, forming a single, dense, spike-like cluster, from May to September. Fruits smooth, 3-sided, seed-like achenes. See p. 424 for conservation status.

American bistort (*B. bistortoides*) is 20–70 cm tall, with showy (at least 1 cm thick) spikes that produce shiny, pale brown achenes (no bulblets). Found in moist to wet meadows and streambanks in subalpine and alpine zones in southern BC and southwestern AB.

Alpine bistort (*B. vivipara*) is 10–25 cm tall, with narrow (5–8 mm thick), white flower spikes producing dull brownish achenes near the tip and vegetative bulblets near the base. Found in moist woods, meadows and streambanks in montane to alpine zones across Canada, except PEI.

Note: In many books these species are still placed in the genus *Polygonum*.

> **WARNING**
> Although no *Bistorta* species is considered poisonous, the sap is often quite acidic, and raw plants can cause intestinal disturbance and diarrhea when eaten in large quantities.

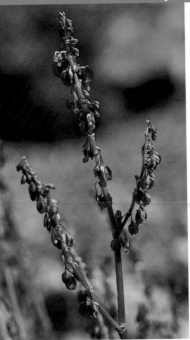

Mountain Sorrel
Oxyria digyna

FOOD: The leaves are tender and rather fleshy, with a sharp, almost vinegary flavour. They make a refreshing, thirst-quenching snack on the trail or a tasty addition to salads and sandwiches. They have also been chopped and soaked in water and then sweetened with sugar to make a drink like lemonade. Mountain sorrel plants are sometimes cooked as a potherb or puréed as a soup thickener. They can make delicious cream soups and purées and can add zip to fish, rice and vegetable dishes. Some indigenous peoples fermented mountain sorrel, which was dried or stored in seal oil for winter use. Others boiled the plants with berries and salmon roe until the mixture thickened. They then poured the mixture about 2 cm thick into frames, where it dried as cakes. These cakes were often an important trade item. The boiled leaves, sweetened with sugar and thickened with flour, are said to taste like stewed rhubarb. These plants will produce succulent leaves year after year if their rhizomes are left undisturbed in the ground. The fruits are also said to be edible. "Sorrel" is derived from the French word *surelle*, meaning "sour," describing the acidity of the leaves; *Oxyria*, the genus name, means "acid-tasting."

MEDICINE: Mountain sorrel is rich in vitamins A, B and C, and it was widely used to prevent and cure scurvy. It was also taken internally or used in poultices and washes to treat diarrhea, sores, ulcers, rashes, itching, ringworm and even cancer. Some recommend the leaves for easing the itch of mosquito bites.

DESCRIPTION: Tufted, hairless, often reddish, perennial herb, about 10–20 cm tall, from fleshy taproots or rhizomes. Leaves mostly basal, long-stalked, kidney-shaped to heart-shaped, 1–4 cm across. Flowers greenish to reddish, to 2.5 mm long, with 4 sepals and no petals, hanging on slender stalks, forming 2–15 cm long, branched clusters, from July to September. Fruits reddish, broadly winged, lens-shaped, seed-like achenes, 3–6 mm wide. Grows on moist, open sites, gravel bars, mudflats, tundra and crevices in rocky outcrops in BC, AB, YT, NT, NU, QC, NS and NL. See p. 424 for conservation status.

> **WARNING**
> These plants should be eaten in moderation. They contain oxalates, which are toxic when consumed in large quantities (see Warning under sheep sorrel, p. 320).

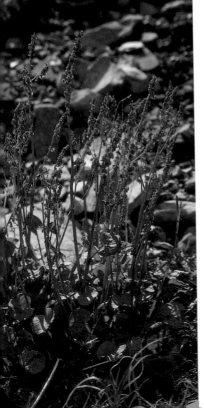

Avens

Geum spp.

FOOD: Water avens was sometimes called chocolate root or Indian chocolate; this was likely due to the practice of making chocolate-like drinks from its aromatic root. The root can also be used as a seasoning. The leaves of large-leaved avens are said to be edible.

MEDICINE: Both large-leaved avens and water avens were used for a variety of medical ailments and were valued for their astringent properties. A decoction of large-leaved avens root was taken to treat stomach pain, excess acid, teething sickness (when combined with other herbs), toothaches and sore throats. The roots were also boiled for a steam bath to treat rheumatism. A poultice of chewed, bruised or boiled leaves was applied to boils and cuts, while a leaf tea was taken as a diuretic and applied as an eyewash. The plant was often chewed during labour, after childbirth to heal the womb and as a contraceptive. Large-leaved avens was chewed by the Quileute and Klallam during labour because the blooming period of these plants coincided with the time that seals gave birth to their pups. Cowichan men in BC would chew leaves and feed them to their pregnant wives to straighten their womb and help with delivery. The roots of water avens were used for spitting of blood, diarrhea, dysentery, coughs (especially in children), fevers, indigestion, hemorrhages, menstrual disorders, intestinal worms and stomach ulcers. The plant was applied externally as a wash to remove spots, freckles and "eruptions" from the face. Water avens has been a popular remedy in pulmonary consumption, simple dyspepsia and diseases of the bowels. A study has shown this species to have antimicrobial properties. *Geum* species contain gein, a phenolic glycoside that may be the antimicrobial principle. Another common name for water avens is cure-all.

OTHER USES: Large-leaved avens has small, brown, hooked fruits that catch easily on clothing and hair; the Nuxalk name for them is lice. The crushed seeds were used as perfume by the Blackfoot. The dried root of water avens is said to repel moths.

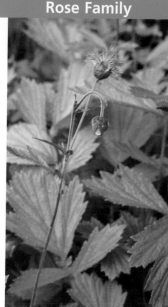

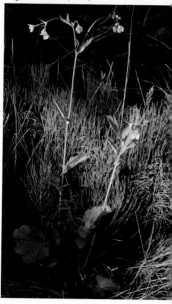

Water avens (above)
Large-leaved avens (below)

DESCRIPTION: Perennial herbs with hairy stems from short rhizomes, to 1 m tall. Basal leaves pinnately divided, stem leaves alternate, smaller, variously toothed or lobed. Flowers 2–2.5 cm across, single or in a few-flowered cluster. Fruits clusters of achenes. See p. 424 for conservation status.

Large-leaved avens (*G. macrophyllum*) has erect flowers with spreading, yellow petals and green sepals. Found in open forests, moist meadows, streamsides, roadsides and thickets across Canada.

Water avens (*G. rivale*) has nodding flowers with orange-pink to yellow and purple-veined petals and purple or reddish sepals. Found in streambanks, marshes and wet ground in all provinces.

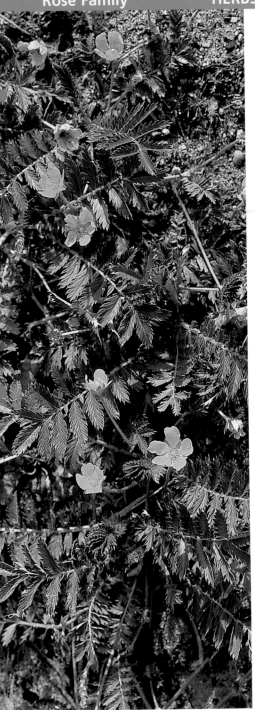

Silverweed

Cinquefoils & Silverweeds

Potentilla spp.

FOOD: The roots of Pacific silverweed were a staple food for all coastal First Nations in BC. They were typically dug in large quantities in autumn (but also in winter and spring), after the leaves had died back. The roots were most commonly dug by women using digging sticks; one woman would have to dig for many days to gather enough roots for the winter's food. Cooking methods included steaming in a box for smaller quantities or pit-cooking for larger quantities (they would cook for 12 hours). The roots would be eaten right away or dried for winter use. To dry them, they would be spread on rocks or mats in the sun. If eaten right away, they would be dipped in oil (eulachon, whale or seal) or eaten with fermented dog-salmon eggs, along with duck, meat or fish, at family meals or large feasts. Pacific silverweed has higher levels of calcium, magnesium, iron, copper and zinc than the common potato. Silverweed was also eaten by indigenous peoples in BC. It was pit-cooked and dried as well and was some-times mixed with sugar and eulachon grease and eaten as dessert.

MEDICINE: White cinquefoil roots were taken by women after childbirth and also used as a treatment for dysentery. The root was dried and powdered, and either moistened and applied to cuts as a poultice or pricked into the temples or placed in nostrils to treat a headache. An infusion of Canadian cinquefoil roots were used to treat diarrhea. A poultice of the boiled roots of Pacific silverweed was mixed with oil and applied to sores and swellings. The root juice was used as wash for inflamed eyes.

OTHER USES: Silverweed and Pacific silverweed were common trade items for indigenous peoples in BC. In some areas, individuals or families owned certain areas of the plants, and passed these down to subsequent generations.

DESCRIPTION: Perennial herbs with leaves basal and on the stem, usually pinnately compound. Flowers solitary or several in small clusters, often yellow, 1.5–2 cm wide. Fruits flattened achenes on a rounded receptacle. These species go by many scientific names; caution is advised. See p. 424 for conservation status.

Silverweed (*P. anserina*) is a herb, to 15 cm tall, with strawberry-like stolons with flowers single on leafless stalks. Leaflets usually covered with long, white, silky hairs, giving it a silvery appearance (leafstalks and stolons hairy too); achenes corky or grooved along back. Found on gravelly shores or flats throughout Canada.

Pacific silverweed (*P. egedii*) is similar to silverweed, and in some books is treated as a subspecies of it. Leaflets usually covered with shorter hairs on the undersurface (leafstalks and stolons usually have no hairs); achenes smooth. Found on coastal sands, salt- and freshwater marshes, river estuaries and floodplains across northern Canada and southward along the coasts.

White cinquefoil (*P. arguta*) is a herb that lacks stolons and has several flowers on leafy stalks. It's a taller plant (30–80 cm tall), the stems covered with fine, sticky, brownish hairs. Found on dry to moist, open sites (meadows, slopes and open forests) across Canada except PEI, NS and NL.

Canadian cinquefoil (*P. canadensis*) is a herb that lacks stolons and usually has a single flower on leafy stalks. It's a smaller plant (5–15 cm tall) with densely silver, hairy stems. Found in dry woods and open fields from ON to NL.

Silverweed

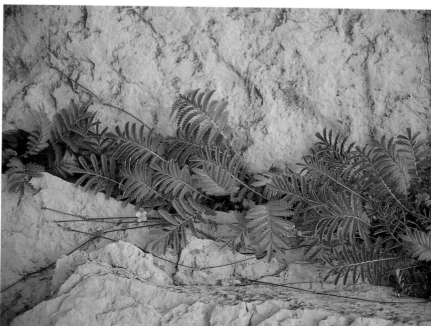

Valerians

Valeriana spp.

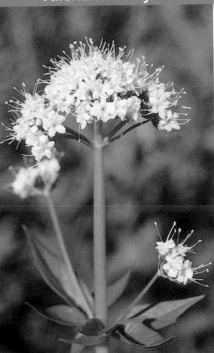

Sitka valerian (all images)

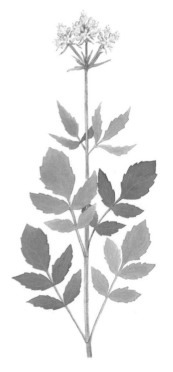

FOOD: Edible valerian was a staple food for some First Nations. The large, sweet-tasting roots were usually buried in fire pits and cooked for about 2 days. They were also boiled for long periods in soups and stews, and cooked roots were sometimes dried and ground into flour. The peculiar smell (like old gym socks, due to the presence of valeric acid) and taste of the raw roots is offensive. Prolonged cooking, however, removes most of this taste and odour. The seeds were sometimes eaten raw but were said to be better parched.

MEDICINE: Valerian root has been used for centuries as a sleep aid and mild sedative with fewer side effects than synthetic sedatives. Pharmacological and clinical studies have shown valerian extracts to be an effective sedative. Valerian is also said to have anti-bacterial, antidiuretic and liver-protective properties. All species can be used in much the same way, but some are stronger than others. Sitka valerian and marsh valerian, for example, are considered much stronger than common valerian, and edible valerian is about half as strong. The Alaskan Tlingit, whose name for this plant means "medicine that stinks," applied crushed roots to a mother's nipples when weaning a child, rubbed them on sore muscles or blew them onto animal traps for luck. Valerian root has generally been recommended for relieving stress-induced anxiety, insomnia and muscle tension. It has also been used to treat menstrual problems, epileptic seizures, Saint Vitus' dance and various ner-

> **WARNING**
> Large doses can cause vomiting, stupor and dizziness. The roots of edible valerian were said to be poisonous unless they had been properly prepared (i.e., cooked for 2 days). Valerian tea should never be boiled. Constant use over a long period of time can cause emotional instability and depression. Many people find the strong odour of these plants (dried, frozen or bruised) nauseating.

vous disorders. Common valerian was widely used during WWII to calm nervousness and hysteria. Native peoples rubbed the chewed or pounded roots onto the head and temples to relieve headaches and applied them to the bodies of people suffering from seizures. The roots were also used in poultices to cure earaches and to heal cuts and wounds. Powdered roots were added to smoking mixtures to relieve cold symptoms. Commercial valerian is standardized to valerenic acid content, although this may not be the main active principle.

OTHER USES: The Shuswap, Gitksan and Carrier peoples used preparations of valerian roots, sometimes mixed with grease, as perfume for the face and hair and as a disinfectant. Hunters washed their bodies with valerian, believing that this smell would make the deer tamer and easier to approach. Some tribes such as the Thompson in BC used dried valerian leaves and roots to flavour tobacco (p. 240). Valerian was used as a perfume in Europe in the 1500s and in the Orient. Cats and rats are said to be very fond of the smell and will dig up the plants and roll on them. Valerians are appreciated in gardens for their ornamental flowers and scent, which also attract butterflies and hummingbirds. Sitka valerian is responsible for the strong, sour odour detected in subalpine meadows after the first frost.

DESCRIPTION: Strong-smelling, perennial herbs with 4-sided stems and opposite leaves. Flowers pinkish to white, tubular, 5-lobed, forming dense (usually), branched clusters. Fruits ribbed, seed-like achenes, 2.5–6 mm long, tipped with many feathery hairs.

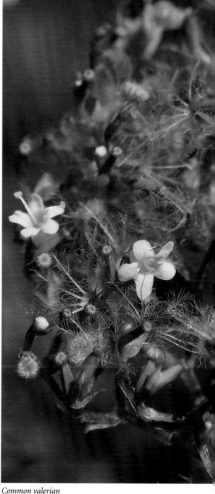

Common valerian

Edible valerian (*V. edulis*) has a thick taproot, thick, parallel-veined leaves and egg-shaped fruits. Grows in moist meadows from southern BC to ON. See p. 424 for conservation status.

These next 3 species have fibrous roots (no taproot), thin, net-veined leaves and lance-shaped to oblong fruits.

Marsh valerian (*V. dioica*) grows 10–40 cm tall, has shorter (1–3 mm long) flowers, undivided basal leaves and 9- to 15-lobed stem leaves. Grows in moist meadows and streambanks at low to high elevations across Canada, but not in NS or PEI. See p. 424 for conservation status.

Common valerian (*V. officinalis*) grows to 1.2 m tall with a smooth, hollow, furrowed stem. Basal and stem leaves pinnate; leaflets in 7–10 pairs, lance-shaped, coarsely serrated. European native naturalized along roadsides and other disturbed sites in southern BC and from MB to NS.

Sitka valerian (*V. sitchensis*) grows 30–90 cm tall, has longer-lobed (4–8 mm long) flowers and 3- to 5-lobed leaves. Grows in moist meadows, streambanks, forests and avalanche tracks at mid- to alpine elevations in central YT, NU, BC, western AB, southern ON, QC and NB. See p. 424 for conservation status.

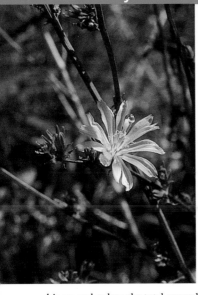

Chicory
Cichorium intybus

FOOD: The leaves can be eaten raw in salads but become very bitter with age and with exposure to sunlight. Green leaves usually require at least 1 change of water during cooking. Chicory is sometimes sold as a tangy (though bitter) flavouring for soups and stews. Young, white, underground parts or young plants grown in darkness are best. Young plants make an excellent cooked vegetable. Belgian endive is a variety of *C. intybus*. Chicory roots can be eaten raw, boiled or roasted. They are said to have a carrot-like flavour when young. More often, however, they are split, dried, roasted until brown throughout and ground to make a coffee substitute. Use about 1½ tsp per cup; if it is mixed with coffee, use 2 parts coffee to 1 part chicory and reduce the total grounds by one-third. The roots are best collected before or well after the plants have flowered. The flowerheads have been added to salads, pickled or cooked in soups and stews. Chicory is grown commercially as a source of fructose and maltol (a sugar enhancer).

MEDICINE: These plants, also called blue sailors, are rich in vitamins A and C. Chicory root tea/coffee is reputed to improve appetite and stimulate bile secretion and urination. Historically, chicory root tea was used to treat liver problems, gout, skin infections, rheumatism, fevers, inflammation, nausea, lung problems, typhoid and cancer. Mashed roots were used in poultices to heal sores from fevers and venereal disease. Studies have shown chicory root extracts lower blood sugar and have slightly sedative, mildly laxative, antibacterial, antimutagenic, liver-protective and anti-inflammatory effects. Chicory slowed and weakened the pulse of test animals, so it has been suggested for study in the treatment of heart problems. The flowers were used in eyewashes for treating inflamed eyelids.

DESCRIPTION: Perennial herb, 30 cm–1.5 m tall, with spreading branches, milky sap and deep taproots. Leaves mainly basal, dandelion-like, 8–20 cm long. Flowerheads blue (rarely white), about 3–4 cm wide, with ray flowers only and 2 rows of involucral bracts, essentially stalkless, single or in twos or threes, from July to October. Fruits hairless, 5-sided, seed-like achenes 2–3 mm long, tipped with tiny scales. This introduced Eurasian weed grows in fields, disturbed ground and roadsides throughout Canada.

> **WARNING**
> Excessive and/or prolonged use of chicory may cause sluggish digestion and damage to the retinas. Some people develop rashes from contact with chicory coffee. People with gallstones should consult a doctor before using chicory.

Salsifies

Tragopogon spp.

FOOD: The thick, fleshy roots of all 3 species included here, collected before the flower stalks appear, can be eaten raw, roasted, fried or boiled, but those of the cultivated species (common salsify) are the largest and tastiest. They are said to taste like parsnips. Salsify roots have also been dried, ground and added to cakes, or roasted until they are dark brown, ground and used as a coffee substitute. Tender young leaves, buds and flowers have been added to salads or served as a cooked vegetable. The young stalks and root crowns can be gently simmered, like asparagus (p. 174) and artichokes (*Cynara scolymus*), respectively. The seeds can be used to make tasty sprouts.

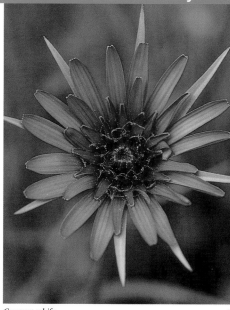

Common salsify

MEDICINE: These plants were used for many years to relieve heartburn and to stimulate urination (especially in the treatment of kidney stones). The milky juice was taken to cure indigestion and was applied to dressings to stop oozing and bleeding of sores and wounds. Common salsify tea was used as a drink or lotion to treat the bites of mad coyotes on both humans and livestock.

OTHER USES: Some tribes gathered the rubbery sap from broken stems and leaves, dried it and rolled it into balls, and chewed it like gum.

DESCRIPTION: Mostly biennial, 20 cm–1 m tall herbs with milky sap. Stems erect, bearing many slender, grass-like leaves 5–50 cm long, with clasping bases. Flowerheads about 5–6 cm across, with ray flowers only and a single row of involucral bracts, borne singly, from April to August. Fruits slender, spiny, seed-like achenes, each with a slender, stalk-like beak bearing a tuft of feathery bristles, forming dandelion-like seedheads to 10 cm wide.

Yellow salsify (*T. dubius*) has enlarged upper stalks, large (25–40 mm long) achenes and about 13 involucral bracts, which are longer than the yellow flowers.

Common salsify or **oyster plant** (*T. porrifolius*) has enlarged upper stalks, large (25–40 mm long) achenes and about 8 involucral bracts, which are longer than the blue flowers.

Meadow salsify (*T. pratensis*) has slender upper stalks, small (15–25 mm long) achenes and about 8 involucral bracts, which are shorter than the yellow flowers.

All 3 species are European weeds that grow on disturbed sites in all provinces, less commonly in the territories.

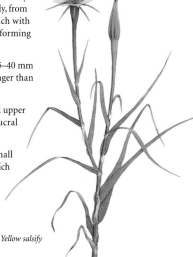

Yellow salsify

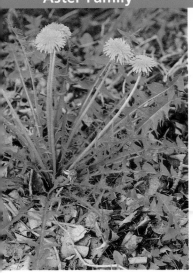

Common Dandelion
Taraxacum officinale

FOOD: All parts of common dandelion are edible. Young leaves have been used in salads (fresh or cooked and chilled) or served hot as a cooked vegetable—scalloped, baked or added to meat dishes and soups. They can also be mixed in a blender with tomato juice, Worcestershire sauce and Tabasco to make a vitamin-rich cold drink. Older leaves or leaves growing in sunny areas are especially bitter. Bitterness can be reduced by growing plants away from light (under straw or baskets), by removing the leaf midveins and by boiling the plants in at least 2 changes of water. The roots, dug in spring or autumn, peeled, sliced and cooked in 2 changes of water with a pinch of baking soda, have been used as a cooked vegetable, similar to parsnips. Dandelion roots can also be used raw in salads or can be dried, roasted slowly until dark brown throughout and ground to make a coffee substitute (though generally considered inferior to coffee made with chicory, p. 330). The flower petals produce a highly esteemed, delicately flavoured, pale yellow wine. They can also make a pretty addition to pancakes. Unopened buds can be eaten raw in salads, cooked in pancakes and fritters or pickled. The chewy seeds (without their fluffy parachutes) have been eaten as a nibble, ground into flour or used to grow sprouts.

MEDICINE: Dandelions are rich in vitamins A, C, E and B-complex, iron, calcium and potassium. Dandelion root or leaf tea was recommended as a mild laxative that would also stimulate urination, salivation and the secretion of gastric juices and bile, improve appetite and generally tone the whole system. It has been used to treat liver, urinary tract and digestive problems. The roots have been reported to lower blood sugar and cholesterol levels, lower blood pressure, reduce inflammation, have antimicrobial effects (against *Candida albicans* in particular) and aid weight loss. They also contain the sugar inulin, which is said to be an immune system stimulant. Historically, dandelion flowers were used to treat jaundice and other liver ailments, perhaps because of their yellow colour. Recently, they have been shown to contain large amounts of lecithin, which has been shown to prevent cirrhosis in chimpanzees. The milky juice, applied 3 times daily for 7–10 days, was said to kill warts.

OTHER USES: Dandelion leaves have been used as a substitute for mulberry leaves for feeding silk worms. The flowers produce a yellow dye, and the roots give a magenta colour.

DESCRIPTION: Perennial herb, to 40 cm tall, with bitter, milky sap and thick taproots. Leaves basal, 5–40 cm long, with triangular, backward-pointing lobes. Flowerheads bright yellow, 3.5–5 cm across, with ray flowers only, borne on hollow, leafless stalks, from May to August. Fruits reddish brown, spiny ribbed, seed-like achenes, 3–4 mm long, tipped with a long-stalked cluster of white hairs, forming fluffy, round heads. This widespread European introduction grows on disturbed, cultivated and waste ground throughout Canada. See p. 424 for conservation status.

WARNING
Never collect dandelions that might have been sprayed with herbicides. The milky sap can cause rashes on sensitive skin.

Sow-Thistles

Sonchus spp.

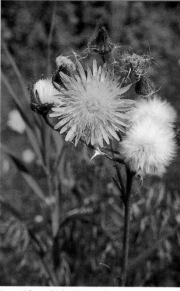

FOOD: Young leaves have been added to salads or cooked as a hot vegetable (served with butter and seasonings or vinegar) or as a potherb. They are sometimes added directly to curries and rice dishes, but they are usually quite bitter and require at least 1 change of water. Older leaves soon become very bitter and tough.

MEDICINE: In the 13th century, sow-thistle was recommended to prolong the virility of gentlemen, perhaps because of its milky sap. It was also believed to increase the flow of milk in nursing mothers. Some herbalists recommend sow-thistle for use in salves for healing hemorrhoids, ulcers and other skin irritations and as a tonic. The dried sap of annual sow-thistle was used to treat opium addiction. Medicinal teas made from perennial sow-thistle have been used

Perennial sow-thistle (all images)

to calm nerves and to treat asthma, bronchitis and coughs. The leaves were used in poultices and washes for relieving swelling and inflammation, and the milky juice was used to treat inflamed eyes.

OTHER USES: The white, milky sap was believed to clear the complexion. It was also dried in balls and chewed like gum. The flowers can be used as a pleasant tasting, gummy chew. Sow-thistles are sometimes given to animals that have lost interest in other forage. Pigs are especially fond of these plants—hence the name sow-thistle—but older European lore often associated sow-thistles with hares, which were said to hide among the plants and eat the leaves to cool their blood after being pursued.

DESCRIPTION: Tall, often bluish green annual, biennial or perennial herbs with milky juice. Leaves usually prickly-edged with bases clasping the stem. Flowerheads yellow, with ray flowers only, forming branched clusters, from July to October. Fruits slightly flattened, ribbed, seed-like achenes, each tipped with a tuft of white, hair-like bristles. All 3 sow-thistles described here are introduced Eurasian species found on disturbed sites throughout Canada (though none are yet recorded for NU).

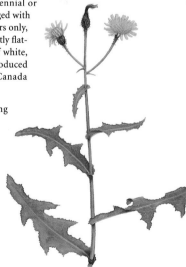

Perennial sow-thistle (*S. arvensis*) is a perennial growing 40 cm–1.5 m tall, from deep, creeping rhizomes, with 3–5 cm wide flowerheads and glandular-hairy involucral bracts.

Prickly sow-thistle (*S. asper*) is an annual (occasionally biennial), growing 10 cm–2 m tall from a short taproot, with smaller (1.5–2.5 cm wide) flowerheads and stiff, spiny, usually unlobed leaves, with rounded basal lobes that clasp the stem.

Annual sow-thistle (*S. oleraceus*) is an annual, growing 10 cm–2 m tall from a short taproot, with 1.5–2.5 cm wide flowerheads and soft, non-spiny, rather dandelion-like leaves, with sharply pointed, clasping lobes.

Wild Lettuces
Lactuca spp.

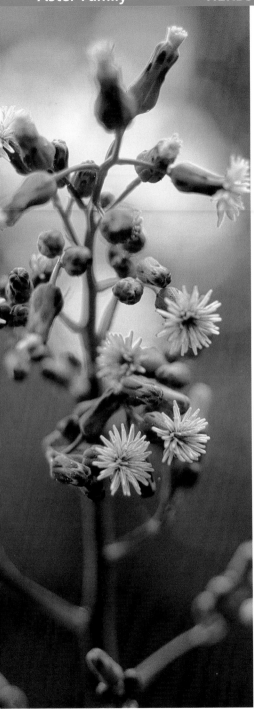

Tall blue lettuce

FOOD: The young leaves can be eaten raw in a salad. They are bitter and leave a bitter aftertaste, so they are better mixed with other greens. Older leaves or leaves collected when the plant is coming into flower are especially bitter, and large quantities can cause intestinal upset. As a potherb, the young leaves can be boiled for 10–15 minutes in 1 change of water and served with butter, vinegar or some other dressing. The young shoots of prickly lettuce can be cooked in the same way as asparagus (p. 174). The developing flowerheads, harvested before the stems unfold, can be added to casseroles. The seeds contain an edible oil, which must be refined before use, that can be used in cooking.

MEDICINE: The milky sap, when collected and dried, forms the drug known as lactucarium, also called lettuce opium because of its sedative and analgesic properties. Used as far back as ancient Egypt, lettuce opium was viewed as a weak alternative to opium, but lacking the side effects of addiction and intestinal upset. It was introduced as a drug in the US and was standardized and described in the 1898 US Pharmacopoeia for use in lozenges, tinctures and syrups as a sedative for dry cough, whooping cough, insomnia, anxiety, neuroses, hyperactivity in children and rheumatic pain. A commercial preparation is available as a pain reliever, and sometimes promoted as a legal psychotropic drug. The European species

WARNING
Cases of poisoning have been reported. Mature plants and those just beginning to flower are slightly more toxic.

L. virosa is probably the richest source of lactucarium, although a superior quality has been obtained from other species, namely *L. scariola* and *L. altissima*. The sedative effects were once attributed to hyoscyamine, although the dried sap was reportedly devoid of this alkaloid. The active compounds are believed to be lactucin and its derivatives, which have demonstrated sedative and analgesic activity comparable or superior to ibuprofen in animal studies. Two major studies, however, have failed to find any significant effects in humans, noting that lactucin and its derivatives were unstable and did not remain long in preparations of lactucarium. Some scientists attribute activity to the placebo effect and warn against taking excessive amounts, especially because there has been at least 1 reported case of a fatality from cardiac paralysis. Homeopathically, the plant has been used for the treatment of chronic catarrh, irritating coughs, swollen liver, flatulence and disorders of the urinary tract. The sap has been applied externally on warts. The fixed seed oil of prickly lettuce is reported to possess antipyretic and sedative properties. A decoction of the root of tall blue lettuce is used to treat body pain, but not pain in the limbs, as well as hemorrhages, heart troubles, diarrhea and vomiting.

OTHER USES: The seed oil is used commercially in soap making, paints and varnishes.

DESCRIPTION: Tall, leafy, annual or biennial herbs, to 2 m tall. Dandelion-like leaves grow scattered along the stems. Numerous (generally 13–40) small, pale, dandelion-like flowerheads, 10–15 mm across, in long, loosely branched clusters. Milky sap.

Tall blue lettuce (*L. biennis*) has a taproot, robust with narrow inflorescence. Flowers bluish to white, occasionally yellow, from July to October. Pappus of bristles is brown. Grows in rich thickets throughout Canada. See p. 424 for conservation status.

Canadian wild lettuce (*L. canadensis*) has a taproot and a slight bloom present on the stems and leaves. Leaves to 30 cm long, variable in shape, from nearly toothless and lance-shaped to deeply lobed. Flowers yellow, numerous, from June to October. Grows in clearings, thickets and forest edges throughout Canada.

Prickly lettuce (*L. serriola*) has fibrous roots. Leaves 5–30 m long, prickly on the midrib and along the margins, pinnately lobed and twisted at the base to lie in a vertical plane. Numerous yellow flowers, from July to September. Grows in fields and disturbed sites throughout Canada, more common in BC and AB.

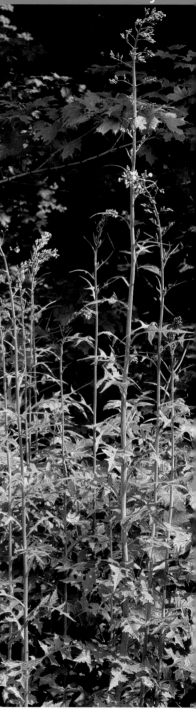

Tall blue lettuce

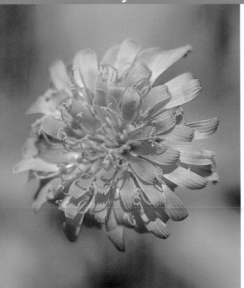

Orange agoseris (above)
Short-beaked agoseris (below)

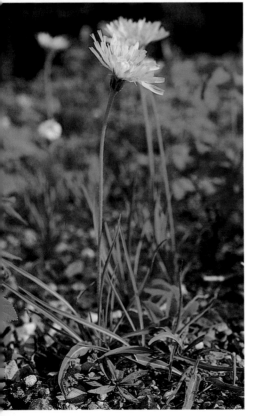

Agoseris
Agoseris spp.

FOOD: The leaves have been eaten raw in salads or cooked as greens. The flowers are also edible raw and can be used to make tea.

MEDICINE: In interior BC, these plants (also called false dandelions) were used to treat sores. In the US, the Navajo used cold tea made from these plants as a lotion and drink to treat arrow and gunshot wounds and "deer infection," and to provide protection from witches. The wet leaves were rubbed on swollen arms, wrists and ankles.

OTHER USES: *Agoseris* sap contains latex (rubbery compounds). The dried juice was collected from broken stems and leaves, rolled into little balls and used as gum. It was chewed for pleasure (like bubble gum) and to clean the teeth and then swallowed. Another name for these plants was Indian bubble gum. The leaves were also dried and then chewed to extract the gum.

DESCRIPTION: Perennial herbs, to 30 cm tall, with milky sap and slender basal leaves 5–35 cm long. Flowerheads with ray flowers and several overlapping rows of slender involucral bracts, borne singly on leafless stalks 10–70 cm tall, from May to September. Fruits smooth, seed-like achenes 5–9 mm long, tipped with a starburst of white hairs on a stalk-like beak.

Orange agoseris (*A. aurantiaca*) has burnt-orange flowers, and achenes have slender beaks more than half as long as the body. Grows on open foothill, montane, subalpine and alpine sites in BC, AB and QC. See p. 424 for conservation status.

Short-beaked agoseris (*A. glauca*) has yellow flowers, and achenes have ribbed beaks less than half as long as the body. Grows in open, grassy foothill and montane slopes in BC and AB.

Ragweeds
Ambrosia spp.

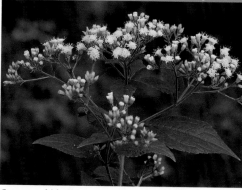

FOOD: Ragweed seeds 4–5 times larger than today's wild species were found in archaeological digs in the Ozark Mountains, suggesting that this plant was selectively bred, perhaps for its seed oil. The seed contains up to 20 percent oil, a small percentage of which is the essential fatty acid, linolenic acid.

Great ragweed (above)
Common ragweed (below)

MEDICINE: The herb was a popular salve for skin problems among several First Nations. The astringent leaves were crushed and smeared on insect bites, minor skin eruptions, hives and infected toes to stop the bleeding and speed healing. A tea of the leaves was once used for prolapsed uterus, leukorrhea, fevers, diarrhea, dysentery, nosebleeds, nausea, mucous discharge and intestinal cramping. A medicinal mouthwash made from leaf tea was used to treat mouth sores. The root was chewed as a folk remedy to allay fears at night, while root tea was used for stroke and menstrual problems. The pollen of both ragweed species listed below is harvested commercially and manufactured into pharmaceutical preparations for the treatment of ragweed allergies.

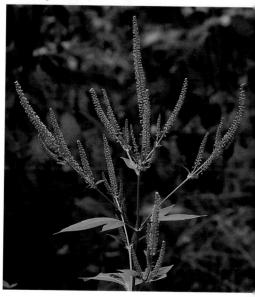

OTHER USES: The seed oil has a reddish tint and was used as a dye. The sap of the plant is also able to stain the skin red.

DESCRIPTION: Coarse, hairy-stemmed, weedy annuals with long clusters of inconspicuous, yellow-green flowers. Grow in cultivated or old fields, waste places and roadsides throughout Canada.

<table>
<tr><td>

WARNING

Pollen causes allergies and is the major cause of hay fever in autumn. Ingesting or touching plants may cause allergic reactions. Pollen from *Ambrosia* is responsible for about 90 percent of pollen-induced allergies in North America.

</td><td>

Common ragweed (*A. artemisiifolia*) is 30 cm–1.5 m tall, with highly dissected, light green leaves, 10 cm long. Male flowers small, borne in heads of 15–20 flowers each, arranged on slender clusters to 15 cm long at the top of the plant. Female flowers stalkless, borne in small clusters at the leaf axils. See p. 424 for conservation status.

Great ragweed (*A. trifida*) is 60 cm–4.5 m tall, similar in appearance to common ragweed, but with long (20 cm) opposite, palmately 3-lobed leaves.

</td></tr>
</table>

Rattlesnake-Weed

Hieracium venosum

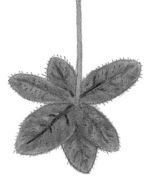

MEDICINE: Rattlesnake-weed was historically used as a snakebite remedy by early settlers in eastern North America. First Nations mixed the root with other herbs and ingredients and made a tea to treat a number of intestinal disturbances, most often chronic diarrhea. Both the root and leaves are astringent and were used in preparations to remedy internal bleeding. An added virtue is that it is a stimulant and promotes circulation to the affected area. Thus, it is useful for uterine hemorrhage, excessive menstruation, bleeding hemorrhoids and spitting of blood. An infusion of the roots or leaves of rattlesnake-weed was applied externally as a poultice to wounds and canker sores and as nasal drops for nasal polyps, nosebleeds and catarrh. Juice from freshly squeezed leaves was applied to warts to speed healing. Modern herbalists recommend using 25 g of rattlesnake-weed root powder or 45 g of the leaf to make 1 litre of infusion, or they can be added along with other ingredients to prepare a sedative syrup.

OTHER USES: Rattlesnake-weed's name may have been derived from its traditional use as a snakebite remedy, or from its segmented underground tubers that resemble the tail of a rattlesnake, or even from the snake-like leaf colouration.

DESCRIPTION: Perennial, hairy, dandelion-like herb, the stems 30–75 cm tall and usually branched, from taproots. Leaves basal (and sometimes a few on the stem), elliptic to spoon-shaped, 4–8 cm long, with reddish purple veins. Flowerheads yellow, 3–10, 1.5–2 cm across, in open clusters topping a long, often leafless floral stalk, from May to July. Grows in dry, open woods and thickets in southern ON. See p. 424 for conservation status.

WARNING
The milky sap resembling that of the narcotic genus *Lactuca* has long been suspected of being toxic.

Joe-Pye Weeds & Boneset
Eupatorium perfoliatum and *Eutrochium* spp.

FOOD: The ash from burnt roots was sprinkled like salt to flavour foods.

MEDICINE: Several of these species were heavily promoted by Joe Pye, a 19th-century American from whom the common name derives, as a treatment for typhus fever. The root tea is a diuretic and used by First Nations to eliminate kidney stones in the urinary tract and to treat urinary incontinence in children. A tea made from the whole herb was used for fevers, colds, chills, diarrhea, gout, rheumatism, asthma, chronic coughs and a variety of kidney and liver ailments. Researchers in Germany have isolated active polysaccharides and sesquiterpene lactones from a number of *Eupatorium* and *Eutrochium* species that are able to boost the immune system, providing support for its traditional uses. Early herbalists believed that the perforated leaves of boneset indicated that the herb was useful in setting bones, and so they were wrapped with bandages around splints. It is also possible that the name is derived from its use in the treatment of dengue, once called "breakbone fever." A tea of boneset leaves was a popular remedy for other fever-inducing diseases such as malaria, typhoid and influenza. First Nations introduced the plant to early settlers as a tonic for general debility and to treat colds, rheumatism and a number of fevers. The temperature at which the tea is

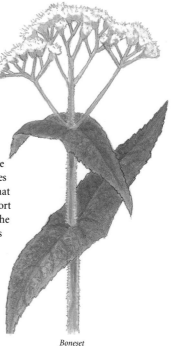

Boneset

administered, however, has different biological effects. When cold, it is a tonic and can be consumed 30 minutes before meals to stimulate appetite and aid digestion. When warm, it induces sweating and is an emetic, used to relieve pains and aches associated with colds and fevers. Hot tea may induce vomiting.

OTHER USES: A pink or red dye was obtained from the fruits. The genus *Eupatorium* was named after the ancient king of Pontus, Mithridates Eupator, who used a closely related plant for medicinal purposes,

DESCRIPTION: Sturdy, erect herbs, to 1.5 m tall. Leaves lance-shaped, toothed, opposite or in whorls. Large, domed cluster of fuzzy, white to pinkish purple flowerheads. Fruits achenes. See p. 424 for conservation status.

Joe-Pye weed (*Eutrochium purpureum*) has green stems with purplish or blackish areas at the leaf joints. Leaves to 25 cm long, in whorls of 3 or 4, and give off an odour of vanilla when crushed. Ray flowers dull, pale pinkish purple, 8 mm long in clusters 10–14 cm wide, from August to October. Grows in damp meadows and thickets across southern Canada.

Spotted Joe-Pye weed (*Eutrochium maculatum*) is similar to *E. purpureum* but with purple or purple-spotted stems. Leaves to 20 cm long, in whorls of 3–5. Flowers from July to September. Grows in damp meadows, thickets and shores across southern Canada.

Boneset (*Eupatorium perfoliatum*) has leaves opposite and united at the base, completely surrounding the stem (perfoliate). Dense cluster of flat-topped, dull white flowers, from August to October. Grows in low woods and wet meadows throughout Canada.

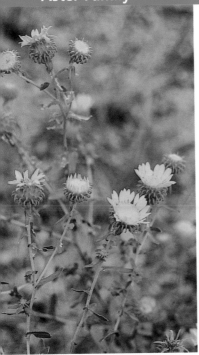

Curly-Cup Gumweed
Grindelia squarrosa

FOOD: Some tribes chewed on gumweed leaves or used them fresh or dried to make an aromatic tea.

MEDICINE: First Nations and early Jesuit missionaries recognized the medicinal value of this plant. Tea made from the resinous flowerheads was taken to relieve indigestion, colic and stomachaches. The leaf tea was used to treat throat and lung problems such as coughs, bronchitis and asthma. It was also widely used as a wash to relieve itching and to heal minor cuts and abrasions, pimples and skin irritations (especially rashes caused by poison-ivy, p. 395). A leaf poultice or the gum from pounded flowerheads was applied to poison-ivy inflammations and minor skin problems. Extracts from the dried flowerheads and leaves are said to have sedative, antispasmodic and expectorant qualities. They were once recommended as a treatment for a wide range of ailments, including headaches, malaria, cancers of the spleen and stomach, gonorrhea, pneumonia, rheumatism, smallpox and tuberculosis. More recently, they have been used in medications for treating asthma and bronchitis, and some herbalists recommend them for treating bladder inflammations caused by fungi or food.

OTHER USES: Plant tops and leaves were used to make washes for healing saddle sores on horses.

DESCRIPTION: Aromatic, biennial or short-lived perennial herb with branched, 20–80 cm tall stems from taproots. Leaves oblong, hairless, lobed to regularly toothed, often clasping the stem and dotted with resinous glands (and sometimes sticky with resin). Flowerheads yellow, 2–3 cm across, with 25–40 yellow ray flowers around a dense cluster of yellow disc flowers and above overlapping rows of backward-curling, sticky involucral bracts, borne in flat-topped clusters, from July to September. Fruits 4- to 5-ribbed, seed-like achenes. Grows on dry, open sites in prairies and foothills in BC and AB.

WARNING
The plant contains the known carcinogen safrole. Large doses of gumweed may cause kidney damage.

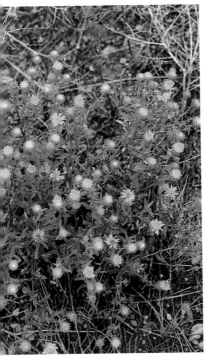

Blessed Thistle

Cnicus benedictus

FOOD: The plant was used as a flavouring agent. Young, unopened flowerheads can be used as a substitute for globe artichoke (*Cynara cardunculus*), but they are much more difficult to eat due to their smaller size. The root can be boiled as a potherb.

MEDICINE: An important herb in homeopathic medicine, blessed thistle was considered a cure-all during the Middle Ages and was widely cultivated throughout Europe. During the black plague, it was used, unsuccessfully, as a remedy. Monks grew the herb as a cure for smallpox. Today, the plant is less widely used but is still a common ingredient in herbal tonics. Its most popular use is as a treatment to promote lactation for nursing mothers. This is not recommended today because its effect on infants is unknown. The plant was also reputed to be a good tonic for girls entering womanhood. A warm infusion of the entire herb was used as a contraceptive and as a treatment for anorexia, poor appetite, depression, dyspepsia, colic, indigestion, diarrhea and liver and gallbladder problems. The herb is approved by the German E Commission as an appetite enhancer. As a remedy for sexually transmitted disease in men, the whole plant was infused in cold water overnight and the liquid drunk 3 times daily, followed by a quick run to encourage sweating. Because the plant is a strong emetic when ingested in large doses, this treatment often caused nausea and vomiting. Its astringent properties were useful in the external treatment of minor skin wounds, ulcers, sores, and burns.

OTHER USES: A good quality oil is obtained from the seed.

DESCRIPTION: Annual herb, to 60 cm tall, with leathery, hairy leaves, to 30 cm long, with spiny margins. Flowerheads deep yellow, surrounded by several spiny basal bracts. This introduced European species grows in disturbed sites and roadsides in southern ON and the Maritimes.

WARNING

Large doses may cause vomiting. People with allergies to flowers in the Aster family should use the plant with caution.

Goldenrods
Solidago spp.

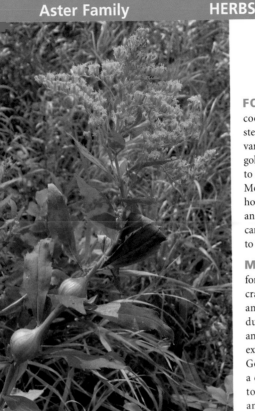

Canada goldenrod

FOOD: Goldenrod plants have been cooked like spinach or added to soups, stews and casseroles. Flavour and texture varies with species, age and habitat. Dried goldenrod leaves or flowers have been used to make pleasant teas (Mormon tea, Blue Mountain tea), usually sweetened with honey. The flowers are edible and provide an attractive garnish for salads. The seeds can be gathered for survival food and used to thicken stews and gravies.

MEDICINE: Goldenrod tea has been used for many years to relieve intestinal gas and cramps, colic and weakness of the bowels and bladder. It is said to reduce the production of mucous in the bronchi, and animal studies have shown that goldenrod extracts increase the production of urine. Goldenrod has been recommended as a cold and flu remedy and as a kidney tonic. Canada goldenrod contains the antioxidant quercetin. The tea was also used as a wash for treating rheumatism, neuralgia (pain along a nerve) and headaches, or it was mixed with grease and applied as a salve to sore throats. The flowers were also chewed to relieve sore throats. Powdered leaves and flowers were sprinkled on wounds to stop bleeding: during the Crusades, goldenrod was called woundwort because of its ability to stop bleeding. Boiled plants provided antiseptic poultices and lotions. The roots were used for treating burns and relieving toothaches and were also made into medicinal teas for treating colds, kidney stones and painful ulcers. Compounds in goldenrod are believed to stimulate the immune system, so these plants might be used to strengthen allergy defences at the beginning of hayfever season (like a vaccine). Some herbalists recommend goldenrod tea for relieving exhaustion and fatigue, while others report that it has hypoglycemic activity and is of great benefit to diabetics. The genus name, *Solidago*, is from the Latin *solidus*, "whole," and *ago*, "to make" (to make whole or cure), reflecting its medicinal use.

> **WARNING**
> Some people are allergic to goldenrod, so these plants should be used with caution, especially if you are allergic to other plants in the Aster family. People with urinary tract disorders should consult a doctor before using goldenrod. If you are retaining fluids because of a heart or kidney disorder, you should not use this plant. Many people point to goldenrod as a cause of hayfever, but the pollen of these showy flowers is too heavy to be carried by the wind and must be transported by insects. Usually, people are reacting to less conspicuous plants, such as ragweeds (p. 337), that grow in the same habitats.

OTHER USES: The sap of Missouri goldenrod is rich in latex, and attempts have been made to breed cultivars that could be used as a source of rubber. Goldenrod flowers produce a yellow dye with alum as a mordant and a gold dye with chrome as a mordant.

DESCRIPTION: Erect, perennial herbs with alternate, simple leaves, from creeping rhizomes or a woody stem base. Flowerheads small (less than 1 cm across), with few (about 8–17) yellow ray flowers around a small cluster of yellow disc flowers, forming branched clusters, from July to October. Fruits nerved, seed-like achenes tipped with a tuft of white, hair-like bristles.

This is a large genus, with at least 30 species in Canada.

Canada goldenrod (*S. canadensis*) has finely hairy upper stems, 30 cm–2 m tall, and lance-shaped leaves. Grows on roadsides, thickets and clearings across Canada.

Giant goldenrod (*S. gigantea*) has bluish green stems that are hairless (though sometimes downy in the inflorescence), 50 cm–2 m tall. Grows in moist, open thickets from AB to the Maritimes. See p. 424 for conservation status.

Missouri goldenrod (*S. missouriensis*) is a smaller plant (20–80 cm tall) with hairless, green stems. Grows in dry prairies and gravel slopes from BC to western ON. See p. 424 for conservation status.

Northern goldenrod (*S. multiradiata*) is another smaller goldenrod (10–50 cm tall) with smaller, elongated flower clusters on clumped, less leafy stems. Well-developed basal leaves hairless, except distinctive fringe of hairs on stalks. Grows in meadows, slopes and open forests at all elevations throughout Canada. See p. 424 for conservation status.

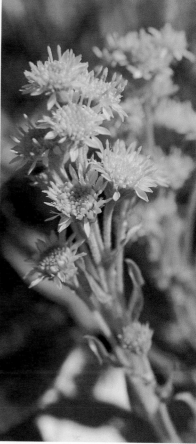

Northern goldenrod (above)
Giant goldenrod (below)

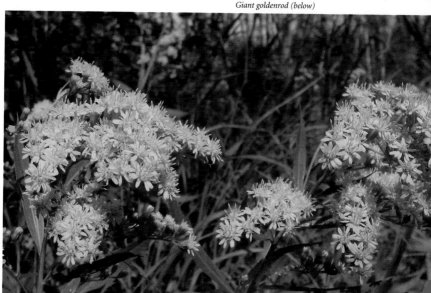

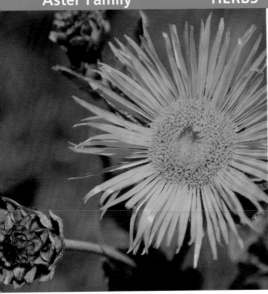

Elecampane
Inula helenium

FOOD: Once a common potherb of ancient Rome, the bittersweet, aromatic leaves are rarely consumed today. The root is listed by the Council of Europe as a natural food flavouring agent but is only approved in the US for use in alcoholic beverages. It can be candied; the root contains up to 44 percent inulin rather than starch, which is broken down to fructose, a natural sugar that does not elicit the same rise in blood sugar that sucrose (table sugar) does. This is of particular importance to diabetics.

MEDICINE: A well-known medicinal plant, elecampane (also known as "horse-heal") root tea has a long history of use as an effective treatment for respiratory complaints, including coughs, pneumonia, asthma, pulmonary tuberculosis, bronchial/tracheal catarrh and bronchitis. It has also been used as a tonic to rid toxins from the body and to stimulate circulation and boost the immune and digestive systems. In China, it is considered a treatment for certain cancers. Studies have demonstrated that an infusion of the root elicits a pronounced sedative effect when administered to mice. The root contains a camphor-smelling volatile oil and the sesquiterpene lactone alantolactone, which is able to reduce blood pressure and, when administered in small doses, decrease blood sugar levels. Larger doses increase blood sugar, at least in experimental animals. Research has demonstrated that alantolactone is also a potent bactericide and fungicide, which supports its traditional use as an antibacterial and antiseptic. In humans, the compound is a strong anthelmintic useful for eliminating roundworm, threadworm, hookworm and whipworm. Alantolactone has also displayed anti-inflammatory activity and is able to reduce mucous secretions, soothe irritated mucous membranes, induce sweating, increase bile secretion and increase urination. An infusion of the roots has been used as an external wash for skin inflammations, facial neuralgia, painful sciatic nerves and varicose ulcers. As a mouthwash, root tea has been recommended for tooth decay and periodontal disease. Herbalists recommend that the root be 2 or 3 years old before harvest and harvested in autumn and dried for later use. The root tea is prepared using 14 g powdered root to 500 ml water.

OTHER USES: A blue dye is obtained from a mixture of bruised and macerated elecampane root, ash and dried bilberry (*Vaccinium myrtillus*).

DESCRIPTION: Perennial herb, 60 cm–1.8 m tall, from a fleshy rhizome. Leaves rough, toothed and white-woolly underneath. Basal leaves, to 50 cm long, have long stalks, while stem leaves are stalkless and clasp the stem. Yellow, sunflower-like heads (5–10 cm wide) with long, narrow, straggly, yellow ray flowers surround a darker central disc atop a tall, hairy stem; bloom from July to September. This introduced European species grows in fields and roadsides in BC (lower Fraser Valley) and from MB to NS.

WARNING
May cause contact dermatitis. Taking elecampane may interfere with existing hyperglycemic and antihypertensive drugs.

Canadian Horseweed

Conyza canadensis var. *canadensis*

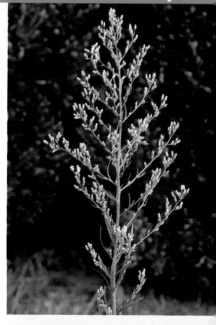

FOOD: Young leaves and seedlings can be boiled or dried for later use as a flavouring agent. The leaves contain essential oils that are used commercially for flavouring sweets, condiments and soft drinks.

MEDICINE: The astringent and styptic properties (the ability to contract blood vessels) of the leaves and seeds have been exploited by First Nations and early settlers as a treatment for a variety of gastrointestinal disorders including diarrhea, dysentery, internal hemorrhages and hemorrhoids. As a diuretic, the herb was used for the treatment of bladder problems, rheumatism, kidney stones, painful urination and nosebleeds. The essential oils occurring in the leaves were considered beneficial for treating sore throats, inflamed tonsils, bronchitis, fevers and coughs. Because the essential oils are volatile, the plant is best used when in flower and used fresh. If dried for later use, it should not be stored for more than a year. The leaves are reputedly very effective for healing bleeding hemorrhoids when applied externally. Some African cultures apply the herb on their skin to treat dermatitis, eczema and tinea (ringworm). Research has demonstrated that the plant possesses hypoglycemic activity, supporting its folk use as an antidiabetic medicine. A tea made from the boiled roots is reportedly a uterine stimulant, supporting its use as a therapy for painful menstruation and other menstrual irregularities by some First Nations.

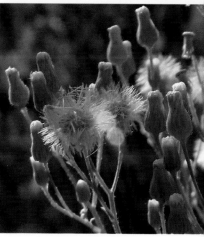

OTHER USES: The essential oils found in the seeds and leaves of this plant (also known as "Canada fleabane") can be distilled and made into perfumes and unusual nuances. The oil's special quality was recognized by some First Nations, who boiled the leaves to make steam for sweat lodges. The smoke from burning dried leaves was used as an insect repellent. The dried leaves were also used as a snuff to promote sneezing during the course of a cold or flu.

DESCRIPTION: Coarse annual or biennial weed, to 2 m tall, with erect, bristly haired stems. Leaves 2.5–10 cm long, linear, hairy and usually slightly toothed. Branching clusters of small, cup-like, greenish white flowerheads, less than 6 mm wide. Small ray flowers white, numerous disc flowers yellow. Fruit tiny and 1-seeded, with several bristles that aid seed dispersal. Found in fields, disturbed sites and roadsides throughout Canada.

WARNING
May cause contact dermatitis.

345

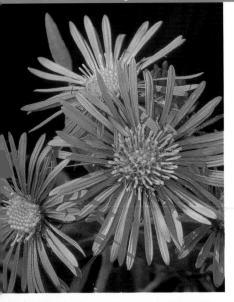

New England Aster

Symphyotrichum novae-angliae

MEDICINE: A decoction of the herb was used as a remedy for all kinds of fevers and to rejuvenate the skin. The mucilage from the root was sniffed to clear the nasal passages of mucous caused by the swelling of the mucous membranes. The root is astringent, increases expulsion of tracheal or bronchial mucous, relieves pain and reduces elevated body temperature. Thus, it was an ideal remedy for colds and fevers. The root tea was used by First Nations as a poultice to treat headaches, body pain and fevers and taken internally to treat diarrhea. Mixed with other herbal ingredients, an infusion of the whole plant was used in a compound medicine to treat mothers with intestinal fevers.

OTHER USES: Considered an aggressive weed by many, New England aster is prized for its attractive flowers and is commonly planted in gardens. New England aster freely hybridizes with other members of the *Aster* and *Symphyotrichum* genera, creating many varieties. It attracts butterflies and moths; it is also a good bee plant, providing nectar in autumn. Perhaps because the flower is noted for attracting wildlife, the Iroquois used the plant as a love medicine. The dried roots were sometimes smoked in a pipe in the belief that it would attract game.

DESCRIPTION: Large, stout, hairy, perennial herb that grows 1–2 m tall. Leaves 4–10 cm long, alternate, lance-shaped, toothless and clasp the stem. Flowerheads clustered at ends of branches, 2.5–5 cm wide, consisting of 50–75 bright lavender to purplish blue ray flowers and 50–110 yellow (becoming purplish) disc flowers, from August to October. Flowerstalks have glandular, sticky hairs. Grows in wet thickets, meadows and swamps across southern Canada from MB to the Maritimes.

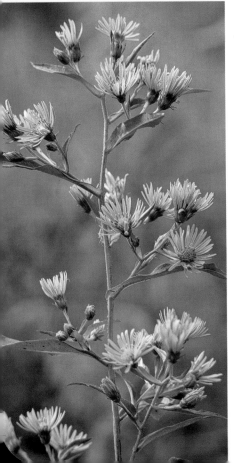

Fleabanes

Erigeron spp.

FOOD: The young plant can be boiled and eaten.

MEDICINE: The name fleabane comes from the mistaken belief that the dried flowers were effective against flea infestations. Traditionally, a tea made from the entire plant was used for fevers, bronchitis, tumours, hemorrhoids and coughs. Colds were sometimes treated with cold root tea. As a diuretic, the plant has been used to treat kidney stones, painful urination, diarrhea, gout and diabetes. Its astringent properties were used to treat hemorrhages of the stomach, intestines, bladder and kidney, as well as nosebleeds and blood-spitting. A poultice of the plant was used by some First Nations to treat headaches, and it was also applied on sores. The Cherokee reportedly used the plant for a variety of menstrual problems and to correct bad vision. The flowers were dried into a powder and used as a snuff for fevers and headaches. The smoke of dried flowers was inhaled for head colds.

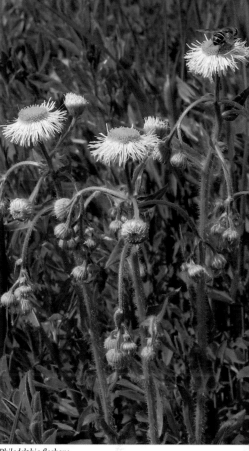

Philadelphia fleabane

OTHER USES: The smoke from dried flowers was used by the Ojibwa to attract deer. If your fleabane doesn't quite match the 2 described below, don't despair: at least 30 species of *Erigeron* have been described for Canada!

DESCRIPTION: Well-branched annual, biennial or perennial herbs, with usually erect stems. Lower leaves oblong and grow in rosettes; stem leaves lance-shaped and stalkless. Stems topped with numerous white, lavender or pink ray flowers and yellow disc flowers. Flowerheads 2.5–4 cm wide. Fruits bristly achenes.

Eastern daisy fleabane (*E. annuus*) is a 30 cm–1.5 m tall annual (occasionally biennial) herb with hairy stems. Leaves hairy, toothed, to 10 cm long. Flowerheads packed with 80 or more white to pale pink ray flowers surrounding the yellow disc flowers from June to August; flowerhead surrounded by a single set of bracts. Grows in fields, disturbed sites and roadsides throughout Canada.

WARNING

May cause contact dermatitis. Fleabanes have reportedly caused miscarriages and should not be taken by pregnant women.

Philadelphia fleabane (*E. philadelphicus*) is a 15–80 cm tall biennial or short-lived perennial herb with hairy basal leaves to 15 cm long, and clasping, smaller leaves on the hairy stem. Flowerheads packed with about 150 pink to purple or white ray flowers surrounding yellow disc flowers from March to June. Grows in thickets, fields and open woods throughout Canada, except NU. See p. 424 for conservation status.

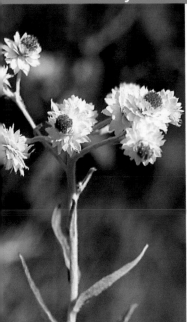

Pearly Everlasting
Anaphalis margaritacea

FOOD: The leaves and young plants have been used as a potherb.

MEDICINE: Pearly everlasting has been reported to have anti-inflammatory and astringent effects and to be a mild antihistamine, expectorant, sedative and diaphoretic (increases perspiration). It has been used in medicinal teas and gargles to treat swollen mucous membranes associated with colds, bronchial coughs, tuberculosis, asthma, throat infections, upset stomachs, diarrhea, bleeding of the bowels and dysentery. First Nations smoked the dried plants to relieve headaches and throat or lung problems, and they used a smudge of pearly everlasting (either alone or mixed with mint) to treat paralysis. Sometimes plants were boiled in water and used to steam rheumatic joints, or they were applied in poultices to rheumatic joints, sores, bruises and swellings. Leaf and flower poultices have been recommended for healing sunburn and moderate burns from heat and friction. Juice from fresh plants was said to be an aphrodisiac.

OTHER USES: Several First Nations smoked pearly everlasting, either alone or mixed with other plants such as tobacco (p. 240). The fuzziest leaves were said to be best. Men chewed the plants and rubbed the paste on their bodies to gain strength, energy and protection from danger. Pearly everlasting smoke was used to purify gifts being left for the spirits and to protect houses from witches. Similarly, a smudge of pearly everlasting and beaver gallbladders was said to revive people who had fainted and to ward off troublesome ghosts after someone in the family died. The flower stalks have a pleasant fragrance, and they also keep their shape and colour when dried, making pearly everlasting an excellent component of dried flower arrangements.

DESCRIPTION: White-woolly, perennial herb with leafy stems, about 20–60 cm tall. Leaves alternate, slender, 3–10 cm long, with a conspicuous midvein and down-rolled edges. Basal leaves small, soon withered. Flowerheads white, to 1 cm across, with showy, papery involucral bracts around smaller, yellow to brownish centres of disc flowers, forming flat-topped clusters, from July to September. Fruits roughened, seed-like achenes tipped with short, white hairs. Grows on open, often disturbed sites across Canada. See p. 424 for conservation status.

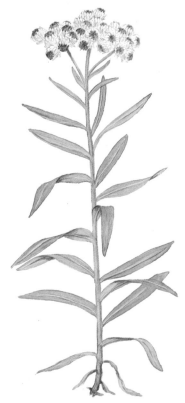

Tall Coneflower & Black-Eyed Susan

Rudbeckia spp.

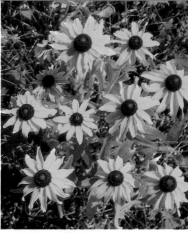

Black-eyed Susan (all images)

FOOD: These plants are often bitter and astringent, but young shoots of tall coneflower were eaten for good health. The hairier black-eyed Susan was not eaten.

MEDICINE: Tall coneflower was generally considered a kidney medicine, and it was sold commercially for use as a tonic, diuretic (for stimulating urination) and soothing balm, especially recommended for long-term inflammation of the mucous membranes of the urinary tract. Its roots were mixed with other herbs in teas for relieving indigestion, and its flowers were included with other plants in poultices for treating burns. Black-eyed Susan was said to increase urination and to have a mild, stimulating effect on the heart. Root tea was taken to treat colds and to expel worms. It was also used as a wash to heal sores, snakebites and swellings. Juice from the root was dropped into the ear to cure earaches. The flowerheads contain antimicrobial thiophenes, and the roots contain thiophenes and highly active thiarubrines. Recent studies report that coneflower root extracts can be more effective at stimulating the immune system than extracts of *Echinacea* species (p. 350), so these plants are being studied as a potential treatment for AIDS.

OTHER USES: Black-eyed Susan was used in colonial times for treating saddle sores on horses. These showy, hardy wildflowers make an attractive addition to sunny gardens.

DESCRIPTION: Biennial or perennial herbs, 30 cm–2 m tall, with erect stems from spreading rhizomes. Stem leaves alternate. Flowerheads usually showy, with few (6–20) ray flowers around a 1–2 cm wide, hemispheric to cone-shaped cluster of disc flowers, long-stalked, 1 to few, from June to August. Fruits hairless, 4-sided, seed-like achenes.

Black-eyed Susan (*R. hirta*) has entire (sometimes toothed) leaves and bright yellow to orange ray flowers surrounding dark, purplish brown disc flowers. Native to the US Great Plains, introduced and widely naturalized in southern Canada on open, often disturbed ground at low to mid-elevations in prairies and open woods in all provinces.

Tall coneflower (*R. laciniata*) has deeply cut leaves and yellow ray flowers surrounding yellow or greyish disc flowers. Grows on moist sites in rich, low grounds in BC (Lion Island, where introduced) and from MB east to the Maritimes, and can be expected as a garden escapee elsewhere. See p. 424 for conservation status.

> **WARNING**
> Some people have an allergic reaction to these plants. Black-eyed Susan tea should be strained to remove the irritating hairs. Poisoning and death of pigs, sheep and horses have been reported following ingestion of tall coneflower.

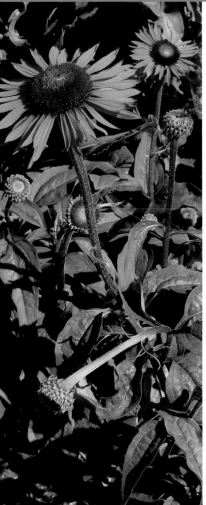

Purple coneflower

Coneflowers
Echinacea spp.

FOOD: The entire plant is edible. Leaves can be used in salads or as a spinach substitute. The deep purple flowers enliven any meal.

MEDICINE: Coneflowers are the most important and internationally recognized native North American medicinal plant. Growing only in central and eastern North America, they have been eagerly adopted into European herbal medicine, Ayurveda and traditional Chinese medicine. Coneflowers' most common use is for the treatment of colds and other upper respiratory tract infections. Their immunostimmulant action is often cited as the mode of action, but recent research shows that they also have an anti-inflammatory action in virus-infected tissue. These plants contain alkamides, polysaccharides and caffeic acid derivatives, which are the active principles. Their clinical activity was an issue of debate, but recent trials suggest that properly formulated products significantly reduce the length and severity of cold symptoms. Coneflower root tea was used externally by First Nations as a treatment for sores, wounds, burns and insect, spider and snake bites. Considered a powerful "blood-purifying" plant, the root tea was ingested for disorders thought to be caused by contaminants in the blood such as colds, fevers, influenza, allergy symptoms, acne, boils, canker sores, herpes sores and eczema. The root was often chewed to relieve toothaches and aid digestion. Modern herbalists do not recommend that the herb be taken for more than 16 days.

DESCRIPTION: Large, perennial herbs, to 70 cm tall, that produce a stout, bristly, hairy stem. Leaves linear to lance-shaped, 8–20 cm long, with the upper leaves stalkless and lower leaves growing on long stalks. Single, daisy-like flower pinkish white to purple with 12–20 large, spreading rays and numerous disc flowers.

Narrow-leaved purple coneflower (*E. angustifolia*) has narrow (linear to lance-shaped) leaves and swept-back ray flowers. Grows in gravelly, sandy and rocky, dry limestone prairies in southern SK and MB. See p. 424 for conservation status.

Purple coneflower (*E. purpurea*) has long, large-toothed, lance-shaped leaves and drooping ray flowers. Grows in moist woods and prairies in southern QC. Also grown as a garden perennial.

WARNING
Echinacea products are not recommended for people with progressive systemic and auto-immune disorders, including AIDS. Additionally, they should not be taken with other drugs known to cause liver toxicity, such as anabolic steroids, amiodarone, methotrexate or ketoconazole.

Cup-Plant & Prairie-Dock

Silphium spp.

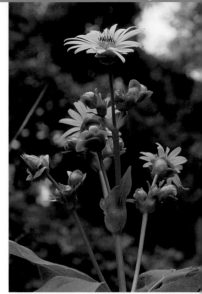

MEDICINE: Members of the genus *Silphium* were regularly used medicinally by prairie First Nations but are rarely used today by modern herbalists. The resin of compass plant (*S. laciniatum*) has a pungent odour similar to urine and has diuretic properties. An infusion of the roots was consumed as a general tonic for debility, coughs, asthma and gonorrhea and to expel worms. A decoction of the smaller roots was used to induce vomiting. An infusion of the leaves also induced vomiting and was once used as a treatment for coughs, asthma and respiratory ailments. The root tea of cup-plant, also emetic, was used for profuse menstruation, to reduce the symptoms of morning sickness and to prevent premature births. It was also used for fevers, internal bruises, debility, ulcers, back and chest pains, lung hemorrhages, liver diseases and enlarged spleens. Topically, it was used as a wash to treat facial paralysis and as a poultice to stop bleeding. The smoke of burning roots was inhaled for head colds, neuralgia and rheumatism.

Cup-plant (above)
Prairie-dock (below)

OTHER USES: The dried resin is chewed as a breath freshener and to clean teeth. The roots of prairie-dock produce various shades of red dyes.

DESCRIPTION: Tall, herbaceous perennials, to 3 m tall, the stems round or slightly angled in cross-section, usually erect and branched, with yellow, sunflower-like flowerheads, to 7.5 cm wide. Ray flowers monoecious, strap-shaped and pistil bearing, disc flowers tubular and sterile, from July to August. Fruit a broad, flat achene with awn-like pappus. Stem exudes resinous juice. See p. 424 for conservation status.

Cup-plant (*S. perfoliatum*) has opposite leaves, to 40 cm long, that envelop its stem, forming a cup-like base around it. Grows in open woodlands, meadows and prairies in southern ON (and introduced in southwestern QC).

Prairie-dock (*S. terebinthinaceum*) has large, oval or heart-shaped basal leaves, to 60 cm long, with very long stalks, and essentially no stem leaves. Grows in prairies in southern ON.

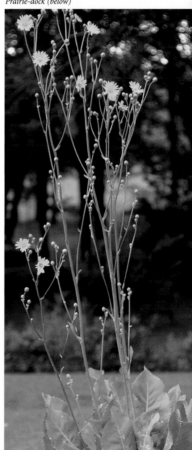

WARNING
There is a report that *Silphium* might be toxic.

Sunflowers & Jerusalem Artichoke

Helianthus spp.

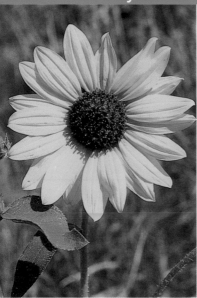

Common sunflower

FOOD: Common sunflower and Jerusalem artichoke were among the very few plants cultivated by First Nations. Sunflower seeds were eaten raw, but most were dried, parched, ground lightly to break their shells and poured into a container of water, where the kernels sank and the shells floated. The shells were skimmed off, roasted and used to make a coffee-like beverage. The kernels were eaten whole or ground into meal, which was boiled in water to make gruel or mixed with bone marrow or grease to make cakes. Crushed seeds were boiled in water, and the oil was skimmed from the surface and used like olive oil. Sunflower seed sprouts are also edible. The tuber of Jerusalem artichoke can be boiled and roasted like a potato but has superior nutritional value. Instead of starch, it contains inulin, a complex carbohydrate that is broken down into fructose, a natural sugar with fewer calories than regular sugar. Raw, the tuber can be sliced and added to salads.

MEDICINE: Common sunflower has been used to treat many ailments, including rheumatism, headaches, kidney weakness, malaria, worms, fatigue, sores, swellings, blisters and even prenatal problems believed to have been caused by an eclipse of the sun. Experimentally, it has been shown to have hypoglycemic activity. Sunflower seed oil was sometimes taken to relieve coughs and laryngitis. The flowers were used to make medicinal teas for treating lung problems, and the leaf tea was given to relieve high fevers. Sunflower leaves were applied as poultices to snakebites and spider bites. To remove a wart, the wart was scratched, and the pith from a sunflower stalk was then burned on top of it.

DESCRIPTION: Coarse, rough-hairy, annual or perennial herbs. Leaves mainly alternate (lowest leaves opposite), stalked, oval to heart-shaped, 10–25 cm long. Flowerheads 5–15 cm wide, with bright yellow ray flowers around a large (2 cm across), reddish brown (rarely yellow) button of disc flowers, borne singly or in open, few-flowered clusters. Fruits thick, 2- to 4-sided, seed-like achenes 5–10 mm long (sunflower seeds).

Common sunflower (*H. annuus*) is an annual plant from fibrous roots that grows to 3 m tall. Wide leaves (to 30 cm wide) and flowerheads 7.5–15 cm wide, enclosed with bracts edged with bristles, and flowers from July to November. Grows in prairies and disturbed sites, is perhaps native from southern BC to MB but is widely cultivated and naturalized over much of the rest of our country.

Prairie sunflower (*H. petiolaris*) is an annual plant from a taproot that grows to 1.8 m tall. Similar to common sunflower but has narrower leaves (rarely more than 10 cm wide) and smaller flowerheads (2.5–5 cm wide). Grows on dry prairie and uncultivated land from southern AB to southern MB, and introduced in BC and ON.

Jerusalem artichoke (*H. tuberosus*) is a perennial plant from rhizomes and tubers that grows to 3 m tall. Larger flowerheads (10–25 cm wide), enclosed with narrow, spreading bracts, flowering from August to October. Probably native to tropical and sub-tropical America, but has escaped cultivation in moist soils and rich thickets over much of southern Canada.

Arnicas

Arnica spp.

MEDICINE: All arnicas can cause severe upset and blistering of the digestive tract and should be used only externally. Flower and rhizome extracts are said to dilate capillaries under the skin and to stimulate the activity of white blood cells. Arnica (also called wolf's-bane) has been used for centuries in liniments, salves, washes and poultices for treating bruises, chilblains, sprains and swollen feet and for stimulating hair growth. These plants should never be applied to broken skin, where toxins could enter the bloodstream. A few people develop severe skin reactions from contact with arnicas.

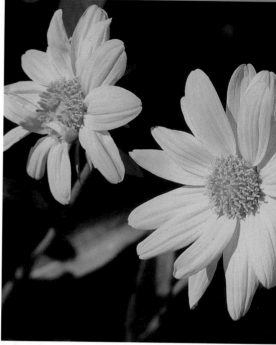

Arnica *species*

DESCRIPTION: Perennial herbs with opposite leaves and yellow, sunflower-like flowerheads. Fruits seed-like achenes with fluffy white or tawny parachutes. See p. 424 for conservation status.

Leafy arnica (*A. chamissonis*) has 5–10 pairs of stem leaves below branched clusters of flowerheads. Each involucral bract tipped with white hairs. Grows in moist meadows and open forests in foothill to sub-alpine elevations from BC to QC, and in YT and NT.

Heart-leaved arnica (*A. cordifolia*) has 2–3 pairs of stem leaves, and basal leaves broad (only 1–3 times as long as broad). Grows on foothill to sub-alpine slopes from BC to ON, and in YT and NT.

Hillside arnica (*A. fulgens*) has 2–4 pairs of stem leaves, and basal leaves narrower (3–10 times as long as broad). Disc flowers white-hairy; old leaf bases often with tufts of brown hairs. Grows in open fields and foothills from BC to MB.

Twin arnica (*A. sororia*), also called bunch arnica, is very similar to hillside arnica, but disc flowers have few or no white hairs, and old leaf bases lack hairs or have at most a few white hairs. Grows in open, often dry sites from the foothills of southern BC to SK.

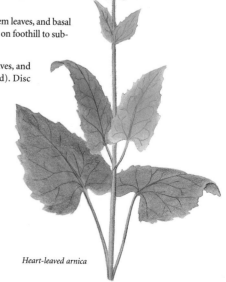

Heart-leaved arnica

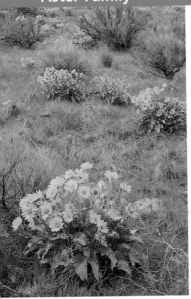

Arrow-Leaved Balsamroot

Balsamorhiza sagittata

FOOD: Balsamroot was one of the most important food resources of the First Nations of interior BC. Young leaves and shoots (often dug before they had emerged from the ground) were eaten raw, boiled or steamed. Immature flower stems and young leaf stalks were peeled and eaten raw, like celery, or were cooked. The peeled roots have been eaten raw, but their bitter, strongly pine-scented sap contains a complex, hard-to-digest sugar (inulin). This sugar is converted to sweet-tasting, easily digested fructose by slow cooking, so roots were usually roasted or steamed in large quantities in pits for several days. Dried, cooked roots were stored and then soaked overnight prior to use.

The small, sunflower-like seeds were dried or roasted and pounded into meal. This meal was mixed with grease and formed into small balls, boiled with fat or grease and made into cakes or mixed with powdered saskatoons and eaten with a spoon. Today, it is added to muffins, breads and granola. These large, distinctive plants provide excellent survival food—all parts are edible, and the roots are available year-round (though they become tough and stringy in summer).

MEDICINE: The large, soft leaves provided poultices for burns, and the sticky sap was used as a topical anesthetic and antiseptic on minor wounds, bites and stings. Balsamroot is said to mildly stimulate the immune system, aid in coughing up phlegm and stimulate sweating. The roots were boiled to make medicinal teas for treating tuberculosis, rheumatism, headaches, venereal disease and whooping cough and for increasing urine flow, purging the bowels and facilitating childbirth. Balsamroot poultices were used to heal sores, wounds, blisters and bruises. The sap has antibacterial and anti-fungal properties, and the roots have been used to treat athlete's foot and other skin infections. Balsamroot smoke or steam was used to cure headaches and to disinfect the rooms of sick people.

OTHER USES: Balsamroot was sometimes burned as incense in ceremonies.

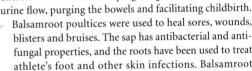

DESCRIPTION: Clumped, velvety grey, perennial herb, 20–70 cm tall, from stout, woody, aromatic taproots. Leaves mainly basal, arrowhead-shaped, 20–30 cm long, 5–15 cm wide, long-stalked. Flowerheads yellow, 5–11 cm across, with 12–22 bright yellow ray flowers around a deep yellow button of disc flowers, borne singly, from April to July. Fruits hairless, 3- to 4-sided, seed-like achenes 7–8 mm long. Grows on dry, often stony slopes in foothills and montane zones of BC and AB.

Quickweeds

Galinsoga spp.

FOOD: Considered a weed in many parts of the world, the plant is also valued as a wild edible plant. It has been used as a food in the Andes since the time of the Incas. The leaves, stem and flowering shoots can be prepared much like spinach, boiled for 10–15 minutes and served with butter or vinegar, added to stews or eaten as a potherb. The cooked vegetable is commonly consumed in Southeast Asia where it has been introduced. The leaves can also be eaten raw, although they are rather bland and should be mixed with other leaves to make a fine salad. Named *guascas* in Colombia and Bolivia, the herb is dried and ground into a powder and added as a flavouring agent to the national dish, *agiaco*. The entire herb can be squeezed and the juice drunk when mixed with tomato or vegetable juice.

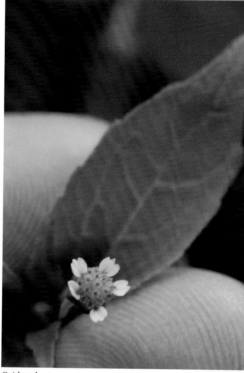

Quickweed

MEDICINE: The herb was used externally to treat stinging nettle (p. 312) stings, and the juice was squeezed onto sores, fresh cuts and wounds. This causes blood to coagulate, reduces inflammation and helps speed healing. In Chinese medicine, a decoction of the flowers is prescribed for cleansing the liver and eyes. In South Africa, the plant was identified by researchers as a potential treatment for high blood pressure. Preliminary findings demonstrate that the extract was able to inhibit the enzyme (angiotensin-converting enzyme) responsible for hypertension.

DESCRIPTION: Slender, slightly hairy, annual herbs from fibrous roots, 20–70 cm tall. Leaves lance-shaped to oval, opposite, 2–5 cm long, margin entire or (usually) toothed. Flowerhead has 3–8 white ray flowers and 15–50 yellow disc flowers, from May to October. Fruit pubescent or glabrous, black achene. Although native to Mexico and Central and South America, these invasive species now have a worldwide distribution. They are prolific seeders, producing several thousand seeds per plant, and can complete a life cycle, from germination to shedding of seeds, in as little as 50 days.

Quickweed (*G. parviflora*) has short, stiff hairs on its leaf stalks and upper stem. Grows in arable, disturbed sites in BC and from MB to NB.

Shaggy quickweed (*G. quadriradiata*) is a shaggier plant, with the leaf stalks and upper stems covered in longer, flexuous hairs and more coarsely toothed leaves. Grows in disturbed sites in all provinces.

WARNING
Quickweed has been reported to be toxic to goats.

Sneezeweed
Helenium autumnale

FOOD: Although no adverse effects have been reported in humans, the plant is poisonous to ruminants and should not be considered palatable. A southern relative, owl's claws (*H. hoopesii*), has resinous roots from which a chewing gum is obtained.

MEDICINE: The common name derives from its traditional use as a snuff to induce sneezing during the course of a head cold or fever. The dried, nearly mature flowerheads were ground and a pinch sniffed to clear nasal passages of mucous and other discharges. When the powder was made into a tea, it was consumed to rid the intestines of worms and other parasites. A tea made from the leaves was taken as a laxative and a tonic to gradually restore health. The roots were mixed with other herbs and the tea administered to prevent menstruation after childbirth. An infusion of the stems was used externally as a compress to reduce a fever. As part of their anticancer screening program, the National Cancer Institute found that helenalin, a lactone occurring in sneezeweed and other *Helenium* species, displayed antitumour activity. The compound is also responsible for the plant's toxicity.

OTHER USES: The toxic properties of the plant have been exploited as insecticide, vermicide (kills worms) and piscicide (kills fish).

DESCRIPTION: Perennial herb from a fibrous root, 60 cm–1.5 m tall, with winged stems. Leaves to 15 cm long, alternate, lance-shaped and toothed, with bases forming winged extensions down the stem. Flowerheads daisy-like, 2.5–5 cm wide with fan-shaped, yellow ray flowers that droop backward, each with 3 lobes at the tip and a globular, greenish yellow button at the centre, from August to September. Grows in swamps, wet meadows and thickets at all elevations from BC to QC and in NT. See p. 424 for conservation status.

WARNING
May cause contact dermatitis.

Yarrow

Achillea millefolium

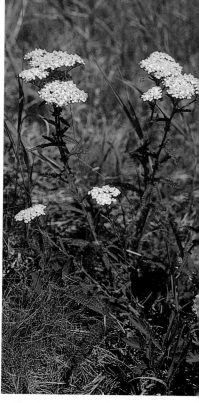

FOOD: Some sources suggest parboiled yarrow as a vegetable, but most consider it too bitter to eat. In Sweden, these plants sometimes replaced hops in beer.

MEDICINE: Yarrow is one of the most widely used medicinal plants in the world. It has been used for thousands of years as a styptic—a plant that stops bleeding. Achilles, the Greek hero for whom this genus was named, was said to have saved the lives of many soldiers by applying yarrow to their wounds. The plant contains alkaloids that have been shown to reduce clotting time and have been used to suppress menstruation. It also has sedative, pain-killing, antiseptic, anti-inflammatory and anti-spasmodic constituents that may help to relieve menstrual cramps. Yarrow leaves have been used in washes, salves and poultices for treating burns, boils, open sores, pimples, mosquito bites, earaches, sore eyes and aching backs and legs. The tea has been taken as a tonic and as a treatment for colds and fevers because it stimulates sweating and lowers blood pressure. The plant also stimulates salivation and the secretion of bile and gastric juices. Yarrow has been used to improve appetite and digestion, to speed labour and heal the uterus after birth and to treat diarrhea, urinary tract infections and even diabetes. Mashed leaves or roots were used as a topical anesthetic on aching teeth.

OTHER USES: Dried yarrow has been used for perfume and bath powder. Fresh leaves can be rubbed on the skin as an effective (though temporary) insect repellent. The hardy, attractive plants are excellent in wildflower gardens, but their spreading rhizomes often creep into areas where they are not wanted. The attractive, spicy-scented dried flowers are lovely in flower arrangements. Yarrow tea is said to make an excellent hair rinse.

DESCRIPTION: Aromatic, perennial herb, 10–80 cm tall, from spreading rhizomes. Leaves alternate, fern-like, 2- to 3-times pinnately divided into fine segments 1–2 mm wide. Flowerheads white (sometimes pinkish), about 5 mm across, with about 5 white ray flowers and 10–30 yellowish disc flowers, forming flat-topped clusters 2–10 cm across, from May to September. Fruits hairless, flattened, seed-like achenes. Grows in open, often disturbed sites in prairie to alpine zones across Canada.

WARNING

People with sensitive skin may react to these plants. Yarrow contains thujone, which is neurotoxic in large doses and can cause miscarriages.

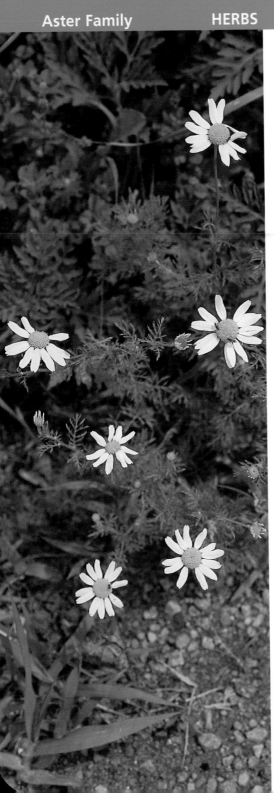

Mayweed
Anthemis cotula

FOOD: This aromatic herb is sometimes used as a flavouring agent. When crushed, the leaves and flowers release a disagreeable odour, so the herb is not commonly used as a food. However, it can be made into a tea much like its close relative, chamomile.

MEDICINE: The herb was used medicinally in much the same way as chamomile, but with far less efficacy. It possesses antispasmodic, astringent, diaphoretic, diuretic, emetic and emmenagogue activity; an infusion of the herb was used to treat a variety of complaints, including rheumatism, dropsy, epilepsy, asthma, diarrhea, colds, fevers and headaches. The tea was also used to induce sweating, menstruation and vomiting. Externally, the leaves were crushed and rubbed on insect bites.

OTHER USES: A gold dye can be obtained from the entire plant. The leaf glands exude an unpleasant odour that reportedly repels mice and fleas, and the plant is sometimes used as an insecticide.

DESCRIPTION: Daisy-like annual, 30–60 cm tall, with white ray flowers around a dome-shaped, yellow disc. Leaves to 6 cm long, thrice-dissected, resembling a fern, with an unpleasant odour and acrid taste. Flowerheads to 2.5 cm wide. This introduced European species grows in waste sites and road-sides throughout Canada. It should not be confused with chamomiles (p. 365).

WARNING
Foliage may cause skin irritation when handled.

Oxeye Daisy
Leucanthemum vulgare

FOOD: The plant most commonly known for the "He loves me, he loves me not" game has leaves that can be eaten raw when young. It has a rather pungent taste, so they should be consumed sparingly or added to mixed green salads. Finely chopped young spring shoots can also be added to salads, as can the root. The unopened buds can be marinated and used like capers as a condiment.

MEDICINE: The flowers are mildly aromatic, and the tea has been used as a treatment for whooping cough, asthma, bronchitis and nervous excitability. The tea is astringent and diuretic and has been used in treatment of stomach ulcers, bleeding hemorrhoids and blood in the urine. As an antispasmodic, it has been employed for colic and general digestive complaints. The tea is a mild tonic and acts similarly to chamomile. When boiled with the leaves and stalks and sweetened with honey, it has been recommended for nightsweats. Nightsweats associated with tuberculosis were treated with a glass of water in which 15–60 drops of the fluid root extract were added. A decoction of the whole herb in ale was used by rural Americans as a folk remedy for jaundice. Externally, a decoction of the flowers was used as a wash for chapped hands, a vaginal douche for ulcerations, an eye lotion for the treatment of conjunctivitis

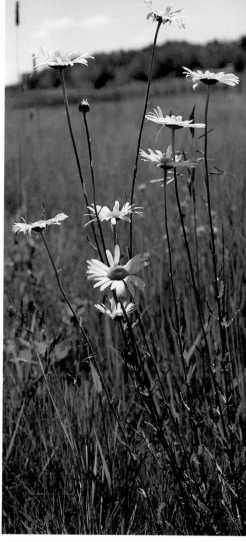

and a skin lotion for wounds, bruises, ulcers and other skin conditions. The flowerheads contain polyacetylenes with antimicrobial activity. Flowers are collected in May and June and can be dried and stored for later use.

OTHER USES: The acrid juice is obnoxious to insects and has been used as an insecticide. Cattle that graze on this plant produce milk with a disagreeable flavour.

DESCRIPTION: Perennial herb from a rhizome, 30–90 cm tall. Leaves dark green, coarsely toothed or pinnately lobed. Basal leaves to 15 cm long, and stem leaves to 7.5 cm long. Flowerheads solitary, 2.5–5 cm wide, atop slender, erect stems, from June to August. Ray flowers white, all female; disc flowers yellow, both male and female. Fruits cylindric, black achenes. This introduced Eurasian species grows in disturbed sites, meadows, pastures and roadsides throughout Canada.

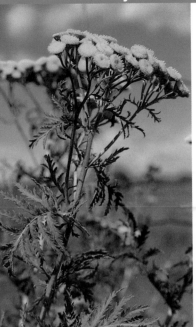

Feverfew & Tansy

Tanacetum spp.

FOOD: Dried feverfew flowers impart a deliciously aromatic, bitter flavour when used to make a tea or in cooking certain pastries. Sweet cakes with snippets of tansy leaves were once popular in Europe as a spring tonic, but they are seldom made today. In small amounts, tansy has been used to replace sage, but this substitution is not recommended (see **Warning**). Tansy is also used as a flavouring agent in certain alcoholic beverages, including chartreuse.

MEDICINE: Since the time of Dioscorides (78 AD), feverfew has gained a credible reputation as a medicinal herb to treat migraine headaches, arthritis, menstrual irregularities, stomachaches and, especially, fevers. It has been traditionally used for the treatment of tinnitus, vertigo, difficult labour, toothaches and insect bites. During the 1970s, feverfew became the alternative therapy of choice for people unable to obtain relief from painful migraines and arthritic pain. Pain intensity and frequency decreased with habitual consumption of only 2 or 3 fresh leaves daily. Considerable evidence supports its reputation. The sesquiterpene lactone constituents, in particular parthenolide, which is thought to be the main active component, possess potent anti-inflammatory activity. It may also provide relief by inhibiting certain prostanoid-producing enzymes associated with migraines and rheumatoid arthritis, as well as reducing the reactivity of the smooth muscles lining cerebral blood vessels to these compounds. The herbal tea in a foot bath provided relief from swollen feet. A tincture of the herb was applied topically to treat bruises and other wounds. A cold extract is said to have a tonic effect.

Tansy (all images)

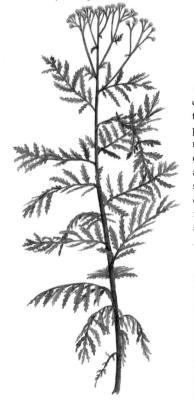

WARNING

The pungent, volatile oils of these plants are poisonous—a small quantity can kill in 2–4 hours. The US Federal Department of Agriculture prohibits the sale of tansy as a food or medicine. People have died from taking tansy oil or drinking tansy tea. People with sensitive skin may develop rashes from contact with tansy.

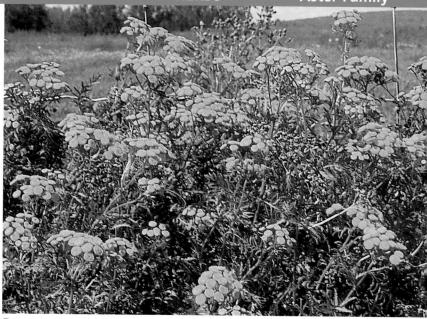

Tansy

Tansy has a similarly long history of use in folk medicine, but as a remedy for worm infestations, especially in children. The dried leaves and flowering tops have been used for upset stomachs, lack of appetite, flatulence, jaundice, suppressed menses, weak kidneys and gout. The physiological action of tansy is due to the volatile oil, which often has a high thujone content (see **Warning**). The oil or strong tea was used to induce abortions, sometimes with fatal results for the woman. Research has shown that aqueous infusions and alcoholic extracts are clinically effective bile stimulants in patients with liver and gallbladder disease. Other studies suggest that tansy may relieve intestinal spasms, fight intestinal worms, reduce blood-lipid levels, influence blood-sugar levels, kill bacteria and fungi, combat tumours and increase resistance to the encephalitis virus. Externally, tansy was used in liniments and cosmetic lotions. Leaf poultices were applied to cuts, bruises, tumours and inflammations. A breath spray made from tansy tea was used for sore throats. However, see **Warning**.

OTHER USES: The dried flower buds of feverfew and tansy were strewn on floors, under mattresses, between blankets and clothing and around food to kill and repel insects. Plants were rubbed on corpses and placed in coffins to mask odours and prevent decay. Feverfew essential oil is used in perfumery.

DESCRIPTION: Aromatic, perennial herbs dotted with pitted glands, with leafy, erect, branched stems. Leaves alternate, blades mostly egg-shaped to oblong. Flowerheads several to numerous, terminal, the lower flowers with longer stems, giving the inflorescence a flattish top. Fruits tiny achenes. These introduced European species can be found in disturbed sites, often as garden escapees.

Feverfew (*T. parthenium*) is a small (30–60 cm tall) plant, with leaf blades 1- to 2-times pinnately lobed. Flowerheads with yellow disc flowers surrounded by stubby white ray flowers, in clusters of fewer than 20 flowers, from June to September. Reported in southern BC and southern ON.

Tansy (*T. vulgare*) is a larger plant (40 cm –1.5 m tall), with much more finely divided, fern-like leaves. Flowerheads deep yellow, button-like clusters of disc flowers only, in clusters of 20–200 flowers, from July to September, across Canada.

Coltsfoots
Petasites frigidus

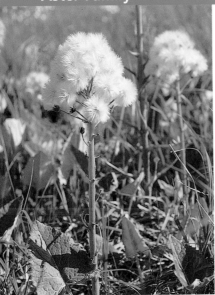

FOOD: These plants have a mild, slightly salty flavour. Young flowering stems can be eaten as a vegetable, either roasted, boiled or stir-fried. The leaves can be cooked like spinach, but they become fuzzy and rather felt-like with age. The salt-rich ash of coltsfoot leaves was widely used as a salt substitute. The leaves were either rolled into tight balls and dried before burning, to increase the consistency of the ash, or they were fired while encased in balls of clay to contain the ash.

MEDICINE: Coltsfoot is said to be soothing and calming because it contains mucilage and compounds with antispasmodic and sedative effects. Dried coltsfoot has been used for hundreds of years to make medicinal teas to relieve coughing and pain between the ribs in chest colds, whooping cough, asthma and viral pneumonia. It has also been smoked to relieve chronic coughs. These plants are reported to contain antihistamines and compounds that impede the nerve impulses triggering coughs. Various coltsfoot extracts have been used to lessen spasms and cramps in the stomach, gallbladder and colon. The leaves were used in poultices and salves for relieving insect bites, inflammation, swellings, burns, sores and skin diseases, and they were also boiled to make a decoction that was applied as a treatment for arthritis. Coltsfoot roots were chewed or made into medicinal teas for treating chest ailments (tuberculosis, asthma), rheumatism, sore throats and stomach ulcers. Crushed roots are said to reduce inflammation, sedate nerves and inhibit bacterial growth, and they have been used in poultices on sprains, bruises, scrapes and cuts. It is recommended that these

Arrow-leaved coltsfoot (above)
Palmate coltsfoot (below)

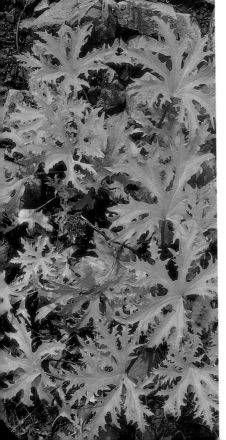

WARNING
Coltsfoot contains alkaloids that may be harmful if eaten in large quantities. Pregnant women should not eat these plants; strong doses may cause miscarriage. Never collect plants from areas where the water may be polluted.

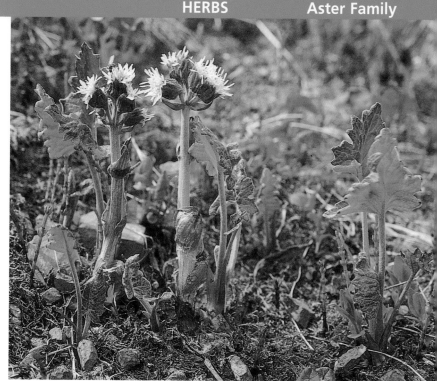

Sweet coltsfoot

poultices be kept on the injury for at least 30 minutes so that their compounds can be absorbed into the skin.

OTHER USES: Dried leaves have been used in a variety of smoking mixtures.

DESCRIPTION: Perennial herbs, 10–50 cm tall, with white-woolly flowering stems from slender, creeping rhizomes. Leaves basal, mostly 10–20 cm wide, long-stalked, often white-woolly beneath. Flowerheads white to pinkish, about 1 cm across, with many white disc flowers and few (or no) white to pinkish ray flowers borne in elongating clusters, from April to July (before the leaves appear). Fruits slender, 5- to 10-ribbed, seed-like achenes, with a tuft of white, hair-like bristles.

The coltsfoots, though very different in appearance because of their distinctive leaf shapes, are none-theless all included as varieties in 1 species, *P. frigidus*. See p. 424 for conservation status.

Sweet coltsfoot (*P. frigidus* var. *frigidus*) has leaves triangular to heart-shaped, lobed or, if toothed, then with few teeth (less than 15 teeth per side). Found in wetlands and wet, open forests, found in tundra or in subalpine and alpine zones from northern BC to SK, and all 3 territories.

Palmate coltsfoot (*P. frigidus* var. *palmatus*) has rounder leaves that are deeply cut into several finger-like (palmate) lobes. Grows on wet sites and roadsides throughout Canada.

Arrow-leaved coltsfoot (*P. frigidus* var. *sagittatus*) has triangular or arrowhead-shaped, shallowly toothed leaves with more than 20 teeth per side. Grows in wet places, shallow standing water or marshy areas, bogs and moist, disturbed areas at all elevations throughout Canada.

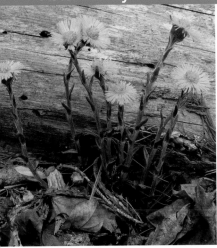

Coltsfoot
Tussilago farfara

FOOD: Dried leaves can be steeped to make an anise-flavoured tea, or burned and the ash used as a salt-like seasoning. The fresh leaves can be eaten raw, added to salads and soups or cooked as a vegetable, but they have a bitter aftertaste and should be washed after boiling. An excellent cough syrup or candy can be made by boiling the fresh leaves and adding 2 cups of sugar per cup of leaf extract. The resulting rich syrup forms a hard ball when dropped in cold water. The slender rootstalk can also be candied in sugar syrup.

MEDICINE: The genus name derives from the Latin *tussis*, meaning "cough," and the plant has a long history of being used to treat this condition. The plant possesses expectorant, antitussive, demulcent and anticatarrhal activity and was traditionally used for asthma, bronchitis, laryngitis and pertussis. Dioscorides, Galen, Pliny, Boyle and Linnaeus, among others, recommend the leaves, blossoms and roots be smoked as a cure for coughs and wheezes. Coltsfoot is the main ingredient in British Herb Tobacco, said to relieve asthma, catarrh and persistent bronchitis. The principal active component of coltsfoot is the mucilage content, and because this is destroyed by burning, no therapeutic value would be obtained by smoking it. Moreover, the effect of smoking itself would further irritate mucous membranes. The throat-soothing mucilage can be more effective for colds and asthma if taken as a decoction sweetened with honey or licorice. However, coltsfoot also contains toxic pyrrolizidine alkaloids, which cause liver toxicity. Because these alkaloids are easily extracted in hot water, a tea made from the fresh plant would presumably contain them. Another compound found in coltsfoot mucilage is tussilagone, a sesquiterpene that has been reported to be a potent cardiovascular and respiratory stimulator. It has also displayed anti-inflammatory and antibacterial activity. Researchers in China reported that 75 percent of patients suffering from bronchial asthma showed some improvement after using coltsfoot; however, the relief was temporary. Given the risk of exposure to pyrrolizidine alkaloids from prolonged use of coltsfoot, people suffering from throat irritations and asthma should consider alternative herbal remedies, such as slippery elm bark (p. 64) or marsh mallow root (*Althaea officinalis*). Externally, a poultice of the flowers is said to have a soothing effect on a variety of skin disorders including eczema, ulcers, sores, bites and inflammations.

OTHER USES: The underside of the leaves has a soft down that can be used as stuffing material. A fine tinder can be made by wrapping the plant in a rag, dipping it in saltpetre and allowing it to dry in the sun.

DESCRIPTION: Perennial, rhizomatous herb, 8–45 cm tall. Leaves basal, 5–25 cm long, broad and heart-shaped, toothed or lobed, whitish-woolly beneath. Flowerheads solitary on a scaly stalk, 2.5 cm wide, with thin, yellow ray flowers surrounding yellow disc flowers, before the leaves from February to June. This introduced European species grows on disturbed sites and roadsides in southwestern BC and from ON to NL.

WARNING

The plant contains low concentrations of pyrrolizidine alkaloids that are potentially toxic if used over a long period of time or in large doses.

Chamomiles
Matricaria spp.

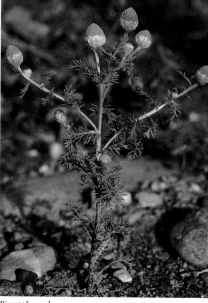
Pineapple-weed

FOOD: Chamomile flowerheads were often gathered for food, especially by children. Today, they are used to make a pale golden tea; pineapple-weed teas have a pineapple-like scent. The flowerheads have also been added to muffins and breads. The plants may be eaten as a trail nibble or salad ingredient, but they can be quite bitter. Powdered plants were sometimes sprinkled on alternating layers of meat or berries to keep flies away and to reduce spoilage.

MEDICINE: German chamomile tea is a well-known herbal remedy for treating nervous tension, irritability and a variety of digestive complaints, such as irritable bowel syndrome, Crohn's disease, peptic ulcers and hiatus hernia. It is especially suited to teething children. A wide variety of pharmacological activity has been documented for German chamomile, including antibacterial, anti-inflammatory, anti-spasmotic, anti-ulcer and antiviral activities. The flowers are used topically for wounds, sunburn, burns, hemorrhoids, mastitis and leg ulcers. Animal studies have demonstrated that ingestion of the oil, at a dose of 0.2 mL/kg, lowered blood pressure and depressed cardiac and respiratory function. In a human study, a chamomile extract administered to patients undergoing cardiac catheterisation induced a deep sleep in 83 percent of the cases. Pineapple-weed tea has been used in a similar manner to German chamomile to treat colds (especially in children), upset stomachs, diarrhea, fevers and menstrual cramps. It was also taken by women to build up their blood at childbirth, to aid in delivering the placenta and to encourage good, healthy milk. As a mild sedative, it helps to expel gas and soothe muscle contractions in the stomach, relieving heartburn and soothing the nerves.

OTHER USES: Native peoples used these aromatic plants as perfume, sometimes mixing them with fir or sweetgrass and carrying this mixture in small pouches to concentrate the fragrance. Pineapple-weed provided a pleasant-smelling insect repellent, and the fragrant dried plants were used to line cradles and stuff pillows.

DESCRIPTION: Hardy, pleasantly aromatic annuals, 5–50 cm tall, from fibrous roots, with 1 or many branched, erect stems. Leaves alternate, divided 1–3 times into linear, narrowly lobed leaflets. Flowerheads with yellowish green disc flowers. Fruits achenes.

German chamomile (*M. chamomilla*) is apple-scented, with white ray flowers and yellow disc flowers, from May to October. This introduced Eurasian species grows in disturbed sites, roadsides and fields throughout Canada.

WARNING

May cause contact dermatitis in people with an existing allergies to members of the Aster family. The flowerheads are reported to act as an emetic in large doses.

Pineapple-weed (*M. discoidea*) is pineapple-scented, with yellow disc flowers from May to September. Grows on disturbed ground, often on roadsides and disturbed sites throughout Canada. It's native to western North America, but because of its weedy nature, its precise native range is unclear.

Burdocks

Arctium spp.

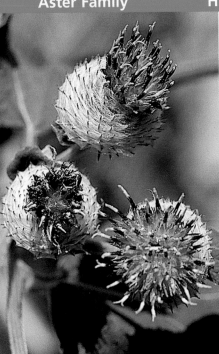

Woolly burdock

FOOD: These large, vitamin- and iron-rich plants were originally brought to North America as food plants. All parts of the plants are edible. Young leaves have been used in salads or boiled as a potherb, though to break down the tough fibres, the leaves may require 1–2 changes of boiling water and the addition of baking soda. They are said to be excellent in soups and stews. The roots of first-year plants have been peeled, diced or sliced and used in stir-fries and soups or served as a hot vegetable. Mashed roots can also be formed into patties and fried. Some First Nations dried burdock roots for winter supplies or roasted and ground them for use as a coffee substitute. The root contains inulin. The white pith of young leaf and flower stalks has been added to salads or cooked as a vegetable. It was also simmered in syrup to make candy or soaked in vinegar and seasonings to make pickles.

MEDICINE: Burdocks were widely used in tonics for "purifying the blood," and they are still recommended as a safe but powerful liver tonic. For centuries, burdock was used in medicinal teas for treating gout, liver and kidney problems, rheumatism, vertigo, high blood pressure, measles and gonorrhea. The leaves provided poultices for healing burns, ulcers and sores, as well as teas and washes for treating hair loss, hives, eczema, psoriasis and skin infections. The seeds, which contain antimicrobial polyacetylenes, were used in washes and poultices to treat abscesses, insect bites, snakebites, scarlet fever and smallpox. They are also said to stimulate urination and have been used to treat water retention and high uric acid levels. The roots were boiled to make an antidote for use after eating poisonous food, especially poisonous mushrooms. In Japan, common burdock is popular because of its reputation for increasing endurance and sexual virility. Studies have shown that burdock can reduce blood-sugar levels, dissolve bladder stones and stimulate liver and bile function. It may also inhibit mutations, slow tumour growth and relieve water retention, rheumatism, skin problems associated with liver dysfunction and high blood pressure.

OTHER USES: The hooked bristles of these bur-like flowerheads are said to have inspired the invention of Velcro.

DESCRIPTION: Robust, biennial herbs with mostly heart-shaped leaves that are thinly white-woolly beneath. Flowerheads bur-like, with slender, tubular, pink to purplish flowers above overlapping rows of hook-tipped involucral bracts, borne in branched clusters, from August to October. Fruits 3- to 5-sided, hairless seed-like achenes. Introduced from Europe.

WARNING

Pregnant women and people with diabetes should not use burdock. In women, it can cause spotting and even miscarriage. It has also shown hypoglycemic activity. People with sensitive skin may develop rashes from contact with these plants.

Great burdock (*A. lappa*) can grow to 2 m tall and has open clusters of large (2.5–4 cm wide) flowerheads on solid, grooved leafstalks. Grows on roadsides, particularly in limey soils, in eastern Canada.

Common burdock (*A. minus*) grows 45 cm–1.5 m tall and has smaller (1.5–2.5 cm wide), stalkless flowerheads that are scattered in elongated groups. Grows in waste sites and roadsides across Canada.

Woolly burdock (*A. tomentosum*) grows 60 cm–1.2 m tall and is easily recognized by its cobwebby flowerheads. Grows on disturbed sites across southern Canada.

Burdocks could be confused with common cocklebur (p. 372), which is reported to have caused poisoning of cattle, sheep, horses and swine. Cockleburs are easily distinguished by their flowerheads, in which the hooked bracts are fused into solid, nut-like burs, and by their leaves, which are rough rather than velvety.

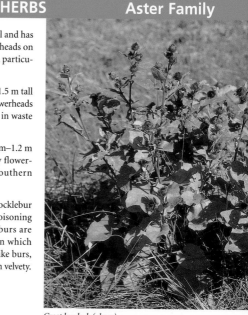

Great burdock (above)
Common burdock (below)

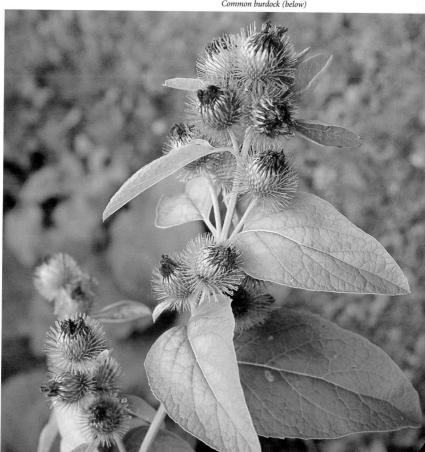

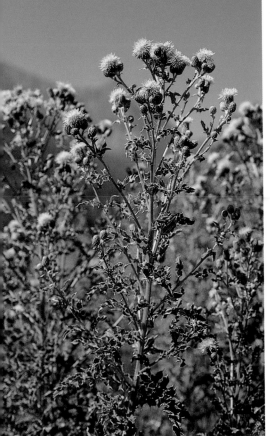

Canada thistle

Thistles

Cirsium spp.

FOOD: Flavour and texture of thistles varies with species, age and habitat, ranging from tender and sweet to tough and bitter. The taproots of young biennial plants (at the end of the first summer and before bolting the following spring) could be eaten raw, but usually they were roasted for several hours in fire pits or were boiled. Cooked roots were sliced and then fried or mashed, dried and ground into flour. Because they contain a relatively indigestible sugar, inulin, raw thistle roots often cause gas, but roots turn sugary when roasted. The stems and leaves are often sweet and juicy, but before they can be eaten, they have to be peeled to remove their prickles—hold the plant upside-down and peel from the bottom to the top with a sharp knife. Peeled parts can then be eaten raw or cooked as a vegetable. The immature flowerheads can be eaten raw or steamed and served with lemon butter. Some say they are better than their well-known relative, the artichoke (*Cynara scolymus*). Because these nutritious plants are so widespread and easily identified, they are an excellent survival food.

MEDICINE: Thistle plants have been used to make medicinal teas to strengthen the stomach, reduce fevers, kill intestinal worms, inhibit conception, increase the chances of conceiving a male child, increase the milk supply of nursing mothers, wash pimples, rashes, ulcers and leprosy sores and "expel superfluous melancholy out of the body and to make a man as merry as a cricket" (Grieve 1931, quoting Culpepper). The root tea was taken to relieve diarrhea and dysentery.

OTHER USES: The seed fluff makes good tinder, pillow stuffing and insulation. Thistle flower petals provide a pleasant substitute for chewing gum. Tough, fibrous older stems can be twisted to make strong twine. Thistle seed oil was used as lamp oil in Europe.

DESCRIPTION: Erect, prickly herbs with alternate, spiny-toothed to deeply lobed leaves. Flowerheads with tubular (disc) flowers above overlapping rows of involu-

WARNING
These spines can injure even the toughest hands. Roots from pastures may harbour harmful bacteria or other parasites and are probably best cooked. Thistles should be eaten in moderation because some contain potentially carcinogenic alkaloids.

cral bracts, few to many, in head-like or spreading clusters. Fruits hairless, ribbed, seed-like achenes, tipped with feathery bristles.

Canada thistle (*C. arvense*) is a perennial growing 30 cm–1.2 m tall with deep, spreading rhizomes. Unlike the other thistles, it has small (12–25 mm wide), pinkish purple flowerheads that are either male or female.

Bull thistle (*C. vulgare*) is easily recognized by its leaves, which are bristly-spiny above, its spiny-winged stem and its wide (about 5 cm), showy, rose-purple flowerheads. Grows 60 cm–1.8 m tall.

Canada thistle and bull thistle are European weeds that grow on disturbed sites throughout Canada. The following 3 species are native thistles.

Indian thistle (*C. brevistylum*) grows 90 cm–2.5 m tall, has leaves with only lightly loose, white-woolly hairs beneath and is weakly spiny. Flowerheads are clustered at the ends of branches. Found in moist meadows and open forests at low to montane elevations in BC.

Leafy thistle (*C. foliosum*) grows to 2.5 m tall and has hairy, slender, tapered involucral bracts. Found in moist meadows and forest openings in foothills to subalpine zones from southern YT and NT south to BC and east to AB. See p. 424 for conservation status.

Hooker's thistle (*C. hookerianum*) grows 40 cm–1.5 m tall and has broad involucral bracts, often with enlarged, fringed tips. Found in moist meadows, roadsides and forest openings at montane to subalpine elevations in BC and AB. See p. 424 for conservation status.

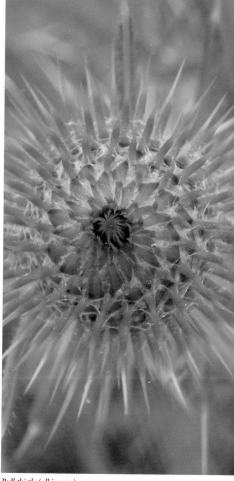

Bull thistle (all images)

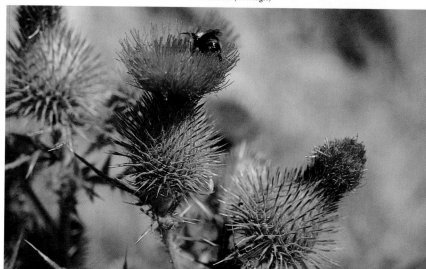

Wild Sages

Artemisia spp.

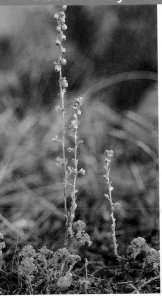

Pasture sagewort

FOOD: Although these aromatic plants are in no way related to the common herb sage (the mint *Salvia officinalis*), they have a similar fragrance and have been used occasionally as a spice with meat or corn. However, their bitterness can be overpowering. The seed-like fruits have been eaten fresh, dried or pounded into meal (see **Warning**).

MEDICINE: Strong, bitter-tasting pasture sagewort tea was taken to treat colds, fevers and Rocky Mountain spotted fever and was used in washes and salves to treat bruises, itching, sores, eczema and underarm or foot odour. The leaves were dried, crushed and used as snuff to relieve congestion, nosebleeds and headaches. Tarragon plants were boiled to make washes and poultices for treating swollen feet and legs and snow blindness. Some tribes called western mugwort women's sage because the leaf tea was taken to correct menstrual irregularity. It was also taken to relieve indigestion, coughs and chest infections. Western mugwort smoke was used to disinfect contaminated areas and to revive patients from comas. Northern wormwood tea was taken to relieve difficulties with urination or bowel movements, to ease delivery of babies and to cause abortions. As the name suggests, it was also used to expel worms—especially pinworms and roundworms. In Eastern Canada, chewed or powdered leaves of *Artemisia* species were often applied to cuts, sores and blisters, and they have been shown to have antibacterial properties.

OTHER USES: Sage plants and smudges repel insects, and these aromatic herbs were also believed to drive away evil. They were widely used in religious ceremonies, both in smoking mixtures and as incense for purifying implements and people. Western mugwort was sometimes spread along the edges of ceremonial lodges and made into protective wreaths and bracelets. If someone committed a taboo, he or she was purified by a whipping with a bundle of western mugwort. The pulverized roots of northern wormwood were used as perfume. It was believed that if you placed them on the face of a sleeping man, he would not wake up and you could then steal his horses. The soft leaves of western mugwort provided toilet paper, sanitary napkins and deodorizing shoe liners, and the leaf tea was used as a hair tonic.

DESCRIPTION: Aromatic, annual and perennial herbs and shrubs with alternate leaves. Flowerheads small, yellowish, with disc flowers only, borne in narrow to open, branched clusters, from June to October. Fruits hairless, seed-like achenes.

Annual wormwood (*A. annua*), to 2.5 m tall, has finely cut, fern-like leaves, with segments oblong to lance-shaped, sharp-toothed or cleft. Flowers tiny, green-yellow and grow in clusters. Grows in waste sites from ON to the Maritimes.

Western mugwort (*A. ludoviciana*) grows to 1 m tall and also has toothless leaves, but they are densely woolly on both sides. Grows in dry, open prairies in BC and AB.

WARNING
Most sages can cause allergic reactions and many are considered toxic, so these plants should always be used with caution. Large doses of tarragon's essential oil caused cancer in experimental animals.

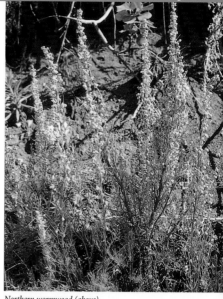

Northern wormwood or **plains wormwood** (*A. campestris*) also grows to 1 m tall, has grey-green (hairy, but not silvery-woolly) foliage and is less strongly scented. Grows on dry slopes in prairies, foothills and montane zones across Canada (except PEI). See p. 424 for conservation status.

Tarragon (*A. dracunculus*) is 50 cm–1 m tall, with essentially hairless, linear (rarely lobed) leaves and 2–4 mm wide flowerheads in open clusters. Grows on dry, open, sandy sites from BC and YT to ON. See p. 424 for conservation status.

Pasture sagewort or **prairie sagewort** (*A. frigida*) is 10–40 cm tall and has densely woolly, feathery leaves that are finely divided 2–3 times into linear segments to 1 mm wide. Grows on dry prairies to subalpine sites from BC to ON. See p. 424 for conservation status.

Mugwort (*A. vulgaris*) is 60 cm–1 m tall, with deeply cut leaves, silvery-downy beneath. Flowerheads erect. This introduced European species grows in open waste sites in southern Canada.

Northern wormwood (above)
Mugwort (below)

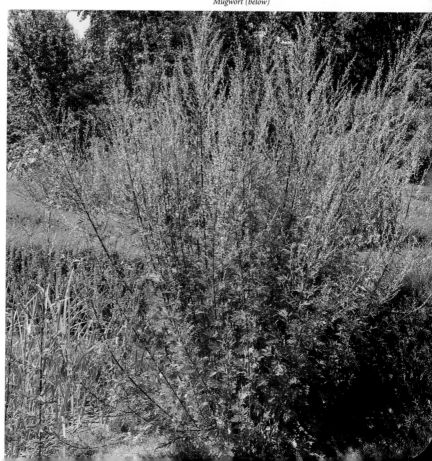

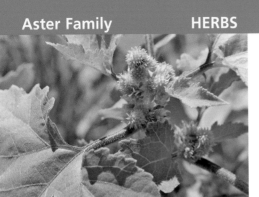

Cocklebur
Xanthium strumarium

FOOD: The leaves and young plants can be eaten cooked, but must be thoroughly boiled and washed before consumption. The seed, eaten raw or roasted, can be ground into a powder and mixed with flour to make bread.

MEDICINE: The root has a long history as a medicinal plant to treat scrofula or struma, a form of tuberculosis characterized by swelling of the lymph nodes, hence the species name. First Nations used an infusion of the leaves to treat kidney disease, rheumatism, rheumatoid arthritis, tuberculosis, diarrhea, constipation, lumbago, leprosy, allergic rhinitis, sinusitis, catarrh and pruritis. The plant was considered therapeutic in treating rabies, fevers and long-standing cases of malaria and was once used as an adulterant for the

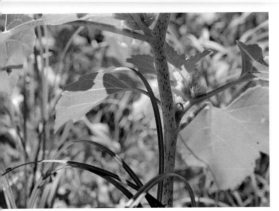

narcotic thorn-apple (*Datura stramonium*). A decoction of the root was used by women to expel afterbirth and in the treatment of high fevers. It is also a bitter tonic and diuretic. The fruits contain biologically active glycosides and phytosterols that possess antibacterial, antifungal, antimalarial, antirheumatic, antispasmodic, antitussive, cytotoxic, hypoglycemic and stomaic activity. The powdered seeds were applied as a salve to open sores. A decoction of the seeds was reportedly useful for bladder complaints.

OTHER USES: The leaves provide a yellow dye, and the seed powder was employed as an ingredient to make blue body paint. The leaves are a source of tannins and were used to repel weevils from wheat stores. Seed oil has been used as lamp fuel. Cocklebur seeds were once fed on by the now extinct Carolina parakeet. Today the plant has become an invasive species worldwide and is poisonous to livestock.

DESCRIPTION: Rough-stemmed annual, 30 cm–1.8 m tall, from a taproot. Leaves alternate, oval to kidney-shaped, 5–15 cm long (including their long stalks). Separate greenish male and female flowerheads in clusters from leaf axils. Female flowers form spiny, non-hairy, egg-shaped burs, 1–3.5 cm long; male flowers on short spikes. Flowers from August to October. Grows in waste places, roadsides and low grounds in all provinces.

WARNING

The plant is poisonous and is avoided by most grazing livestock. Symptoms appear within a few hours after ingestion and include weakness, vertigo, depression, nausea and vomiting, convulsions of the neck muscles, rapid and weak pulse, loss of breath and, eventually, death.

Chufa

Cyperus esculentus

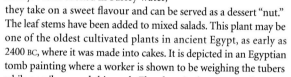

FOOD: The species name *esculentus* means "edible" in Latin, referring to the tubers, which have an excellent, slightly sweet, nutty flavour. They can be eaten raw, but they are hard, rather chewy and have a tough skin. They are generally soaked in water before they can be eaten but taste best when they are dried. Once dried, they can be ground into flour or roasted to a dark brown and ground into coffee. A milky drink can be made from the ground tuber, water, wheat and sugar, and a refreshing cool drink made from the ground tuber, water, cinnamon, sugar, vanilla and ice. Soaking the tubers in water for several days, then crushing them in fresh water and straining them through cheesecloth makes a tasty drink once sweetened with sugar or honey. When cooked in barley water, they take on a sweet flavour and can be served as a dessert "nut." The leaf stems have been added to mixed salads. This plant may be one of the oldest cultivated plants in ancient Egypt, as early as 2400 BC, where it was made into cakes. It is depicted in an Egyptian tomb painting where a worker is shown to be weighing the tubers while a scribe records his work. Elsewhere in the same tomb appear instructions on how to prepare the ground tubers as confectioneries. They are cultivated today in Spain to make *horchata de chufas*, a milky beverage made from chufa tubers, water and sugar. The tubers are very nutritious and rich in minerals, especially phosphorus and potassium, with a fat composition similar to that of olive oil: 18 percent saturated (palmitic and stearic) and 82 percent unsaturated (oleic and linoleic) fatty acids.

MEDICINE: The tubers are regarded as a digestive tonic and prescribed for all manner of intestinal disturbances. In Ayurveda, they are considered to have a heating and drying effect on the intestinal lining and are employed as a remedy for flatulence, indigestion, colic, diarrhea, dysentery and excessive thirst. Traditionally, First Nations used them as a ceremonial emetic, as a cough medicine and to stimulate urine production or menstruation. Externally, the chewed root was applied as a poultice on snakebites.

OTHER USES: Pieces of chewed root were sometimes placed inside a horse's nostrils to stimulate them. The tubers may be a potential oil crop for the production of biodiesel because they contain 20–36 percent oil. Leaves were used for weaving hats and matting.

DESCRIPTION: Perennial, grass-like plant, 20–90 cm tall, with solitary stems growing from stolons and tubers. Stems triangular in cross-section and bear slender leaves 3–10 mm wide. Flower branches radiate from the top of the stem, with yellow-green scales, in clusters perpendicular to the branch, like a bottle brush. This introduced Eurasian species grows in damp, sandy soil in southwestern BC, and from ON to NS; it's considered an intrusive weed in lawns and gardens. See p. 424 for conservation status.

Bulrushes

Schoenoplectus spp.

FOOD: The juicy young shoots and lower stalks have been eaten raw as a thirst-quenching snack or cooked as a vegetable. The starchy rhizomes are best collected in autumn or early spring. Growing tips of the rhizomes have been eaten raw, roasted like potatoes or added to soups and stews. Dried rhizomes were crushed to remove their fibres and then ground into flour for making bread, muffins and biscuits. Similarly, fresh rhizomes have been boiled into a gruel and then dried and ground into flour or used wet in pancakes and breads. Young rhizomes were crushed and boiled to make a sweet syrup. Pollen was pressed into cakes and baked, or it was mixed with flour and meal to make bread, mush or pancakes. The seeds can be eaten raw or parched. They were added to stews, breads and mush or ground into meal and used as a flour supplement or thickener. Some tribes gathered the sweet, dried sap or "honeydew" exuded by the stems and rolled it into balls for storage.

MEDICINE: Plants were boiled to make medicinal teas for treating nervous, fretful, crying children and for washing weak legs.

OTHER USES: The long, flexible stems of bulrushes were woven into baskets and mats by many west coast First Nations. They can also be twisted to make the seats of rush-bottomed chairs. They were often used with or instead of cattail leaves (p. 316).

DESCRIPTION: Slender, pale green, aquatic herbs with round, 50 cm–3 m tall stems from scaly, creeping rhizomes. Leaves mostly reduced to bladeless sheaths. Flowers tiny, in finely hairy, oval spikelets, forming a branched, 5–10 cm long cluster from the base of an erect, stem-like bract, from June to September. Fruits 2-sided, oval, seed-like achenes about 1.5–3 mm long, with 4–6 slightly barbed bristles from the base.

Hard-stemmed bulrush or **tule** (*S. acutus*) has firmer, less easily crushed stems. Spikes grey-brown, and spikelets usually clustered. See p. 424 for conservation status.

Soft-stemmed bulrush (*S. tabernaemontani*) has soft, spongy stems that are easily crushed. Spikes reddish brown, and spikelets often solitary. See p. 424 for conservation status.

Both species grow in shallow, calm water throughout Canada.

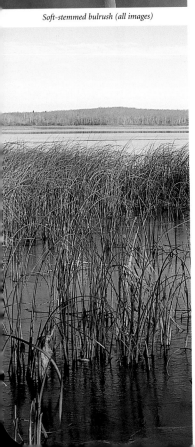

Soft-stemmed bulrush (all images)

Wild Rice

Zizania spp.

FOOD: Although wild rice is now sold as a luxury food in natural health food stores, it was used for millennia by central and eastern First Nations as a valuable staple food. Traditionally, wild rice was eaten plain, boiled or steamed, or roasted and eaten dry; it was cooked in soups, boiled with meat, fish, roe, beans, corn or squash, grease or maple sugar or with blueberries or other fruits. Wild rice is very nutritious; it is high in protein and fibre and low in fat.

Wild rice was traditionally harvested by canoe. Standing stalks of wild rice would be gathered and tied in bundles by indigenous peoples (often women). They would travel in twos; one would pole the canoe, while the other would pull the grass bundles over the canoe and gently beat the plant with a stick to loosen the mature kernels. The rice was then dried or cured, sometimes on mats set on a scaffold over a fire. The awned hulls were thrashed off, often by the men, by trampling or dancing on the grain. The grains would then be winnowed, sometimes by tossing them in a tray in a breeze, so the chaff would be removed from the grain. The rice was often stored in sacks or birchbark containers, sometimes in underground caches, for future use or sale. Wild rice harvesting has become a commercial activity to meet the increasing demand for this grain. SK is the largest producer in Canada.

OTHER USES: Wild rice is an important food for wild birds and waterfowl.

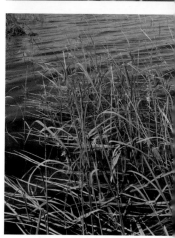

Northern wild rice (all above)
Wild rice (below)

DESCRIPTION: Annual herb with erect stems, thick, spongy and hollow, to 3 m tall. Leaves flat, to 1 m long and 4 cm wide, smooth, margins sharply toothed, leaf markings purple, thick midrib often nearer 1 margin than the other. Flowers ranging from white to purple, with long, stiff, twisted, barbed awns at stem tip and branches and branchlets to 40 cm long; lower branchlets drooping (male flowers), upper branchlets pointing stiffly upward (female flowers), blooming early August. Seeds purplish black when ripe, 12–19 mm long, mature in late summer (late August to early September); upon maturity, the hulls with enclosed grains easily "shatter" or drop into the water.

Wild rice (*Z. aquatica*) has dull, flexible, hairy lemmas, aborted pistillate spikelets less than 1 mm wide, and the branches bearing pistillate spikelets spread widely from the stem. See p. 424 for conservation status.

Northern wild rice (*Z. palustris*) has shiny, stiff lemmas that are hairless or have rows of hairs, aborted pistillate spikelets usually more than 1 mm wide, and the branches bearing pistillate spikelets mostly pressed up against the stem.

Both species are found on the margins of lakes and streams, preferring non-stagnant water, often covering large areas. Wild rice is native to southern ON and southern QC, and northern wild rice may also be native to the Maritime provinces.

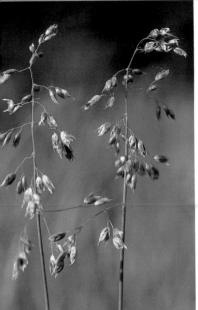

Common Sweetgrass

Hierochloe odorata

FOOD: Although sweetgrass grains are edible, they do not appear to have been used as food. These plants are rich in coumarin and should not be eaten (see **Warning**). An essential oil from the leaves has a strong vanilla-like flavour and is used as a food flavouring in sweets and soft drinks.

MEDICINE: The plants were used to make medicinal teas for treating coughs, sore throats, fevers, venereal infections, chafing, windburn and sore eyes. They were also taken to alleviate sharp internal pains, stop vaginal bleeding, help with childbirth and expel afterbirth. Sweetgrass smoke was inhaled to relieve colds.

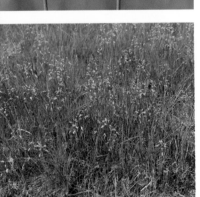

OTHER USES: Common sweetgrass leaves were collected in autumn and used to perfume clothing and to repel insects. Some women wove sweetgrass into their hair or soaked the leaves in water to make a sweet-smelling hair rinse. Sweetgrass was also soaked in water with gelatin from boiled horse hooves to make a hair lotion. Saddlesores on horses were treated with sweetgrass leaves. Sweetgrass is a very important and well-respected plant to many First Nations in Canada. It is commonly braided, dried and burned as incense; its smoke is used to cleanse and purify people, often within spiritual ceremonies, and to bring blessings and protection. Interwoven strands of sweetgrass are a symbol to some of life's growth and renewing powers. It was chewed to extend endurance during ceremonies involving prolonged fasting. Sweetgrass was sometimes ceremonially smoked with tobacco (p. 240), and it was often used within ceremonial regalia. Silvery or golden sweetgrass flower clusters make a lovely, sweet-smelling addition to dried bouquets. The grass blades were also used for making mats, baskets or as a sewing material. The long, creeping rhizomes stabilize unstable slopes and roadsides.

This plant goes by several scientific names and is included in some treatments in the genus *Anthoxanthum*.

DESCRIPTION: Sweet-smelling, vanilla-scented, perennial grass, 30–60 cm tall, from slender rhizomes. Leaves mainly basal, flat, usually about 3–5 mm wide. Flowers in shiny, bronze to purplish, pyramid-shaped clusters of flattened, 3-flowered, tulip-shaped spikelets 4–6 mm long, produced from May to July. Grows in open, moist to dry, often disturbed ground in prairies to subalpine zones across Canada.

WARNING
Sweetgrass contains the sweet-smelling compound coumarin, which delays or prevents blood from clotting.

Quackgrass
Elymus repens

FOOD: The rhizomes can be cooked and eaten or roasted and drunk as a coffee substitute; they have been dried, ground into a powder and used in bread or boiled down into syrup, which was sometimes brewed into beer. The leaves and shoots are edible and can be eaten fresh in salads; they are best gathered early in spring when the leaves are less fibrous and tough. The seeds are edible, and a cereal mash can be made from them; they have 18.5 g protein in 100 g of fresh weight.

MEDICINE: Quackgrass has a long history of medicinal use in Europe, since the classical period. The rhizome is the part of the plant used medicinally and has most often been used to treat kidney, liver and urinary problems such as inflamed bladders, painful urination, "thick" urine (when combined with twigs of alders, p. 151) and water retention. It is valued for its antiseptic and laxative properties as well as its ability to soothe irritated tissue. The rhizome has also been used as a worm expellant and to treat poor eyesight, chest pain, fever, syphilis, jaundice and swollen and rheumatic limbs.

OTHER USES: Sick dogs and cats have been known to dig up and eat the rhizomes or leaves, which is likely the source of one of its common names, dog grass. Quackgrass is considered a troublesome weed, especially by farmers. It is well known for its ability to spread quickly through its rhizomes and survive in any soil or weather conditions. The words "quack" and "couch" (couchgrass is another common name for this plant) are derived from the Anglo Saxon cwice or cwic, meaning "vivacious," owing to its reputation as a persistent weed. Quackgrass was placed under and over food in pit cooking. A grey dye can be obtained from the roots. An infusion of the whole plant can be used as liquid plant feed.

DESCRIPTION: Perennial herb, to 1 m tall, from pale yellow, long, creeping rhizomes. Stems often hairy at leaf sheaths. Leaves flat, firm, hairy to hairless, 5–10 mm wide, very short ligules. Flowers borne in a long spike (7–15 cm long), stalkless, alternate and flat against spike, closely crowded and overlapping. This introduced plant is found in disturbed sites, fields, lawns, meadows, waste areas and on roadsides in all provinces as well as NT.

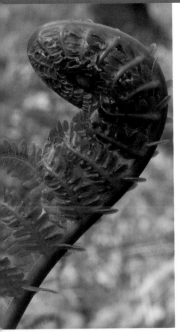

Ostrich Fern

Matteucia struthiopteris

FOOD: Fiddleheads, the coiled fronds of the young fern, are a traditional dish in QC and NB; they are an excellent wild edible that is sold commercially in some regions. (They're called fiddleheads because of their resemblence to the scroll of a violin.) The NB village of Tide Head, located on the south bank of the Restigouche River, bills itself as the "Fiddlehead Capital of the World." Fiddleheads have also been part of the traditional diets in parts of Asia, Australia and New Zealand. In Japan, ostrich fern sprouts, called *kogomi*, are considered a delicacy. Fiddleheads are collected mid-spring when they are less than 15 cm high and still tightly curled. The brown scales do not need to be removed. Fiddleheads can be sliced up raw and added to salads (but see **Warning**) or cooked for 10–15 minutes. Their taste is often compared to that of asparagus (p. 174). They should be served at once with a little butter because the quicker they are eaten, the more delicate their flavour. When harvesting, no more than 3 tops (roughly half) per plant should be taken. Over-picking depletes the rhizome's energy reserves and kills the plant. There are reports that the rhizome, once peeled and roasted, is also edible.

MEDICINE: First Nations in east-central SK drank a decoction of the leaf stalk base from the sterile frond for back pain and to speed expulsion of the afterbirth.

OTHER USES: Ostrich fern is a popular ornamental plant in gardens.

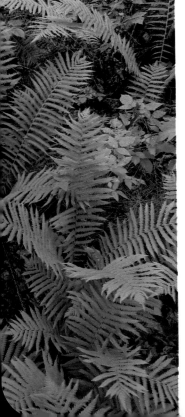

DESCRIPTION: Large, perennial fern from a stout, scaly rhizome. Fronds of 2 types: sterile fronds deciduous, green, plume-like, long tapering to the base but short tapering to the tip, growing in graceful, vertical, vase-like crowns, 50 cm–1.5 m tall and 15–30 cm wide; and fertile fronds smaller, 40–60 cm tall, stiffly erect, brown when ripe, developing in autumn and persisting over winter to release spores in early spring. Fiddleheads tightly coiled, rich emerald green, covered with large, papery, brown scales. Grows in rich, moist or wet soils near streambanks, riverbanks, open woods and swamp edges throughout Canada (except NU). See p. 424 for conservation status.

WARNING
A food-borne illness outbreak in BC in 1990 was caused by the consumption of either raw or lightly cooked fiddleheads. Although the toxin was not identified in ostrich fern fiddleheads, it is strongly advised that they be thoroughly cooked before eating.

Christmas Fern & Sword Fern

Polystichum spp.

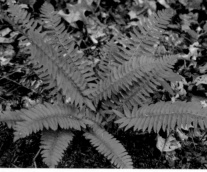

Christmas fern

FOOD: The fiddleheads of Christmas fern are eaten in much the same way as those of ostrich fern (p. 378), although it is prudent to thoroughly boil them for 10 minutes in 2 changes of water to remove any potential toxins (see **Warning**). The rhizomes of sword fern were peeled and baked like potatoes, but this was considered a famine food by First Nations. The rhizomes were harvested in spring before the appearance of sprouts.

MEDICINE: Christmas fern was used medicinally by several First Nations for a wide array of disorders. An infusion of the plant was taken for rheumatism, chills, fevers, toothaches, cramps in children and diarrhea and as a blood purifier for venereal disease. The rhizomes were used as an ingredient in an emetic preparation for dyspepsia and tuberculosis, as a cold infusion for stomach and intestinal pains and chewed raw for hoarseness. They were also mixed with other ingredients and massaged with warm hands on rheumatic areas of the body. A footbath of infused, mashed rhizomes was a remedy for rheumatic pain in the back and legs. A poultice of the wet, pulverized rhizomes was applied to the backs and heads of children for convulsions and red spots and of babies for spinal trouble and sore backs. Children were given a decoction of the rachis with small leaves to alleviate fevers. Young sword fern sprouts were chewed or eaten to treat sore throats, tonsillitis and cancer of the womb, and women chewed mature fronds to facilitate childbirth. A poultice made from an infusion of the fronds was applied to boils and sores, and a decoction of the rhizomes used as a remedy for dandruff. The spores were rubbed on the skin to relieve the pain from stinging nettle (p. 312) exposure.

OTHER USES: The dark green fronds of sword fern were used as lining for boxes and fruit drying racks. They were also used as a stuffing material in bedding.

DESCRIPTION: Shiny, vase-like, evergreen ferns with 30 cm–1.5 m long fronds, sprouting from stout, creeping rhizomes. Leaves lustrous, leathery, tapering.

Christmas fern (*P. acrostichoides*) has bristle-tipped, strongly eared pinnae with incurved teeth. Fronds grow to 80 cm long, with spores produced on smaller fertile fronds, the sori (spore clusters) growing together into a single large mass. Grows in wet woods and on rocky slopes from ON to NS. See p. 424 for conservation status.

Sword fern (*P. munitum*) has a small, upward-pointing lobe at the base of each pinna, with the edges toothed with bristly tips. Fronds grow to 1.5 m long, with spores produced on any fronds (no specialized fertile fronds), the sori occupying 2 discrete rows on either side of the midrib of each pinna. Grows in moist, coniferous forests, and occasionally on rocks, at low to montane elevations in BC.

> **WARNING**
> Although the toxicity of *Polystichum* is unknown, many ferns contain known carcinogens. *Polystichum* also contains thiaminase, an enzyme that breaks down the B vitamin thiamine (see **Warning** on p. 383).

Sword fern

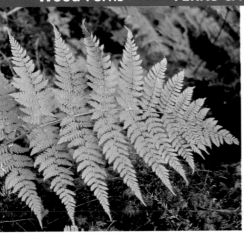

Broad spiny woodfern

Woodferns
Dryopteris spp.

FOOD: The bitter rhizomes of narrow spiny woodfern and broad spiny woodfern become sweeter when cooked, and some indigenous peoples gathered them for food. Cooking involved several hours of boiling in pots, roasting in or over coals or steaming in pits. Cooked rhizomes were peeled and eaten with grease or fermented salmon roe. Their flavour has been likened to that of sweet potatoes (*Ipomoea batatas*). The fleshy rhizomes were usually gathered in late autumn or early spring (before the leaves developed). Only rhizomes edged with round, fleshy, light green fingers of new growth were eaten, not those that were dark inside. Although considered edible, consumption is not recommended (see **Warning**).

MEDICINE: Oil from the rhizomes of male fern has been used to expel tapeworms from humans and animals. The patient was put on a fat-free diet for 2–3 days and then given a single dose of male fern. Compounds in the resins would paralyze the worms and force them to release their hold on the intestine. A salty laxative would then flush them from the system. Male fern was also said to cause abortions. Mashed rhizomes were sometimes applied to skin to heal cuts and ulcers. Some native peoples recommended woodfern rhizomes as an aid for losing weight and a cure for paralytic shellfish poisoning. A tea made from crested woodfern rhizomes was used to treat stomach trouble.

OTHER USES: Woodfern leaves were soaked in water to make a hair rinse.

DESCRIPTION: Large, perennial, clumped, deciduous or evergreen ferns, 30–90 cm tall, from brown-scaly, stout rhizomes covered with old leaf bases. Fronds feathery with dark brown-scaly stalks. Dots of spore-containing sori line the veins, each partly covered by a thin, horseshoe-shaped to kidney-shaped flap (indusium).

Narrow spiny woodfern (*D. carthusiana*) has more elongate leaves with a mostly symmetrical lowermost pair of leaflets. Grows in wet woods, on moist wooded slopes and on streambanks at low to subalpine elevations in all provinces except SK and MB. See p. 424 for conservation status..

Broad spiny woodfern (*D. expansa*) has triangular leaves with an asymmetrical lowermost pair of leaflets. Found in cool, moist woods and rocky slopes in all provinces and territories except NU. See p. 424 for conservation status.

Crested woodfern (*D. cristata*) has 2 types of twice-divided leaves: fertile fronds narrow and erect, 25–60 cm long, and vegetative fronds shorter, broader and floppier, 15–40 cm long, with widely spaced leaflets tilted out to the plane of the blade. Found in swamps, moist to wet woods or open, shrubby wetlands in all provinces. See p. 424 for conservation status.

Male fern (*D. filix-mas*) has twice-divided leaves with blunt teeth. Found on moist talus slopes and dense woods at montane to subalpine elevations in BC, AB, SK, ON, QC, NB, NS and NL. See p. 424 for conservation status.

WARNING
Raw rhizomes are bitter, strongly laxative and potentially toxic.
Overdoses cause muscular weakness, coma and, most frequently, blindness.
Male fern will irritate sensitive skin.

Polypodies

Polypodium spp.

FOOD: The sweet, licorice-flavoured rhizomes of some *Polypodium* species contain sucrose and fructose, as well as osladin, a compound that is said to be 300 times sweeter than sugar. Although these tough rhizomes have seldom been used as food (for some, only in times of famine), they were occasionally used for flavouring, and they were often chewed as an appetizer or candy. Chewing polypody rhizomes before drinking water was said to make the water taste sweet, and the rhizome was chewed to "make the mouth sweet." The rhizome also served as a dietary aid; it was kept in the mouth to prevent hunger and thirst.

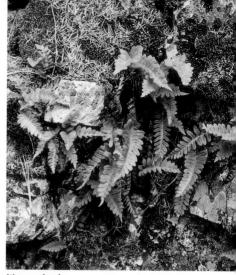

Western polypody

MEDICINE: The creeping rhizomes of *Polypodium* species were chewed (raw or roasted) to soothe sore throats and coughs, treat vomiting blood and relieve cold symptoms. They were also boiled to produce medicinal teas for treating dysentery, diarrhea, stomachaches, heart disease, internal ailments, pleurisy, shortness of breath, sore gums, gas and venereal complaints, for washing chapped hands and dislocated joints and for expelling intestinal worms. Because of their sweet, licorice flavour, licorice fern rhizomes were sometimes used to mask the taste of other bitter medicines. Present-day herbalists have recommended western polypody rhizomes for reducing inflammation caused by allergic reactions. A decoction of the rock polypody plant was used to treat tuberculosis and as an expectorant and laxative.

OTHER USES: Some settlers used western polypody rhizomes to flavour tobacco (p. 240).

DESCRIPTION: Evergreen, perennial ferns with leaves scattered along creeping, reddish brown, scaly rhizomes. Leaves (fronds) lance-shaped in outline, pinnately divided into 5–18 opposite or offset pairs of blunt lobes. Leaf stalks 1–12 cm long, smooth, straw-coloured, shorter than the blade. Spores borne in large, rounded dots (sori) on the underside of leaflets, midway between the edge and the central vein.

Licorice fern (*P. glycyrrhiza*) has leaves to 75 cm long, not very leathery; with an intensely licorice-flavoured creeping stem. Found on cliffs and rocky slopes or commonly epiphytic on tree trunks or branches along the coast of BC and YT.

WARNING

All ferns should be used with caution and never during pregnancy because the toxicity of most species is not known. Some *Polypodium* species contain methyl salicylate, a compound with aspirin-like effects, so people who are allergic to aspirin or who have blood-clotting disorders should not use these plants.

Western polypody (*P. hesperium*) has leaves to 35 cm long, somewhat leathery. Grows in crevices and ledges on rocks at low to subalpine elevations in BC and extreme southwestern AB (Rocky Mountains). See p. 424 for conservation status.

Rock polypody (*P. virginianum*) has leathery leaves to 40 cm long. Grows on cliffs and rocky slopes at low to subalpine elevations from AB and NT across to NL. See p. 424 for conservation status.

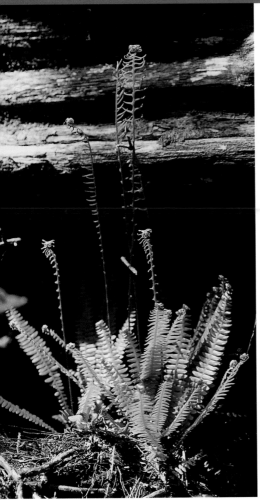

Deer Fern

Blechnum spicant

FOOD: The plant was generally eaten as a starvation food when nothing else was available. The young, tender stalks were peeled and the centre portion eaten. Young shoots and rhizomes can be cooked. When people were lost in the woods, the fronds were eaten to relieve hunger, and the young stems chewed to alleviate thirst. The fronds were placed under items cooked in steaming pits to give them flavour.

MEDICINE: The leaflets were chewed to treat internal tumours and respiratory and gastric complaints. A tonic to relieve general ill health was made from a decoction of the leaves. A decoction of the rhizome, alone or mixed with other plants, was taken for diarrhea. Alternatively, diarrhea could be treated with the rhizome held in the mouth. The fronds were also applied externally to skin sores.

OTHER USES: Leaves were used by First Nations for bedding. Today, the plant is used as an indoor and outdoor ornamental, providing good groundcover in the shade of trees.

DESCRIPTION: Tufted evergreen fern from a short rhizome, with slender stems, short-creeping or ascending. Leaves dimorphic; fertile fronds more erect and with narrower pinnules than sterile leaves, withering soon after the spores are shed. Fertile and sterile fronds both generally 10–50 cm long, lance-shaped (the fertile blade more narrowly so), coarsely scaly at the base. Sori linear, like 2 lines, 1 on either side of the midrib of fertile pinnae. Grows in moist to wet, coniferous forests, bogs and streamsides at low to mid-elevations in western BC.

> **WARNING**
> No reported poisonings have been documented, but caution is advised because numerous ferns contain carcinogens. They also contain the enzyme thiaminase, which breaks down the B vitamin thiamine. Ingesting large quantities can cause the thiamine deficiency beriberi. In 1860–61, the first Europeans to cross Australia south to north, Robert O'Hara Burke and William John Wills, ate the baked nardoo-fern (*Marsilea drummondii*) on their return trip and died of beriberi, the baking not having been sufficient to deactivate the enzyme.

Lady Fern
Athyrium filix-femina

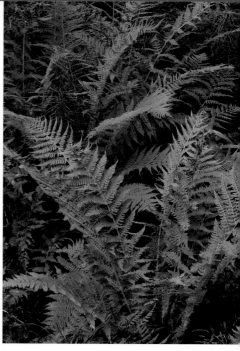

FOOD: First Nations often used the large leaves of lady fern to lay out or cover food, especially when drying out berries. In early spring, the fiddleheads, when they are 7–15 cm tall, can be boiled, baked and prepared like asparagus (p. 174). There are reports that the rhizome centres were eaten once peeled and roasted, but this has been disputed as a case of mistaken identity with a similar-looking species, broad spiny woodfern (p. 380).

MEDICINE: As the common name suggests, lady fern was considered particularly useful for complaints specific to women. A decoction of the pounded stems was taken to ease labour, and that of the rhizomes to ease breast pain associated with childbirth. An infusion of the rhizomes was used to stimulate milk flow in patients with caked breasts. When combined with the entire herb of New England aster (p. 346), it was used by mothers for intestinal fevers. A tea made from the plant was used as a diuretic and anthelmintic, and that of the boiled rhizomes taken as a tonic for general body pains. The young, unfurled fronds were eaten for internal disorders such as cancer of the womb. The dried powdered rhizome was applied to sores to speed healing, and a decoction of the rhizomes was used as a wash for sore eyes. The oil extracted from the rhizomes has been used since the times of Theophrastus and Dioscorides as a remedy for worms, although some herbalists note that the effect is not as powerful as that of male fern (p. 380). This remedy was used on both humans and livestock, with a single strong dose considered sufficient to expel the worms. However, if the dose is too strong, it can cause muscular weakness, coma and blindness.

OTHER USES: First Nations used the fronds as covering for fungus that was placed on hot stones to produce a red dye. When travelling through the mountains, the sight of lady ferns signified the presence of water.

WARNING

Fresh shoots contain the enzyme thiaminase, which breaks down the B vitamin thiamine, rendering it unavailable for human absorption. Although the small concentrations found in the plant are not sufficient to cause any real harm, consuming large quantities can cause severe health problems. Adequate cooking and drying deactivates this enzyme.

DESCRIPTION: Deciduous, perennial fern, to 1.8 m tall, from creeping to erect, scaly rhizomes. Leaves erect, 40–90 cm long, 10–35 cm wide, narrowly to widely lance-shaped, tapered at both ends, divided 2–3 times, growing in circular clumps. Pinnae lance-shaped, pointed, short-stalked to stalkless. Stalks straw-coloured to brownish red, fragile, grooved and scaly near base. Sori kidney- to horseshoe-shaped on underside of pinnae. Grows in moist, shaded areas throughout Canada. See p. 424 for conservation status.

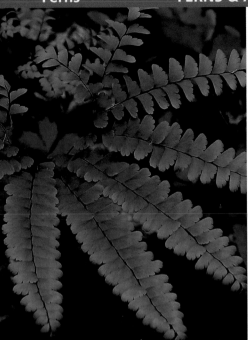

Western maidenhair fern

Maidenhair Ferns
Adiantum spp.

MEDICINE: Maidenhair ferns were employed to treat a variety of cold-related and respiratory ailments, such as coughs, colds, hoarseness, sore throats and asthma, to soothe mucus membranes of the throat and to loosen phlegm. The smashed wet fronds were used for snakebites and venereal disease and as a wash for sores. The whole plant was chewed to stop wounds from bleeding and to treat shortness of breath. Maidenhair ferns were also used to treat fevers, fits, labour pains and children with cramps or sore backs; a strong infusion of the whole plant was used as an emetic. The rhizome was used as "bitters," to treat excessive menstruation, as a stimulant and for rheumatism (internally or externally with a rhizome decoction massaged into the joints). Maidenhair ferns were historically exported to Europe and used by herbalists to make cough medicine. They were boiled with sugar to make a syrup called "capillaire," which has emetic properties. The Hesquiat used the leaves for strength and endurance (e.g. dancers in winter, to make them light-footed).

OTHER USES: Maidenhair ferns are popular ornamental ferns. The frond stems were used in basketry. The leaves can be used as a lining for carrying or storing fruits in baskets and on berry-drying racks. The name maidenhair may refer to the plants' glossy, hair-like stalks, their masses of dark root hairs, or perhaps their traditional use as a rinse to make hair shiny. Some say it works best in the hair when combined with chamomile (p. 365) or yarrow (p. 358). The genus name *Adiantum* means "unwetted"; raindrops roll right off the fronds, leaving the fronds nearly dry.

DESCRIPTION: Delicate, palmately branched, perennial fern from scaly rhizomes. Leaves solitary or few, 15–60 cm tall, blade 10–40 cm across, at almost right angles to leaf stalk, each leaflet with oblong or fan-shaped segments, with dark brown to purplish black stripes. Sori oblong on the edges of upper lobes of the leaflets.

These 2 species look very similar and until recently were considered a single species. Fortunately, their ranges are generally quite different, so unless you're in southern QC, you should be all right with the identification.

Western maidenhair (*A. aleuticum*) has the ultimate leaflet lobes separated by sinuses to 4 mm deep. Found in rich, moist to wet areas (wooded ravines, talus slopes, near waterfalls, on limestone) in BC, AB, QC and NL. See p. 424 for conservation status.

Canada maidenhair (*A. pedatum*) has the ultimate leaflet lobes separated by shallower sinuses to 2 mm deep. Found in rich, deciduous woodlands at low elevations from ON to NS.

Bracken

Pteridium aquilinum

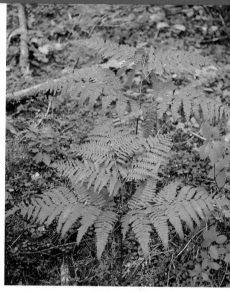

FOOD: Historically, young coiled leaves (fiddleheads), 10–15 cm tall, were collected in spring and rubbed free of hairs. They were then either soaked in salt water to reduce bitterness and eaten raw (but see **Warning**) or boiled for 30 minutes in 2 changes of water and eaten as a hot vegetable. The rhizomes were an important traditional food of some First Nations; they were roasted or pit-steamed. Cooked rhizomes were peeled and then pounded to separate the whitish, edible part from the fibres and outer black "bark." Some people simply chewed small chunks until the starch was gone and spat out the fibres. Bracken rhizomes were often eaten with oily foods, such as animal grease, fish grease or salmon eggs because these rhizomes were said to be constipating. Dried rhizomes were ground into flour, then mixed with water to make dough, formed into cakes and roasted. Warabi starch, extracted from bracken rhizomes, has been used in candies. Bracken rhizomes were also used to make ale.

MEDICINE: Bracken rhizomes were used in teas to treat rickets, stomach cramps, diarrhea and worms. Salves (made by boiling the leaves in fat) or boiled, mashed rhizomes were applied to burns, sores and "caked" breasts. The leaves were smoked to relieve headaches.

> **WARNING**
> Bracken contains the carcinogen ptaquiloside, which has little taste or odour and was not detected as a toxin by traditional peoples because of the long latency for carcinogenesis. Recent research from Latin America shows that it causes cancer in grazing animals, and the carcinogen is transmitted in milk, causing stomach cancer in people. Direct consumption of cooked bracken fern is a known risk factor for stomach cancer in Japan. In view of this, **bracken fern should not be consumed**. Sheep, pigs, cattle and horses have been poisoned by eating large amounts of mature bracken leaves. The leaves contain thiaminase, an enzyme that disturbs thiamine (vitamin B1) metabolism.

OTHER USES: Bracken tea was sometimes used in rinses to stimulate hair growth. The tannin-rich leaves were used for tanning leather. They were also used to dye wool yellow-green and to dye silk grey. Burning leaves provided mosquito-repellent smudges. These large, abundant leaves resist decay, so they have been used in many ways, including as thatching, bedding and packing material for produce. Rhizomes lather in water and have been used as a soap substitute.

DESCRIPTION: Coarse fern, 50 cm–2 m tall, with single, spreading to horizontal, long-stalked leaves from deep, spreading rhizomes. Leaves triangular in outline, the blades 30 cm–1 m long, 2- to 3-times pinnately divided into firm, round-toothed leaflets, turning a bright rusty colour after freezing in autumn. Spores borne in a continuous band under down-rolled leaf edges. Found at low to subalpine elevations in fields, meadows, bogs and open woods, and often on disturbed ground, in all provinces except SK, but not as far north as the territories. See p. 424 for conservation status.

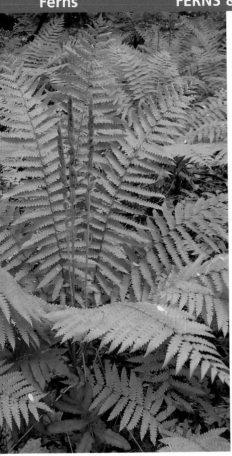

Cinnamon Fern
Osmunda cinnamomea

FOOD: The genus name is derived from the Saxon god Osmunder the Waterman (the Saxon equivalent of the Norse god Thor) who, according to legend, hid his family from danger in a clump of these ferns. This would be quite the ideal hiding place because cinnamon ferns form huge clonal colonies, while at the same time providing a source of nourishment that would be crucial for survival. The fiddleheads are reminiscent in taste of asparagus (p. 174) once cooked. They can be eaten as is or added to soups. First Nations used the frond as a nibble and ate the white base of the plant raw. The frond tips were simmered to remove ants and added to soup stock.

MEDICINE: First Nations applied a compound decoction of the rhizome with warm hands to an area affected with rheumatism. To treat a wound, a person would first chew and swallow a portion of the rhizome, then apply the rest to the injury. A decoction of the plant, most likely the rhizome, was taken internally to treat colds, chills, headaches, joint pain, rheumatism and malaise and to promote the flow of milk in nursing mothers while preventing caked breasts. The young shoots were perceived as a sort of spring tonic that cleansed the body after a winter of eating nothing but stored foods.

OTHER USES: Cinnamon ferns are sometimes planted as ornamentals. The rhizome is massive, with densely matted, wiry roots. These are used in the horticultural industry as a substrate for several epiphytic plants such as orchids. First Nations used the plant as a hunting aid, believing that the fern shoot, when eaten before a hunt, would give them the same scent as that of the shoot-eating deer, thereby hiding their human scent and reducing the likelihood that the deer would be frightened away.

DESCRIPTION: Deciduous, herbaceous, perennial fern, 30 cm–1.5 m tall, with separate fertile and sterile fronds. Sterile fronds erect, light green turning to yellow in autumn, oval to lance-shaped, with broadly oblong and deeply lobed pinnae, 5–10 cm long, 2–2.5 cm wide, and a persistent tuft of rusty, woolly hairs on upper surface at base. Fertile fronds shorter and narrower, bright green turning to a rich cinnamon brown, with much smaller, nonphotosynthetic pinnae that wither after sporulation. Fiddleheads large, showy, with silver-white hairs that turn rusty as the fronds unfurl. Grows in bogs, peatlands, thickets, wet woods, swamps and on streambanks from ON to NL.

WARNING
As with most other ferns, cinnamon fern may contain some carcinogens and the B vitamin inhibitor thiaminase. This enzyme, however, is destroyed by heat, so thorough cooking is advised.

Rattlesnake Fern

Botrychium virginianum

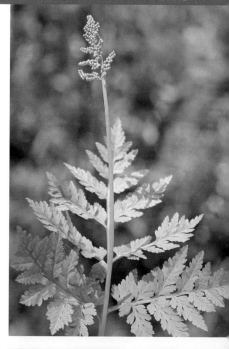

MEDICINE: The rhizome of rattlesnake fern was used medicinally. A poultice was applied to cuts and snakebites. Rattlesnake fern has properties that soothe irritated tissues and, because of this, is said to be good for respiratory illnesses. A cold infusion of the rhizome mixed with liquor was taken for consumption cough. A tea made from the rhizomes was taken as an emetic, to induce sweating and as an expectorant. A decoction of rattlesnake fern was given to sick children.

OTHER USES: The genus name *Botrychium* comes from the Greek word *botrus*, "grape," because the fruit resembles a cluster of grapes. The species name is derived from the location it was first discovered, Virginia. This fern acquired its common name from the resemblance of the fruiting stem to a rattlesnake's rattle.

DESCRIPTION: Perennial herb, 10–50 cm tall, arising from stout rhizomes. Three fronds arranged evenly around the stem, with fertile stalk sticking straight up from the centre. Fronds bright green, 25–30 cm long, membraneous and broadly triangular, with thin, lacy blades, usually 3- or 4-times pinnate. Fertile stalk branched, bearing many spherical, bright yellow spore cases, the spore cluster 2–15 cm long. Fronds seasonal, appearing in early spring and dying in late summer. Found in wetlands, moist to wet forests and on streambanks. See p. 424 for conservation status.

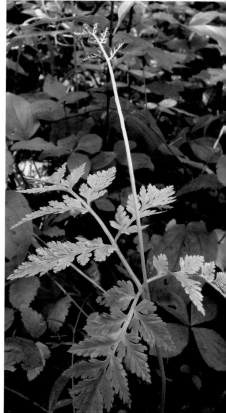

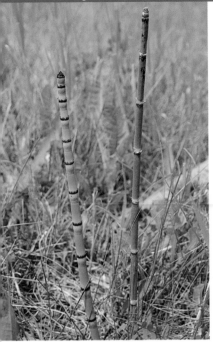

Common scouring-rush (all images)

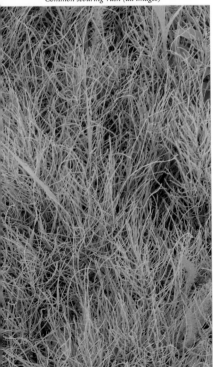

Horsetail & Scouring-Rush

Equisetum spp.

FOOD: The rhizomes and small, brown, fertile shoots of common horsetail have been eaten fresh or boiled, but they should be used only in moderation, if at all. The tough outer fibres are either peeled off or chewed and discarded. Young, green, tightly compacted bottlebrush shoots were cleaned of their sheaths and branches and eaten occasionally, but consumption is not recommended (see **Warning**).

MEDICINE: Horsetails and scouring-rushes have been used as medicines in much the same manner, though scouring-rushes were often considered stronger. Teas made from these plants were usually taken to treat bladder and kidney problems, water retention and constipation, but they were also used for treating gout, gonorrhea, stomach problems, menstrual irregularities, bronchitis and tuberculosis and were applied as washes to stop bleeding and combat infection. Plants were used in poultices to relieve bladder and prostate pain and to heal wounds and sores. Also, their ashes were applied to mouth sores. Horsetails and scouring-rushes may have some antibiotic properties, and glycosides in some plants have

> **WARNING**
> Horsetails have caused deaths of horses and cattle through the action of the enzyme thiaminase, which destroys thiamine (vitamin B1). Cooking destroys thiaminase, and B-vitamin supplements reverse its effects. Some horsetails also contain alkaloids, such as nicotine and palustrine, which are toxic in large quantities. Large amounts of silica may irritate the urinary tract and kidneys. Horsetails readily absorb heavy metals and chemicals from the soil, so plants from contaminated soil should never be used for food or medicine. People with high blood pressure and related problems should not use horsetails.

a weak diuretic action. Some present-day herbalists value these plants for their highly absorbable silica and calcium content. These minerals are said to maintain the health and resilience of cartilage and connective tissues, to promote circulation in the scalp and to strengthen bones. Horsetails and scouring-rushes have been recommended for preventing osteoporosis, for strengthening fingernails and for treating bursitis (inflamed connective tissue around joints), tendonitis (inflamed tendons), baldness, bone fractures, mouth infections, offensive perspiration and various eye, teeth, nail and skin problems. However, there is still controversy over the efficacy of these plants and the potential dangers associated with their use.

OTHER USES: These plants are embedded with abrasive silica crystals, so they can be used as polishers, facial scrubs and disposable pot scourers. First Nations gathered scouring-rushes to polish pipes, bows and arrows, and European housewives used these abrasive plants to brighten tins, floors and woodenware. Before they could be used as such, the stems were bleached by repeatedly wetting and drying them in the sun. Boxes of scouring-rush segments are still sold for shaping clarinet and oboe reeds. Teething babies were given horsetail rhizomes to chew on, and older children used common scouring-rush stems to make whistles (though their elders warned them that blowing the whistles could attract snakes). Tea made from these plants was used as a hair rinse to reduce baldness and kill lice.

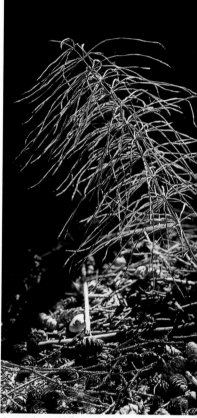

Common horsetail (all images)

DESCRIPTION: Perennial, evergreen herbs with hollow, jointed, vertically ridged stems from creeping rhizomes. Branches forming whorls at the nodes ("horsetails") or not ("scouring-rushes"). Leaves reduced to small scales, fused into sheaths on the stem. Spores borne in cones (strobili) at the stem tips.

Common horsetail (*E. arvense*) produces 2 types of plants—brownish, unbranched, fertile plants, 10–20 cm tall (in spring) and green, bottlebrush-like, sterile plants, 10–80 cm tall (in summer). Grows in disturbed sites, alluvial forests, fields, marshes, tundra and on roadsides throughout Canada.

Common scouring-rush (*E. hyemale*) has stiff, unbranched, 18- to 40-ridged, evergreen stems 4–8 mm thick and 30 cm–1.2 m tall, with 3–10 mm long sheaths that have 2 black bands. Grows in moist, alluvial forests, forest edges and disturbed ground (roadsides, clearings) throughout Canada (though apparently absent from NU).

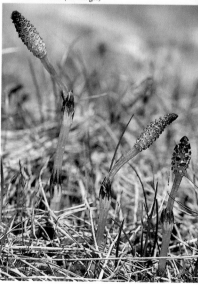

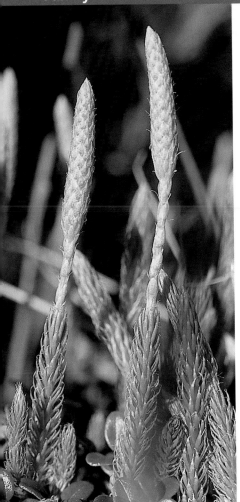

Running clubmoss

Clubmosses
Lycopodium and *Huperzia* spp.

FOOD: These plants have been used occasionally for food, but they are described as rather unappetizing, and they can be toxic (see **Warning**).

MEDICINE: Clubmoss spores have been used as dusting powder on wounds and surgical incisions and as treatment for various skin problems, including eczema, herpes, rashes and chafed skin. Animal and test tube studies have shown that clubmosses contain alkaloids that can increase urine flow, relieve spasms, stimulate bowel movements, vomiting and estrogenic activity (including uterine contractions), reduce fever, pain and inflammation and combat bacteria and fungi. Running clubmoss plants were used to treat several ailments, including kidney problems (especially those associated with high uric acid concentrations), postpartum pain, fever, weakness, rheumatism and even rabies. The spores were used to stop bleeding and to treat diarrhea, dysentery, rheumatism and indigestion. They were also believed to be an aphrodisiac. Northern clubmoss was recommended for treating a variety of complaints, including uterine problems, knee problems, swollen thighs and water retention. More recently, it has been found to contain the alkaloid huperzine, which has been shown to increase the efficiency of learning and memory in animals by inhibiting the breakdown of acetylcholine, an essential neurotransmitter. Northern clubmoss is now being studied for use in the treatment of myasthenia gravis (a disease in which muscles become increasingly weak and easily tired) and Alzheimer's disease.

OTHER USES: Clubmoss spores are rich in oil and are highly flammable. At one time, they were used by photographers as flash powder. Theatre performers used them to produce special effects such as lightning and explosions. The fine yellow spores shed water and have been used as baby powder. They have also been used to untangle and delouse matted hair, to prevent pills or suppositories from sticking together and as a powder on condoms and rubber gloves.

WARNING
Running clubmoss and northern clubmoss contain toxic alkaloids. Clubmoss spores can irritate mucous membranes and sensitive or damaged skin. People exposed to large amounts of these spores (e.g., in factories where spores are used in dusting powder) have developed asthma.

DESCRIPTION: Low, evergreen, perennial herbs, often trailing on the ground, with erect, leafy, bottlebrush-like stems 5–30 cm tall. Leaves firm, shiny, needle-like, 3–10 mm long, in usually 6 or 8 dense, vertical rows. Sporangia either in the axils of the ordinary leaves (*Huperzia*) or aggregated in terminal cones (*Lycopodium*).

Stiff clubmoss (*L. annotinum*) has pointed leaves on unbranched to twice-forked shoots from creeping, irregularly rooted stems to 1 m long. Spores borne in single, stalkless, 12–35 mm long cones (strobili) at the stem tips. Grows in dry to moist forests, bogs and open areas in foothill, montane and subalpine sites in all provinces and territories.

Running clubmoss (*L. clavatum*) is similar to stiff clubmoss, but young leaves tipped with a slender, hair-like bristle, and fertile stems have 2 or more strobili on a long stalk. Grows in similar habitats over a similar range as stiff clubmoss. See p. 424 for conservation status.

Northern clubmoss (*H. selago*) is a tufted species, about 5–10 cm tall, with spore clusters in the axils of upper leaves (rather than in terminal cones). Grows in open areas (including lakeshores) and swampy forests at low to montane elevations in alpine and subalpine zones from northeastern BC and eastern YT across Canada's boreal forest to NL. Across most of high-elevation BC and YT, the very similar **alpine clubmoss** (*H. haleakalae*) is found in moist meadows and heath at subalpine and alpine elevations. Aside from the different habitats, the shoots of northern clubmoss have weak annual constrictions, and those of alpine clubmoss have none. See p. 424 for conservation status.

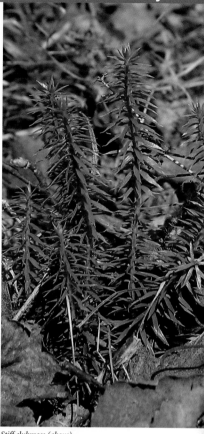

Stiff clubmoss (above)
Northern clubmoss (below)

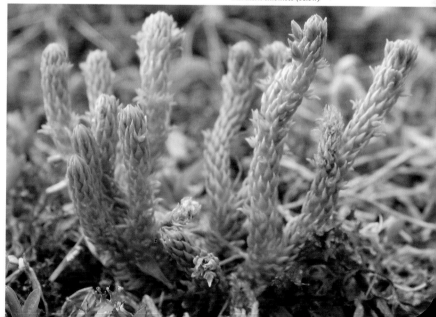

Poisonous Plants

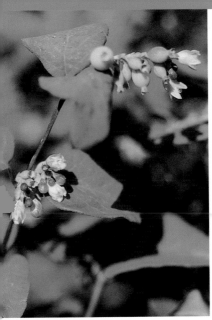

Common snowberry

This section describes some of the most common toxic plants in Canada, but it is by no means a complete guide to the country's poisonous plants. Many potentially toxic species in this book are not found in this section. Some have been widely used by humans and are discussed in the main body of the book, with notes about toxicity in the Warning boxes. For example, many of the drugs produced by plants can be deadly poisons when improperly prepared or administered.

Plants have developed a wide array of protective strategies to compete against other plants and to avoid infection and predation (being eaten or otherwise used) by animals. Many of these protective mechanisms are dangerous to humans, but as with most natural systems, the effects can vary greatly from plant to plant and from person to person. There are very few deadly poisonous plants in Canada. In most cases, you would have to inject large quantities to be fatally poisoned, but even though these plants may not kill you, you may wish you were dead when you experience their effects.

Toxins are rarely distributed evenly throughout all parts of a plant. For example, you may enjoy eating cherries, but did you know that all parts of these trees and shrubs, with the exception of the flesh of the cherries, contain hydrocyanic acid, which causes cyanide poisoning? Many of us enjoy rhubarb, but only the leaf stalks are edible. The broad, green leaf blades contain toxic concentrations of oxalates. Toxicity often changes as plants grow. Some species are most poisonous when they are young, whereas others grow increasingly toxic with age, often concentrating poisons in their seeds.

The toxicity of most wild plants has yet to be studied, but many are known to be poisonous. People can be harmed by plants in many ways.

1. Ingestion of plant toxins

Plant toxins are generally most effective when they are taken into the body in plants or plant extracts (e.g., as teas or tinctures) and absorbed into the system through the digestive tract. Types of toxins in this group include the following.

(a) Alkaloids are bitter-tasting chemicals that tend to be mildly alkaline. Many alkaloids affect the nervous system. This group includes some of our most powerful drugs, such as morphine, mescaline, caffeine, nicotine and strychnine.

(b) Glycosides are two-parted molecules composed of a sugar such as glucose and a non-sugar or aglycone. Usually, glycosides become poisonous when they are digested and the sugar is

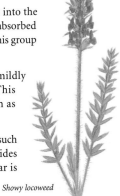

Showy locoweed

separated from its poisonous aglycone. Some of the more common aglycones include cyanide, cardioactive steroids (which affect the heart), saponin and mustard oil (which irritate the digestive tract) and coumarin (a powerful anticoagulant).

(c) Organic acids are carbon-based acids that lack nitrogen. Our only common organic acid, oxalic acid, causes ionic imbalances, internal bleeding and kidney damage. It is present in many plants, but seldom in toxic concentrations.

(d) Alcohols: all alcohols are somewhat toxic, but some are more poisonous than others. The deadly poison of water-hemlock (p. 411), cicutoxin, is an unsaturated alcohol that causes convulsions and death in a few minutes to a few hours.

(e) Resins and resinoids are a varied group of chemicals, many of which are phenolic compounds. Some phenolic resins, such as tetrahydrocannabinol of marijuana (p. 314), affect the nervous system. Others cause skin reactions. Urushiol in poison-ivy (p. 395) can cause rashes and blistering, and hypericin in St. John's-wort (p. 227) can cause reactions when skin is exposed to sunlight.

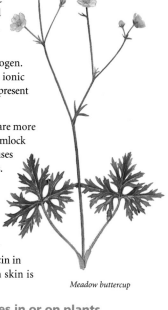

Meadow buttercup

2. Ingestion of bacteria and other parasites in or on plants

Not all poisonings result from substances produced by the plants. Bacteria, protozoa, nematodes and other animals growing in soil or water can adhere to plants, and they cause parasitic infections when plants are eaten raw without proper cleaning. This situation is most common with aquatic plants growing in polluted water. Some fungi that infect plants can also be toxic to humans. One of the best-known examples of toxic fungi is ergot (*Claviceps*), a group of parasitic fungi that infects the grains of grasses (pp. 375-377) and causes ergotism when eaten by humans.

WHAT TO DO

Proper treatment for cases of poisoning requires more information than this guide provides. It is usually best to induce vomiting, but in some cases, vomiting can do more harm than good. If a person is believed to have been poisoned, consult a doctor. If you suspect that a certain plant (or plants) is responsible for the problem but do not know the plant's identity, take samples (preferably whole plants, with roots and flowers or fruits) that can be examined later for positive identification.

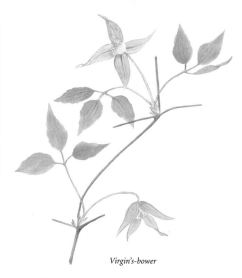

Virgin's-bower

3. Ingestion of chemical pollutants in or on plants

Soil, water and air can become polluted with chemicals from factories (often widespread), vehicle exhaust (along roadsides) or herbicides and pesticides (in parks and school yards and along roads). These compounds may be absorbed by plants or may simply coat the plant stems and leaves. Many pollutants are not removed by washing and are ingested when plants from polluted environments are eaten. Not all harmful chemicals are synthetic. For example, when selenium is present in the soil, some plants (e.g., paintbrushes [*Castilleja* spp.]) take it up and concentrate it to toxic levels in their tissues, making them poisonous. Similarly, many plants can accumulate toxic amounts of nitrates or molybdenum.

Common snowberry

4. Contact with irritating plants

Human skin is sensitive to contact with many plants that do not affect other animals. Sensitivity varies greatly from person to person. For example, most people develop rashes from contact with poison-ivy (p. 395), but a few people can handle these plants with impunity. Skin reactions may be caused by plant toxins or may simply result from irritation caused by protective hairs and spines.

Many plants, such as lady's-slipper orchids (*Cypripedium* spp.) and scorpionweeds (*Phacelia* spp.), are covered with stiff, protective hairs that irritate the skin when the plant is touched or eaten. These hairs cause allergic reactions (dermatitis) in some people, but they have no effect on others. A few species have developed specialized hairs to irritate potential grazers. The hairs of stinging nettles (p. 312) act like miniature hypodermic syringes, injecting droplets of acid under the skin and causing a burning sensation in everyone.

Stiff bristles, spines and thorns are obvious protective mechanisms that can damage skin. Some plants have barbs that help them to catch onto passers-by and to work their way into tender tissues around the mouth and eyes of grazing animals. These structures can also cause serious wounds and obstructions in the digestive tract.

A few plants produce irritating resins that stick to hair and clothing and cause rashes and blisters when they come into contact with skin. Poison-ivy (p. 395) is one of the best-known plants in this group. Other compounds, such as furanocoumarins in common cow-parsnip (p. 297), cause dark blotches, rashes and even blisters when plants are eaten and the skin is then exposed to light.

5. Contact with plant allergens

Allergy-producing materials are life-threatening to relatively few people, but in these cases, their effects can be as dangerous as those of any toxin. Allergic reactions vary greatly from person to person and plant to plant. Air-borne spores and pollen go unnoticed by most of us, but in people with allergies, specific types of pollen and spores can cause anything from a runny nose to a severe asthma attack. Similarly, foods that most of us enjoy everyday can cause fatal reactions in people who have developed allergies to a specific ingredient (e.g., peanuts). Most skin reactions (including poison-ivy rashes) are allergic reactions.

Poison-Ivy & Poison-Oak

Toxicodendron spp.

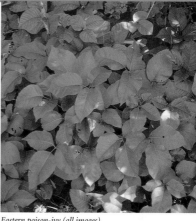

Poison-ivy and poison-oak plants contain an oily resin (urushiol) that causes a nasty skin reaction in most people, especially on sensitive skin and mucous membranes. The allergic contact dermatitis appears with some delay after exposure. Sensitization can lead to more severe reaction after re-exposure. Urushiol is not volatile and therefore it is not transmitted through the air, but it can be carried

Eastern poison-ivy (all images)

to unsuspecting victims on pets, clothing and tools and even on smoke particles from burning poison-ivy plants. The resin is also ejected in fine droplets when the plants are pulled. The resin can be removed by washing with a strong soap. Washing can prevent a reaction if it is done shortly after contact, and it also prevents transfer of the resin to other parts of the body or to other people. The liquid that oozes from poison-ivy or poison-oak blisters on skin does not contain the allergen. Ointments and even household ammonia can be used to relieve the itching of mild cases, but people with severe reactions might need to consult a doctor.

DESCRIPTION: Trailing to erect, deciduous shrubs, forming colonies. Leaves bright glossy green, divided into 3 oval leaflets, scarlet in autumn. Flowers cream-coloured, 5-petalled, 1–3 mm across, forming clusters, from May to July. Fruits whitish, berry-like drupes, 4–5 mm wide.

Poison-oak (*T. diversilobum*) has round-tipped leaflets that are usually lobed (hence the reference to "oak") and shorter than poison-ivy's (to 7 cm long, vs. to 15 cm or more in poison-ivy). Grows on dry, rocky slopes at low elevations on southeastern Vancouver Island and the nearby Gulf Islands.

Eastern poison-ivy (*T. radicans*), 10–25 cm tall, has well-developed stems and often forms thickets. Leaflets irregularly toothed or slightly lobed. Grows in sandy or rocky soil in dry, open woods in southern ON, southwestern QC, NB and NS. See p. 424 for conservation status.

Western poison-ivy (*T. rydbergii*), to 2 m tall, spreads mainly by stolons and forms distinct patches. Leaflets entire (neither toothed nor lobed). Grows on dry, rocky slopes across southern Canada from BC to QC.

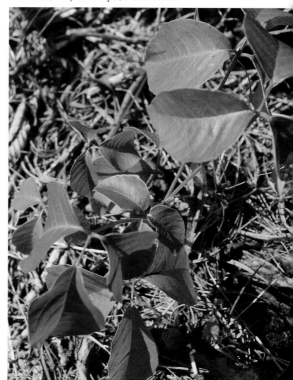

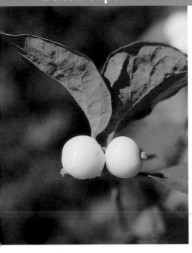

Common Snowberry

Symphoricarpos albus

Some sources report that these berries are edible, though not very good. However, snowberries are mildly poisonous and in large quantities can be toxic. The branches, leaves and roots are also poisonous. These plants contain the alkaloid chelidonine, which can cause vomiting, diarrhea, depression and sedation. One child who ate the berries reportedly became nauseous, delirious and fell into a semi-comatose state. Most tribes considered snowberries poisonous. Some believed they were the ghosts of saskatoons (p. 109), part of the spirit world and not to be eaten by the living.

DESCRIPTION: Erect, deciduous shrub, usually 50–75 cm tall, with pale green, opposite, elliptic to oval leaves, 2–4 cm long. Flowers pink to white, broadly funnel-shaped, 4–7 mm long, borne in small clusters at the stem tips, from June to August. Fruits white, waxy, berry-like drupes, 6–10 mm long, persisting through winter. Grows on rocky banks and roadsides from BC and YT to QC. See p. 424 for conservation status.

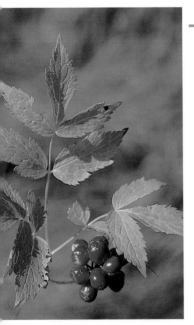

Baneberry

Actaea rubra

Baneberry poisoning is usually attributed to an unknown essential oil, but some sources say these plants contain the glycoside ranunculin. All parts are poisonous, but the roots and berries are most toxic. Eating 2–6 berries can cause severe cramps and burning in the stomach, vomiting, bloody diarrhea, increased pulse, headaches and/or dizziness. Severe poisoning causes convulsions, paralysis of the respiratory system and cardiac arrest. No deaths have been reported in North America, probably because the berries are so bitter. Baneberry is related to the phytomedicine black cohosh (*Cimicifuga racemosa*), and indigenous peoples used baneberry root tea in a similar way to treat menstrual and postpartum problems, as well as colds, coughs, rheumatism and syphilis. Some herbalists have used baneberry roots as a strong antispasmodic, anti-inflammatory, vasodilator and sedative, usually for treating menstrual cramps and menopausal discomforts.

DESCRIPTION: Branched, leafy, perennial herb, 30 cm–1 m tall, from a woody stem base and fibrous roots. Coarsely toothed leaves alternate, divided 2–3 times, in threes. Flowers white, with 5–10 slender, 2–3 mm long petals, forming long-stalked, rounded clusters, blooming from May to July. Fruits glossy red or white berries, 6–8 mm long. Grows in deciduous forests, mixed coniferous forests, streambanks and swamps at low to montane elevations across Canada.

Nightshade & Bittersweet

Solanum spp.

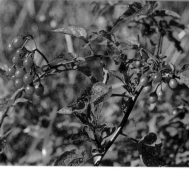
European bittersweet

The immature (green) berries and leaves of European bittersweet contain toxic alkaloids that can cause vomiting, dizziness, weakened heart, liver damage, convulsions, paralysis and even death. Cattle and sheep have been poisoned by eating these bitter plants, but livestock deaths are rare. The ripe berries contain only small amounts of alkaloids and are not considered a threat if eaten in moderation, but large amounts could prove toxic. Stem extracts of European bittersweet have been taken internally as a sedative and pain reliever, for increasing urination and for treating asthma, gout, rheumatism, whooping cough and bronchitis, but pharmacological evidence does not support these uses. Extracts are reported to have antibiotic activity, which could be useful in salves and lotions for combatting infection. These plants have been used for many years to treat skin diseases, sores, swellings and inflammations around nails. Recent research has shown that European bittersweet contains beta-solanine, a tumour-inhibiting compound that may prove useful for treating cancer.

DESCRIPTION: Rhizomatous, annual or perennial herbs and vines, often somewhat woody; stems leafy, 1–3 m tall or long, erect or tending to climb, scramble or sprawl on other vegetation. Flowers with a yellow cone projecting from the centre of 5 back-curved, white to blue petals, borne in loose, branched clusters. Fruits round to oblong berries, 8–11 mm wide.

Black nightshade (*S. americanum*) is an erect, annual, taprooted herb with white flowers and black berries. This species, introduced to Canada from the southern and eastern US, grows in disturbed sites (roadsides, thickets) in all provinces.

European bittersweet (*S. dulcamara*) is a perennial vine, trailing or climbing on other vegetation, with blue-violet to purple flowers and bright red berries. This Eurasian species can be found in thickets and clearings near habitation in all provinces.

False Azalea

Menziesia ferruginea

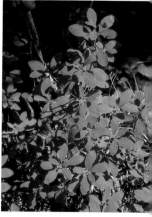

Although these plants are less toxic than many other members of the Heath family, they do contain andromedotoxins. These alkaloids can cause watering of the mouth, nose and eyes, headaches, vomiting, weakness and eventually paralysis when consumed in sufficient quantities. Poisonings and deaths of sheep as a result of eating false azalea have been reported. Symptoms include weakness, salivation, vomiting, difficulty breathing and paralysis.

DESCRIPTION: Erect, sometimes skunky-smelling, deciduous shrub with fine, rust-coloured, glandular-sticky twigs. Leaves dull blue-green, elliptic, with the midvein protruding at the tip, broadest above the middle, 3–6 cm long, crimson-orange in autumn. Flowers peach-coloured, urn-shaped, 6–8 mm long, nodding in small, loose clusters, from May to July. Fruits oval capsules, 5–7 mm long. Grows on moist, wooded slopes in foothills and montane zones in BC and AB.

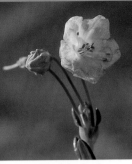

Bog-Laurels
Kalmia spp.

These plants contain alkaloids called andromedotoxins, which can cause watering of the mouth, nose and eyes, headaches, vomiting, weakness and eventually paralysis when consumed in sufficient quantities. Symptoms may appear 3–14 hours or more after the plant has been eaten. Poisoning and death of cattle, sheep, goats and horses have been reported. Even the honey made from bog-laurel nectar is said to be poisonous.

Western bog-laurel

DESCRIPTION: Slender, evergreen shrub. Leaves 1–5 cm long, glossy, green, simple, lance-shaped and arranged spirally on the stems. Flowers rose-pink, saucer-shaped, in dense clusters around the stem. Fruit a 5-lobed capsule containing numerous seeds.

Sheep-laurel or **lambkill** (*K. angustifolia*) grows 30–90 cm tall, has oblong, flat, thin leaves, 3–5 cm long, dark green above and pale beneath when mature. Flowers from May to August. Grows in dry or wet, sandy or sterile soil in bogs or old fields from ON eastward. See p. 424 for conservation status.

Western bog-laurel (*K. microphylla*) grows 5–40 cm tall, has oval to elliptic-oblong, thick, leathery leaves, generally less than 2 cm long, dark green above and glandular-hairy beneath when mature, with down-rolled edges. Flowers from June to September. Grows in bogs, bog forests and meadows in moist to wet, open sites at all elevations in YT, NT and from BC to ON. See p. 424 for conservation status.

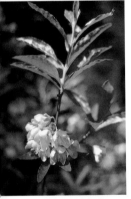

Rhododendrons
Rhododendron spp.

Rhododendrons contain alkaloids called andromedotoxins, which can cause watering of the mouth, nose and eyes, headaches, vomiting, weakness and eventually paralysis and death when consumed in sufficient quantities. Children have been poisoned by eating the leaves and flowers of white rhododendron, and sheep and occasionally cattle have died from eating these bitter shrubs.

DESCRIPTION: Deciduous or evergreen shrubs, with slender, reddish-hairy (when young) branches. Leaves alternate, crowded near the branch tips. Flowers bell- or cup-shaped, in clusters in leaf axils or terminal. Fruits woody, oval, glandular-hairy capsules.

White rhododendron

White rhododendron (*R. albiflorum*) is 50 cm–2 m tall. Leaves deciduous, green above but pale beneath, narrowly elliptic to lance-shaped, 2–9 cm long. Flowers white, cup-shaped, 5-petalled, 1.5–2 cm across, nodding in clusters of 1–4 from leaf axils, from June to August. Grows in moist to wet forests and parkland in montane and subalpine zones in BC and southwestern AB.

Rhodora (*R. canadense*) is a scrambling shrub, to 1 m tall, with grey-green, hairy, deciduous leaves and showy, pink or lavender flowers. Grows in moist woodlands and swamps at higher elevations from QC to NL.

Lapland rosebay (*R. lapponicum*) is a low, branching, dwarf shrub, usually no more than 10 cm tall (but taller in protected sites). Flat, leathery, elliptical, evergreen leaves, 4–12 mm long. Fragrant, purple-pink, 5-petalled flowers, 5–15 mm wide, appear in clusters of 1–5 (usually 3). Grows on tundra, rocky or gravelly areas, slopes and in dry meadows in all territories and the northern parts of most provinces to NL, but not in the Maritimes.

Flowering Spurge
Euphorbia corollata

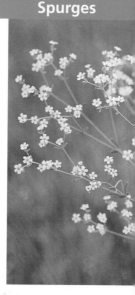

The milky latex is extremely caustic and irritating to the skin, especially in contact with mucous membranes such as the eyes, nose and mouth. Animal experiments found that the compounds in the latex were 10,000 to 100,000 times more irritating than capsaicin, the main ingredient in pepper spray. Redness, swelling, blisters and photosensitivity occur after some delay after coming into contact with the plant. If ingested, it causes nausea, vomiting and diarrhea. The plant has been used traditionally as a laxative and was used in the 1800s as an emetic and cathartic, but this was abandoned because it was too potent, causing nausea. Some First Nations used an infusion of the bruised roots to treat urinary diseases and a decoction of the whole plant as an ingredient in an herbal anticancer medicine. Ironically, several of the compounds that occur in the latex are found to cause cancer.

DESCRIPTION: Erect, herbaceous perennial, 25–90 cm tall, with a slender stem and milky juice. Leaves oblong, symmetrical, entire, about 3.8 cm long, mostly alternate but whorled just below flower cluster. Flowers in an umbellate cluster, each flower having 5 round, white bracts, 9 mm wide, surrounding a group of minute, true flowers, from June to October. Grows in dry, open woods, fields and on roadsides from SK to ON.

Leafy Spurge
Euphorbia esula

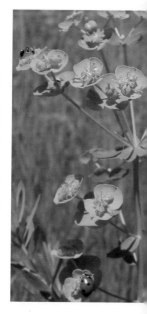

The acrid, milky juice (latex) of leafy spurge can inflame and blister sensitive skin. Most animals (including humans) do not eat these plants. Symptoms of poisoning include burning in the mouth and throat, swelling around the mouth and nose, abdominal pains, vomiting, diarrhea and fainting spells. Even honey made from the nectar of some spurges is mildly poisonous. Sheep are relatively resistant to the toxins, so they have been used, in conjunction with beetles, in biological control programs. However, large quantities can kill sheep. Spurge toxins are not neutralized by drying, so these plants remain toxic in hay. Non-fatal internal doses can cause skin reactions in people, sheep, cattle and horses after exposure to sunlight. Deep rhizomes and prolific seed production make leafy spurge difficult to control, and it is considered a noxious weed in many regions.

DESCRIPTION: Erect, bluish green, perennial herb, 20–90 cm tall, with milky juice. Leaves alternate, linear, 2–6 cm long. Flowers yellowish green, tiny, but borne above showy pairs of heart-shaped, yellowish green bracts that resemble petals. Fruits round, finely granular capsules, about 2 mm wide. This European species grows at low to montane elevations on disturbed sites, roadsides, in stream valleys and open woodlands throughout Canada.

Blue Flags
Iris spp.

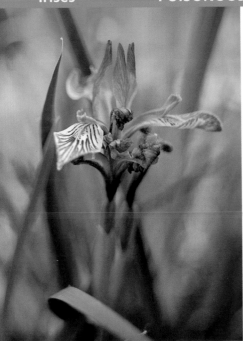

Blue flag rhizomes, roots and young shoots are toxic and should never be taken internally, but their sharp, bitter taste usually prevents the consumption of sufficient quantities to cause poisoning. Irises contain the acrid, resinous substance irisin, which irritates the digestive tract, liver and pancreas. Symptoms include stomach upset with a burning sensation, difficulty breathing, vomiting and diarrhea. Some people develop severe allergic skin reactions from handling iris plants and iris rhizomes in particular. Some indigenous peoples placed a mashed piece of western blue flag rhizome on tooth cavities or gums to kill the pain. Poultices of northern blue flag root were used to reduce swelling and soothe burns or sores. Northern blue flag is the provincial flower of QC (and, perhaps, the inspiration for the *fleur de lys*).

Western blue flag (all images)

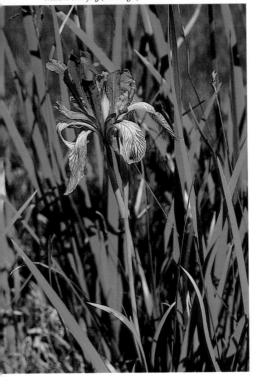

DESCRIPTION: Clumped, rhizomatous, perennial herbs with sword-shaped leaves. Flowers pale to deep blue, about 6–7 cm across, with 3 backward-curved, purple-lined sepals, 3 erect, narrower petals and 3 flattened, petal-like style branches, borne in groups of 2–3, from May to July. Fruits 3–5 cm long capsules.

Western blue flag (*I. missouriensis*) is 20–50 cm tall, with narrow leaves (less than 1 cm wide). Grows on wet (at least in spring) sites (streambanks, marshy meadows) in prairies, foothills and montane zones in southeastern BC and southwestern AB. See p. 424 for conservation status.

Northern blue flag (*I. versicolor*) is 20–80 cm tall, with wider leaves (1.3–2.5 cm wide). Grows on wet, open sites (marshes, roadsides) from southeastern MB to NL.

Green False-Hellebore

Veratrum viride

False-hellebores are violently poisonous and can cause birth defects in animals. The rhizomes, roots and young shoots are the most toxic. They contain steroidal alkaloids that slow heartbeat and breathing and lower blood pressure. Cardiac and respiratory stimulants (e.g., atropine) are used in treatment. Symptoms include frothing at the mouth, nausea, blurred vision, lockjaw, vomiting and diarrhea. People have reported stomach cramps after drinking water in which this plant was growing. Cattle, sheep, poultry and mice have been poisoned by false-hellebores. Powdered false-hellebore has been used in insecticides and in salves and shampoos for treating scabies, herpes, ringworm, lice and mites.

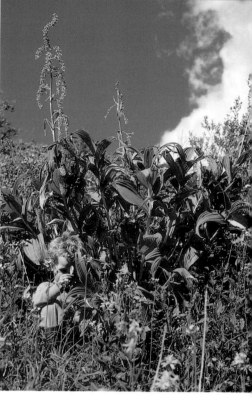

MEDICINE: Green false-hellebore is recognized by all indigenous groups in northwest BC as an extremely poisonous plant. This was a highly respected plant by many First Nations and used to treat a number of ailments; it was believed that green false-hellebore could cure almost any disease. A decoction of the bulb was taken for stomach pains, chronic cough, constipation, high blood pressure, gonorrhea, to break open boils, for toothaches, internal back and chest pain and as a sedative. An infusion of the plant was taken for indigestion, and the plant was often employed as an emetic. The roots were often used as compresses for sprains, bruises, swellings, fractures and rheumatism. A poultice of a compound containing the bulb was applied to the chest for heart trouble. The roots were taken as a snuff to treat headaches, to induce sneezing and to treat tuberculosis. The plant was used for skin washes. The juice was taken by women to bring about an abortion. Leaves were chewed by children for drooling. The roots were ingested to commit suicide. The plant has been used in purification rituals for hunting and trapping. The smoke from the plant was used to assist the spirits of sleepwalkers to return to their bodies. The roots were put on the ends of arrows by the shaman to shoot toward "disease spirits."

DESCRIPTION: Robust, perennial herb from rhizomes and bulbs with leafy, unbranched stems 70 cm–2 m tall. Leaves alternate, clasping, elliptic, 10–30 cm long, prominently parallel-veined or accordion-pleated. Flowers green to yellowish, 6-petalled, about 2 cm across, musky-smelling, forming open clusters 30–70 cm long, with tassel-like branches, from June to September. Fruits straw-coloured to brown, egg-shaped capsules 2–3 cm long. Two disjunct varieties are recognized, one (var. *eschscholtzianum*, with inflorescence branches spreading to drooping and flowers erect) in western Canada (BC, western AB, YT and NT) and the other (var. *viride*, with inflorescence branches ascending to spreading and flowers generally spreading) in eastern Canada (QC, NB and NL).

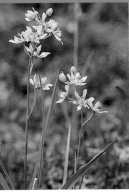

Death-Camases
Zigadenus spp.

All parts of these plants contain steroidal alkaloids (e.g., zygacine, zygadenine) that are more toxic than strychnine. Two bulbs, raw or cooked, can be fatal. Severe poisoning causes digestive upset and vomiting followed by loss of muscle control, lowered blood pressure and temperature, difficulty breathing and eventually coma and death. If someone has eaten this plant, induce vomiting and get medical help. Sheep (herds of as many as 500), cattle and horses have died from eating these plants. Meadow death-camas is about 7 times more poisonous than mountain death-camas, but both are dangerous.

Mountain death-camas

DESCRIPTION: Grey-green, perennial herbs from oval, blackish-scaly bulbs, to 80 cm tall, with grass-like leaves. Flowers whitish, bell-shaped, 6-petalled, with 6 glands near the centre, forming elongated clusters, from June to August. Fruits erect, 3-lobed capsules.

Mountain death-camas (*Z. elegans*) has 2 cm wide flowers, with heart-shaped glands. Grows on moist to dry grasslands, riverbanks and lakeshores, in bogs and coniferous forests from BC to NB. See p. 424 for conservation status.

Meadow death-camas (*Z. venenosus*) has 1–1.5 cm wide flowers, with round to oblong glands. Grows on dry to mesic, rocky slopes, in grasslands and open forests at lower elevations from BC to SK.

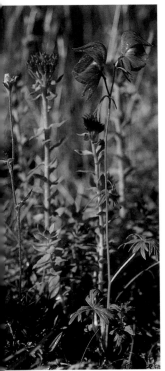

Monkshoods

Aconitum spp.

All parts of these plants contain the poisonous alkaloid aconitine, plus other toxins. The roots are most poisonous—ingestion of less than 500 g can be fatal to a horse. The flowers are harmless to handle but violently poisonous if eaten. Symptoms include anxiety, vomiting, diarrhea, weakness, salivation, dizziness, numbness and prickling, impaired speech and vision, weak pulse, convulsions, paralysis of the lower legs and respiratory system and coma. Death can occur in a few hours. The sap causes numbness and tingling on the skin.

DESCRIPTION: Erect, perennial herbs from tuberous roots with palmately divided leaves. Flowers in terminal clusters, dark blue to purple, flattened sideways, with a large hood over 2 parallel side wings and 3 small lower petals. Fruits erect pods to 2.5 cm long.

Columbian monkshood (*A. columbianum*) is often more than 80 cm tall, with deeply lobed leaves (not divided to the very base). Grows in spring-fed bogs, meadows, seep areas and other moist areas in the mountains (montane to subalpine elevations) in southern BC.

Mountain monkshood (*A. delphiniifolium*) is usually less than 80 cm tall, with separate, short-stalked leaflets (leaves divided to the very base). Grows in meadows, thickets, open forests and alpine tundra at higher elevations (montane to alpine) in YT, western NT, northern BC and west-central AB. See p. 424 for conservation status.

Mountain monkshood

Columbines
Aquilegia spp.

All columbines are probably poisonous. The flowers are said to be sweet and edible in small quantities, but consumption is not recommended. All other parts of these plants can be quite toxic. The seeds and roots are most poisonous. In Europe, columbines were used to treat many ailments, including heart palpitations, boils, ulcers, gallstones or kidney stones and jaundice. However, some children died from overdoses of the seeds, and medicinal use was discontinued. Some First Nations in Canada used the plant as a good luck charm or rubbed the plant on people's legs to increase stamina before a race.

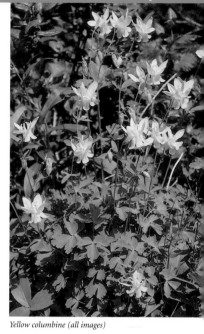

DESCRIPTION: Erect, perennial herbs from woody stem bases and taproots, 20 cm–1 m tall. Leaves alternate, divided 2–3 times in threes, with broad, round-lobed leaflets 2–5 cm long. Flowers with 5 spreading, petal-like sepals and 5 smaller petals that extend back from the base as spurs, nodding in small, loose clusters.

Yellow columbine (all images)

Blue columbine (*A. brevistyla*) has flowers with blue spurs and white blades with pale blue spots. Found in open woods, meadows and on rocky slopes in YT and NT and from northern BC to northern ON.

Wild columbine (*A. canadensis*) has flowers with red spurs and red blades that are usually yellow or yellow-green inside. Found in thickets and open woods throughout the boreal forest from southeastern SK to NL (but not on PEI).

Yellow columbine (*A. flavescens*) has flowers with yellow spurs and cream-coloured blades. Found on moist mountain meadows and alpine slopes in BC and western AB (Rocky Mountains).

Red columbine (*A. formosa*) has flowers with red spurs and yellow blades. Found in mesic to moist meadows, clearings, roadsides and open woods in southern YT, BC and western AB (Rocky Mountains). See p. 424 for conservation status.

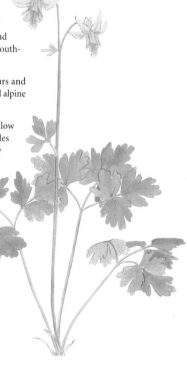

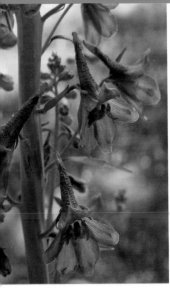

Larkspurs
Delphinium spp.

These plants contain many toxic alkaloids. Symptoms of poisoning include burning in the mouth, tingling skin, nausea and cramps, weak pulse, difficulty breathing, nervousness and depression or excitement. Some people develop skin reactions from contact with larkspurs. The seeds are particularly poisonous. Toxicity decreases as the plants age. Many cattle have been poisoned by larkspurs. Fatal poisoning usually requires eating plants equivalent to at least 3 percent of an animal's body weight. Sheep tolerate high levels of these toxins, and tall larkspur can provide fair-to-good forage for them. Teas and tinctures made from larkspur seeds were used for many years to kill lice and to cure scabies, but these extracts are now considered too dangerous to use. The Blackfoot gave an infusion of the plant to children with diarrhea, frothy mouth and fainting spells; they used the flowers as a light blue dye for quills.

Tall larkspur

DESCRIPTION: Erect, perennial herbs with palmately divided leaves. Flowers mostly purplish, with 5 spreading, petal-like sepals below 4 small petals. Fruits erect clusters of pods with spreading tips.

Low larkspur (*D. bicolor*) has solid, 10–50 cm tall stems, with small clusters (3–12 flowers) of blue-and-white flowers. Grows in a range of habitats from open woods and grasslands to subalpine scree in BC, AB and SK. See p. 424 for conservation status.

Tall larkspur (*D. glaucum*) has hollow, 60 cm–2 m tall stems, with larger clusters (10–90 flowers) of purplish blue flowers. Grows on streambanks, in meadows and moist, open woods at higher elevations (montane to subalpine zones) in NT, YT and from BC to MB. See p. 424 for conservation status.

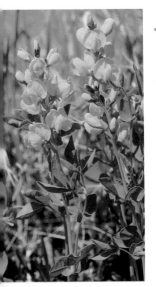

—— *Prairie Goldenbean*
Thermopsis rhombifolia

Goldenbeans contain toxic alkaloids, as well as anagyrine, which causes calf deformities when eaten by pregnant cows. Mountain goldenbean (*T. montana*, a species of the western US) has poisoned cattle and horses, with as little as 500 g of ripe seeds constituting a lethal dose. The toxicity of prairie goldenbean is less studied. Some sources report that prairie goldenbean is only suspected of poisoning children, but others say that in some regions it causes more human poisonings than any other plant and that large doses can be fatal.

DESCRIPTION: Perennial herb from a woody rhizome, 20–40 cm tall. Leaves alternate, with 3 oval leaflets and 2 large, leaflet-like basal lobes. Flowers pea-like, bright yellow, to 2.5 cm long, 10–30 in terminal clusters. Fruits pea-like pods, 4–8 cm long, curved. Grows in dry prairies and meadows from southern BC to southern MB, and is reportedly introduced to Churchill, MB. See p. 424 for conservation status.

Milk-Vetches

Astragalus spp.

The milk-vetches comprise a large, complex group of plants, including both edible and extremely poisonous species. Because some milk-vetches are high in protein and also fix nitrogen in the soil, they are valued as forage and soil-building crops. Species of *Astragalus* have the name "milk-vetch" from the belief that milk supply was increased when goats ate these plants. However, a number of species can become toxic by absorbing harmful chemicals from the soil—excess selenium causes depression, diarrhea, increased urination, hair loss and even death from lung and heart failure; molybdenum causes poor growth, brittle bones and anemia. Some milk-vetches contain the alkaloid locoine, which causes locoism (see *Oxytropis* spp., p. 408), and consequently, milk-vetches are often called locoweeds. Timber milk-vetch contains miserotoxin, which can cause acute poisoning (with death a few hours after ingestion) or chronic toxicity (with liver and nerve damage, local bleeding in the brain and difficulty breathing). Grazing livestock have been poisoned by ingesting the whole plant, and honeybees have been poisoned by consuming timber milk-vetch nectar. American milk-vetch may or may not be poisonous. First Nations ate the roots in small quantities only as a famine food. The Cree chewed the roots of American milk-vetch and swallowed the juice if they had stomachaches, cramps or stomach flu. The Cree name for this plant includes the word for "rattle" because the ripe seeds rattle noisily in their inflated pods; they were used as noisemakers in ceremonies and also given to babies as a rattle. The traditional Chinese medicine *huang qi* (prepared from *A. propinquus*) is used to treat fatigue and strengthen vital energy. It is now cultivated in Canada and widely used.

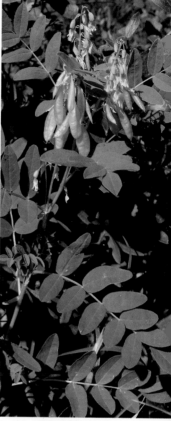

American milk-vetch (above)
Timber milk-vetch (below)

DESCRIPTION: Perennial herbs with leafy stems. Leaves pinnately divided into 7–21 leaflets. Flowers white to lilac with blue lines, pea-like, 8–12 mm long. Fruits thin, hanging, stalkless pods. This is a large genus with more than 40 species in Canada.

American milk-vetch (*A. americanus*) is a 30 cm–1 m tall, erect plant with unbranched stems. Found along streambanks and in moist, open woods, bogs, fens, forest openings and riverbanks from southeastern YT south through western Canada, with limited spread into ON and QC. See p. 424 for conservation status.

Timber milk-vetch (*A. miser*) is a smaller, sometimes scrambling plant, 10–40 cm tall, the stems often branched. Grows in grasslands, moist meadows and dry ridges at low to alpine elevations in southern BC and southwestern AB. See p. 424 for conservation status.

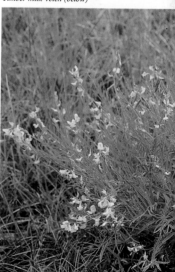

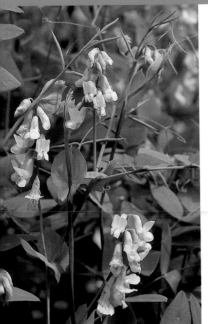

Creamy peavine (above)
Beach pea (below)

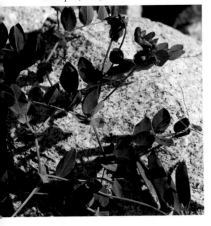

Peavines

Lathyrus spp.

There are many many similar-looking *Lathyrus* species (over 100 species scattered throughout the North Temperate Zone, with 19 species in Canada), often extending over the same range as these species. Because most of these other species are of unknown edibility, harvesting should be undertaken with caution. Many plants of this genus have been used for food (as greens and as peas) and for forage. However, peavines are generally viewed with suspicion because the seeds of some species contain peculiar non-protein amino acids that poison nerve cells (neurotoxins). Eaten in moderation, peavines can provide a nutritious food, but if the diet consists almost exclusively of peavine for 10 days to 4 weeks, a type of cumulative poisoning called "lathyrism" can result as human proteins are denatured by incorporating the unusual amino acids. Even the common garden pea (*Pisum* spp.) can cause nervous disorders if large amounts are eaten regularly over long periods of time. Lathyrism causes a progressive loss of coordination, which in extreme cases can end in irreversible paralysis. Evidence of this can be found during famine times when people were forced to eat peavines almost exclusively. Nutritionally, the shelled peas of beach pea are high in both protein and vitamins A and B. The Dena'ina ate beach pea seeds raw or boiled and preserved in seal oil. The Iroquois harvested young shoots in spring. In early summer, the tender pods were eaten whole, and in late summer, shelled peas were gathered. *Lathyrus* is from the Greek word *lathouros,* meaning "something exciting," from the belief that the seeds had some medicinal value.

DESCRIPTION: Perennial herb from slender rhizomes, 30 cm–1.5 m tall or long, angled stems, trailing or climbing on or over other plants. Leaves compound with an even number (6–12) of leaflets and tipped with curling tendrils; leaflets opposite, to 7 cm long. Flowers pea-like, about 10–15 mm long. Fruits slender pods, 4–7 cm long.

Beach pea (*L. japonicus*) flowers reddish purple to blue, pea-like, to 3 cm long, in loose clusters of 2–8. This plant was called raven's canoe by the Haida because of the shape of its seed pods, which are also black when ripe, and hairy. Grows on sandy or gravelly beaches and dunes along the shores of oceans and large lakes (e.g., Lake Winnipeg, Great Lakes) across Canada. See p. 424 for conservation status.

Creamy peavine (*L. ochroleucus*) flowers yellowish white, to 1.5 cm long, in loose clusters of 6–14. Seed pods brown when ripe, hairless. Grows in moist prairies and open woods, thickets and clearings, from BC and YT to QC. See p. 424 for conservation status.

Lupines
Lupinus spp.

These plants can be especially dangerous because their pods look like hairy garden peas, and children may assume that they are edible. Some lupines are edible (see p. 259), but many contain poisonous alkaloids, and even botanists can have difficulty distinguishing poisonous and non-poisonous species. Poisonous lupines (especially their flowers, pods and seeds) contain the alkaloids lupanine, lupinine and/or sparteine. Large amounts must be eaten in a short time to cause poisoning, but these toxins are not destroyed by drying, so hay with lupine plants can be poisonous to livestock. Silvery lupine and silky lupine are known to have killed sheep, goats, cattle and horses. Both lupines (especially their seeds, pods and young leaves) contain the glycoside anagyrine in concentrations 2–3 times higher than those known to cause birth deformities in calves, kids and lambs. Lactating goats pass anagyrine in their milk. At least 1 child was believed to have been born with deformed limbs because her mother drank milk from goats that were grazing on lupines. A few European lupines are grown as a substitute for peas, but our wild lupines are not used in this way. Some edible lupine seeds are sold in health-food stores, but these seeds must be soaked and then boiled in several changes of water to remove bitter toxins, or they can cause dizziness and incoordination. Lupine poisoning may also slow breathing and heart rate.

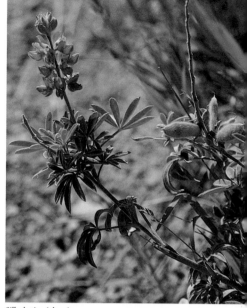

Silky lupine (above)
Silvery lupine (below)

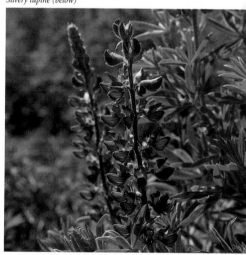

DESCRIPTION: Large, complex group of mostly perennial herbs with round, alternate leaves divided into 7–9 lance-shaped, finger-like leaflets. Flowers mostly blue or purple, pea-like, borne in whorls in showy, elongated clusters. Fruits pea-like pods, mostly hairy, about 2–3 cm long.

Silky lupine (*L. sericeus*) is a silky-hairy plant, to 70 cm tall, and has larger flowers (generally more than 1 cm long), with hairs over most of the upper (back) surface of its top petal and upper leaf surfaces. Grows in dry prairies to montane slopes in southern BC and southwestern AB.

Silvery lupine (*L. argenteus*) is a similar plant, but with smaller flowers (generally less than 1 cm long), with an essentially hairless top petal and upper leaf surfaces. Grows in dry prairies to montane slopes from southern BC (Okanagan Valley) to SK. See p. 424 for conservation status.

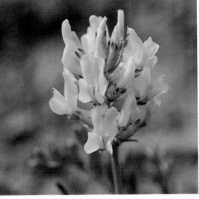
Silky locoweed

Locoweeds
Oxytropis spp.

Many locoweeds are poisonous to horses, sheep and cattle. These plants contain toxic alkaloids, and some ostensibly edible species also take selenium from the soil, which can render them toxic to some animals. After eating large quantities of locoweed for several weeks, cattle, horses and sheep develop locoism, a disease that mainly affects the nervous system. Some animals grow to like these plants, and many have died as a result. Symptoms include depression, a lack of coordination and excitability. Locoweeds also cause heart disease, fluid retention, diarrhea, birth deformities and miscarriages. Cattle usually die after eating an equivalent of 300 percent of their body weight, but eating only 30 percent of their body weight can be fatal to horses. Because no comprehensive study has been undertaken to determine exactly which species contain the poisonous alkaloid locoine and which species are non-poisonous, it is best to avoid using these plants altogether.

DESCRIPTION: Tufted, perennial herbs, to 35 cm tall, usually from taproots, with basal, pinnately divided leaves. Flowers about 1–2 cm long, pea-like, the lower 2 petals forming a pointed keel. Fruits pea-like pods, about 1–2 cm long.

Lambert's locoweed (*O. lambertii*) has bright rose-purple flowers and flat-lying, parallel hairs. Grows in prairies, on bluffs and in badlands, preferring clay, limestone or loess soils in a band along southern AB, southeastern SK and southern MB. See p. 424 for conservation status.

Silky locoweed (*O. sericea*) has whitish to pale yellow flowers. Pods different from other locoweeds in that they become leathery, hardened and bony when mature. Grows in prairies to subalpine meadows and on slopes in YT, BC, AB, SK and southwestern MB. See p. 424 for conservation status.

Showy locoweed (*O. splendens*) is a greyish, silky-hairy plant with showy dark blue to pinkish purple flowers. It can be distinguished, when not in flower, by its leaflets, which are arranged in whorls of 2–6. Grows in open woods, clearings and on riverbanks; common in prairie and parkland, less so in the north, where it can inhabit low elevation grasslands and rocky, south-facing slopes from northeastern BC, YT and NT to SK, MB and western ON. See p. 424 for conservation status.

Showy locoweed

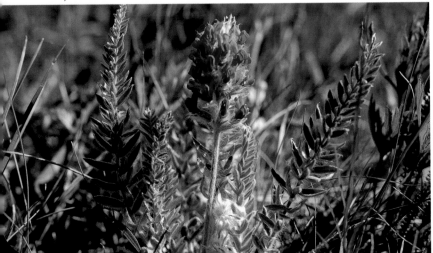

American Vetch

Vicia americana

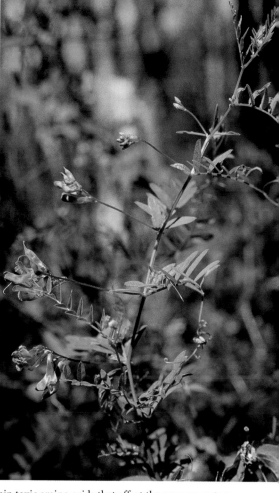

The toxicity of vetches varies from person to person and species to species (there are at least 12 species of vetches in Canada). Some vetches contain the toxic alkaloids vicine and convicine. These alkaloids produce oxidants that attack the red blood cells of people who lack the enzyme glucose-6-phosphate dehydrogenase. Eating the beans or inhaling the pollen of toxic species can cause headaches, weakness, dizziness, vomiting, fever, jaundice, anemia and even death in susceptible people. This enzyme deficiency is genetically controlled and is most common in a small percentage of people of Mediterranean or African origin. Domestic broad beans (*V. faba*) cause this reaction (favism), and large quantities of broad beans have poisoned pigs and chickens. Some vetches contain chemicals that produce hydrocyanic acid, and some contain toxic amino acids that affect the nervous system. Vetch seeds are attractive to young children because they resemble small peas. Young shoots and tender seeds of American vetch have been boiled or baked for food, but these plants should be used with caution, if at all, considering the history of their relatives. This common plant was not widely used by native peoples in the boreal or western regions. However, in the East, Iroquois women reportedly made a tea from the roots as a love medicine. The name "vetch" is from the Latin *vicia*, which is thought to be derived from the Latin verb *vincio* (to bind), in reference to the climbing habit of these plants.

DESCRIPTION: Slender, vine-like, perennial herb that grows to 38 cm, with tangled, angled stems. Leaves pinnately divided into 8–12 leaflets, tipped with tendrils. Flowers reddish purple, pea-like, 15–20 mm long, in loose clusters of 2–9. Fruits flat, hairless pods, 2–4 cm long. Grows in open forests, thickets, meadows and on damp or gravelly shores in YT and from BC to western QC. See p. 424 for conservation status.

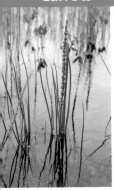

Seaside Arrow-Grass
Triglochin maritima

Arrow-grasses contain 2 cyanogenic glycosides (triglochinin and taxiphillin) that release hydrocyanic acid when the plants are chewed. These compounds are most concentrated in young flowering stalks. Also, water-stressed plants can be 5–10 times more poisonous than plants growing in water. Dried plants remain poisonous. Doses of only 0.5 percent of body weight can be lethal. Ruminants are most commonly poisoned. Many cattle and sheep have died from eating seaside arrow-grass. Symptoms include nervousness, trembling, salivation, vomiting, convulsions and death from respiratory failure. Some Aboriginal peoples in BC gathered the sweet, white stem bases of these plants (the green upper parts were discarded) in spring and ate them raw, cooked or canned. The white part is said to taste like cucumber. Some people preferred the leaf bases of the vegetative, non-flowering plants, while others ate both. Those who preferred vegetative plants stated that the flowering plants caused headaches. They were gathered in large quantities and stored in jars for winter. Some indigenous names for arrow-grass (translated into English) are "goose tongue" and "little spruce." The seeds were also parched and eaten or used as a coffee substitute. A decoction of the plant was drunk to relieve diarrhea with blood in the stool. The seeds and stem bases have relatively low glycoside concentrations, but arrow-grasses should be used with caution, if at all.

OTHER USES: The ashes of the plant can be used in making soap because they are high in potassium.

DESCRIPTION: Clumped, perennial herb, to 75 cm tall, with fleshy, basal, grass-like leaves about 2 mm wide, growing from woody rhizomes. Flowers inconspicuous, 3–4 mm long, 6-petalled, greenish, with feathery, red stigmas, forming 10–40 cm long spikes, from May to August. Fruits oval capsules, about 5 mm long . Grows in salt marshes, estuarine flats and freshwater marshes and shores across Canada, but is most common in NT, BC, AB and SK. See p. 424 for conservation status.

Poison-Hemlock
Conium maculatum

All parts of this plant are extremely poisonous. The toxic alkaloid (coniine) is most abundant in young plants, leaves and flowers. The toxin directly affects the nervous system, causing numbness and paralysis of the lower limbs, followed by paralysis of the arms and chest. Symptoms include nervousness and confusion, weakness, vomiting and diarrhea, weak pulse, difficulty breathing and finally death from suffocation. If a person has eaten this plant, induce vomiting, administer a strong laxative and consult a physician. Fatal doses vary by animal and by person. Low concentrations can cause birth defects. Some people develop a rash from contact with poison-hemlock, so wash your hands carefully if you must handle this plant. These plants have been mistaken for wild carrot, anise or parsley, with fatal results. Poison-hemlock was the plant that reputedly killed Socrates.

DESCRIPTION: Musty-smelling, hairless, biennial herb with branched, leafy, purple-blotched stems, 50 cm–3 m tall. Leaves lacy, fern-like, 15–30 cm long. Flowers small, white, occur in twice-branched, flat-topped clusters above a whorl of small, lance-shaped bracts. Fruits oval, slightly flattened, about 2 mm long, with raised, often wavy ribs. This weedy European species has spread to disturbed sites across Canada, except for YT, NT, NU and NL.

Water-Hemlocks

Cicuta spp.

These are among our most poisonous native plants. All parts of these plants contain the highly poisonous toxin cicutoxin, and it is most concentrated in the rhizomes. Small amounts of the plant can be deadly: for example, a couple of small pieces may be fatal to humans; 100 g is fatal to sheep, 3 times that amount is fatal to horses, and 4 times that amount is fatal to cattle. Even pea-shooters and whistles made from hollow water-hemlock stems have been shown to be poisonous, particularly to children. Cicutoxin, a polyacetylene, acts on the central nervous system, and it can take effect within 15 minutes of ingestion. Symptoms include stomachache, excess salivation, nausea, vomiting, diarrhea, difficulty breathing, tremors and violent convulsions. If a person has eaten water-hemlock, induce vomiting, administer a strong laxative and consult a doctor.

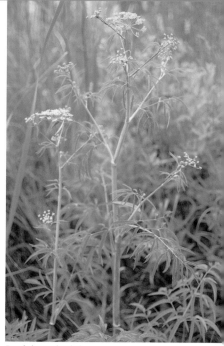

Douglas' water-hemlock

DESCRIPTION: Perennial herbs with foul-smelling, oily, yellow sap and thickened, chambered stem bases and/or roots. Leaves alternate and 2–3 times divided into leaflets. Flowers small, white to greenish and form twice-branched, flat-topped clusters (with few or no bracts). Flowers typically bloom from June to August. Fruits flattened and contain round to oval seeds, with thick, corky ribs.

Bulbous water-hemlock (*C. bulbifera*) grows to 80 cm tall with linear, 0.5–4 mm wide leaflets and small bulblets in its leaf axils. Grows in wet soils throughout all provinces and territories (except NU). See p. 424 for conservation status.

Douglas' water-hemlock (*C. douglasii*) grows to 2 m tall and has lance-shaped to oblong leaflets, whose veins end at the tooth bases (remember, "vein to the cut, pain in the gut"). Grows in wet areas (stream edges, marshes) of prairies to subalpine zones throughout BC and in southwestern NT and western AB.

Spotted water-hemlock (*C. maculata*) grows to 2 m tall and is highly branched with magenta-streaked stems and white, dome-shaped, compound umbel flower clusters. Toothed, lance-shaped leaflets have sharp tips and are divided into 2 parts, with veins ending at the tooth bases. Grows in wet places (streams, marshes, ditches) throughout Canada (except NU and NL).

Bulbous water-hemlock

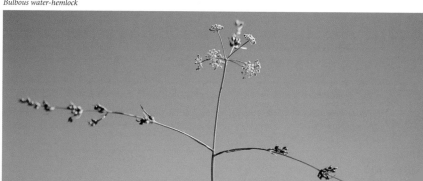

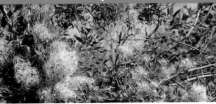

Virgin's-Bowers & Clematis
Clematis spp.

White virgin's-bower

The sap of these plants contains the glycoside ranunculin. Some people develop severe skin reactions and swollen, inflamed eyelids from contact with them. If virgin's-bower is eaten, it can cause stomach upset, internal bleeding, nervousness, depression and even death. It has been used to treat nervous disorders, migraines and rashes. The stalk and roots of white virgin's bower were used to make a women's contraceptive, and the plant was often used as a head-wash. The seed fluff was used in diapers.

DESCRIPTION: Perennial, woody vines with opposites leaves divided into 3–7 stalked leaflets. Flowers with 4 petal-like sepals and no petals. Fruits seed-like achenes tipped with feathery styles, forming fluffy heads when mature. See p. 424 for conservation status.

White virgin's-bower (*C. ligusticifolia*) grows to 30 cm tall, has leaves 1- to 2-times pinnate, and clusters of 6–10 mm wide, cream-coloured flowers, blooming from June to September. Found in moist, open sites (streambanks, forest edges, ditches, riparian deciduous woodlands) at steppe to montane elevations from southern BC to southern MB.

Virgin's-bower (*C. virginiana*) climbs to 5 m tall, has 3 stalked, oval to lance-shaped leaves, and clusters of 1–2 cm wide, cream-coloured flowers, blooming from June to September. Found in open, moist, disturbed sites (streamsides, roadsides) at low to subalpine elevations from MB to the Maritimes.

Purple clematis (*C. occidentalis*) climbs or trails 25 cm–3.5 m, has 3 stalked, oval to lance-shaped leaves and single, nodding flowers, with purple sepals 3.5–6 cm long, blooming from April to June. Found on rocky bluffs and in open forests in foothills and montane zones in all provinces except MB, PEI and NL.

Pasqueflowers
Anemone spp.

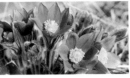

Prairie crocus

These plants are in the same genus as the anemones, but are separated here because their long, feathery achene beaks give them a very different appearance in fruit. All parts are poisonous if taken internally and irritating if applied externally. The sap contains the glycoside ranunculin. Some First Nations applied crushed pasqueflower leaves to rheumatic joints as a counter-irritant. Homeopaths have used minute doses of prairie crocus to treat eye problems, rashes, rheumatism, menstrual obstruction, bronchitis, asthma and coughs. Some herbalists recommend alcohol extracts from western pasqueflower as an antidepressant sedative. Overdoses cause lowered blood pressure, nausea, salivation and dizziness. This extract should not be used during pregnancy or by people with an abnormally slow heart rate. Prairie crocus is the provincial flower of MB.

DESCRIPTION: Silky-hairy, perennial herbs from taproots, with finely divided leaves. Flowers with 5 petal-like sepals and petals reduced or absent, single, above a whorl of stem leaves. Fruits tiny, seed-like achenes, each tipped with a long, feathery style, forming fluffy heads when mature.

Western pasqueflower (*A. occidentalis*) is a 10–60 cm tall, white-flowered species of moist meadows and forest openings in montane, subalpine and alpine zones in BC and AB (Rocky Mountains).

Prairie crocus or **common pasqueflower** (*A. patens*) is a 5–30 cm tall, blue-flowered species found in dry, open woods, prairies and on hillsides in steppe to alpine zones from BC to western ON and in all territories. See p. 424 for conservation status.

Anemones

Anemone spp.

All anemones are somewhat poisonous, but toxicity varies greatly with habitat and between species. The sap contains the glycoside ranunculin (see buttercups, p. 414). Small amounts of mashed anemone leaves were sometimes used as counterirritants for treating bruises and sore muscles. The primary active ingredient, protoanemonin, is volatile, so dried or thoroughly cooked plants are said to be harmless.

DESCRIPTION: Perennial herbs from woody stem bases with alternate, divided leaves. Flowers usually white, with 5 petal-like sepals and no petals. Fruits tiny, beaked, seed-like achenes in dense heads.

Round-lobed hepatica (*A. americana*) is 5–20 cm tall. Basal leaves 3–15, deeply divided, often purplish underneath. Flowers solitary, white, pink or bluish, with bracts underneath flowers, blooming in spring. Found in mixed woods at all elevations in MB, ON, QC, NB and NS. See p. 424 for conservation status.

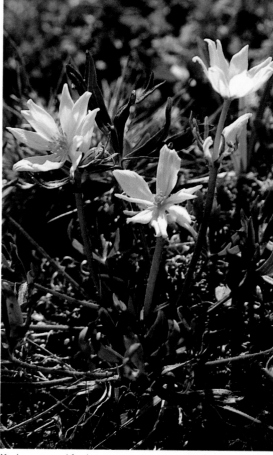

Narcissus anemone (above)

Canada anemone (*A. canadensis*) is 20–80 cm tall, with hairy stems. Basal leaves 1–5, deeply divided. Flowers 1–3, white, blooming spring and summer. Achenes hairy. Found in open forests, moist meadows and thickets at montane elevations in all provinces and NT. See p. 424 for conservation status.

Cut-leaved anemone (*A. multifida*) is 20–60 cm tall. Basal leaves finely divided, palmately lobed. Woolly achenes and 1 to several, white (sometimes reddish-tinged) flowers above a whorl of stem leaves, blooming in summer. Grows on rocky slopes and in meadows in all provinces and territories except PEI. See p. 424 for conservation status.

Narcissus anemone (*A. narcissiflora*) is 5–60 cm tall. Basal leaves with 3 deeply divided lobes. Flowers creamy white with bluish tinge, 1 per stem or in clusters of 2–5. Found in meadows, on grassy or rocky slopes and in heath at subalpine to alpine elevations in northern BC, YT and western NT.

Canada anemone

413

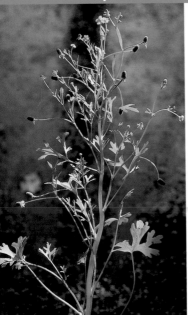

Buttercups
Ranunculus spp.

All buttercups are somewhat poisonous, but toxicity varies greatly with habitat and species. Meadow buttercup and cursed buttercup are among the most toxic. Buttercup sap contains the glycoside ranunculin, which is converted into an irritating yellow oil, protoanemonin, when the plant is damaged. Protoanemonin can cause intense pain and burning of mucous membranes (e.g., in the digestive tract) and may raise blisters on sensitive skin. Glycoside concentrations are highest during flowering. Fresh buttercups blister the mouths of grazing animals and can cause salivation, abdominal pains, diarrhea, slow heartbeat, muscle spasms, blindness and, rarely, death. Buttercups also have a narcotic effect on cattle and give a bitter taste to their milk. Human poisonings are rare (probably because the most toxic plants are so acrid), and they usually result only in digestive upset. In the past, meadow buttercup juice was used as a counter-irritant for treating rheumatism, arthritis and neuralgia (severe pain along a nerve), and it was applied to blister or eat away warts, pimples and plague sores. Beggars sometimes used it to raise blisters and gain sympathy from passers-by. The English believed that the smell of buttercup flowers could drive a person mad and induce epileptic seizures. In the first century AD, the Roman scholar Pliny warned that if people ate Illyrian buttercup (*R. illyricus*), they would burst into gales of laughter, ending in death. The only antidote was a mixture of pineapple kernels and pepper dissolved in wine. Protoanemonin is volatile, so dried or thoroughly cooked plants are said to be harmless. The dried, ground fruits and cooked roots and leaves of some buttercups have been used for food, but this practice is not recommended.

Cursed buttercup (above)
Meadow buttercup (below)

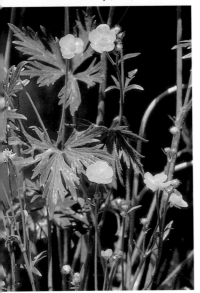

DESCRIPTION: Low, perennial herbs with alternate, variously divided leaves. Flowers usually yellow, with 5 sepals and 5 petals, each petal with a nectar-bearing spot at the base, blooming from March to September. Fruits tiny, seed-like achenes in dense, round to cylindrical heads. *Ranunculus* is a large genus, with at least 40 species in Canada.

Meadow buttercup (*R. acris*) grows 30 cm–1 m tall and has palmately 3- to 5-lobed basal leaves and shiny, deep yellow petals 8–16 mm long. Common introduced Eurasian weed of roadsides and meadows in lowland to montane zones across Canada.

Cursed buttercup (*R. sceleratus*) is 20–60 cm tall and has succulent, deeply lobed leaves and small, 2–4 mm long, pale yellow petals. Grows in wet ground (ponds, mudflats and marshes) in lowland to steppe zones in all provinces and territories. See p. 424 for conservation status.

Groundsels
Senecio spp.

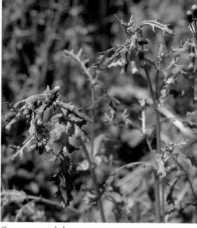

Some groundsels (e.g., common groundsel, western groundsel) contain pyrrolizidine alkaloids that cause irreversible liver damage after long-term exposure and may cause liver cancer. Alkaloid concentrations are highest in the flowers and lowest in roots and young leaves, but levels vary greatly from species to species and plant to plant. These toxins are not destroyed by drying. Horses and cattle have died from eating common groundsel. Young animals are most susceptible. Unfortunately, liver damage is usually severe before outward signs are noticeable. Some people use groundsel in teas

Common groundsel

and herbal remedies. Extended use of groundsel tea or use of flour contaminated with groundsel seed has caused loss of appetite, vomiting, bloody diarrhea, sleepiness, weakness, staggering and jaundice, with liver damage and even death. Some people develop rashes from contact with these plants. Pregnant women should not use groundsel tea because it could harm the fetus. The bitter-tasting honey made from groundsel nectar contains high levels of pyrrolizidine alkaloids. These toxins are also passed in the milk of dairy animals. Some species (e.g., arrow-leaved groundsel) are recommended as wild greens, but without further information it is probably best to view all members of this genus with suspicion.

DESCRIPTION: One of the largest and most diverse genera in the world, with more than 35 species in Canada and 77 species in North America. Ours are mostly annual or perennial herbs with alternate leaves, few to many small, yellow flowerheads with disc flowers and with or without ray flowers, involucral bracts in a single row and seed-like fruits (achenes) with fluffy, white "parachutes."

Western groundsel (*S. integerrimus*) is a perennial species that grows to 30 cm tall, with toothless leaves and black-tipped involucral bracts; flowers in spring. Grows in grasslands, shrublands, meadows and forest openings from YT and BC to MB.

Canadian groundsel (*S. pauperculus*) grows 10–60 cm tall, has lance-shaped to elliptic leaves and hairless stem bases. Flowers few to several in terminal clusters; yellow ray flowers, usually fewer than 20 on flowerheads, appear from May to June. Found in peatlands and gravels, pastures, on roadsides and in meadows in all provinces and territories.

Arrow-leaved groundsel (*S. triangularis*) is a taller plant (to 1.2 m tall), with sharply toothed, triangular leaves, and flowers in summer. Found in damp places and open woodlands at low to alpine elevations (sometimes as a major species in low alpine meadows) from YT and NT to BC and AB.

Common groundsel (*S. vulgaris*) is an annual species that grows to 45 cm tall, with inconspicuous flowerheads that lack ray flowers, in bloom from spring to autumn. This introduced weed grows on disturbed ground and roadsides throughout Canada.

Arrow-leaved groundsel

415

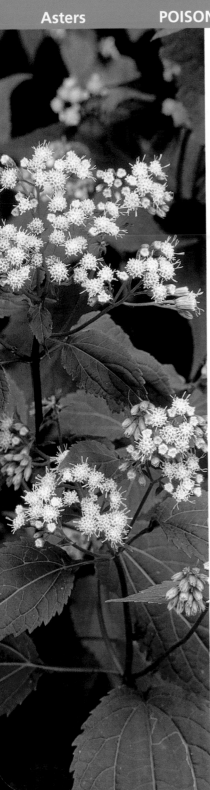

White Snakeroot
Ageratina altissima

FOOD: Herbivores avoid this herb as a food source because of its bitter and toxic foliage. Cattle sometimes eat it in over-grazed pastures, causing the fatal disease "staggers."

MEDICINE: A decoction of the root has been used as a treatment for "ague," diarrhea, painful urination, fevers and kidney stones. A poultice of the root was applied on snakebites. The plant is best known for its toxic properties, however, and was used by some First Nations to poison their enemies. No other plant has poisoned more animals and people in North America; during the colonial era, "milk sickness" decimated entire villages. Tremetol, a fat-soluble alcohol, accumulates in animals that consume the plant. Because tremetol is excreted in milk, humans are affected, but lactating animals are less susceptible to being poisoned. Milk contaminated with tremetol is toxic to non-weaned animals and those who consume milk and butter. Milk sickness in humans begins as weakness, loss of appetite, abdominal pain and violent vomiting followed by constipation, severe thirst, vomiting, tremors, acetone breath, prostration, delirium, coma and death. The modern practice of pasteurization does not inactivate tremetol, but milk sickness is uncommon today because of current practices of animal husbandry and the pooling of milk from many producers.

OTHER USES: The smoke of the burning herb was used to revive unconscious patients.

DESCRIPTION: Perennial herb, 50–80 cm tall, with solitary or clustered firm stems. Leaves 6–18 cm long, opposite on slender stalks, heart-shaped with toothed margins. Flat-topped clusters of small, fuzzy, white flowerheads about 5 mm long and 4 mm wide. Fruits tiny, seed-like and bear white bristles. Grows in rich woods and thickets from southern SK to NS. See p. 424 for conservation status.

Corydalises
Corydalis spp.

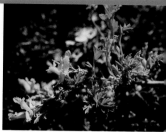

Corydalis species are most common in disturbed areas and often behave as weeds. In northern regions, they are most abundant after disturbances such as wildfire. They apparently bank their seeds in the forest floor for decades or even centuries until germination is triggered by disturbance, exposure and warming of the soil. *Corydalis* species are classified as poisonous because they contain

Golden corydalis

isoquinoline and other alkaloids. Some poisoning of cattle and sheep has been reported.

DESCRIPTION: Annual or biennial herbs with low, often prostrate stems, 10–40 cm long, soft, with watery juice, much branched, hairless, from a taproot. Leaves alternate, much divided. Flowers in many-flowered, loose-end clusters; irregular; petals 10–18 mm long. Fruits pod-like capsules, spreading or somewhat drooping, constricted between seeds, usually curved; seeds black, shiny.

Golden corydalis (*C. aurea*) has yellow flowers, with capsules 20–25 mm long. Prefers open woods, clearings, banks, shores and roadsides in moist to dry, sandy or rocky places at low to subalpine elevations from BC to QC and in YT and NT. See p. 424 for conservation status.

Pink corydalis (*C. sempervirens*) has pink flowers with yellow tips, and capsules 30–45 mm long. Prefers open woods, dry meadows and clearings, often following a burn, at low to subalpine elevations in all provinces and territories.

Dutchman's Breeches & Pacific Bleeding Heart
Dicentra spp.

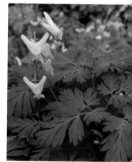

These plants contain a number of isoquinoline alkaloids, including aporphine and protopine (which is also found in the opium poppy, *Papaver somniferum*). Experimental feeding of Dutchman's breeches to cattle caused the animals to "become nervous, run back and forth, violently eject stomach contents, tremble, convulse, and fall down with

Dutchman's breeches

the legs extended and rigid." Happily, the cattle were eventually able to stand up and recover from their ordeal. The most common symptom of poisoning by this herb is a staggering gait, giving this plant its other common name, staggerweed. The underground tubers of this plant are considered more toxic than the flowers and leaves. The common name Dutchman's breeches refers to the flowers, which resemble a pair of breeches hung up to dry. The roots of Pacific bleeding heart were both chewed to relieve toothaches and taken internally to expel worms. Rinses made of the crushed plants were believed to help hair grow.

DESCRIPTION: Lacy, delicate, perennial, hairless herbs. Flowering stems 10–40 cm tall. Leaves basal or alternate, long-stalked, broadly triangular, finely divided into many linear segments, bluish green. Nodding flowers in terminal clusters. Fruits brown, pod-like capsules.

Dutchman's breeches (*D. cucullaria*) has white to pinkish flowers, tipped with pale yellow, with 4 petals, the 2 outer petals joined at the base and widely crested. Found in fresh to moist hardwood forests and rich woodlands at low to subalpine elevations from MB to the Maritimes. See p. 424 for conservation status.

Pacific bleeding heart (*D. formosa*) has pinkish purple, heart-shaped flowers. Found in moist forests and on streambanks at low to montane elevations in southern BC, most commonly near the coast.

GLOSSARY

achene: a small, dry fruit that doesn't split open; often seed-like in appearance; distinguished from a nutlet by its relatively thin wall.

alkaloid: any of a group of bitter-tasting, usually mildly alkaline plant chemicals. Many alkaloids affect the nervous system.

allergen: a substance that causes an allergic reaction.

alternate: situated singly at each node or joint (e.g., as leaves on a stem) or regularly between other organs (e.g., as stamens alternate with petals).

anaphylaxis: increased sensitivity to a foreign substance (often a protein) resulting from previous exposure to it (as in serum treatment).

andromedotoxin: a toxic alkaloid derived from a diterpene.

annual: a plant that completes its life cycle in one growing season.

anthelminthic: an agent that expels worms.

anticoagulant: an agent that stops or slows coagulation.

antimicrobial: an agent that destroys or prevents the growth of microorganisms.

antimutagenic: an agent that inhibits mutations.

arbutin: a glycoside found in plants of the Heath family (Ericaceae).

aril: a specialized cover attached to a mature seed.

astringent: an agent that contracts body tissues and checks secretions, capillary bleeding, etc.

axil: the position between a side organ (e.g., a leaf) and the part to which it is attached (e.g., a stem).

balm: a healing or soothing ointment.

bannock: a flat bread, traditionally unleavened but now made with flour, fat and baking soda.

barbiturate: an organic derivative of barbituric acid that depresses the central nervous system, respiration, heart rate, blood temperature and blood pressure.

beak: a prolonged, more or less slender tip on a thicker organ such as a fruit or seed.

berry: a simple fleshy fruit with an outer skin.

biennial: a plant that lives for two years, usually producing flowers and seed in the second year.

boil: a painful, localized inflammation of the lower layers of a skin gland or hair follicle, producing a hard central core and pus; usually caused by a bacterial (staphylococcus) infection.

bolt: to send up long, erect stems (usually elongating flower/fruit clusters) from a basal rosette.

bract: a specialized leaf with a flower (or sometimes a flower cluster) arising from its axil.

bulb: a short, vertical underground stem with thickened leaves or leaf bases (e.g., an onion).

bulblet: a small, bulb-like structure produced in a leaf axil or replacing a flower.

bur: the rough, prickly case or covering of the seeds of certain plants.

burl: a hard, often round, woody outgrowth on a tree.

bursitis: inflammation of a pad-like sac (bursa) in connecting tissue; usually around joints.

calyx: the outer (lowermost) circle of floral parts; composed of separate or fused lobes called sepals; usually green and leaf-like.

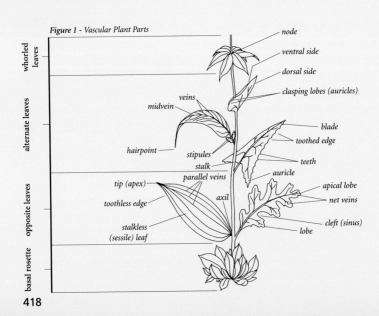

Figure 1 - Vascular Plant Parts

cambium: the thin growing layer; responsible for producing new stem cells.

candidiasis: an infection of skin or mucous membranes caused by a species of the yeast-like fungus Candida.

carbuncle: a painful localized inflammation of skin and deeper tissues with several openings for the discharge of pus and with sloughing of dead tissue.

cardiac; cardio: of the heart.

catkin: a dense spike or raceme of many small, unisexual, naked flowers that lack petals but have a bract.

cellulose: the polysaccharide that comprises most of plant cell walls.

chiggers: the six-legged, parasitic larvae of mites in the family Trombiculidae; also called redbugs.

chlorophyll: the pigment that gives most plants their green colour and the means of manufacturing sugars and starches through photosynthesis.

chronic: persistent; of long duration.

cirrhosis: loss of function of an organ; usually applied to progressive liver dysfunction because of development of dense nodules and fibres.

clasping: embracing or surrounding; usually in reference to a leaf base around a stem.

cone: a dry, elongated multiple fruit composed of woody scales, with naked seeds on the surface of the scales.

corm: a swollen stem base containing food material and bearing buds in the axils of the scale-like remains of leaves from the previous season.

corolla: the second circle of floral parts, composed of separate or fused lobes called petals; usually conspicuous in size and colour but sometimes small or absent.

coumarin: a white, crystalline lactone with the sweet smell of new-mown hay; a potent anticoagulant.

counter-irritant: an agent for producing irritation in one part to counteract irritation or relieve pain or inflammation elsewhere.

cultivar: a plant or animal originating in cultivation.

cyst: a closed sac containing fluid, semi-fluid or solid material; usually an abnormal growth caused by developmental anomalies, duct obstruction or parasitic infection.

decoction: a solution produced by boiling a plant substance in water.

delirium tremens: a psychic disorder, usually associated with withdrawal from alcohol, producing visual and auditory hallucinations.

dermatitis: inflammation of the skin, with redness, itching and/or lesions.

digitalis: the powdered leaves of common foxglove (*Digitalis purpurea*), containing glycosides that act as a powerful heart stimulant.

disc floret: a small, tubular flower in a flowerhead of the Aster family; usually clustered at the centre of the head.

diuretic: an agent that increases the flow of urine.

Doctrine of Signatures: a medical theory first popularized in the 14th century in which each plant displays a clear sign or "signature" of the purpose for which it was intended: plants with heart-shaped leaves are good for the heart, those resembling hair are good for the hair, etc.

dropsy: an obsolete term for edema.

drupe: a fruit with an outer fleshy part covered by a thin skin and surrounding a hard or bony stone that encloses a single seed (e.g., a plum).

drupelet: a tiny drupe; part of an aggregate fruit such as a raspberry.

dysentery: intestinal disorders, especially of the colon, caused by infection and characterized by severe bloody diarrhea.

eczema: a disease of the skin characterized by inflammation, itching and the formation of scales.

Figure 2 - Underground Parts

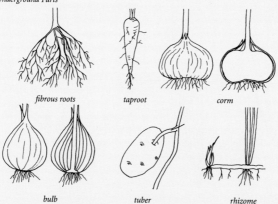

fibrous roots   taproot   corm

bulb   tuber   rhizome

edema: the abnormal accumulation of excessive amounts of fluids in body tissues.

emmenagogue: an agent that assists or promotes menstrual flow.

emphysema: a condition (usually of the lungs) characterized by air-filled expansions within tissues that may damage the tissue structure.

endocrine: pertaining to a gland that secretes directly into the bloodstream.

enema: an injection of liquid into the rectum and colon via the anus.

ergot: a fungal disease of grasses caused by *Claviceps purpurea*, with black to dark purple fruiting bodies containing several powerful alkaloids.

excelsior: fine, curled wood shavings; often used for packing fragile items.

expectorant: an agent that facilitates removal (coughing-up) of mucous from the respiratory tract.

febrifuge: an agent that reduces fever.

flavone: a colourless, crystalline ketone found in many primroses; flavone derivatives often occur in yellow pigments and are used in dyes.

floret: a small flower, usually one of several in a cluster.

follicle: a dry, pod-like fruit that splits open along a single line on one side.

forb: a broad-leaved flowering plant distinguished from grasses, sedges, etc.

frond: a fern leaf.

fructose: fruit sugar; a five-carbon monosaccharide found in corn syrup, honey, fruit juices, etc.

fumigant: smoke, vapour or gas applied to kill pests or combat infection.

gingivitis: gum disease producing redness, swelling and a tendency to bleed.

glume: one of a pair of bracts at the base of a grass spikelet, often persisting after the seeds have fallen.

glycoside: a two-parted molecule composed of a sugar and an aglycone, usually becoming poisonous when digested and the sugar is separated from its poisonous aglycone.

gout: a hereditary metabolic disorder; a form of acute arthritis with painful inflammation of joints (usually in the knees or feet).

Gram-positive: retaining the purple colour when stained with gentian violet in the Gram's test; usually pertaining to bacteria.

gravel: crystalline dust or stones in the kidney; composed of phosphate, calcium, oxalate and uric acid.

gruel: thin porridge.

haw: the fruit of a hawthorn, usually with a fleshy outer layer enclosing many dry seeds.

hemorrhoid: a mass of dilated, twisted veins in the lower rectum or upper anus.

hip: the fleshy fruit of a rose.

histamine: a compound that dilates capillaries and contracts smooth muscles; often released during allergic reactions.

hives: itchy weals caused by an allergic reaction.

hybrid: a cross between two species.

hyperglycemia: too much sugar in the blood.

hyperthyroidism: excessive secretion by the thyroid glands, resulting in an increased metabolic rate.

hypoglycemia: too little sugar in the blood.

incontinent: unable to retain bodily discharges such as urine or feces.

inflammation: redness, pain, heat, swelling and/or loss of function of some part of the body as a result of injury, infection, irritation, etc.

infusion: a liquid extract made by steeping a substance in water that is initially boiling.

involucre: a set of bracts closely associated with one another, encircling and immediately below a flower cluster.

involuntary muscle: a muscle controlling a reflex action and not under direct, voluntary control; especially a smooth muscle.

Figure 3 - Parts of an Aster (Asteraceae) Flowerhead

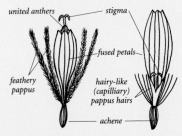

united anthers • stigma
fused petals
feathery pappus
hairy-like (capilliary) pappus hairs
achene

tubular (disc) floret • strap-like (ray) floret

ray florets
disc florets
buds
involucral bract
achenes
receptacle
stalk (penduncle)

radiate flowerhead

420

irregular: usually referring to bilaterally symmetrical flowers in which the upper half is unlike the lower, while the left half is a mirror image of the right; occasionally regarding flowers in which one or more sets of organs differ among themselves in size, shape or structure.

iso-: of equal or homogeneous form.

jaundice: an abnormal condition caused by increased bile pigments in the blood; characterized by yellowish skin, yellowish whites of the eyes, weariness and loss of appetite.

keel: a sharp, conspicuous longitudinal ridge, like the keel of a boat; the two partly united lower petals in a pea flower.

lactation: the secretion of milk.

latex: milky plant juice containing rubbery compounds.

lecithin: a fatty substance (phospholipid) found in blood, bile, nerves and other animal tissues.

legume: the seed pod of a Pea family plant.

lemma: the lower of the two bracts immediately enclosing a grass flower.

lenticel: a slightly raised pore on root, trunk or branch bark.

lignin: the substance that bonds with cellulose to form woody cell walls and to cement these cells together.

liniment: a liquid medication applied externally by rubbing or by applying on a bandage.

linoleic acid: an unsaturated fatty acid that is essential for the nutrition of some animals.

lipid: any of a group of fat-like substances (including true fats, lipoids and sterols) that are insoluble in water and soluble in fat solvents such as alcohol.

lupus: any of a group of diseases characterized by skin lesions.

melanoma: a malignant, darkly pigmented tumour or mole.

meprobamate: a bitter tranquilizer used to relieve anxiety.

mordant: a substance used to fix colour when dyeing; often a metallic agent that combines with a dye to form an insoluble, coloured compound.

mucilage: a sticky, gelatinous plant substance.

mutagen: an agent that causes genetic mutations.

narcotic: producing stupor or sleep and reducing pain.

neuralgia: severe pain along the course of a nerve or in its area of distribution.

neurotoxin: a nerve poison.

nutlet: a small, hard, dry, one-seeded fruit or part of a fruit; does not split open.

opposite: situated across from each other at the same node (not alternate or whorled); or situated directly in front of another organ (e.g., stamens opposite petals).

oxalate: a salt or ester of an oxalic acid.

oxalic acid: a strong, poisonous acid; often used in white, crystalline powder form as a bleach or stain remover.

oxytocin: a pituitary hormone that stimulates contraction of the uterus and secretion of milk.

palea: the upper of the two bracts immediately enclosing a grass flower.

palmate: divided into three or more lobes or leaflets diverging from a common point, like fingers on a hand.

palpitation: strong, rapid pulsation, such as a fast throbbing or fluttering of the heart.

panicle: a loosely branched cluster of stalked flowers or spikelets, blooming from the bottom up.

pappus: a modified calyx forming a crown of bristles, hairs, awns, teeth or scales at the tip of the seed; often aids in seed dispersal.

parch: to toast under dry heat.

Figure 4 - Parts of a Female Willow (Salix) *Shrub*

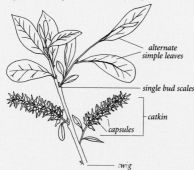

alternate simple leaves

single bud scales

catkin

capsules

twig

Figure 5 - Branching Patterns

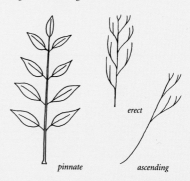

erect

pinnate

ascending

pectin: a water-soluble substance that binds adjacent cell walls together, producing a gel.

pemmican: a mixture of finely pounded dried meat, fat and sometimes dried fruit.

perennial: a plant that lives for three or more years, usually flowering and fruiting for several years.

perigynium: a modified bract forming a sac around the pistil (achene) of a sedge (*Carex*) flower.

pharmacology: the science of drugs, their properties and reactions, especially those related to therapeutic use.

photosynthesis: the process of manufacturing sugars and starches using chlorophyll, carbon dioxide, water and energy from the sun.

pinnate: with branches, lobes, leaflets or veins arranged on both sides of a central stalk or vein; feather-like.

pinole: flour made from finely ground, parched corn.

plaque: a localized, abnormal patch on skin or mucous membranes, often referring to abnormal fatty deposits in arteries.

platelets: minute discs in the blood that play an important role in blood coagulation.

pome: a fleshy fruit with a core (e.g., an apple) comprised of an enlarged hypanthium around a compound ovary.

postpartum: after childbirth.

poultice: a soft, moist mass of cloth, bread, meal or herbs; applied as a remedy for sore or inflamed parts of the body.

prostaglandin: any of a group of compounds derived from saturated fatty acids and found in many body tissues, having hormone-like actions including control of uterine contractions and blood pressure.

psoralen: any of a group of plant substances, some of which are phototoxic (causing skin reactions when applied to skin and then exposed to ultra-violet radiation).

psoriasis: a chronic skin disease characterized by scaly, reddish patches.

purgative: causing watery evacuation of the bowels.

quinine: a bitter, white crystalline alkaloid derived from cinchona bark.

raceme: an unbranched cluster of stalked flowers on a common, elongated central stalk, blooming from the bottom up.

ray floret: a small, flattened, strap-like flower of a flowerhead in the Aster family; often radiating from the edges of the head.

receptacle: an expanded stalk tip at the centre of a flower, bearing the floral organs or the small, crowded flowers of a head.

rhizome: a thickened horizontal underground stem, usually bearing stems above and roots below.

rickets: a deficiency disease in which lack of sunlight and vitamin D results in insufficient assimilation of calcium and phosphorus into newly formed bones, causing abnormalities in bone shape and structure.

ringworm: an itchy, red-ringed, painful, scaly fungal infection of the skin.

rosette: a cluster of crowded, usually basal leaves in a circular arrangement.

salicin: a glycoside found in willows and poplars, related to salicylic acid and used, like aspirin, for relieving pain and fever.

saponin: any of a group of glycosides with steroid-like structure, found in many plants, that causes diarrhea and vomiting when taken internally but is used in detergents.

scabies: a contagious skin disease caused by a parasitic mite (*Sarcoptes scabiei*) that burrows under the skin to deposit eggs, causing intense itching.

schizocarp: a fruit that splits into two or more parts at maturity (e.g., fruits of the Carrot family, Apiaceae).

sciatica: any painful condition in the region of the hips and thighs, especially neuritis of the long nerve.

scrofula: tuberculosis of the lymph nodes, especially in the neck.

scurvy: a deficiency disease caused by lack of vitamin C; characterized by bleeding and abnormal formation of bones and teeth.

Figure 6 - Fruits

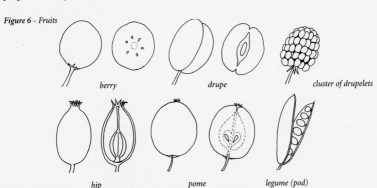

berry   drupe   cluster of drupelets

hip   pome   legume (pod)

sepal: one segment of the calyx; usually green and leaf-like.

shingles: a disease caused by reactivation of the chickenpox virus (*Herpes zoster*); characterized by painful, inflamed eruptions along a peripheral nerve, usually on the trunk of the body but occasionally on the head.

sitz bath: a tub for sitting in, with water covering the hips.

smudge: a smoldering mass, placed on the windward side to produce smoke and/or heat for protection from insects, frost, etc.

snoose: a small wad of tobacco held between the gums and the lip or cheek.

spike: a simple, unbranched flower cluster with (essentially) stalkless flowers arranged on an elongated axis.

spikelet: a small or secondary spike, as in the flower-heads of grasses and sedges.

sporangium: a structure in which spores are produced; a spore-case.

spur: a hollow appendage on a petal or sepal, usually functioning as a nectary.

steroid: any of many compounds containing a 17-carbon, 4-ring structure including D vitamins, saponins, glucosides of digitalis and certain hormones and carcinogens.

sterol: a solid steroidal alcohol (such as cholesterol) found in plant and animal fats.

stipules: a pair of bract-like or leaf-like appendages at the base of a leaf stalk.

stolon: a slender, prostrate, spreading branch, rooting and often developing new shoots and/or plants at its nodes or at the tip.

style: the part of the pistil connecting the stigma to the ovary; often elongated and stalk-like.

tallow: the solid, nearly tasteless fat rendered from cattle and sheep fat.

tannin: a soluble, astringent phenol found in many plants; used in tanning, dyeing and medicine.

taproot: a root system with a prominent main root, directed vertically downward and bearing smaller side roots, sometimes becoming very swollen with stored food material (e.g., starch or sugar).

tartar: an encrustation on the teeth, created by food, saliva and salts such as calcium carbonate.

tendonitis: inflammation of a tendon.

tendril: a slender, clasping or twining outgrowth from a stem or leaf.

tepal: a sepal or petal, when these structures are not easily distinguished.

throat: the opening into a corolla tube or calyx tube.

tincture: an alcohol or alcohol-and-water solution containing animal, plant or chemical drugs.

tooth: a small, sharp-pointed lobe on the edge of a plant organ (usually on a leaf).

tuber: a thickened portion of a below-ground stem or root, serving for food storage and often also for propagation.

tubercle: a small swelling or projection on an organ.

ulcer: an inflamed lesion of the skin or of a mucous membrane, with sloughing dead tissue and often pus.

umbel: a round- or flat-topped flower cluster in which all flower stalks are of approximately the same length and arise from the same point.

vasoconstrictor: an agent causing constriction of blood vessels.

vasodilator: an agent causing dilation of blood vessels.

vein: a strand of conducting tubes (a vascular bundle), especially if visible externally, as in a leaf.

whorl: a ring of three or more similar structures (e.g., leaves, branches or flowers) arising from one node.

wing: a thin, flattened expansion on the side(s) or tip of an organ; the side petals of most flowers of the Pea family (Fabaceae).

winnow: to remove lighter material, such as chaff, using wind currents.

Figure 6 (cont.) - Fruits

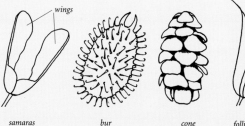
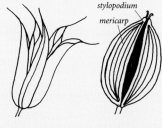

samaras   bur   cone   follicles   schizocarp

PLANT CONSERVATION STATUS

TABLE 1. *Plant conservation status according to the Committee on the Status of Endangered Wildlife in Canada (COSEWIC). Plants are listed in alphabetical order. Apparently secure (4) or secure species (5) are not included in this table.*

1: Critically Imperilled—*Critically imperilled in the province because of extreme rarity (often 5 or fewer occurrences) or because some factor(s) such as very steep declines make it especially vulnerable to extirpation from the province.*

2: Imperilled—*Imperilled in the province because of rarity resulting from very restricted range, very few populations (often 20 or fewer), steep declines or other factors making it very vulnerable to extirpation from the province.*

3: Vulnerable—*Vulnerable in the province because of a restricted range, relatively few populations (often 80 or fewer), recent and widespread declines or other factors making it vulnerable to extirpation.*

4: Apparently Secure—*Uncommon but not rare; some cause for long-term concern because of declines or other factors.*

5: Secure—*Common, widespread and abundant in the province.*

H: Possibly Extirpated (Historical)—*Species or community occurred historically in the province and there is some possibility that it may be rediscovered. Its presence may not have been verified in the past 20–40 years.*

U: Unrankable—*Currently unrankable because of lack of information or substantially conflicting information about status or trends.*

X: Presumed Extirpated—*Species or community is believed to be extirpated from the province. Not located despite intensive searches of historical sites and other appropriate habitat, and virtually no likelihood that it will be rediscovered.*

Scientific Name	CAN	BC	AB	SK	MB	ON	QC	NB	NS	NL	LB	PE	YT	NT	NU
Acer nigrum							3								
Aconitum delphiniifolium			3												
Acorus americanus		2–3	3							1–2		3–4			
Adiantum aleuticum			2				2			3					
Agastache nepetoides							1								
Agastache urticifolia	3	3													
Ageratina altissima									1						
Agoseris aurantiaca							1								
Alisma triviale										1–2			1		
Allium canadense							2	1							
Allium cernuum				1–2	2										
Allium geyeri	2		2	1											
Allium schoenoprasum									2						
Allium textile					3										
Allium tricoccum					1		3	2	1						
Ambrosia artemisiifolia			3												
Amelanchier alnifolia							3								
Amelanchier canadensis							3	3				1			
Anaphalis margaritacea	3–5			2						3–5	3–5		1		

PLANT CONSERVATION STATUS

Scientific Name	CAN	BC	AB	SK	MB	ON	QC	NB	NS	NL	LB	PE	YT	NT	NU
Anemone americana					1		3–4	2	1						
Anemone canadensis		2–3							2	2		1			
Anemone multifida							3–4	2–3	1						
Anemone patens						1									
Angelica arguta			3–4												
Angelica atropurpurea							3–4		3–5			2–3			
Angelica genuflexa			3												
Apios americana												1			
Apocynum cannabinum			3												
Aquilegia formosa													2		
Aralia hispida										3–5	U				
Aralia nudicaulis										3–5			2–3		
Aralia racemosa				2									3–4		
Arctostaphylos uva-ursi										3–5	2–3				
Arisaema triphyllum					2										
Arnica chamissonis							1						3		
Arnica cordifolia				3	1	1									
Arnica fulgens					2										
Arnica sororia			3	1											
Artemisia campestris								3	1						
Artemisia dracunculus						1							2		
Artemisia frigida						2–3									
Artemisia tridentata			2												
Asarum canadense					3		3–4								
Asclepias incarnata									3			1			
Asclepias speciosa			3												
Asclepias syriaca				1											
Asimina triloba	3					3									
Astragalus americanus					3	H	1								
Astragalus miser			3												
Athyrium filix-femina													2–3		
Atriplex spp.	3–4						2–3		1			1–3			
Berberis repens			3												
Betula alleghaniensis									2–3						
Betula lenta	1					1									
Betula papyrifera										3–5	3–5				
Bistorta bistortoides		3–4	3												
Bistorta vivipara				1–2				1	1						
Botrychium virginianum										3	1	3–4	2		
Calochortus apiculatus			3												
Caltha leptosepala			3										2		
Caltha palustris									2		1				
Camassia quamash	3		2												
Camassia scilloides	2					2									
Cardamine diphylla												1			
Cardamine pensylvanica										3–5	2–3				
Carya ovata							3								

425

Scientific Name	CAN	BC	AB	SK	MB	ON	QC	NB	NS	NL	LB	PE	YT	NT	NU
Castanea dentata	3					2									
Caulophyllum giganteum							3–4								
Caulophyllum thalictroides					2		3	3			2				
Ceanothus americanus							2								
Ceanothus velutinus			3												
Celastrus scandens				1			3–4	X							
Cephalanthus occidentalis								1–2	2–3						
Chelone glabra					2–3										
Chenopodium album	1–3														
Chenopodium capitatum							3								
Chimaphila menziesii		3–4													
Chimaphila umbellata				3											
Cicuta bulbifera		3–4							3–5				2		
Cirsium foliosum		3–4	3										2		
Cirsium hookerianum		3													
Claytonia lanceolata				2–3											
Claytonia megarhiza		3											1		
Clematis ligusticifolia	3–5				1										
Clematis occidentalis				2			3	3	1						
Clematis virginiana					2										
Clintonia borealis										3–5	3–5				
Clintonia uniflora		3													
Cornus canadensis							·			3–5	3–5				
Cornus sericea										3–5	3–5				
Corydalis aurea							2								
Corylus americana							H								
Crataegus chrysocarpa												1			
Crataegus crus-galli							1								
Crataegus douglasii			3	2											
Crataegus succulenta				1				2				3–4			
Cyperus esculentus					U		3								
Cypripedium acaule			3								U				
Delphinium bicolor				2–3											
Delphinium glaucum				1–2											
Dicentra cucullaria					1							1			
Drosera rotundifolia										3–5	3–5				
Dryopteris carthusiana		3–4									U		2		
Dryopteris cristata		2–3	1	3											
Dryopteris expansa							3–4			H	3–5		2–3		
Dryopteris filix-mas			1	1			2	1	3	3–4					
Echinacea angustifolia	3–4			3	3										
Elaeagnus commutata							2								
Epilobium latifolium					3										
Equisetum hyemale										U					
Ericameria nauseosa			3												
Erigeron philadelphicus									2			1	2		
Erythronium oregonum	3														

PLANT CONSERVATION STATUS

Scientific Name	CAN	BC	AB	SK	MB	ON	QC	NB	NS	NL	LB	PE	YT	NT	NU
Euonymus atropurpureus	3					3									
Eupatorium perfoliatum												2–3			
Eutrochium maculatum			1–2												
Eutrochium purpureum			U			3									
Fritillaria camschatcensis													1		
Fritillaria pudica			3												
Galium aparine					U										
Galium boreale									2			1			
Galium triflorum											2–3		3		
Gaultheria hispidula			3							3–5	3–5				
Gaultheria humifusa		3–4	3												
Gaultheria procumbens					3–4					1–2					
Gaylussacia baccata							3–4			3–5					
Gentiana calycosa	3	2–3	3												
Gentiana quinquefolia						2									
Gentianella amarella								2	1						
Gentianopsis detonsa			1			H									
Geranium robertianum								2				3			
Geum macrophyllum										3–5	3–5				
Geum rivale		3–4								3–5	1–2				
Glaux maritima ssp. *obtusifolia*						3									
Glycyrrhiza lepidota		2				3									
Goodyera oblongifolia			3	2			3–4	2	2–3	H		1			
Gymnocladus dioicus	2					2									
Hamamelis virginiana							3					1			
Hedeoma pulegioides							3	2	2–3						
Hedysarum alpinum							3			3–5	1–2				
Hedysarum boreale							1								
Helenium autumnale			3												
Helianthemum canadense						1	1		1						
Heracleum maximum										3–5					
Heuchera americana	2					2									
Hieracium venosum						2									
Huperzia haleakalae			2												
Hypericum scouleri			1												
Impatiens capensis										3–5					
Impatiens pallida							3–4	2	1–2		2				
Iris missouriensis	1		1												
Juglans cinerea	3–4					3	3–4	3							
Juniperus communis												3–4			
Juniperus horizontalis										3–5	3–5	3–4			
Juniperus scopulorum	3–4		3	1											
Juniperus virginiana							2								
Kalmia angustifolia										3–5	3–5				
Kalmia microphylla					1–2	2									
Lactuca biennis			2	2						3–5			1		
Larix occidentalis			2												

427

PLANT CONSERVATION STATUS

Scientific Name	CAN	BC	AB	SK	MB	ON	QC	NB	NS	NL	LB	PE	YT	NT	NU
Lathyrus japonicus										3–5	2–3		1		
Lathyrus ochroleucus							2						2		
Ledum glandulosum			3												
Ledum groenlandicum										3–5	3–5				
Lepidium virginicum		3–4													
Lewisia rediviva			1												
Lilium canadense						1			2–3						
Lithospermum canescens						3									
Lithospermum incisum		3–4			3	1									
Lithospermum ruderale				1											
Lobelia cardinalis					H			3							
Lobelia inflata												2–3			
Lomatium cous	1		1–2	1–2											
Lomatium dissectum			3	1											
Lomatium triternatum			3												
Lonicera dioica							3								
Lonicera involucrata							3–4								
Lupinus argenteus			3	3											
Lupinus littoralis	3	3–4													
Lupinus nootkatensis			3										1–2		
Lycopodium clavatum			3							3–5					
Lycopus americanus		3								2					
Lycopus uniflorus			3	3						3–5	3–5				
Maianthemum canadense										3–5	3–5				
Maianthemum racemosum					2										
Maianthemum stellatum										3–5	3–5	3			
Marah oreganus	2–3	1													
Matricaria discoidea		U													
Matteucia struthiopteris		3–4	3							3–4					
Mentha arvensis	3–5								U	3–5	2–3	U			
Mentzelia decapetala			3		H										
Mitchella repens										2		1			
Monarda fistulosa							3								
Moneses uniflora										3–5	3–5				
Monotropa uniflora			3							3–5	1–3				
Morus rubra	2					2									
Myrica gale			3–4												
Nymphaea odorata				1	2					3–4		1			
Oplopanax horridus			3			1							1–2		
Opuntia fragilis						3									
Osmorhiza claytonii					2							2			
Osmorhiza longistylis			2				3	2	2			1			
Ostrya virginiana					2										
Oxycoccus oxycoccos										3–5	3–5				
Oxyria digyna									1	2					
Oxytropis lambertii				2	3–4										
Oxytropis sericea					1										

PLANT CONSERVATION STATUS

Scientific Name	CAN	BC	AB	SK	MB	ON	QC	NB	NS	NL	LB	PE	YT	NT	NU
Oxytropis splendens						3									
Panax quinquefolius	2–3					2	2								
Panax trifolius							3–4	2	3			2			
Pedicularis canadensis							3	1							
Pentaphylloides floribunda										3–5	2–3	1			
Penthorum sedoides					1–2		2								
Perideridia gairdneri		3–4	3	2											
Petasites frigidus var. frigidus			3												
Petasites frigidus var. palmatus										3–5		2			
Petasites frigidus var. sagittatus							3								
Phryma leptostachya					3			2							
Phytolacca americana							1			U					
Picea rubens						3									
Pinus albicaulis			2												
Pinus banksiana		2–3									1	3			
Pinus monticola			U												
Pinus strobus					2					3					
Podophyllum peltatum							1								
Polygala senega		1	3	3–4			2	2							
Polygonum douglasii	3–5		3				2								
Polypodium hesperium		3–4	1–2												
Polypodium virginianum										U	2–3	1			
Polystichum acrostichoides												2–3			
Pontederia cordata												1			
Populus balsamifera ssp. balsamifera												2			
Populus deltoides			3												
Populus tremuloides												2–3			
Potentilla anserina										3–5					
Potentilla arguta							3–4	3							
Potentilla canadensis						U									
Potentilla egedii					2										
Prunella vulgaris			3	1											
Prunus americana			2												
Prunus pensylvanica										3–5	2–3				
Ptelea trifoliata	3					3									
Pteridium aquilinum			3												
Pyrola elliptica		2–3	3							2–3					
Pyrola rotundifolia					2			3–4		3–5					
Quercus alba							3								
Quercus bicolor							2								
Ranunculus sceleratus							3–4	1	1–2						
Rhamnus alnifolia			3						3			3			
Rhodiola integrifolium			3												
Rhodiola rosea							3–4	3		3–5	3–5				
Rhus glabra		3–4		1		H									
Rhus trilobata			3												
Rhus typhina												2			

PLANT CONSERVATION STATUS

Scientific Name	CAN	BC	AB	SK	MB	ON	QC	NB	NS	NL	LB	PE	YT	NT	NU
Ribes americanum							3								
Ribes aureum	3–5		3	2											
Ribes hudsonianum							2–3								
Ribes inerme			3												
Ribes lacustre										3–5	2–3				
Ribes lobbii													1		
Ribes oxyacanthoides							1								
Ribes triste										3–5		3			
Rorippa palustris												2			
Rosa acicularis								1							
Rosa woodsii						U							2		
Rubus chamaemorus							3			3–5	3–5	2			
Rubus occidentalis							2								
Rubus pedatus													1		
Rubus pubescens										3–5	3–5				
Rudbeckia laciniata							3–4		2–3						
Rumex triangulivalvis						H			2						
Sagittaria cuneata												U	2		
Sagittaria latifolia			1							1–2					
Salicornia rubra		3–4													
Salix arctica						3	3–4			1–2					
Sanguinaria canadensis					2		3–4		3–4						
Sanicula marilandica		3–4								2–3		2			
Schoenoplectus acutus										2–3					
Schoenoplectus tabernaemontani										1–2					
Scutellaria galericulata										3–5	2–3		2–3		
Scutellaria lateriflora		3–4								2					
Shepherdia canadensis								2	2	3–5	U				
Silphium perfoliatum	2					2									
Silphium terebinthinaceum						1									
Sisyrinchium angustifolium		U					2	H	3						
Sium suave										3–5			2		
Smilax herbacea							3–4								
Smilax rotundifolia						2									
Solidago gigantea												3–4			
Solidago missouriensis						2									
Solidago multiradiata								1	1–2	3–5	3–5				
Sorbus americana										3–5					
Sorbus scopulina				2											
Sorbus sitchensis			3										1		
Stachys palustris												2			
Streptopus amplexifolius					3					3–5					
Symphoricarpos albus							3								
Symplocarpus foetidus								2	3						
Taraxacum officinale				2											
Taxus brevifolia			1												
Taxus canadensis					3										

PLANT CONSERVATION STATUS

Scientific Name	CAN	BC	AB	SK	MB	ON	QC	NB	NS	NL	LB	PE	YT	NT	NU
Thermopsis rhombifolia		1			2										
Thuja occidentalis									1–2						
Thuja plicata			1–2												
Tilia americana							3–4								
Toxicodendron radicans							3	2							
Triglochin maritima										3–5	3–5				
Trillium erectum									3						
Trillium grandiflorum							3–4								
Trillium ovatum		1	3												
Triosteum aurantiacum							3	2				2			
Triosteum perfoliatum						1									
Triteleia grandiflora	3														
Tsuga heterophylla			1												
Typha angustifolia				1											
Typha latifolia													2		
Urtica dioica													3–4		
Vaccinium angustifolium										3–5	3–5				
Vaccinium caespitosum					2			3	2	3	3–5		3–4		
Vaccinium membranaceum						1							2		
Vaccinium ovalifolium			2			2	3–4		1	3–5			2–3		
Vaccinium uliginosum			3					1	2	3–5	3–5	1			
Vaccinium vitis-idaea												3			
Valeriana dioica							3–4	1							
Valeriana edulis	2–3				1										
Valeriana sitchensis					2										
Veratrum viride										U					
Verbena hastata				1–2					3						
Veronica americana													3–4		
Veronica serpyllifolia			3	1											
Viburnum acerifolium							3–4	1							
Viburnum alnifolium												2–3			
Viburnum edule									3–5			2			
Viburnum lentago			2				3–4	1							
Viburnum opulus			3												
Viburnum trilobum		3–4								3–5					
Vicia americana							2						2		
Viola adunca							3								
Viola canadensis							1–2	1					2–3		
Viola nuttallii				3–4											
Vitis riparia				3–4											
Xerophyllum tenax			3–4												
Zanthoxylum americanum							3–4								
Zigadenus elegans							3–4	1							
Zizania aquatica								2							
Zizia aurea									1–2						

REFERENCES

Alberta Agriculture. (1983). Outdoor Plants Harmful or Poisonous to Humans. In *Agdex* (666-2). Edmonton, AB: Alberta Tree Nursery and Horticulture Centre.

Andre, Alestine, Amanda Karst and N.J. Turner. (2006). Arctic and Subarctic Plants. In D.H. Ubelaker, D. Stanford, B. Smith and E.J.E. Szathmary (Eds.), *Smithsonian Institution Handbook of North American Indians: Environment, Origins and Population* (Vol. 3, pp. 222–235). Washington, DC: Smithsonian Institution.

Arnason, T., R.J. Hebda and T. Johns. (1981). Use of plants for food and medicine by Native Peoples of eastern Canada. *Canadian Journal of Botany 59*(11), 2189–2325.

Brill, S. and E. Dean. (1994). *Identifying and Harvesting Edible and Medicinal Plants in Wild (and Not So Wild) Places*. New York, NY: Hearst Books.

Chambers, B., K. Legasy and C. Bentley. (1996). *Forest Plants of Central Ontario*. Edmonton, AB: Lone Pine Publishing.

Coffey, Timothy. (1993). *The History and Folklore of North American Wildflowers*. New York, NY: Facts On File.

Coombes, Allen J. (2000). *Dorling Kindersley Handbooks: Trees*. New York, NY: Dorling Kindersley Inc.

Deur, Douglas and N.J. Turner (Eds.). (2005). *Keeping it Living: Traditions of Plant Use and Cultivation on the Northwest Coast of North America*. Vancouver: UBC Press.

Duke, James A. (1986). *Handbook of Northeastern Indian Medicinal Plants*. Lincoln, MA: Quarterman Publications.

Elias, Thomas S. and P. A. Dykeman. (1990). *Edible Wild Plants of North America Field Guide*. New York, NY: Sterling Publishing Company.

Erichsen-Brown, Charlotte. (1979). *Medicinal and Other Uses of North American Plants*. New York, NY: Dover Publications.

Fernald, M.L. and A. C. Kinsey. (1958). *Edible Wild Plants of Eastern North America*. Revised by R. C. Rollins. New York, NY: Harper and Brothers Publishers.

Foster, S. and James A. Duke. (1990). *Eastern/Central Medicinal Plants*. Peterson Field Guide Series. Boston, MA: Houghton Mifflin Company.

Grieve, M. (1931). *A Modern Herbal*. Harmondsworth, England: Penguin Books.

Hutchens, A. R. (1991). *Indian Herbology of North America*. Boston, MA: Shambhala Publications, Inc.

Johnston, A. (1987). Plants and the Blackfoot. Occasional Paper No. 15. Lethbridge, AB: Lethbridge Historical Society.

Johnson, Derek, *et.al.* (1995). *Plants of the Western Boreal Forest and Aspen Parkland*. Edmonton, AB: Lone Pine Publishing.

Kerik, J. and S. Fisher. (1982). *Living With the Land: Use of Plants by the Native People of Alberta*. Edmonton, AB: Provincial Museum of Alberta.

Kershaw, Linda. (1991). *The Plants of Northwestern Canada, with Special Reference to the Dempster Highway, Yukon and Northwest Territories*. Unpublished manuscript.

Kershaw, Linda. (2000). *Edible & Medicinal Plants of the Rockies*. Edmonton, AB: Lone Pine Publishing.

Kershaw, Linda, Andy MacKinnon and Jim Pojar. (1998). *Plants of the Rocky Mountains*. Edmonton, AB: Lone Pine Publishing.

Kindschner, K. (1987). *Edible Wild Plants of the Prairie: An Ethnobotanical Guide*. Lawrence, KS: University Press of Kansas.

Kirk, Donald R. (1975). *Wild Edible Plants of Western North America*. Happy Camp, CA: Naturegraph Publishers.

Kozloff, Eugene N. (1995). *Plants and Animals of the Pacific Northwest: An Illustrated Guide to the Natural History of Western Oregon, Washington, and British Columbia*. Seattle: University of Washington Press.

Krochmal, Arnold and Connie Krochmal. (1984). *A Field Guide to Medicinal Plants*. New York, NY: Times Books.

Kuhnlein, H.V. and N.J. Turner. (1991). Traditional Food Plants of Canadian Indigenous Peoples: Nutrition, Botany and Use. In S. Katz (Ed.), *Food and Nutrition in History and Anthropology* (Vol. 8). Philadelphia, PA: Gordon and Breach Science Publishers.

Kunkel, G. (1984). *Plants for Human Consumption: An Annotated Checklist of the Edible Phanerogans and Ferns*. Koenigstein, Germany: Koeltz Scientific Books.

REFERENCES

Langshaw, R. (1983). *Naturally: Medicinal Herbs and Edible Plants of the Canadian Rockies.* Banff, AB: Summerthought Publications.

Legasy, K. (1995). *Forest Plants of Northeastern Ontario.* Edmonton, AB: Lone Pine Publishing.

Little, Elbert E. (1990). *The Audubon Society Field Guide to North American Trees.* New York, NY: Alfred A. Knopf, Inc.

Lust, J. (1974). *The Herb Book.* New York, NY: Bantam Books.

MacKinnon, Andy, Jim Pojar and Ray Coupé. (1992). *Plants of Northern British Columbia.* Edmonton, AB: Lone Pine Publishing.

Marles, R.J., C. Clavelle, L. Monteleone, N. Tays and D. Burns. (2000). *Aboriginal Plant Use in Canada's Northwest Boreal Forest.* Vancouver, BC: UBC Press.

Moerman, D. E. (1998). *Native American Ethnobotany.* Portland, OR: Timber Press.

Mulligan, G. A. and D. B. Munro. (1990). Poisonous Plants of Canada. Publication 1842/E. Ottawa: Agriculture Canada.

Naegele, T.A. (1996). *Edible and Medicinal Plants of the Great Lakes Region.* Davisburg, MI: Wilderness Adventure Books.

Newall, C.A., L.A. Anderson and J.D. Phillipson. (1996). *Herbal Medicines: A Guide for Health-care Professionals.* London: The Pharmaceutical Press.

Niering, W. A. (1993). *The Audubon Society Field Guide to North American Wildflowers.* New York, NY: Alfred A. Knopf, Inc.

Peirce, A. (1999). *The American Pharmaceutical Association Practical Guide to Natural Medicines.* New York, NY: The Stonesong Press, William Morrow and Co.

Peterson, L.A. (1977). *A Field Guide to Edible Wild Plants of Eastern and Central North America.* Peterson Field Guide Series. Boston, MA: Houghton Mifflin.

Pojar, Jim and Andy MacKinnon. (1994). *Plants of Coastal British Columbia.* Edmonton, AB: Lone Pine Publishing.

Robinson, Peggy. (1979). *Profiles of Northwest Plants: Food Uses, Medicinal Uses, Legends.* Portland, OR: Far West Book Service.

Schofield, Janice J. (1989). *Discovering Wild Plants: Alaska, Western Canada, the Northwest.* Anchorage, AK: Alaska Northwest Books.

Scoggan, H.J. (1978–79). Flora of Canada (Parts 1–4). In *Botany* (No. 7). Ottawa, ON: National Museum of Natural Sciences.

Szczawinski, A.F. and G.A. Hardy. (1971). Guide to Common Edible Plants of British Columbia. *British Columbia Provincial Museum Handbook* (No. 20). Victoria, BC: British Columbia Provincial Museum.

Szczawinski, A.F. and N.J. Turner. (1978). Edible Garden Weeds of Canada. *Edible Wild Plants of Canada* (No. 1). Ottawa, ON: National Museum of Natural Sciences, National Museums of Canada.

Szczawinski, A.F. and N.J. Turner. (1980). Wild Green Vegetables of Canada. *Edible Wild Plants of Canada* (No. 4). Ottawa, ON: National Museum of Natural Sciences, National Museums of Canada.

Taylor, Ronald J. (1990). *Northwest Weeds: The Ugly and Beautiful Villains of Fields, Gardens and Roadsides.* Missoula, MT: Mountain Press Publishing Company.

Tilford, Gregory L. (1997). *Edible and Medicinal Plants of the West.* Missoula, MT: Mountain Press Publishing Company.

Turner, N.J. (1995). Food Plants of the Coastal First Peoples. *Royal British Columbia Museum Handbook.* Vancouver, BC: UBC Press.

Turner, N.J. (1998). Plant Technology of First Peoples in British Columbia. *Royal British Columbia Museum Handbook.* Vancouver, BC: UBC Press.

Turner, N.J. (2004). *Plants of Haida Gwaii.* Winlaw, BC: Sono Nis Press.

Turner, N.J. and Fiona Hamersley Chambers. (2006). Northwest Coast and Plateau Plants. In D.H. Ubelaker, D. Stanford, B. Smith and E.J.E. Szathmary (Eds.), *Smithsonian Institution Handbook of North American Indians: Environment, Origins and Population* (Vol. 3, pp. 251–262). Washington, DC: Gordon and Breach Science Publishers.

Turner, N.J. and Harriet V. Kuhnlein. (1982). Two important "root" foods of the Northwest Coast Indians: springbank clover (*Trifolium wormskioldii*) and Pacific silverweed (*Potentilla anserina* ssp. *pacifica*). *Economic Botany*, 36(4), 411–432.

Turner, N.J. and A.F. Szczawinski. (1991). *Common Poisonous Plants and Mushrooms of North America.* Portland, OR: Timber Press.

REFERENCES

Turner, N.J. and A.F. Szczawinski. (1979). Edible Wild Fruits and Nuts of Canada. *Edible Wild Plants of Canada* (No. 3). Ottawa, ON: National Museum of Natural Sciences, National Museums of Canada.

Turner, N.J. and A.F. Szczawinski. (1978). Wild Coffee and Tea Substitutes of Canada. *Edible Wild Plants of Canada* (No. 2). Ottawa, ON: National Museum of Natural Sciences, National Museums of Canada.

Turner, N.J., J. Thomas, B.F. Carlson and R.T. Ogilvie. (1983). Ethnobotany of the Nitinaht Indians of Vancouver Island. Occasional Paper No. 23. Victoria, BC: British Columbia Provincial Museum.

Turner, N.J., L.C. Thompson, M.T. Thompson and A.Z. York. (1990). Thompson Ethnobotany. Memoir No. 3. Victoria, BC: Royal British Columbia Museum.

Tyler, V. E. (1993). *The Honest Herbal: A Sensible Guide to the Use of Herbs and Related Remedies.* New York, NY: Pharmaceutical Products Press.

Willard, T. (1992). *Edible and Medicinal Plants of the Rocky Mountains and Neighbouring Territories.* Calgary, AB: Wild Rose College of Natural Healing.

Websites

Canadian Biodiversity: http://canadianbiodiversity.mcgill.ca/english/species/plants/index.htm

Evergreen Native Plant Database: http://www.evergreen.ca/nativeplants/search

Flora of North America, from the Flora of North America Association website: http://www.fna.org/FNA

Germplasm Resources Information Network, from the United States Department of Agriculture: Agricultural Research Service website: http://www.ars-grin.gov

Native American Ethnobotany: A Database of Foods, Drugs, Dyes and Fibers of Native American Peoples, Derived from Plants, from the University of Michigan at Dearborn website: http://herb.umd.umich.edu

Natural History of the North Woods: http://www.rook.org/earl/bwca/nature/

Natureserve: http://www.natureserve.org/explorer/

Plants Database, from the United States Department of Agriculture: Natural Resources Conservation Service website: http://plants.usda.gov

Plants for a Future: edible, medicinal and useful plants for a healthier world, from the Plants for a Future website: http://www.pfaf.org

PHOTO CREDITS

INDEX TO COMMON AND SCIENTIFIC NAMES

INDEX

INDEX

INDEX

ABOUT THE AUTHORS

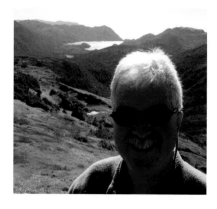

ANDY MACKINNON is a professional biologist who lives in Metchosin, BC, with his beautiful wife, two handsome sons and mandolin. Andy is a research ecologist with the BC Forest Service, and also an adjunct professor at the School of Resource and Environmental Management at Simon Fraser University. He is the author of four Lone Pine books on the plants of Western Canada and the Pacific Northwest.

An avid naturalist since childhood, **LINDA KERSHAW** finally focused on botany at the University of Waterloo, earning her master's degree in 1976. Following her education, she has worked as a consultant and researcher in northwestern Canada and as an editor/author in Edmonton, while pursuing two favourite pastimes—photography and illustrating. Linda hopes that through her books people will glimpse some of the beauty and fascinating history of wild plants, and will recognize the intrinsic value of nature's rich mosaic.

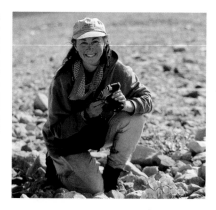

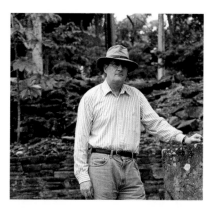

JOHN THOR ARNASON is professor of biology at the University of Ottawa, where he is director of the phytochemistry and ethnopharmacology laboratory. His laboratory has contributed to the study of North American botanicals such as American ginseng, echinacea, goldenseal and many other species. In collaboration with indigenous elders, he and his students have undertaken ethnobotany and ethnopharmacology studies to better understand traditional science and its relation to modern science. Currently, his research is focused on antidiabetic, immunomodualtory and anxiolytic plants.

ABOUT THE AUTHORS

PATRICK OWEN obtained his PhD in human nutrition from McGill University and has a background in botanical sciences. His interests lie in the use of traditional medicinal and food plants for the treatment of chronic diseases such as cardiovascular disease and type 2 diabetes in areas of the world undergoing modernization. His studies have brought him to various parts of the world including Canada, Tibet, India, Mexico and Papua New Guinea. He was the first recipient of the Richard E. Schultes Research Award granted by the Society for Economic Botany.

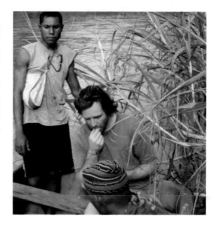

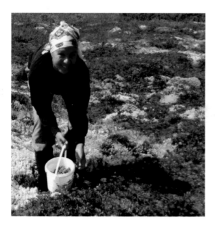

AMANDA KARST has always been fascinated by the relationship between people and plants. She has worked on a range of projects in ethnobotany and plant ecology in British Columbia, Saskatchewan, Quebec and Newfoundland and Labrador. She received her M.Sc. in ethnobotany/plant ecology from the University of Victoria in 2005. She now lives in Winnipeg and has been a Research Associate at the Centre for Indigenous Environmental Resources (CIER) since 2006.

FIONA HAMERSLEY CHAMBERS is passionate about ethnobotany, plants and the natural world. She attributes this passion to spending much of her childhood in and around coastal BC. She holds an honours B.A. from the University of Victoria in French and Environmental Studies, a Masters of Environmental Design from the University of Calgary and a Masters of Science in Environmental Change and Management from Oxford University. Fiona teaches environmental studies part-time at the University of Victoria, consults in the fields of natural resource and community-based co-management and enjoys travelling and working abroad. She currently lives on a farm outside Victoria with her two small boys who also love plants, animals and bugs.

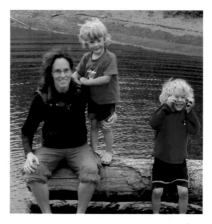